To Dan Jacobs,
whose encouragement
and support
made this book
become a reality

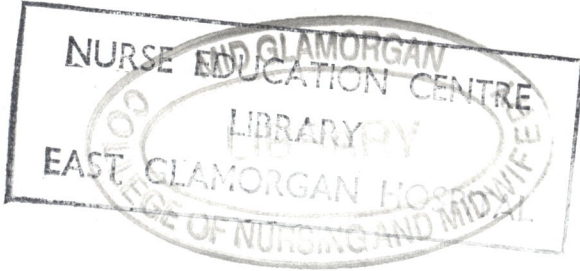

Signs
and
Symptoms
in

3

d Management

Edited by
Margaret Meier Jacobs, R.N.C., M.S.N.
Clinical Nurse Specialist, Primary Care Instructor
Adjunct Instructor, School of Nursing
University of Michigan
Ann Arbor, Michigan
and
Wilma Geels, R.N., M.S.
Nutrition Clinical Nurse Specialist
University Hospital
University of Alabama
Birmingham, Alabama

Signs and Symptoms in Nursing

Interpretation and Management

22 Contributors

J.B. Lippincott Company
Philadelphia
London
Mexico City
New York
St. Louis
São Paulo
Sydney

Sponsoring Editor: Eleanor Faven
Manuscript Editor: Mary K. Smith
Indexer: Deana Fowler
Art Director: Tracy Baldwin/Earl Gerhart
Designer: Arlene Putterman
Production Supervisor: Kathy Dunn
Production Coordinator: Charles W. Field
Compositor: Circle Graphics
Printer/Binder: R. R. Donnelley & Sons

6 5 4 3 2 1

**Library of Congress Cataloging in
Publication Data**
Main entry under title:

Signs and symptoms in nursing.

Bibliography: p.
Includes index.
1. Nursing.   2. Symptomatology.
3. Diagnosis.
I. Jacobs, Margaret Meier.   II. Geels, Wilma.
[DNLM: 1. Nursing Process.   WY 100 S578]
RT48.S56 1984   610.73   84–12609
ISBN 0–397–54391–3

The authors and publisher have exerted
every effort to ensure that drug selection and
dosage set forth in this text are in accord
with current recommendations and practice
at the time of publication. However, in view
of ongoing research, changes in government
regulations, and the constant flow of
information relating to drug therapy and
drug reactions, the reader is urged to check
the package insert for each drug for any
change in indications and dosage and for
added warnings and precautions. This is
particularly important when the
recommended agent is a new or infrequently
employed drug.

Contributors

Violet H. Barkauskas, R.N., Ph.D.
Associate Professor of Nursing, School of Nursing, University of Michigan, Ann Arbor, Michigan

Howard Beckman, M.D.
Residency Coordinator, Primary Care, Internal Medicine Training Program, Assistant Professor of Medicine, School of Medicine, Wayne State University, Detroit, Michigan

Barbara Kersten Campbell, R.N., M.S.
Instructor, School of Nursing, University of Michigan, Ann Arbor, Michigan

Cynthia S. Darling–Fisher, R.N., M.S.
Doctoral Student, School of Nursing, University of Michigan, Ann Arbor, Michigan

Susan De Rosa, R.N., M.S.
Instructor, School of Nursing, University of Rochester, Rochester, New York

Sue Fink, R.N., M.S.
Assistant Professor, School of Nursing, University of Michigan, Ann Arbor, Michigan

Wilma Geels, R.N., M.S.N.
Nutrition Clinical Nurse Specialist, University Hospital, University of Alabama, Birmingham, Alabama

Pamela Heiple, R.N., M.S.
Instructor, Clinician II, School of Nursing, Psychiatric, Mental Health/Gerontology, University of Rochester, Rochester, New York

Judith Holcombe, R.N., M.S.N.
Assistant Professor, School of Nursing, University of Alabama, Birmingham, Birmingham, Alabama

Margaret Meier Jacobs, R.N.C., M.S.N.
Clinical Nurse Specialist, Primary Care, University of Michigan Hospitals; Adjunct Instructor, School of Nursing, University of Michigan, Ann Arbor, Michigan

Joyce Jenkins, R.N., M.P.H.
Assistant Professor, Primary Care Nursing, University of Michigan, Ann Arbor, Michigan

Marilyn Doerman Kellum, R.N., M.S.N.
Nurse Practitioner, Student Health Service, University of Michigan, Ann Arbor, Michigan

E. Suzanne McAuliffe, R.N., M.S.
Formerly Assistant Professor, School of Nursing, University of Michigan, Ann Arbor, Michigan

Deborah McNeil, R.N., M.S.N., C.S.
Assistant Professor of Nursing, Eastern Kentucky University, Richmond, Kentucky

Patricia E. Natale, R.N.C., M.S.N.
Clinical Nurse Specialist, Coordinator Primary Care Nursing Service, Detroit Receiving Hospital/University Health Center; Adjunct Assistant Professor, College of Nursing, Wayne State University, Detroit, Michigan

Mary Niemeyer, R.N., M.S.N.
Clinical Nurse Specialist, University of Michigan Hospitals, Ann Arbor, Michigan

Elizabeth M. Nolan, R.N., M.S.
Clinical Nurse Specialist, University of Michigan Hospitals, Assistant Professor, School of Nursing, University of Michigan, Ann Arbor, Michigan

Penelope Paul, R.N., D.S.N.
Associate Professor, School of Nursing, University of Alabama, Birmingham, Birmingham, Alabama

Carol J. Schaupner, R.N., M.S.
Staff Nurse, Stanford University Hospital, Palo Alto, California

Karen Kellam Smith, R.N., M. Ed. M.S.
Assistant Professor, Psychiatric/Mental Health Nursing, Nazareth College, Kalamazoo, Michigan

Terry Vandenbosch, R.N., M.S.
Clinical Nurse Specialist, University of Michigan Hospitals, Assistant Professor, School of Nursing, University of Michigan, Ann Arbor, Michigan

Margie Van Meter, R.N., M.S.N.
Nursing Coordinator, Michigan Headache and Neurological Institute, Ann Arbor, Michigan

Preface

Nursing practice often involves caring for patients with signs and symptoms (e.g., fever, confusion, constipation) that may or may not be specifically related to a medical problem and that may have a strong psychosocial component. The clinical interpretation and management of these signs and symptoms often are the primary responsibility of the nurse. Nurses who practice in a wide variety of settings, with diverse patient populations, may encounter patients with these same signs and symptoms. Unable to find a nursing reference textbook that could provide easily accessible information about these problems, we wrote SIGNS AND SYMPTOMS IN NURSING to fill this void.

The purpose of SIGNS AND SYMPTOMS IN NURSING is to provide an easy-to-use reference book to help both practicing nurses and nursing students to care for adult patients with these problems. The book provides a practical guide for the interpretation and subsequent nursing management of selected signs and symptoms that all nurses can use, regardless of the practice setting. We believe that SIGNS AND SYMPTOMS IN NURSING is useful to both undergraduate and graduate students, nurse specialists and generalists, and that it is relevant to both inpatient and outpatient settings.

SIGNS AND SYMPTOMS IN NURSING is a multicontributor book. Each chapter addresses one or two related signs or symptoms and is written by a nurse with expertise involving the problem(s). There are many signs and symptoms the book could address; however, we selected those signs and symptoms that are frequently encountered in most settings. The book begins with topics that are primarily psychosocial in nature: confusion, depression, anxiety, impairment of body image, and fatigue. The next three chapters address selected types of pain: chronic pain, low back pain, and headache. Chapters 9 through

17 address topics involving different body systems: dizziness and vertigo; communication deficits; impaired mobility; fever; skin changes; diarrhea and constipation; nausea, vomiting, and dehydration; urinary incontinence; and dyspnea and cough. The last four chapters are problems demonstrating a collection of signs and symptoms that are commonly seen in a wide variety of settings: allergy, obesity, menopause, and chemical dependency. Although most of the signs and symptoms discussed are not life-threatening, they can be difficult management problems for the health care provider, whether he or she is managing the patient independently or as part of a team.

The organizing framework of the book is the Nursing Process, which is a cognitive, scientifically based process that the nurse uses in professional nursing practice. It involves collecting and assessing data, making a nursing diagnosis, setting goals for nursing management, planning and carrying out interventions, and evaluating the effectiveness of the interventions and the need for further interventions. Each chapter follows the same format: a brief introduction of the problem, followed by sections headed Mechanisms, Nursing Assessment, Nursing Diagnosis, and Management. The introduction for each chapter describes the area of concentration and its limitations. Definitions helpful to understanding the sign or symptom are provided, and, if appropriate, a historical perspective is given. The Mechanism section provides information on normal anatomy and physiology, critical pathophysiology and the mechanisms involved, discussion of possible causes, psychosocial aspects of the symptom, and any other influential variables needed to make a nursing assessment and diagnosis and to provide nursing management. The Nursing Assessment section consists of subjective data, which includes descriptive information regarding the complaint (quality, location, quantity, onset, chronology, aggravating and alleviating factors, and associated symptoms); family history; pertinent medical history; and objective data obtained from the physical examination and the paraclinical data. The Nursing Diagnosis section includes a summary of potential nursing judgments regarding the patient's sign or symptom. The section does not follow any one classification system of nursing diagnoses. The content varies between chapters and may also include discussion of indicators of a stable or an acute process, relationship to possible medical diagnoses, and differentiation between those conditions needing physician or other referral and those cared for primarily by the nurse. The management section includes nursing interventions, common medical interventions, effectiveness and rationale for those interventions, referrals, and patient education. Nursing interventions for these signs and symptoms are rarely based on research-proven methods, but rather on experience, trial and error, and anecdotal data. Therefore, many chapters conclude with suggestions for areas of nursing research.

The depth to which each nurse assesses and manages a sign or symptom varies according to area of practice and level of expertise. It is our intent to provide information to meet the needs of both the inexperienced and the experienced nurse. However, we assume that the reader has previous knowledge of the basics of history-taking and physical examination skills, and therefore we do not discuss methodology, except where necessary. This book, then, provides the nurse in the clinical setting with a practical guide for comprehensive nursing care of patients with complex signs and symptoms.
(Note: For ease of expression, we have used "he" to indicate patient, and "she" to indicate the nurse.)

Margaret Meier Jacobs, R.N.C., M.S.N.
Wilma Geels, R.N., M.S.

Contents

Confusion

Pamela Heiple

Confusion, by its very nature, is one of the most difficult symptoms that nurses must interpret. One reason for this is the lack of a clear and consistent definition for the term *confusion*. Because of this ambiguity, the labeling of a patient as *confused* is often a subjective process, one that is affected by social and environmental factors relevant to both the patient and the nurse. Indeed, sometimes labeling a patient *confused* reveals more about the nurse than the patient.

A review of medical and nursing literature indicates that various terms are used to indicate confusion: acute brain failure, acute confusional state, delirium, toxic confusional state, acute (recent) confusion, acute brain syndrome, disorientation, acute organic psychosis, and organic memory loss. Wolanin and Phillips, nurses who have done the most extensive work on confusion, describe it as "...a label for behaviors that caregivers recognize as being deviant from those expected from the client in a certain place and at a certain time."[57] In an earlier study, Wolanin looked at the terms used to define confusion by nurses in a long-term care setting. Using data gathered from written records and taped interviews with staff members, she classified the patient behaviors labeled as confused into two categories: 1) cognitive inaccessibility and 2) social inaccessibility. Terms used to describe confused behaviors that prevented the patient from interacting with his environment according to expectations (cognitive inaccessibility) included forgetful, lost, not aware of surroundings, mixed up, delusional, uses poor judgment, cannot understand directions, withdrawn, and zombie. Terms used by the nurses to describe confused behaviors that were institutionally disruptive (social inaccessibility) were: uncooperative, agitated, violent, combative, wanders, suspicious, into other possessions, and difficult to manage.[57]

For the purpose of this chapter, *confusion* is broadly defined as a change in mental state characterized by disturbances of cognitive functioning that affect the person's ability to interact effectively with his environment. Confusion is treated as a symptom of a disturbance in physiological, psychological, or social equilibrium, and these areas will be emphasized in the discussions of nursing assessment and intervention techniques.

Dall suggested that health care professionals readily apply the term *confused* to the elderly, but are more likely to call younger people *anxious* or *delirious*.[15] Older people are more at risk for the development of acute and chronic confusion due to a combination of physiological, psychological, environmental, and iatrogenic factors. Therefore, this chapter will focus on the causes and management of confusion in the elderly.

MECHANISMS OF CONFUSION

Figure 1-1 lists some of the causes of confusion due to a reversible, acute process, or an irreversible, chronic illness. The medical term *delirium* is used to describe the sudden, rapid, reversible changes in mental status that usually indicate a toxic state resulting from drugs or other physiological imbalance. The term *dementia* refers to a chronic, global cognitive decline that is characterized by impairment in most aspects of functioning and is usually due to an irreversible neurologic illness. However, some reversible causes of confusion (e.g., depression or hypothyroidism) may present as a chronic dementia.

Determining the etiology of a patient's confusion is a challenging task because, as Figure 1-1 illustrates, the factors producing confusion are complex and varied. One type of confusion that frequently goes undiagnosed and untreated is a reversible, sometimes acute confusion superimposed on a chronic, progressive dementia. This is illustrated by the patient with Alzheimer's disease who is unable to prepare meals and becomes delirious due to dehydration, or the patient with a multi-infarct dementia who, aware of his failing memory, develops a depression that aggravates his cognitive disabilities. Recognizing and treating the source of secondary confusion in these patients is vital.

REVERSIBLE CAUSES OF CONFUSION

Physiological Causes

Infection The tendency for central nervous system (CNS) infections such as encephalitis and meningitis to cause confusion is obvious. What is less obvious is that systemic disease such as pneumonia or urinary tract infections can also cause a confusional state characterized by disturbances of attention, concentration, and disorientation.[31] Confusion, not fever, can be the presenting symptom of infection in the elderly, due to aging changes in the temperature-regulating mechanism.

Diseases of the urinary tract are frequent causes of confusion in the elderly. Diminished renal function and an increased blood urea nitrogen (BUN) level are common with aging.[38] The presence of an infection may worsen a chronic mild nephritis, and the patient may become uremic. Mental status changes characteristic of uremia are depression associated with a variable delirium, shortened attention span, irritability, and psychotic behavior.[46,57] The mental changes are usually reversible if the cause of the uremia responds to treatment.

Temperature Imbalance

Hypothermia Mental status changes are characteristic of both hypothermia and hyperthermia (fever). Wolanin and Phillips state that accidental hypothermia occurs when the patient's deep rectal temperature is below $95°$ F ($35°$ C).[57] The people most at risk for the development of hypothermia are those who do not have the normal physiological response to cold (shivering) such as elderly persons with diabetes or atherosclerosis, those who take drugs that interfere with the thermal regulatory apparatus (alcohol, phenothiazines, sedative, and hypotensives), those who are bedridden and unable to generate heat, and those with metabolic prob-

```
                                        Confusion
                                            |
                  +-------------------------+-------------------------+
                  |                                                   |
              Reversible                                        Irreversible
                  |                                                   |
      +-----------+-----------+                   +-----------+-----------+-----------+
      |                       |                   |           |           |           |
Physiological           Psychological      Alzheimer's  Multi-infarct  Other    Benign
                                            Disease      dementia       dementias senescent
Infection               Depression                                               forgetfulness

Temperature             Stress/anxiety
imbalance

Metabolic               Sensory alteration
disturbances

Lack of vitamins        Iatrogenic
and minerals
                        Drugs
Hypoxia
                        Self-fulfilling
Intracranial problems   prophecy
```

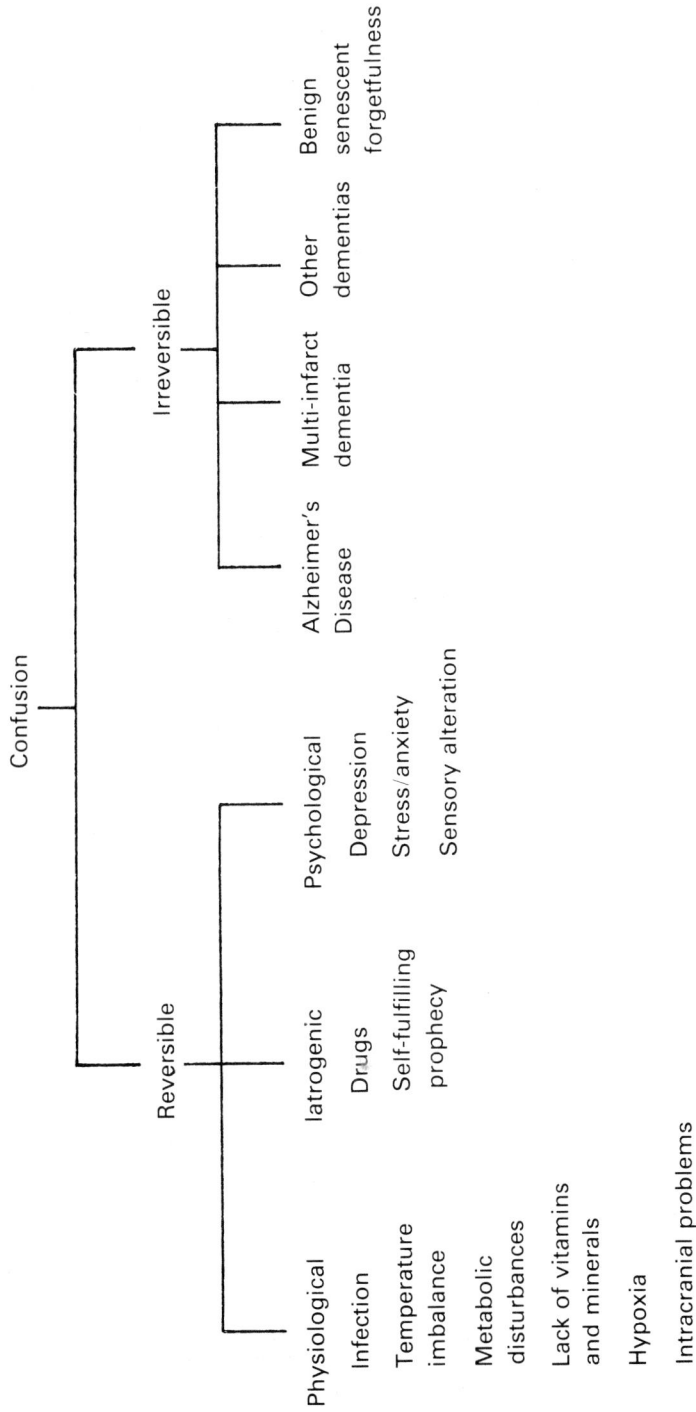

FIG. 1-1 Causes of confusion.

lems. Others at risk are those undergoing surgical procedures and those prone to falling.

When the core temperature is lowered, cardiac, respiratory, renal, and cerebral functions are all affected. Shivering occurs between body temperatures of 35° to 36° C, confusion and disorientation between 34° to 35° C, amnesia between 33° to 34° C, and cardiac arrthymias at 33° C. Undertake rewarming the patient slowly and carefully to prevent the vasodilation that could lead to fatal hypotension.[57] Suspect hypothermia when an elderly person presents with confusion, especially in cold weather.

Hyperthermia Hyperthermia, or a core temperature of 37.7° C or above, may be caused by the body's reaction to infection or a high ambient temperature that prevents the loss of heat by convection.[57] Again, the elderly are a high-risk group because the diminished number of sweat glands prevents cooling by evaporation.

One mental status change characteristic of a rise in temperature above 37.7° C is apathy. As the temperature increases further, clouded sensorium, irritability, diminished attention span and concentration, and increased forgetfulness become apparent. Auditory or visual hallucinations may be present at higher levels of temperature, although in the elderly they can be present at temperatures as low as 37.7° C.[57]

Those at risk for the development of confusion secondary to hyperthermia are people with infections, people with circulatory problems that interfere with vasodilation, and those who are dehydrated.

Metabolic Disturbances

Thyroid Mental status changes characteristic of hyperthyroidism are depression, dementia, irritability, or apathy. Hypothyroidism also is associated with depression, apathy, and lethargy, including slowness of thinking. Habot and Libow state that hypo-thyroidism represents the classic clinical situation in which the elderly person is misdiagnosed as being demented and report that treatment does improve mental functioning in many cases; however, recovery may be prolonged.[23]

Glucose Metabolism Hyperglycemia associated with ketoacidosis is associated with mental status changes of mental obtundation and progressive lethargy that will progress to coma if untreated. This condition is usually easily recognized. The confusion due to mild hypoglycemia is more insidious. An example is an elderly person who continues to take his oral hypoglycemic agent but decreases his caloric intake. If hypoglycemic episodes are more severe, prolonged, or repeated, irreversible brain damage may be the result.[23]

Calcium Imbalance Hypercalcemia may occur in patients with metastatic carcinoma (especially of the lung or breast), Paget's disease, hyperparathyroidism, or hypervitaminosis. People who are immobilized for a long period of time are especially at risk for the development of hypercalcemia because weightbearing is related to the retention of calcium in the bone. Signs and symptoms, which include apathy, lethargy, changes in affect and coordination, anorexia, nausea and vomiting, and skeletal muscle weakness, are related to the effects of increased calcium on nerves and muscles.[57] Hypocalcemia due to hypoparathyroidism, malabsorption states, excessive ingestion of antacids, or inadequate dietary intake may present as senile dementia in the elderly.[38]

Fluid and Electrolyte Imbalance The elderly, those on diuretics or purgatives, those who are depressed, those who are exposed to heat, and especially those who are restrained and dependent on others to provide fluids all are at risk for the development of confusion related to dehydration. Hypernatremia is a hyperosmolar state that indicates fluid depletion. Water is drawn from interstitial and intracellular compartments, including brain cells, in an effort to maintain normal osmolarity, which produces mental confusion, lethargy, and profound weakness.[57] Diarrhea, vomiting, and severe burns are other causes of hypernatremia.

Hyponatremia is a hypo-osmolar syndrome and can produce confusion, lethargy, anorexia, headache, and mental sluggishness. It can be due to diuretics or inappropriate antidiuretic hormone (ADH) secretion caused by drugs, bronchogenic carcinoma, pneumonia, cerebral vascular accidents (CVA), and skull fractures. Severe pain, such as is found in arthritis, can also cause inappropriate secretion of ADH, and there is some evidence that patients with organic brain disease have a high susceptibility to this syndrome.[20] Thus, the older person with painful arthritis and a mild dementia who becomes acutely confused should be assessed for hyponatremia.

Hypokalemia which can result from vomiting, diarrhea, diuretics, and conditions of stress, can produce muscle weakness and apathy.

Lack of Vitamins and Minerals The elderly are particularly at risk for the development of iron-deficiency anemia due to either poor nutrition or undetected slow bleeding from chronic aspirin use, and the achlorhydria common to the elderly that restricts the absorption of dietary iron. Symptoms of iron deficiency anemia include loss of energy and fatigue with minimal exertion, along with the confusion that results from the diminished supply of oxygen to the brain.

Pernicious anemia, a macrocytic anemia, has its highest incidence in people between 60 and 70 years old. The disease is due to malabsorption of vitamin B_{12} in the lower ileum and is usually unrelated to dietary practices. People at risk are those who have had a total gastrectomy, which interferes with the stomach lining's ability to produce intrinsic factor. Depression may be the presenting symptom of pernicious anemia; however, it is usually associated with dementia or a fluctuating confusional state and may be misdiagnosed as presenile or senile dementia.[46]

A deficiency in thiamine can cause apathetic confusion, ataxia, oculomotor disturbances (Wernicke's triad), and the memory deficit and confabulation characteristic of Korsakoff's syndrome.[23] Alcoholics are particularly at risk for these disorders. Confusion, apathy, and irritability are found in nicotinic acid deficiency, and mental status changes have also been attributed to deficiencies in vitamins A and C.[23]

Hypoxia

Cardiac Disease   Arrhythmias, embolic disease, or congestive heart failure affect cardiac output, which in turn can lead to diminished cerebral blood flow (CBF) and symptoms of confusion. In older people, confusion may be the only symptom of an acute myocardial infarction.[23] The hypoxia related to cardiac failure can produce confusion, disorientation, agitation, and restlessness.[57]

Respiratory Disease   Respiratory infections can present as confusion and can lead to further mental impairment in a patient who already is suffering from a chronic dementia. Ventilatory problems such as chronic obstructive pulmonary disease, and an accumulation of secretions due to anesthesia, can also produce restlessness, decreased concentration, and confusion as a result of hypoxia. Respiratory problems can also cause inappropriate ADH secretion.

Hypotension   Hypotension can result from cardiac disease, prolonged bed rest or immobilization, postural changes with inadequate baroreceptor sensitivity, or drugs. Confusion results from lack of cerebral perfusion. Hypotension can also precipitate falling, which can lead to head injuries and subsequent confusion. Those at risk for the development of confusion secondary to hypotension include people with cardiac failure, arrhythmias, electrolyte disturbances, people receiving vigorous treatment with antihypertensive medications, phenothiazines, or antidepressants, and those who use alcohol along with antianginal or antihypertensive drugs.[57] Those people taking psychoactive agents (especially phenothiazines and tricyclic antidepressants) are at risk for the development of postural hypotension, especially if the drugs are given in one large dose at bedtime.

Intracranial Problems Changes in mental state often are associated with intracranial problems. Drowsiness, slowness of speech, restlessness, fluctuating level of consciousness, and lack of concentration can be signs of increased intracranial pressure resulting from space-occupying lesions, head injury, or cerebral edema.

Tumors Patients with intracranial tumors present with behavior changes in 50% to 70% of cases.[23] Dementia, memory disturbance, and affective lability can be a result of tumors in the frontal lobes, thalamus, third ventricle, temporal lobes, or corpus callosum.[45] Personality changes such as apathy, irritability, and social inappropriateness are more characteristic of diseases of the frontal lobe.[48]

Trauma Subdural hematomas may result from a head injury, such as one sustained in a fall, which damages a blood vessel and causes hemorrhage. Alcoholics have a high incidence of subdurals. Fluctuating symptoms of confusion and a history of falls are diagnostic indicators of subdurals, along with forgetfulness, loss of judgment, dull headache, or mild vertigo. In the elderly, symptoms related to cerebral tumors or subdural hemorrhage often occur later than usual because of the increased intracranial space available as a result of age-related cerebral atrophy.[38] A careful history and physical examination is essential to establish the acuteness of the change.

Normal Pressure Hydrocephalus Normal pressure hydrocephalus (NPH) is a condition that may follow trauma, subarachnoid hemorrhage, chronic meningitis, accompany neoplasms, or appear as an idiopathic condition.[23] In NPH the absorption of cerebrospinal fluid (CSF) is impaired. The ventricles enlarge in an attempt to compensate; the cerebral tissues are compressed, and normal pressure is found in the CSF. The classic symptoms of NPH are progressive dementia, incontinence, and gait disturbance. Treatment of NPH with shunting has been only inconsistently effective.

Iatrogenic Causes of Confusion

Drugs Wolanin and Phillips discuss six possible ways drugs can produce confusion: they can alter the metabolic environment of the brain cells, interfere with the CBF or reduce cardiac output, reduce blood glucose, depress the respiratory center and interfere with oxygen supply to the brain, alter brain neurotransmitters, and alter or compete with the vitamins or amino acids (needed substances by the brain).[57]

Table 1-1 depicts the mechanism by which some frequently used drugs cause confusion. People who take psychotropic drugs are especially at risk.

Although drug toxicity is usually associated with florid delirium, chronic confusion or a dementia may also result from some of the medications many older people take on a long-term basis. For example, there is a 40% increase in the half-life of digoxin in the el-

TABLE 1-1
DRUGS ASSOCIATED WITH CONFUSION

DRUG	DEPRESSES CNS	ACTS AS HYPOTENSIVE	ACTS AS ANTICHOLINERGIC
Alcohol	X		
Barbiturates	X		
Benzodiazepines (chlordiazepoxide, diazepam)	X		
Phenothiazines (chlorpromazine, thioridazine)		X	X
Butyrophenones (haloperidol, thiothixene)		X	X
Tricyclic antidepressants (amitriptyline, doxepin)		X	X
Scopolamine (found in over-the-counter sleeping aids)			X
Propoxyphene (Darvon)	X		
Sympatholytic antihypertensives (methyldopa, Ismelin)		X	
Antiparkinsonian agents			X

(Material reproduced and adapted with permission from Kayne R: Drugs and the Aged. In Burnside I (ed): Nursing and the Aged, 1st ed, pp 442–448. New York, McGraw–Hill, 1976)

derly, which contributes to a higher incidence of drug toxicity. Cardiac arrhythmias, mental confusion, depression, and extreme fatigue often precede the usual gastrointestinal and visual symptoms of toxicity in the elderly, and can make toxicity more difficult to diagnose.[37] This is illustrated by a situation described by Wolanin in which a geriatric nurse practitioner who assumed the care of elderly men on a geriatric unit questioned their need for digitalis. After discovering that their serum digoxin levels were above normal, she discontinued the drug and the men became alert and responsive, with improved equilibrium and mobility.[56] Other drugs commonly used by the elderly that can cause confusion are bromides. Raskind and colleagues report that older people show signs of bromide toxicity (memory impairment, irritability, psychomotor retardation, and emotional lability) at levels significantly lower than usual.[43]

Libow reports that another commonly used medication, chlorpropamide, sometimes is associated with a specific syndrome of water intoxication and senile dementia due to its tendency to increase ADH activity.[38]

Although most health care providers are aware of the risk of confusion with psychoactive agents, antihypertensive drugs, and sedatives/barbiturates, most prescription or over-the-counter medications can cause confusion in an older person by mechanisms not yet completely understood. Drugs should be immediately suspected when an elderly person presents with a change in mental status.

The complex interaction of anesthesia

and the stress of surgery can also produce confusion in people of all ages, although the elderly are at greater risk. Sensory deprivation and overload associated with hospitalization are also factors and will be discussed in another section. Postoperative delirium in cardiac surgery patients occurs fairly frequently. This delirium may develop 2 to 5 days postoperatively, with symptoms continuing for weeks.[1] Strub and Black state that "elderly patients most sensitive to subtle changes in homeostasis frequently become confused post-operatively when electrolytes are out of balance and strong analgesics have been administered for pain."[48] Libow terms this phenomenon *postoperative senile dementia* and reports that it can be weeks or months before the confusion clears.[38]

Self-fulfilling Prophecy A major cause of iatrogenic confusion is the low expectation placed on those who may be just mildly confused, or hard of hearing, or just old. Elderly people who have a hearing loss tend to be treated as if they are confused; without adequate stimulation and attention to communication techniques, their cognitive functioning will likely deteriorate. People who are limited by a chronic dementia need to use as many of their abilities as frequently as possible to maintain an optimal level of functioning and prevent the "excess disabilities" associated with this disease.[7]

The most disastrous form of iatrogenic confusion is labeling someone with a reversible form of confusion as "demented" or "senile," and exposing them to the medications and environment of the chronically confused. The combination of drugs and lack of stimulation will ensure that their confusion will become progressive and irreversible.

Psychological Causes of Confusion

Depression Kiloh identified endogenous depression as the condition most likely to be misdiagnosed as dementia.[34] The term *pseudodementia* is used to describe the syndrome in which a functional psychiatric illness, such as depression, mimics the signs and symptoms of dementia. This is particularly common in the elderly. It has been reported that 9% of older people with a diagnosis of senile dementia referred to a geriatric outreach program were, instead, clinically depressed.[31] It was thought formerly that the only way of determining whether a confused patient was depressed or suffered a dementia was to treat the patient for depression (e.g., with antidepressants) and watch for improvement. However, on the basis of his experiences with ten patients suffering from pseudodementia, Wells identified several clinical features that can help differentiate dementia from depression.[54] The onset of dementia is usually difficult to determine since it occurs gradually, whereas the onset of pseudodementia usually can be determined with some precision, occurring sometimes after a major loss or change. A personal or family history of depression is common in pseudodementia, and the symptoms of depression often precede those of cognitive failure, as opposed to dementia, in which the patient becomes depressed as a reaction to his cognitive decline. The patient with pseudodementia communicates his distress and concern about his memory deficit and highlights his failures, whereas the patient with dementia does not show concern and attempts to conceal his impairment. "Near-miss" answers and confabulation are characteristics of dementia; the patient with depression does not attempt a response to questions but replies "I don't know." Attention and concentration are usually intact in depression; however, there is marked memory loss for both recent and remote events. In dementia, attention and concentration are usually impaired along with memory, but remote memory usually is preserved better than memory for recent events. The most pronounced characteristic of pseudodementia is the inconsistency of behavior and performance on tasks of similar difficulty. Wells also states that dependency may be a symptom and suggests that "pseudodementia might thus be viewed as an effective means of communicating a sense of helplessness."[54]

Pseudodementia due to depressive illness can be treated successfully, usually with antidepressants or electroconvulsive therapy.[42] It is imperative that treatment be initiated as soon as possible, before the patient is stereotyped and treated as "senile."

Depression can also be present concurrently with dementia. It is not uncommon for depression to occur in the early stages of Alzheimer's disease, when the patient begins to be aware of his cognitive decline. Depression is also commonly associated with cerebrovascular disease such as stroke and multi-infarct dementia.

Stress or Anxiety   Inability to think clearly when anxious or stressed is a common experience for most people. A period of mild confusion is commonly associated with bereavement and other major life changes. People at risk for the development of confusion resulting from anxiety are those who have a chronic but well-compensated dementia. This state of an acute confusion superimposed on a dementia has been termed *beclouded dementia* and is thought to be related to environmental, physiological, or psychological stressors. Frequent forgetfulness, periodic depression or anxiety, and a limited adaptability to new situations are thought to be predisposing factors.[45]

Stress can also cause confusion in people who do not have dementia. Habot and Libow report that post-traumatic confusional states occur in some elderly persons who have suffered physical trauma unrelated to the head.[23] Kral described a phenomenon that he terms *acute confusional states of the aged*.[35] These states develop in response to an acute stress in older people who have not previously shown signs of dementia. The onset and duration of these states depend on the severity of the stressor and the patient's defenses. The symptoms are clouded consciousness, perceptual disorders, decreased attention span, disorientation to time and place with preservation of personal orientation, severely impaired recall and recent memory but with preservation of remote memory. Kral believes that acute confusional states of the aged are caused by the impact of corticosteroids on the hypothalamus. He recommends treating this condition by a daily slow infusion of 5% glucose solution combined with high vitamin and protein feedings to increase the patient's stress resistance.

The stress of relocation is commonly associated with the development or worsening of confusion. Many elderly people with a chronic dementia are able to maintain themselves adequately in their own homes, using memory cues and keeping to familiar patterns and routines. The disruption of routine, loss of cues, depersonalization, and changes in sensory input associated with hospitalization or entrance into a nursing home can lead to disorientation, forgetfulness, and behavior changes. One study examined the prevalence of confusion in hospitalized patients aged 60 and above. It was found that 55 of the 99 patients studied during two study periods were considered acutely confused; however, only 5 of these 55 patients were labeled confused on admission; the others became confused about 6½ days after admission. The stresses of relocation, combined with the effects of illness, drugs, or surgery, almost guarantee confusion.

Sensory   Alteration   Studies   have shown that a person with a hearing or vision

Decreased sensory input → Total cognitive breakdown
due to ↓ in efficiency
of sensory receptors

Isolation

Brain receives less stimuli

↑ Blockage of
reception of stimuli

Atrophy of brain cells

Depression and apathy

Diminished ability to
manipulate environment

Sense of failure

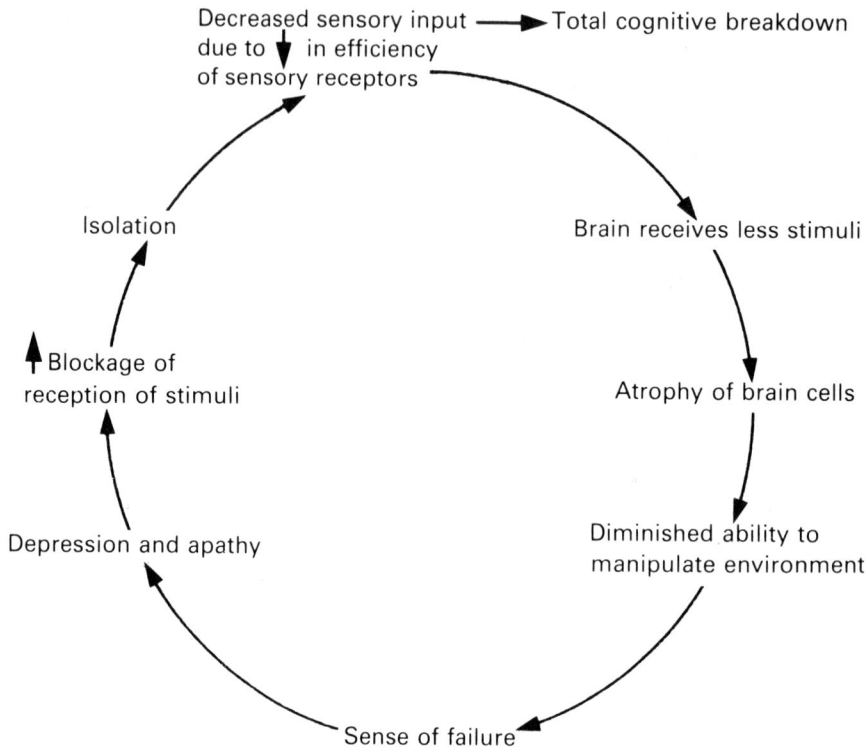

FIG. 1-2 *The relationship of sensory deprivation to confusion in the elderly (Data from Ernst P et al: Isolation and the symptoms of chronic brain syndrome. Gerontologist 18, No. 5:468–474, 1978)*

deficit is at high risk for the development of confusion.[27] Sensory impairment interferes with effective communication and the person's ability to assimilate and respond to environmental stimuli. People with hearing and vision impairments may be prone to suspiciousness and the development of illusions (misperceptions), which may be mistaken for hallucinations.

Ernst and co-workers state that sensory deprivation and environmental factors play a vital role in the development of the symptoms of organic brain syndrome.[16] They cite a study that found a clear correlation between sensory loss and the manifestation of organic brain syndrome in nursing home residents.

Their model for cognitive failure as a result of sensory deprivation is diagrammed in Figure 1-2. It is thought that brain cells atrophy due to lack of stimulation. This atrophy precipitates failure, which leads to depression, producing isolation, further deprivation, and eventually, total cognitive breakdown.

Sensory alteration also is produced by: perceptual deprivation, the reduction of meaningful stimuli for the person; immobilization, the confinement and dependence on others for stimulation; social isolation, isolation from people or a familiar environment; and sensory overload, a condition of very intense stimuli that does not have a pattern.[8]

The CNS screens and organizes sensory

input, all of which is potentially overwhelming. The sensory threshold, which varies among individuals, determines which stimuli are perceived and which go undetected. Not only must the stimuli be strong enough to exceed the sensory threshold, they must also be perceived as being meaningful to the person. Sensory alteration occurs when there is an increase or decrease in the intensity or amount of variation in the stimuli (sensory deprivation or overload), with subsequent changes in relevance for the person (perceptual deprivation).[40]

Anyone in an institutional environment is at risk for the development of confusion secondary to sensory alteration. For example, an older person who is hospitalized experiences both sensory deprivation and overload related to the hospital environment (page systems, monitors, intrusions by strangers, and decreased visual stimuli), perceptual deprivation due to the separation from meaningful objects, immobilization, and dependence on others due to his confinement to bed, along with being isolated from friends and family. It is not surprising that confusion is such a common occurrence in patients on medical wards and intensive care units.

Phillips reports that inability to concentrate, difficulty controlling the direction of thoughts, difficulty with recall, and regression into fantasy are the most common effect of sensory alteration on cognition.[40] She also identified several factors that influence the person's ability to handle sensory alteration; the person's capacity for self-stimulation, intelligence, and the degree of dependence. Apparently people who enjoy solitude and do not rely on outside sources of stimulation (such as nonsmokers), those with average or below average intelligence, and those who have traits of dependence and low impulsivity are better able to tolerate sensory deprivation.

IRREVERSIBLE CAUSES OF CONFUSION
Alzheimer's Disease

Alzheimer's disease, or primary degenerative dementia, is the most common cause of dementia, accounting for as many as 100,000 to 120,000 deaths annually in the United States.[47] Although the onset of the disease is usually in persons aged 70 or older it may begin earlier. Formerly, it was thought that "presenile dementia" was different than the type occurring later in life; however, studies have indicated identical morphological changes regardless of age of onset.[53] The present trend is to label both early and late dementia as Alzheimer's disease.

Alzheimer's disease is characterized by structural changes in the brain, consisting of senile plaques, neurofibrillary tangles, and granulovacular degeneration. Although these changes are also found in the brains of normal elderly persons, they occur in greater numbers and in different sites in Alzheimer's disease.[53] The brains of Alzheimer's disease patients also show a marked cortical atrophy with some ventricular dilation. Neuronal loss is evident, especially in the frontal, parietal, and temporal lobes.

The cause of Alzheimer's disease is unknown. Studies have demonstrated that there are lower levels of choline acetyltransferase and acetylcholinesterase in the brains of Alzheimer's disease patients.[47] Research presently is being done to determine if the administration of choline precursors (lecithin) has a beneficial effect. Other studies have indicated that increased levels of aluminum may play a role in the development of neurofibrillary tangles.[47] Another study indicated that heredity may be a factor since relatives of 125 people with Alzheimer's disease showed an excess of dementia consistent with genetic transmission.[26]

Alzheimer's disease is an incurable disease. The average time from the onset of the disease to death is 5 years, although it usually is difficult to determine an exact time of onset due to its insidious nature.[44] Hayter described three stages of Alzheimer's disease.[25] The first stage has a duration of approximately 2 to 4 years. The patient at this point may be able to conceal his difficulties because his ability to think logically is greater than his memory. Occasionally, family members assume tasks previously performed by the patient (such as balancing the checkbook) to deny the fact that something may be wrong. Disorientation to time, lack of spontaneity, and especially memory loss are the most prominent symptoms in the first stage.

The second stage, which can extend over many years, is characterized by increased memory impairment and the neurologic symptoms of aphasia, apraxia, and agnosia. Perseveration, a tendency to wander, and muscular twitching are common. Bulimia and hyperorality occur in the early part of this stage, which progresses to indifference towards food in the latter part. In the first stage and early part of the second stage, the patient looks healthy and strong and may be able to function minimally in social situations. This makes it difficult for friends and relatives, who do not have extended contact with the patient, to believe that something is wrong. Several wives of Alzheimer's disease patients have shared with this author the anguish they felt when told by other family members, "There's nothing wrong with him. Maybe you should see a psychiatrist."

The third stage is terminal. Patients become cachectic, increasingly apractic, spastic, and bedridden. Grand mal seizures can occur during the last 6 months of life, and patients generally succumb to infections, particularly bronchopneumonia.[25]

Multi-infarct Dementia

The symptoms of multi-infarct dementia, which is the second most common type of dementia, are caused by multiple infarcts scattered throughout the brain. Hypertension and a history of stroke usually are associated with this. Multi-infarct dementia is characterized by a step-wise deterioration of certain functions (such as memory and intellectual functions) as opposed to the gradual global deterioration of Alzheimer's disease. The sudden appearance of focal neurologic signs is also characteristic of multi-infarct dementia. Patients with this type of dementia exhibit classic aphasias due to infarcts in the speech centers in the brain.[44] Other features of this disease are emotional lability, preservation of personality and social skills and episodes of acute confusion occurring with each new infarct. Multi-infarct dementia is more common in men than women.[44] The presence of hypertension is the most significant predisposing factor.

Other Dementias

Pick's disease is an irreversible dementia clinically similar to Alzheimer's disease, and is characterized by profound personality changes, blunting of emotions, disinhibition, and lack of insight and social awareness.[57] Pathologically, the disease is characterized by the presence of Pick and Hirano bodies and the absence of neurofibrillary tangles and senile plaques.[31] The onset of Pick's disease is insidious and usually begins in the mid-fifties, with a lifespan of 7 years after diagnosis.

Jakob–Creutzfeldt disease usually occurs between the ages of 40 and 60.[45] Its distinguishing feature is a very rapid onset that is first evident in motor or sensory disturbances. This is followed by rapid deterioration; the patient may be blind, deaf, severely ataxic, and hemiplegic within weeks. Myoclonus and tremors may occur. There is deterioration of language, emotions, and intellect, all of which may occur within 4 to 8 months.[47] Neuropathologically, the cerebral cortex takes on a spongelike appearance giving rise to the term *spongiform encephalopathy*. Research into the cause of this disease indicates that transmission of a slow virus infection may be involved.

Benign Senescent Forgetfulness

Normal aging involves some degree of memory impairment. Research has shown that there is no aging decline in primary memory, which refers to material which is "still in mind, still being rehearsed, still at the focus of conscious attention."[11] Immediate repetition of a digit span involves the use of primary memory. Primary memory is relatively short and generally assumed to be limited to 2 to 4 items.[58] *Secondary memory* (sometimes called *long-term memory*) exceeds the capacity of primary memory and involves both acquisition and recall of information. Studies indicate that older subjects show deficits in their ability to put information into secondary memory (*acquisition*) and get it out when necessary (*retrieval*). Older people also show more difficulty with attention and in manipulating or reorganizing stored information.[11] Some older people are able to compensate for these difficulties by using different methods of cuing (see section on forgetfulness). However, sometimes this memory impairment combined with the chronic low grade anxiety common to the elderly may lead to a misdiagnosis of early dementia.[31]

NURSING ASSESSMENT

The assessment of a confused patient requires skilled clinical observation as well as a mental status and physical examination. Table 1-2 outlines the components of the assessment process. These guidelines can be modified according to the character of the patient's confusion and the setting in which the evaluation is done. For example, a hospitalized patient who develops acute confusion the day after surgery needs a medical evaluation more than a functional assessment. However, an elderly patient who becomes confused several days after admission to a nursing home requires a comprehensive assessment of factors influencing his ability to adjust to a new environment.

INTERVIEWING THE CONFUSED PERSON

The outcomes of a successful interview with a confused patient are twofold: the nurse obtains the necessary information and the patient maintains his dignity and sense of self-esteem. The interview situation can be very threatening for the patient who is aware of his confusion and he may react with suspiciousness or manipulative behavior to "having his mind examined." Ideally, the interview should take place in an environment familiar to the patient, such as his own home or hospital room. The author has seen marked improvement in performance on tests of mental functioning when they were administered to patients in their own homes as opposed to the clinic situation. A familiar setting may also reinforce the patient's sense of control.

Interviewing the confused elderly patient takes time. The elderly patient fatigues easily and may be anxious. In addition, reminiscing, a helpful technique if the patient's mental functioning permits, is time-consuming. Reminiscing provides an opportunity to assess the patient's flow of thought and past coping mechanisms, as well as remote memory.

Questions about mental functioning can be included in an assessment of the patient's overall health. Comfort recommends that the mental status examination be included with

(Text continues on page 16)

TABLE 1-2
GUIDELINES FOR NURSING ASSESSMENT OF CONFUSION

I. **DESCRIPTION OF CONFUSED BEHAVIOR (FROM RESPONSIBLE PERSON)**
   A. Characteristics of behavior
      Disorientation
      Emotional lability
      Memory loss
      Lethargy
      Wandering
      Withdrawal
      Confabulation
      Hallucinations
      Fluctuating level of awareness
      Anxiety
      Delusional thinking
      Inability to manage finances
   B. Onset of confused behavior or change in level of functioning
   C. Where does behavior occur?
   D. When does it occur (morning, evening)?
   E. How frequently does behavior occur?
II. **MEDICAL HISTORY**
   A. History of falls or dizziness
   B. Alcohol use
   C. Medications: dosage and frequency
      1) Prescription
      2) Over-the-counter drugs
   D. History of hypertension
   E. History of stroke
   F. History of cardiac problems
   G. History of renal problems
   H. History of thyroid problems
   I. History of diabetes
III. **PSYCHOLOGICAL AND SOCIAL DATA**
   A. Previous problems with confusion/depression
   B. Family history of mental illness
   C. Personality style
   D. History of coping with stressors
   E. Education and occupation
VI. **MENTAL FUNCTIONING ASSESSMENT**
   A. Appearance
   B. Behavior
   C. Communication (note hearing and vision impairments)
      1) Language
      2) Comprehension
   D. Cognitive capacity screening examination
      1) What day of the week is this?
      2) What month?

TABLE 1-2
GUIDELINES FOR NURSING ASSESSMENT OF CONFUSION (continued)

      3) What year?
      4) What place is this?
      5) Repeat the numbers 8,7,2
      6) Say them backwards
      7) Repeat the numbers 6,3,7,1
      8) Listen to these numbers: 6,9,4. (Count 1 through 10 out loud, then repeat 6,9,4. (Help if it is needed: then use numbers 5,7,3)
      9) Listen to these numbers: 8,1,4,3. Count 1 through 10 out loud, then repeat 8,1,4,3
    10) Beginning with Sunday, say the days of the week backward.
    11) 9 + 3 is
    12) Add 6 to the previous answer
    13) Take away 5 (from 18)
    14) Repeat these words after me and remember them; I will ask for them later: hat, car, tree, twenty-six
    15) The opposite of fast is slow. The opposite of up is?
    16) The opposite of large is?
    17) The opposite of hard is?
    18) An orange and a banana are both fruits. Red and blue are both?
    19) A penny and a dime are both?
    20) What were those words I asked you to remember? (hat)
    21) Car
    22) Tree
    23) Twenty-six
    24) Take away 7 from 100, then take away 7 from what is left and keep going: 100 − 7 is:
    25) Minus 7
    26) Minus 7
    27) Minus 7
    28) Minus 7
    29) Minus 7
    30) Minus 7
  E. Remote memory
  F. Knowledge of current events
  G. Constructional ability
      1) Ask patient to copy these figures

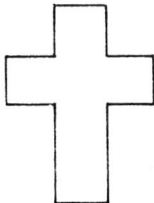

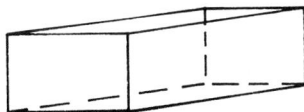

      2) Clock drawing
  H. Emotional behavior
  I. Judgment

(continues)

TABLE 1-2
GUIDELINES FOR NURSING ASSESSMENT OF CONFUSION (continued)

    J. Insight
    K. Social functioning
V. *FUNCTIONAL ASSESSMENT*
    Independence/dependence in:
    A. Toileting
    B. Bathing
    C. Dressing
    D. Ambulation
    E. Eating
    F. Ability to take medication
    G. Ability to use telephone
    H. Shopping
    I. Transportation
    J. Food preparation
    K. Housekeeping
    L. Ability to handle finances
VI. *COMPLETE PHYSICAL*
VII. *LABORATORY DATA*
    Routine tests
        Complete blood count with differential
        Electrolytes, glucose, BUN, creatinine, liver function
        Urinalysis
        Serum B_{12} and folate
        Serologic test for syphilis (VDRL)
        Chest x-ray
        Skull films
        Electrocardiogram
        Electroencephalogram
        CT scan
    Optional tests (done if indicated)
        Lumbar puncture
        Brain scan
        Cisternography
        Psychological testing
        Toxic screen

(Cognitive capacity screening examination reprinted with permission from Jacobs J, Bernhard M, Delgado A et al: Screening for organic mental syndromes in the medically ill. Ann Int Med 86, No. 1:40–46, 1977)

other components of the neurologic assessment (such as reflexes).[13] Gurland states that mental status testing should not be attempted at the end of the interview and recommends that the patient be given as much control as possible.[22]

Some patients will refuse to attempt an answer to questions due to a fear of failure. This may have diagnostic importance (see section on depression). It is important to praise the patient's attempts and minimize his failures.

If the patient's confusion is compounded by sensory losses, special care must be taken to ensure effective communication. The interviewer should sit in front of the patient and speak slowly and clearly. Touch can be an effective facilitator of communication with the sensory impaired person. If the patient has a hearing loss, speaking into the "good" ear is more effective than shouting. (For more information the reader is referred to the chapter on communication deficits.)

Interviewing the severely confused patient requires skill and sensitivity. Patients with disturbances of attention cannot tolerate lengthy interviews and will do better with several brief contacts. Special care must be taken to eliminate distracting stimuli that may tax the patient's attention span further. Nonverbal communication, such as touch and gesturing, is necessary for those with impairment in verbal language.[5] Simple measures (e.g., addressing the patient by his surname and making sure he is wearing his glasses and dentures) are often overlooked but are essential to the development of a therapeutic relationship.

HISTORY

The history should be obtained from a reliable person (relative or friend) who has been in recent contact with the patient. Relatives are usually more candid and honest about their concerns when interviewed alone, rather than in the presence of the patient. This may also be less threatening to the patient. The following are items that should be included in the history (see Table 1-2).

DESCRIPTION OF CONFUSED BEHAVIOR

It is important for the relative or friend to describe the behavior of the patient in specific detail; for example is he disoriented, anxious, forgetful, preoccupied with the past?

How does he react when reality information is given? Does he confabulate or refuse to answer questions? When, where, and how often does the confused behavior occur? Confused behavior occurring only in the early morning or late afternoon may indicate hypoglycemia, while disorientation and illusions occurring only at night, in the dark, suggests a sensory or perceptual problem. Confusion occurring only in a specific place may be due to environmental factors.

Accurate information about the onset of the confusion is crucial. The appearance of acute confusion usually can be dated fairly precisely, while the dementias have a more insidious onset. It is important to inquire into recent changes or loss that may have precipitated the confusion, and to remember that even seemingly inconsequential events can be perceived as stressful by the patient.

Many times, the best information can be obtained by inquiring into the patient's ability to perform activities of daily living and other functions. For example, sometimes insidious confusion can be dated by the patient's inability to pay bills or balance the checkbook. Some people will stop fixing complete meals and serve sandwiches instead. Wearing the same clothing every day because of inability to do laundry may be another sign that something is wrong. It is the *change* from a higher to lower level of functioning that is a diagnostic clue. If the patient presents with acute confusion, the nurse should evaluate the patient's prior level of functioning to determine whether an acute confusional state is superimposed on a progressive dementia. An example of this is: "Mother has been failing for several years, but has managed adequately with help only for shopping. She has been forgetful and sometimes has trouble expressing herself. Since Dad died last month, however, she's been disoriented, agitated, and totally unable to do anything for herself."

MEDICAL HISTORY

Two important questions to ask are if the patient has a history of falls or alcohol abuse. It is important to remember that subdural hematomas can develop slowly in the elderly. The acutely confused patient with a history of alcohol abuse needs to be evaluated for delirium tremens. Chronic alcohol abuse can lead to Wernicke–Korsakoff's syndrome. Other important data are history of hypertension, stroke, cardiac, pulmonary, renal, or neurologic problems. A history of the patient's use of prescription and over-the-counter drugs is essential, including the schedule and method used to take the medications. Impaired vision or confusion can lead to errors in taking medication. Occasionally a home visit may be necessary to obtain accurate information.

PSYCHOLOGICAL AND SOCIAL HISTORY

The nurse should ask whether any of the patient's blood relatives ever suffered a mental illness (schizophrenia, depression) or a dementia, because there may be a genetic component to these diseases. Information about personality styles may also be helpful because dependence may be a factor in the development of pseudodementia, and compulsiveness and difficulty adapting to new situations are common traits found in people who develop dementia.[52,54] The patient's means of coping with major and minor losses and his job history should be explored.

MENTAL FUNCTIONING ASSESSMENT

Appearance

The patient's body weight (frail or obese) should be noted. Grooming and appropriateness of dress (such as wearing a coat in winter) can reflect cognition and mood. Assess for signs of neglect (both shoes tied, all buttons buttoned), which may indicate a neurologic disturbance.

Behavior

The patient's behavior includes motor activity (psychomotor retardation, agitation, fidgeting) and the appropriateness of the patient's behavior to his situation.

Communication

Assessment of hearing and vision should be performed as part of the physical examination; however, impairments should be noted because of their impact on the patient's ability to communicate effectively. The characteristics of the patient's speech should be noted; for example, is it logical, coherent, rambling, rapid, monotonous, grammatically correct? Is the patient aphasic? Broca's aphasia is characterized by telegraphic, nonfluent, poorly articulated speech with retention of auditory and reading comprehension. The speech of a patient with Broca's aphasia consists mostly of nouns and verbs with a paucity of verbal fillers. Conversely, Wernicke's aphasia is characterized by fluent, effortless, well-articulated but paraphrasic speech combined with a severe impairment in auditory comprehension.[48] This patient's speech lacks substantive words and is often inappropriate due to the problems with comprehension.

Comprehension can be assessed in someone who is confused by asking him to respond to yes or no questions (e.g., "Is it raining today?") or by asking him to point to objects (pencil, chair, etc). The patient's nonverbal communication techniques (e.g., gesturing) and his attempt to compensate for a communication problem should be noted.

Cognitive Functioning

This portion of the assessment is adapted from the Cognitive Capacity Screening Examination (CCSE) developed by Jacobs and colleagues (see Table 1–2).[30] The CCSE was developed as an easily administered, efficient method of screening for organic mental symptoms on medical wards. The tool has been found to discriminate between functional illness and diffuse organic brain syndromes in hospitalized psychiatric patients, although the authors caution that cultural or educational variances may affect the results of the test. A score of 19 or less on the original 30 items indicates organic mental dysfunction. Questions 1 to 4 assess orientation, 6 to 10 immediate recall, 12 to 14 calculations, 14 and 20 to 23 new learning ability, 15 to 19 abstract thinking, and 24 to 30 attention and calculations.

Remote memory is tested by asking the patient previously learned information such as his birthday, mother's maiden name or other information which is *relevant to him.* Sometimes historical data are used, for example, "Who bombed Pearl Harbor?", or "What happened to President Kennedy?" If historical questions are used, cultural and educational factors must be taken into account. Asking elderly patients to give the names and ages of their grandchildren can be useful, and more pleasant for them.

Knowledge of current events is assessed by asking the patient if he keeps up with the news, and if so, by asking more specific questions about major current events.

Constructional ability is a higher cognitive function that involves integration of occipital, parietal, and frontal lobe functions. Because these abilities involve so many parts of the brain, they can be a good indicator of early brain damage, particularly the diffuse cortical atrophy seen in Alzheimer's disease. Tests of constructional ability are considered good screening measures for older people with vague psychiatric or neurologic complaints, because of the high incidence of constructional impairment in dementia. Constructional ability is assessed by having the patient copy drawings such as a cross and three-dimensional cube (see Table 1–2) and asking him to draw a picture of a clock with the hands showing a specific time, for example, 10 minutes after 11 o'clock.

Emotional Behavior

The assessment of depression is covered in Chapter 2 and will not be discussed here. The confused patient's mood or prevailing emotional state, and range of affect should be noted. Emotional lability or a rapid fluctuation of emotional responses is suggestive of frontal lobe disease or some types of delirium, whereas blunting of emotions is characteristic of Alzheimer's disease. It is also important to differentiate the apathy that may be associated with an organic brain disease, from depression. Suicide assessment should always be performed if depression is suspected (see Chap. 2). Sometimes caregivers assume that patients with dementia cannot "get it together" to carry out a plan to kill themselves. *Never assume that a patient is too confused to commit suicide,* particularly if he is in the early stages of dementia (especially multi-infarct type) and is aware of his intellectual decline. Sometimes patients in long-term care facilities with more advanced dementia attempt suicide in more passive ways, such as by refusing to eat. This possibility always needs to be explored.

Judgment

This is an important area to assess, particularly when trying to determine the chronically confused patient's ability to live independently. Typical questions used to assess judgment are, "What would you do

if you found a library book on the street?"
or "What would you do if you were in a
theater and detected a fire?" It is, however,
more appropriate to ask questions relevant
to the patient, such as, "What would you
do if there was a fire in your kitchen?"
and, "What would you do if you fell during
the night?"

Insight

Insight refers to the patient's self-knowledge,
his awareness of his illness, and the ability to
understand its origin. Some patients, when
asked the reason for their evaluation by a
mental health professional, reply, "My family thinks there is something wrong, but
there is nothing wrong with me." A follow-
up question to this response could be "why
do you think your family believes there is
something wrong with you?" Preservation of
insight is common in the early states of
multi-infarct dementia.

Social Functioning

The patient's eye contact, response when the
nurse offers her hand, and the manner in
which he relates are indicators of social functioning. Social skills may be preserved in the
early states of dementia and some patients
are quite expert at covering their cognitive
deficits. These patients should not be confronted with their obvious deficits because
this may result in severe anxiety and a catastrophic reaction (total disintegration of the
personality).[50]

FUNCTIONAL ASSESSMENT

The best indicator of a mental functioning
problem in an elderly patient may be a subtle
change in level of physical functioning. The
relative or friend should be asked about the
patient's independence or need for assis-

tance in matters of physical self-maintenance
(first 5 items of functional assessment in
Table 1-2), and ability to maintain themselves in the home (remaining items). Again,
the important clue is not as much the patient's level of functioning, if it has remained
stable, but a recent *change* in ability to perform activities of daily living or other necessary functions.

PHYSICAL ASSESSMENT

A complete physical examination should be
performed with special attention paid to the
neurologic examination. Several primitive
reflexes have been associated with diffuse
cerebral dysfunction.[22]

The *palmomental reflex* is elicited by
having the patient look straight ahead (at the
examiner's nose) while the thenar eminence
of the hand is stroked. This contracts the
ipsilateral mentalis muscle (muscle of the
chin) which causes the chin to wrinkle. This
reflex is found in 54% of elderly persons
with organic brain syndrome, and 52% with
neurologic impairment.[23]

The *snout reflex* is elicited by a sharp tap
on the closed lips of the patient. A positive
response is the puckering of the lips. One
study found the snout reflex in 72% of patients with organic brain syndrome.[23]

The *suck reflex* is elicited by stroking
the oral region. A positive response is demonstrated by the sucking movement of the
lips, tongue, and jaw.

The *grasp reflex* is elicited by stroking
the palm of the hand, especially the area between the thumb and index finger.

Another addition to the traditional neurologic examination may be the administration of a perceptual sensory test such as the
face–hand test.[17] The face–hand test, developed by Fink and colleagues, may be a useful
adjunct to the mental functioning examina-

tion because it may help to distinguish psychotic patients from those with brain damage. This test is based on the patient's ability to recognize simultaneous tactile stimulation to the cheek and palm of the hand. Although psychotic patients may have cognitive dysfunctions similar to patients with dementia, they are usually able to identify the location of the stimulation.[33] The reader is referred to Fink's article for information on administration and scoring.

PARACLINICAL DATA

The tests identified in Table 1-2 are necessary to rule out an acute brain syndrome or a treatable cause for a dementia (e.g., thyroid disorder, vitamin deficiency). Consultation with a physician is needed to determine which laboratory tests are appropriate. The EEG is commonly used because it is noninvasive and usually available. Progressive slowing of the dominant alpha frequency and the appearance of slow waves in the theta or delta range is common in older people and not necessarily indicative of pathology. There is diffuse slowing in dementia usually more marked in presenile dementia than dementia of later onset.[51] The EEG can help to diagnose the presence of brain lesions; however, a normal EEG does not rule out the possibility of brain damage. Skull x-rays are also widely available and are useful for detecting evidence of a skull fracture, increased intracranial pressure, and some space-occupying masses.

Computerized tomography of the brain (CT scan), has made the use of risky and invasive procedures (e.g., pneumoencephalography and angiography) unnecessary in most cases. The CT scan can be useful in differentiating Alzheimer's disease from multi-infarct dementia, NPH, and in identifying focal lesions.[51]

Other tests that are not done routinely, but are useful in specific circumstances, are the lumbar puncture (if neurosyphilis or infection is suspected); the brain scan, which aids in the localization of lesions or cerebral injuries due to trauma; cisternography, which can aid in the detection of NPH; and psychological testing, which can be useful in differentiating cognitive dysfunction due to depression (pseudodementia) from a true dementia. A screen of urine and blood for toxic levels of drugs (such as digoxin) is done if indicated.

NURSING DIAGNOSIS

Unfortunately the nursing diagnosis of confusion usually is applied casually, after only brief observations of the patient's behavior, and little or no systematic investigation into possible causes. It is essential that any change in mental status or functional ability be identified and investigated promptly. Remember that confusion is always symptomatic of an underlying physiological, psychological, or socioenvironmental problem, many of which can be ameliorated.

The first task is to determine if the patient's confusion indicates an acute or chronic process. Table 1-3 summarizes some behavioral characteristics of dementia and delirium. The next step is to determine the source of confusion. Collaboration with a physician may be necessary to help identify the cause. The nursing diagnosis should be as specific as possible. A few examples of nursing diagnoses include: confusion due to a reversible physiologic imbalance (such as hypoxia or infection), confusion related to depression, confusion due to sensory deprivation, wandering due to Alzheimer's disease, or confusion related to the use of methyldopa.

TABLE 1-3
CHARACTERISTICS OF DELIRIUM AND DEMENTIA

	DEMENTIA	DELIRIUM
Predisposing factors	Age > 70 yrs	Recent illness or surgery Medications Alcohol abuse
Onset	Insidious	Rapid
Behavior	↓ Psychomotor activity ↓ State of alertness Gradual ↓ in level of functioning Incontinence Nocturnal restlessness[*]	↑ Psychomotor activity[*] State of alertness fluctuates Overactivity of autonomic nervous system functions (sweating)[†] Vivid visual hallucinations Variable performance
Mental functioning	Progressive decline of cognitive functioning Progressive decline of memory, especially for recent events Disorientation to person, place, time Confabulation Difficulty in use of names and numbers	Fluctuating symptoms and level of confusion Patchy memory, often good up to time of illness Gross disorientation in presence of alertness and vigilance Sometimes anxious when unable to find a correct response Displacement (correct name, wrong address)

[*]Anderson D: Confusion in the elderly: A protocol to determine acute organic brain syndrome vs. chronic organic brain syndrome. In Wollanin M, Phillips L (eds): Prevention and Care. St. Louis, CV Mosby, 1981
[†]Adams R, Victor H: Delirium and other acute confusional states. In Isselbacher K, Adams R, Braunweld E et al (eds): Harrison's Principles of Internal Medicine. New York, McGraw–Hill, 1980

MANAGEMENT

NURSING MANAGEMENT OF CONFUSION SECONDARY TO PHYSIOLOGICAL IMBALANCE

Nursing care of the patient with confusion resulting from a reversible physiological imbalance is directed toward correcting the cause. Physician consultation often is needed in the management because the administration of IV fluids, antibiotics, or oxygen may be indicated. Careful observation is needed for the patient whose confusion results from an acute neurologic problem. The reader is referred to neurologic nursing books for specific guidelines.

Patients with confusion resulting from a physiological imbalance are often delirious. Hallucinations, especially visual ones, are common in delirium. Frequent reality testing should be done, and potential sources of perceptual misinterpretations, illusions, (such as poor lighting, IV poles) should be identified and corrected. The characteristics of the environment should be described to make it meaningful to the patient. Nursing measures to relieve anxiety and prevent agitation should be instituted (see next section). Safety is a concern with patients who are delirious; therefore, potentially harmful objects should be removed. Physical restraints should be the last course of action; however, occasionally they are necessary to protect the safety of the patient and others. Use them for the briefest time possible, and remove the patient's limbs from the restraints and exercise them hourly, one at a time. Explain the purpose of the restraints to the patient in easily understood terms. ("These are for your safety. We need to help you control your behavior. We will remove them as soon as we can.") He should be told that he will be checked every 10 or 15 minutes by a nurse who will offer him fluids or food. It is essential to maintain nutrition, hydration, and an adequate level of stimulation to prevent further deterioration.

NURSING MANAGEMENT OF CONFUSION FROM IATROGENIC FACTORS

Drugs

Prevention is the key to nursing management of the patient with confusion secondary to drug use. When any medication is prescribed, the patient's comprehension of the frequency, dosage, and method of administration needs to be carefully assessed, taking into account auditory, visual, or language deficits. Nursing measures should always be tried before the administration of such potentially hazardous drugs as tranquilizers or sedatives (see section on agitation). If medication is necessary, give it in the smallest dose possible, remembering that older people take longer to reach a therapeutic level of many drugs. Too often, medications are increased too rapidly, resulting in confusion and other untoward effects (e.g., hypotension). Multiple drug interactions need to be avoided. Some authorities recommend that older people be given periodic drug "holi-

days" to prevent the accumulation of drug metabolites.

Older people are especially vulnerable to the effects of drugs because of aging changes that affect absorption, distribution, and excretion of substances. Consequently, preventive efforts are sometimes ineffective and confusion secondary to toxic reactions may occur. These situations require medical management.

Self-fulfilling Prophecy

A comprehensive assessment and careful diagnosis of confusion should prevent the occurrence of confusion secondary to self-fulfilling prophecy. Other preventive measures include placing reasonable expectations for functioning on the confused person, providing adequate stimulation, and ensuring good communication.

NURSING MANAGEMENT OF CONFUSION RESULTING FROM PSYCHOLOGICAL FACTORS

Depression

Depression aggravates preexisting memory loss and confusion, leading to further perceived loss of control by the patient, which in turn increases his depression. The use of memory cues, adequate stimulation, and interventions to promote control may prevent some of the depression that is frequently secondary to memory loss. (See Chap. 2 for an in-depth discussion of nursing interventions for the depressed patient.)

Patients whose depression presents as a dementia (pseudodementia) are very challenging. Antidepressant treatment usually is indicated, with psychotherapy or counseling after the confusion clears. Tricyclic antidepressants, such as imipramine (Tofranil) or doxepin (Sinequan), are commonly used. If the patient is living alone, family members or a public health nurse must be recruited to ensure that he is taking the medication as ordered. The patient should be monitored carefully for side-effects, the most troublesome of which is orthostatic hypotension. The patient should be encouraged to make slow position changes and dangle his feet over the edge of the bed before arising. Blurred vision, constipation, urinary retention, and dry mouth are other common side-effects resulting from the anticholinergic properties of these drugs. The drowsiness that often occurs with these medications can be advantageous if the full dosage is given at bedtime.

Anxiety

Anxiety can worsen preexisting confusion by putting an added strain on already compromised brain functioning. Promoting orientation, using good communication techniques, and insuring an adequate level of stimulation helps to prevent anxiety. Perhaps the most important preventive measure for anxiety is to give the patient as much control as possible over his environment. Allow patients who have any type of tube or catheter to touch and explore it under the guidance of the nurse. Continue the patient's usual patterns and routines as much as possible. An increase in compulsive behavior is a defense against anxiety and should be respected. Patients admitted to any institution are at high risk for depersonalization; the only things that may have meaning for them are their routines for bathing, eating, and so forth. Patients' routines should not be changed for the convenience of the nurse. Maintain consistency in nursing staff as much as possible. The confusion secondary to relocation anxiety may be prevented if patients bring personal objects, family pictures, or other items, such as a favorite shawl, with them when they are hospitalized or enter a nursing home. Helping the patient to reminisce about

his home, and arranging his room in a similar pattern to that at home (e.g., moving the bed so that the bathroom is on the same side as it is at home) can also be helpful.

Sometimes nursing measures to relieve anxiety need to be combined with the use of antipsychotics. Haloperidal (Haldol) and thioridazine (Mellaril) are commonly used in very small doses because they have less tendency to cause hypotension. Benzodiazepines such as diazepam (Valium) should not be used in older patients because they tend to remain the bloodstream longer and cause confusion. Most of the major tranquilizers and anti-anxiety drugs can cause or worsen confusion.

Sensory Alteration

Good communication is essential to working with the patient who has a sensory impairment. It is important to sit within the patient's field of vision, to speak slowly and clearly (without shouting), and to use touch liberally, if the patient does not perceive this as an intrusion. It is easy to overlook such details as whether the patient's glasses are clean enough to see through, or if his hearing aid batteries work; however, these details are essential for effective communication. It must be kept in mind that suspiciousness often is associated with sensory loss.

Patients must be assessed for their ability to tolerate the sensory overload or deprivation characteristics of the hospital environment. Nursing measures should be directed toward alleviating the cause of sensory distortion and providing for a more consistent level of stimulation which has meaning for the patient.

NURSING MANAGEMENT OF IRREVERSIBLE CONFUSION

This section focuses on the prevention and management of some of the problem behaviors associated with chronic, irreversible confusion.

Agitation

Agitation is one of the most common and most difficult behaviors to manage. The patient who pulls out the urinary catheter, fights attempts to bathe him, and yells late at night can disrupt an entire hospital or nursing home unit. Two nursing actions used for the management of agitation, the administration of tranquilizers and the application of restraints, frequently will increase this behavior. The major tranquilizers (antipsychotic medications such as phenothiazines and butyrophenones) can cause akathisia (difficulty sitting still), which can be mistaken for an increase in agitation. The usual sequence of events is an increase in the tranquilizer dose, which leads to further akathisia and so on. Restraints can be frightening and can reinforce the patient's sense of loss of control, which will increase his agitation.

Agitation can be prevented in many cases by taking steps to minimize anxiety and promote control (see section on anxiety). The patient should be given as many opportunities as possible to make decisions, no matter how small they may seem. If the patient becomes agitated about a specific task (e.g., bath), letting him choose what time he has his bath may increase his sense of control and willingness to participate in his care.

If agitation does occur, frequent supportive contacts should be given. Touch can be effective; however, some patients, when agitated, perceive touch as an intrusion. Sometimes music can be helpful; staff in one nursing home found that a patient's nighttime screaming was alleviated by a radio tuned to a station that played quiet, soothing music. Others have experimented with using tape-recorded messages from family members. This is a promising idea for patients who are not psychotic and are able to reality test.

Sometimes, in spite of good nursing interventions, the patient's agitation progresses to panic. "Panic is a temporary disorganization of the personality manifested by hyperactive behavior and disorientation without a physiological basis".[9] The patient in state of panic requires prompt, decisive nursing intervention. Guidelines for managing panic are:

1. Remain calm. The patient will pick up on your anxiety and become more panicked. He must be reassured that someone is in control of the situation.
2. Reduce all stimuli. Get rid of excess noise (radio, TV) and people.
3. Calmly approach the patient from the side (never approach a panicked patient from the front because he may feel threatened and strike out). Identify yourself and attempt to get eye contact.
4. Continue speaking to the patient in a calm, monotonous voice, reassuring him that you have control of the situation and are there to help.
5. Provide reality testing if he is hallucinating or delusional.
6. If possible, hold the patient from the side and use a rocking motion, relaxing your body as you rock. This rocking can have a calming effect on the patient.[9]
7. Bring the patient to his room or another quiet place and stay with him until he is calm.
8. If medication must be administered, prepare the patient using simple, clear language.

Confused patients are especially at risk for the development of agitation because most stimuli are potentially overwhelming, and patients' perceptions of control are tenuous. Wolanin and Phillips state that agitation is almost always a result of loss of control or perceived loss of control by the patient.[57] Patients at risk for the development of perceived loss of control (patients with catheters or other tubes, patients with sensory losses, patients with compulsive traits, or anyone entering an institutional setting) need to be identified so that preventive measures can be instituted early.

Paranoia

Paranoid features can occur in people with a progressive dementia who have had a lifelong tendency toward suspiciousness. Hearing loss is a predisposing factor, as is social isolation.[50] These persons may feel threatened when they develop symptoms of cognitive decline. They deny this fear and project it onto others.

Another common paranoid behavior of a confused person is to accuse others of stealing from him when in reality the patient misplaced the object (often money) due to forgetfulness. Fear of loss of control is often the mechanism behind the development of paranoia. A characteristic of the delusions seen in people with dementia is a lack of systematization and sophistication, reflecting their intellectual dysfunction. The content is also variable and inconsistent.[50]

Nursing management of the confused, paranoid patient requires a great deal of skill. The first and most difficult task is to build a trusting relationship with the patient. This can be facilitated by giving him more control over his contacts with you (e.g., "I would like to come see you next week. Is Wednesday or Thursday better for you?") and listening attentively while he describes the injustices against him. It is important, however, to maintain some degree of distance and not relate to him in an overly friendly manner, because this leads to mistrust. Delusional material should not be reinforced; however, the patient's feelings can be acknowledged; for example "That must be very frightening for you. How has it affected your sleep, appe-

tite, nerves?" Although medications can be helpful, the majority of paranoid patients will refuse medication. Presenting the medication in the context of helping one's general health and well-being is sometimes effective; for example, "All the things that are happening are making you very nervous, and hard for you to sleep. This is not good for your health. This medicine can help your nerves." Sometimes family members will tell the patient that the antipsychotic medication is really a vitamin or tonic; this is neither ethically or therapeutically warranted.

Helping the patient to feel a sense of control in as many aspects of his life as possible, and at the same time ensuring his safety and that of others, is one of the goals of nursing intervention with confused, paranoid patients. A complicating factor in this type of illness is the amount of attention these patients receive from community agencies, the police, and everyone who becomes involved with them.[6] This secondary gain reinforces the patient's behavior and can make it difficult for him to give it up. Giving him attention for other, positive aspects of his life and encouraging more appropriate methods of obtaining social contact can be helpful.

Hoarding

Most caregivers who work in long-term care facilities are familiar with the chronically confused older patient who hoards various objects, (eating utensils, food, cigarettes) under the mattress, in dresser drawers, or in various other places in the room. The hoarding of objects may be a means of gaining control for a person who feels as if he is losing control over his life. The type of object hoarded is usually an enigma for the caregiver, but may have some meaning for the patient. Hoarding may serve a useful purpose for the patient, but it may be problematic if he is taking things from other people, does not have enough room to store his posses-sions, or, as in the case of food, creates a health hazard. Behavior modification tech-niques may be useful in these situations (see below). More research needs to be done in this area.

Compulsiveness

Excessive orderliness, list-making, and writ-ing everything down are ways of trying to maintain control and diminish the sense of loss for confused patients with compulsive traits. These persons have a very strong need to feel in control and are especially threat-ened by the loss of cognitive abilities. The compulsive behavior, as frustrating as it may be for the caregiver, is an adaptive method of coping with loss and should be supported.

Communication Difficulties

Communicating with the cognitively im-paired can be a time-consuming, sometimes frustrating task for the caregiver. This sets up a vicious cycle in which the patient is avoided and subsequently understimulated, which leads to even more confusion. The communication techniques previously dis-cussed should be used.

One of the most difficult tasks can be to get and keep the patient's attention. Porter and colleagues suggest that touch be used to initiate eye contact.[41] Once eye contact is ob-tained, the nurse should smile broadly to keep the patient's attention. The use of touch and nonverbal messages with cognitively im-paired patients cannot be overemphasized. One study found a significant increase in the use of nonverbal responses (smiling, im-proved eye contact) by elderly nursing home residents when they were touched on the arm by the nurse.[36] The study suggests that touch enhances the relationship aspect of communication. When verbal communica-tion is used, the messages given should be

kept brief and simple, and repeated until the nurse is sure that they are understood. In giv-ing instructions to a confused patient, it is often helpful to combine verbal and non-verbal messages, for example, gesturing with the hand while saying "Come with me."

"Sundowner's Syndrome"

Sundowning, or the increase in confusion that occurs in the evening, is a common phe-nomenon in long-term and acute care facili-ties. The phenomenon has been sadly ne-glected in research, however; only two studies were found in the literature. One ex-plored the effect of varying doses of caffeine in promoting relaxation and sleep in patients who were prone to sundowner's syndrome; however, this method was not found to be helpful.[19] The other study, which was per-formed in 1941, attempted to replicate the symptoms of "nocturnal senile delirium" in patients by exposing them to conditions sim-ilar to nighttime (darkness, diminished sen-sory input).[10] This researcher suggested that the memory impairment of the patient with dementia interferes with his ability to pre-serve spatial images, and thus in the dark he is not able to locate himself in space. He be-comes disoriented and subsequently agi-tated. Some have suggested that sundowner's syndrome is due to fatigue resulting from the stimulation of daytime events, but Cameron suggests that darkness is the causative factor. However, because this syndrome is a com-mon occurrence in the late afternoon at change of shift, it would seem likely that fac-tors other than darkness play a role. Perhaps the decrease in stimulation usually found in the evening in institutions is a significant factor. This is also an area that needs more research.

Some nursing measures that can prevent sundowner's syndrome are use of a night-light in the patient's room, maintaining orientation during the day, and providing brief, frequent orienting contacts during the late afternoon and continuing throughout the evening. If nursing measures are not effective, the administration of a very small dose of a tranquilizer such as haloperidol (Haldol) or thioridizine (Mellaril) 1 hour before the confusion and disorientation occurs is sometimes helpful.

Wandering

Wandering is one of the most problematic behaviors seen in confused patients. It is problematic for the patient living in the community because it can precipitate his admission to a long-term care facility even though otherwise he may be able to care for himself. It is also troublesome for the caregiver because neither of the common ways of dealing with the wandering patient (having soneone follow him around all day or tying him in a chair) are appropriate. Wandering is another area for which research is needed.

Wandering usually is considered to be nonpurposeful; however, in a detailed study of the wandering patterns of three nursing home residents, Hussian found that: 1) they consistently spent more stationary time in stimulating places (open rooms, windows); 2) they consistently kept to the same routes, even when taken to another floor with identical floor plans but different personnel; and 3) daily periods of free ambulation significantly decreased time spent in wandering, and the distance traveled.[29] This research indicates that one way of preventing or minimizing wandering is to provide the opportunity for exercise and adequate stimulation. Some long-term care facilities have locked units that provide a safe place for confused wanderers. Cornbleth found that a protected unit area (open to a courtyard but locked to the rest of the facility), which permitted freedom of movement, may have positive effects on some aspects of physical functioning (e.g., range of motion) in wanderers.[14]

If the person is living at home, the family may be able to recruit neighbors to keep an eye out for the wanderer on his walks. Because wanderers usually keep to the same routes and use environmental cues to orient themselves, this may be an adequate safety measure.

Serious consideration must be given to the hazards involved in physically restraining the wanderer. Wandering can be dangerous, but so can the increased confusion, decreased self-esteem, skin breakdown, and other physical disorders caused by physical restraints. Providing adequate environmental cues and helping the patient to become accustomed to a safe route can minimize the hazards of wandering and permit the patient to remain independent for as long as possible. Some families have tried using double bolt locks, which require a key, or installing a bell, which rings when the door is opened, to prevent their confused relatives from wandering.

Forgetfulness

The process of aging affects secondary memory, which involves the acquisition and recall of information. Attempts to improve memory in older people by the use of visual imagery or organizing strategies have been successful. Zarit also believes that many older people tend to exaggerate their concerns about memory because of belief in age stereotypes and low morale. He suggests that education about the effects of aging on memory, reassurance that occasional forgetfulness does not mean senility, and improving morale in those who are depressed are strategies to help improve memory in the elderly.[58]

Those patients with chronic dementia can also benefit from the use of memory cues, although in a more limited way. Making lists, tacking the bills on the calendar on the date when they must be paid, and setting out daily pills in egg containers are several techniques that may be helpful. Having the patient keep an appointment book with his name, address, telephone number, and other essentials in his pocket can assist his memory while preserving his dignity. The forgetful patient should write appointments and other information down immediately. Some persons can think of creative ways to help their memory; one elderly nursing home resident tied a bright red bow on the railing outside her door so she would be able to find her room.

Repetitiveness

Repetitiveness is a particularly annoying behavior for caregivers and family members. The patient asks the same question over and over again, without ever seeming to hear the response. Arie describes repetitiveness as "...the expression of a wish for reassurance which, however, often it is given, is never able to be assimilated."[4] Promoting a sense of security and other interventions used to prevent anxiety may be helpful. It is important for family members to understand that this behavior is not a deliberate attempt by the patient to drive them crazy, but comes from their need to know that they will be taken care of and are safe.

Disorientation

The ability to know where one is, who one is, and have a sense of time is essential for even the most basic functioning. Patients with a chronic dementia frequently are disoriented to time and place. Clocks and calendars within easy access of the patient may be the most important means of promoting orientation. In their study of confusion among elderly hip fracture patients, Williams and co-workers found that the presence of a timepiece was associated with higher levels of mental clarity.[55] Ensuring that the patient is wearing his own clothing is a very basic, but sometimes overlooked, means of promoting orientation to person. The patient's personal articles and family pictures displayed within the patient's visual field can also help.

Reality orientation is a popular technique used to promote orientation in nursing homes. This technique usually consists of two parts; daily reality orientation (RO) classes for patients, involving a structured orientation to time, place, and person, naming common objects, describing the weather; and 24-hour reality orientation, which is a concerted effort by all personnel to orient the patient to the environment, emphasizing time, place, and person. A clock and calendar are at the patient's bedside.[28] Reality orientation boards that give the name and address of the institution, date, and next meal, among other information, are used in the classes. Several studies have attempted to measure the effectiveness of RO; however, objective measures have failed thus far to show that structured RO is beneficial. Staff reports in one study indicated that a RO program improved the appearance, confidence, disposition, and interest in activities of its participants.[18] Another study that attempted to evaluate the patient's level of confusion by a questionnaire before and after a RO program found no significant difference in scores of the patients who had been involved in the program and a control group. Informal observations, however, indicated that the patients in the experimental group appeared to become less confused and more alert.[28] It would be difficult to determine, however, if the positive effects noted in this study were due to the content or social aspects of the RO sessions, or to the extra attention given during the 24-hour RO program.

Hussian proposes a modified form of RO that teaches the patient skills that he could generalize to other situations and environments instead of just learning verbal responses.[29] He also identifies three types of patients who are not appropriate for RO: 1) the patient with a rapidly progressing terminal illness, 2) the very old patient who has been totally disoriented and withdrawn for more than 2 years, and 3) the patient who becomes very anxious or panicky when pushed to become oriented to the present. An individualized assessment, which includes an assessment of the patient's coping skills, needs to be performed before structured RO is initiated.

Behavioral Techniques

Behavior modification techniques have been used successfully with confused older people to deal with problem behaviors such as refusal to ambulate, diminished social interaction, and self-destructiveness. The type of behavior modification used with chronically confused patients is based on the fact that behavior that is reinforced (rewarded) will occur more frequently than behavior that is not. For example: a confused elderly man used abusive language towards the nursing staff. This always elicited a great deal of attention as staff tried to make him see the error of his ways. When they began to ignore his abusiveness and made it a point to spend a couple of minutes talking with him when he was sitting quietly, his verbal abusiveness decreased markedly, and he became more socially appropriate, conversant, and less anxious.

Behavioral problems are usually symptomatic of underlying conflicts and no behavior modification program should be initiated without a careful investigation into the possible causes of the behavior and the purpose it serves.[39] The following guidelines may be used to plan a behavior treatment program:

- *Identify the problem behavior.* This must be a *specific* behavior, one that is simple and amenable to change. Once the behavior is identified, it must be determined for whom it is a problem, the patient or the staff. Some behaviors may serve a useful purpose for the patient and merely be annoying to the staff. Other behaviors, such as verbal and physical abusiveness, may lead to social isolation and the use of physical restraints.
- *Record the baseline of the problem behavior.* When does the behavior occur? Where does the behavior occur and how frequently? Does anything precede the behavior? The nurse may find that the verbal abuse occurs only in the evening when the patient is fatigued and dealing with sensory changes, or that social withdrawal occurs only on visiting days when the patient is depressed about his lack of visitors.
- *Identify the desired behavior.* It is very important to be realistic and start with small goals, or both the nurse and the patient will be frustrated by the lack of progress. For example, a goal of "patient will walk to dining room with walker only by the end of the week" is not realistic for a woman who has refused to get out of her chair for months. Having the woman touch the walker or perhaps stand with it by her chair is a more realistic initial goal. This process of breaking a behavior down into a sequence in which the patient masters one step before progressing to the next is called *shaping.*
- *Decide on a reinforcer.* A reinforcer is given to the patient immediately after the desired behavior occurs. Social contact and touch usually are very effective reinforcers for confused patients. Sometimes the social re-

inforcer is paired with another reward, like candy. As the desired behavior occurs with greater frequency, the candy is gradually withdrawn and only the social reinforcer is used. It is important to choose a reinforcer that will be effective for the patient.

• *Begin the behavior modification program.* The program is carried out by *immediately* providing reinforcement for the desired behavior. The program will not work if the reinforcer is given one half hour after the desired behavior. If the patient's reinforcer is going for a walk with the nurse or something which cannot be carried out immediately, the patient should be given something to symbolize this, such as an I.O.U. after the desired behavior occurs.

The effectiveness of the behavior program is continually monitored. If it does not seem to be working, perhaps the reinforcer is not effective or is not being given consistently. The program must be reevaluated and changed if necessary. If it is successful, the reinforcer is applied less frequently and gradually withdrawn.

The success of a behavioral treatment program depends on the appropriateness of the goals, the meaning of the reinforcer for the patient, and the consistency of the staff in administering the reinforcer. Occasionally, identifying something that is rewarding to the patient can be a difficult task. Family members can assist with this. One of the biggest obstacles in carrying out a behavioral program is the lack of consistency of the staff, which may be due to shift rotation, floating to other units, unwillingness to spend the extra time with the patient, or skepticism regarding the effectiveness of the program. Staff members must be given a great deal of support and encouragement, especially in the early stages of the program.

Several ethical problems have been raised regarding the use of behavior treatment programs in patients with dementia.[24] These center on the use of punishment, the ability of the patient to give informed consent to such a program, and whether institutions have the right to initiate such programs for patients who do not give consent, but are potentially harmful to self or others. These issues are difficult to resolve and must be dealt with on an individual basis. Generally speaking, the use of punishment is *not* appropriate, either ethically or therapeutically, for confused patients. The amount of attention obtained by disruptive behaviors in institutions is so rewarding that ignoring this behavior and reinforcing a more appropriate one is usually effective.

It is usually a good idea to include family members in planning the program even if the patient is able to give consent, because their assistance in carrying out the program may be crucial. The consequences of permitting the problem behavior to continue should be explored (e.g., social withdrawal may lead to depression, refusal to walk may lead to muscle atrophy and skin breakdown), and other possible methods of treatment discussed.

The topic of behavior modification is too broad and complex to be dealt with adequately in this chapter. The reader is referred to one of the many available books on the subject before attempting to implement a behavior program for a confused patient.

MEDICAL MANAGEMENT OF IRREVERSIBLE CONFUSION

Several drugs have been introduced which, by their different actions on the brain, are thought to alleviate or prevent cognitive decline and the associated behavioral symptoms. Dihydroergotamine mesylate (Hydergine), a drug that affects brain metabolism, is one of the most widely used of these drugs. Some studies have indicated that dihydro-ergotamine is effective in reducing somatic complaints and improving mood, attitude, sense of well-being, and activities of daily living. However, changes in memory performance as measured by objective techniques are difficult to demonstrate.[44] Dihydroergot-amine is usually most effective in patients with mild cognitive impairment. Papavarine and cyclandelate, both drugs with vasodi-lator properties, have also been shown to be more effective than placebo in ameliorating some of the behavioral symptoms associated with mild dementia in some patients; how-ever, results have not been consistent.[44]

Hyperbaric oxygen (HBO) initially showed some promising results in the treat-ment of patients with dementia; however, successive studies have not replicated the re-sults of the original study.[21,49] In fact, Gold-farb and colleagues found that their subjects (patients with Alzheimer's disease) actually became more aggressive, restless, and occa-sionally paranoid with HBO treatment.

IMPLICATIONS FOR NURSING RESEARCH

Although there has been a recent surge of research into the causes of Alzheimer's dis-ease and other types of dementia, there has been very little research in the area of man-agement of the behaviors seen with these dis-eases. Because nurses are the people who are most familiar with the behaviors and behav-ior problems associated with confusion, they are the ones who need to begin systematic-ally to investigate possible approaches and management techniques. Two of the behav-iors that cause the most disruption in a hos-pital or nursing home environment, that is, wandering and sundowner's syndrome, are

behaviors about which little is known. Part of the problem has been that institutions that deal with the chronically confused are typi-cally understaffed, and it is easier and faster at first to rely on techniques of medical management, such as the administration of tranquilizers or application of restraints. However, these techniques can create more problems than they solve, which may be even more time-consuming in the long run.

Research also must be done in the area of environmental causes of confusion, in partic-ular, the characteristics of the hospital and nursing home environment. If we knew more about the causes, nurses could take steps to prevent the confusion that frequently occurs in older people who are hospitalized or relo-cated.

Finally, although some work has been done, more research is needed to help iden-tify the characteristics of people who are at risk for the development of confusion.[57] More data regarding populations at risk would facilitate the institution of preventive mea-sures.

REFERENCES

1. Adams M, Hanson R. Norkoal D et al: Psychological responses in critical care units. Am J Nurs 78:1504–1512, Sept 1978
2. Adams R, Victor H: Delirium and other acute con-fusional states. In Isselbacher K, Adams R, Braun-weld E et al (eds): Harrison's Principles of Internal Medicine, 122–126. New York, McGraw–Hill, 1980
3. Anderson D: Confusion in the elderly: A protocol to determine acute organic brain syndrome vs. chronic organic brain syndrome. In Wolanin M, Phillips, L (eds): Confusion: Prevention and Care. St. Louis, CV Mosby, 1981
4. Arie T: Confusion in old age. Age Ageing 1 (Suppl): 72–76, 1978
5. Bartol MA: Nonverbal communication in patients with Alzheimer's disease. J Gerontol Nurs 5:21–31, July, Aug, 1979
6. Berger K, Zarit S: Late life paranoid states: Assess-

ment and treatment. Am J Orthopsychiatry 43, No. 8:528–536, 1978

7. Brody E, Kelban H, Lowton MP et al: Excess disabilities of mentally and impaired aged: Impact of individualized treatment. Part I. Gerontologist 11:124–133, 1971

8. Bruen D: The relationship between the presence of sensory deprivation and the development of acute confusion in elderly hospitalized patients. Master's thesis, unpublished, University of Rochester, 1981

9. Burwell DM: Working with the patient in panic. Presented at the 5th Annual Meeting of the Ontario Psycho-geriatric Association, London, Ontario, September 24–27, 1978

10. Cameron D: Studies in nocturnal senile delirium. Psychiatr Q, 15, No. 1:47–54, 1941

11. Craik F: Age differences in human memory. In Birren J, Schail KW (eds): Handbook of the Psychology of Aging pp 384–420. New York, Van Nostrand Reinhold, 1977

12. Chisolm S, Deniston L, Igrisan R et al: Prevalence of confusion in elderly hospitalized patients. J Gerontol Nurs 8, No. 2:87–97, Feb 1982

13. Comfort A: Non-threatening mental testing of the elderly. J Am Geriatr Soc XXVI, No. 5:261–262, 1979

14. Cornbleth T: Effects of a protected hospital ward area on wandering and non-wandering geriatric patients. J Gerontol 32, No. 5:573–577, 1977

15. Dall J: Management of confusional states. Age Ageing (Suppl) 7:77–78, 1978

16. Ernest P, Beran B, Safford R et al: Isolation and the symptoms of chronic brain syndrome. Gerontologist 18 No. 5:468–474, 1978

17. Fink M, Green M, Bender M: The face–hand test as a diagnostic sign of organic mental syndrome. Neurol 2, No. 48:46–58, 1952

18. Folsom JC: Reality orientation for the elderly mental patient. J Geriatr Psychiatry, 1, No. 291:307, Spring 1968

19. Ginsburg R. Weintraub A: Caffeine in the sundown syndrome. J Gerontol 31, No. 4:419–420, 1976

20. Glick F: Changes in behavior, mood or thinking in the elderly: Diagnosis and management. Med Clin North Am 60, No. 6:1297–1314, Nov 1976

21. Goldfarb A, Holkstadt N, Jacobson JH: Hyperbaric oxygen treatment of organic mental syndrome in aged persons. J Gerontol 27:212–217, 1972

22. Gurland B: The assessment of the mental health status of older adults. In Birren J, Sloane RB (eds): Handbook of Mental Health and Aging, pp 671–700. New Jersey, Prentice–Hall, 1980

23. Habot B Libow L: The interrelationship of mental and physical status and its assessment in the older adult: Mind–body interaction. In Birren J Sloane R: Handbook of Mental Health and Aging. New Jersey, Prentice–Hall, 1980

24. Harris S, Snyder B, Snyder R et al: Behavior modification therapy with elderly demented patients: Implementation and ethical considerations. J Chronic Dis 30:129–134, 1977

25. Hayter J: Patients who have Alzheimer's disease. Am J Nurs 74, No. 8:1460–1463,Aug 1974

26. Heston L, Mastri A, Anderson V et al: Dementia of the Alzheimer type: Clinical genetics, natural history, and associated conditions. Arch Gen Psychiatry 38:1085–1090, Oct 1981

27. Hodkinson HM: Mental impairment in the elderly. J R Coll Physicians Lond 7, No. 4:305–317, July 1973

28. Hogstel J: Use of reality orientation with aging confused patients. Nurs Res 28, No. 3:161–165, May/June 1979

29. Hussian R: Geriatric Psychology. New York, Van Nostrand Reinhold, 1981

30. Jacobs J, Bernhard M, Delgado A et al: Screening for organic mental syndromes in the medically ill. Ann Int Med 86, No. 1:40–46, 1977

31. Jarvick L: Diagnosis of dementia in the elderly: A 1980 perspective. In Eisdorfer C (ed): Annu Rev Gerontol Geriatr, Vol 1, pp 180–203. New York, Springer Publishing, 1980

32. Jenkyn L, Walsh D, Culver C et al: Clinical signs in diffuse cerebral dysfunction. J Neurol Neurosurg Psychiatry 408, No. 8:956–966, 1977

33. Kane R, Kane R: Assessment in Long–Term Care. Lexington, Mass, Lexington Books, 1981

34. Kiloh LG: Pseudo-dementia. Acta Psychiatr Scand 37:336–351, 1961

35. Kral VA: Confusional states. In Howells JE (ed): Modern perspectives in the psychiatry of old age, pp 356–363. New York, Bruner/Mazel, 1975

36. Langland R, Panicucci C: The effects to touch on communication with elderly confused clients. J of Gerontol Nurs 8, No. 3:152–156, Mar 1982

37. LaPorte H: Reversible causes of dementia: A nursing challenge. J Geront Nurs 8, No. 2:74–81, Feb 1982

38. Libow L: Senile dementia and pseudosenility: Clinical diagnosis. In Eisdorfer C, Friedel R (eds): Cognitive and Emotional Disturbance in the elderly. Chicago, Year Book Medical Publishers, 1977

39. Oberleder M: Managing problem behaviors of elderly patients. Hosp Community Psychiatry 27, No. 5:325–330, May 1976

40. Phillips LR: Care of the client with sensoripercep-

tual problems. In Wolanin MD, Phillips LR (eds): Confusion: Prevention and Care. St. Louis, CV Mosby, 1981

41. Porter J, Rasmussen T, Burnside I: Developing a working relationship with a confused client. Nursing and the Aged. New York, McGraw–Hill, 1981

42. Post R: Dementia, depression and pseudodementia. In Benson BF, Blumer D (eds): Psychiatric Aspects of Neurological Disease, pp 99–120. New York, Grune & Stratton, 1975

43. Raskind M, Kitchell M, Alvarez C: Bromide intoxication in the elderly. J Am Geriatr Soc XXVI, No. 5: 222–224, 1979

44. Raskin MA, Storrie MC: The organic mental disorders. In Busse EW, Blazer DG (eds): Handbook of Geriatric Psychiatry, pp 305–329. New York, Van Nostrand Reinhold, 1980

45. Ropper A: A rational approach to dementia. Canadian Medical Association Journal 121:1175–1190, Nov 1979

46. Salzman C, Shader R: Clinical evaluation of depression in the elderly. In Raskind A, Jarrick L (eds): Psychiatric Symptoms and Cognitive Loss in the Elderly. Washington, Hemisphere Publishing, 1979

47. Schneck M, Reisberg N, Ferris S: An overview of current concepts of Alzheimer's disease. Am J Psychiatr 139, No. 2:165–171, Feb 1982

48. Strub RL, Black FW: The Mental Status Examination in Neurology. Philadelphia, FA Davis, 1977

49. Thompson LW, Davis GC, Obrist WD: Effects of hyperbaric oxygen on behavioral and physiological measures in elderly demented patients. J Gerontol, 31:23–28, 1976

50. Verowerdt A: Clinical Geropsychiatry. Baltimore, Williams & Wilkins, 1976

51. Wang H: Diagnostic procedures. In Busse E, Blazer D (eds): Handbook of Geriatric Psychiatry, pp 285–304. New York, Van Nostrand Reinhold, 1980

52. Wang H, Busse E: Dementia in old age. In Wells C. (ed): Dementia: Contemporary Neurology Series. Philadelphia, FA Davis, 1971

53. Wells C: Chronic brain disease: An overview. Am J Psychiatr 135, No. 1:1–12, Jan 1978

54. Wells C: Pseudodementia. Am J Psychiatr 136, No. 7: 895–900, July 1979

55. Williams M. Holloway J, Winn M et al: Nursing activities and acute confusional states in elderly hip-fractured patients. Nurs Res 28, No. 1:25–35, Jan/Feb 1979

56. Wolanin MD: Physiologic aspects of confusion. J Gerontol Nurs 7, No. 4:236–242, Apr 1981

57. Wolanin MD, Phillips LR: Confusion: Prevention and Care. St. Louis, CV Mosby, 1981

58. Zarit S: Helping an aging patient to cope with memory problems. Geriatrics 34:82–90, Apr 1979

2

Depression

Deborah McNeil

The existentialists propose that depression, anxiety, and loneliness are inherent in human existence. A person is born alone, exists subjectively alone, and must die alone. To know the soaring of elation, one must experience sadness. Likewise, to be truly alive requires an awareness of one's possibly imminent death.[28,35,36,49] The human life cycle ebbs and flows with seasons of ecstasy and agony. The focus of this chapter is the sadness, depression, and loneliness that plague all people in the course of existence.

Depression is defined as a dysphoric lowering of mood state. Psychodynamically, depression is usually conceptualized as a response to loss and is, therefore, closely related to grief (a normal and time-limited response to loss).

Grief may be considered a tribute to someone or something loved and lost. The something might be a body part, prized belief, or cherished position. Whatever the loss, depression colors the grief process. Friends and loved ones traditionally draw near to support and nurture the afflicted. Through the mist of pain, healing begins. As the person works through feelings about the loss, symptoms decrease. With time, the loved person or object may be fondly remembered without pain. Life continues and pleasure is again experienced.

Depression may be conceptualized as a dynamic phenomenon existing on a continuum ranging from mild, transient sadness to a severe psychotic experience.[48] The depression will vary depending on its depth, the personality of the individual, and the environment. The primary focus of this chapter is adults suffering mild or moderate depression. These people are encountered by the nurse in all clinical settings and in personal interactions. Because of this emphasis and the dynamic conceptualization, we will not address psychiatric diagnosis, psychopharmacology, and electroconvulsive therapy. This information is readily available in many excellent psychiatric texts.

Loneliness, a phenomenon considered a part of depression by most researchers up until the 1960s, is also discussed. Various measures of loneliness have been significantly correlated repeatedly with various measures of depression in a variety of populations. These findings indicate that depression and loneliness do tend to occur together. Despite these correlations, plus pleas from some nursing leaders that loneliness is fertile ground for nursing intervention, most texts address the phenomenon only in passing. Loneliness is emphasized in this chapter in the hope that an increased understanding will augment the nurse's ability to provide holistic care to the depressed patient.

The organizing framework in this chapter is the depression continuum, the holistic person (i.e., emotional, intellectual, physical, social, and spiritual elements), and the nursing process. The framework creates some arbitrary divisions of depression and the person for the sake of simplification. Depression is determined by viewing the totality of the experience, not a piece of it. A disturbance or change in any realm of being affects the whole person, not some isolated segment. The nursing process further organizes the information into subjective and objective assessment, nursing diagnosis, and management strategies.

MECHANISMS OF DEPRESSION

PSYCHODYNAMICS AND PATHOPHYSIOLOGY: A THEORETICAL EXPLANATION

Theory consists of a group of interrelated concepts that describes and explains phenomena for the purpose of understanding.[26] Scientists have formulated an impressive body of theory related to depression; however, there is no one universally accepted or totally satisfying explanation of depression. In this section, key ideas from a variety of leading theories are described briefly. The theories provide varied perspectives for understanding the mechanisms of depression.

A Theory of Grief

From the analysis of interviews with over 200 terminally ill patients in the famous Chi-

cago seminars, Kübler–Ross outlined a stage theory of dying.[28] Later, the theory was proposed to be descriptive of the grief response to any loss.[29] The theory's five stages are denial, anger, bargaining, depression, and acceptance.

Denial, a defense against fear and isolation, buffers the news of loss. Usually a temporary reaction, denial gives way to the less radical defense of anger. Anger is sometimes referred to as "impotent rage" and is associated with feeling out of control and powerless.[29] Bargaining, the third stage, presents as promises and attempts to complete unfinished business. Much like a young child, the grieving person often offers good behavior in exchange for an extension of time or assistance through a painful period. Taking care of unfinished business includes such behaviors as handling legal affairs and sharing those things that need to be said to special people.[30]

Depression, the fourth stage in the grief process, is the specific response to the loss. Reactive depression, or grief for past loss, occurs first, followed by preparatory depression, or grief for future loss. Marked withdrawal and intense grief characterize preparatory depression, which is reflected in decathexis or withdrawal of energy invested from the object that will be lost. For the dying, the object may be loved ones and the world itself. The final stage, acceptance, is defined as "facing finiteness, living a different quality of life marked by joy in the present day, with little worry about tomorrow."[30] Hope, which is nurturing, may be and should be maintained throughout the stages. The stages often occur in linear sequence, but not always. They may also overlap.

Psychoanalytic Theory

Freud emphasized loss as the central issue in grief and depression. He compared and contrasted mourning and melancholia, which can be equated generally with grief and depression. He stated: "In grief, the world becomes poor and empty; in melancholia, it is the ego itself."[16] Freud was referring to the internal nature of the loss in depression, with its sharp lowering of self-regard. In mourning, the person gradually withdraws libidinal cathexis (sexual energy) from the real, lost love object. Later, this energy is transferred to a new attachment object to restore psychic balance of libidinal forces. In melancholia, the loss, which may be real or symbolic, reactivates feelings experienced with a much earlier significant loss. In childhood, the future melancholic experiences a primal loss because of disappointment with a loved person. Instead of the libido being transferred to a new love object, as in grief, the libido is withdrawn into the ego. The original love object (which was both loved and hated) is incorporated into oneself. The internalized object then becomes the target of the hatred that would have been directed at the original object. When reactivation occurs later in life, the melancholic patient's anger is directed at the internal object representation, which has now become fused with the patient's ego. The rage may be so great as to result in suicide. This process offers an explanation of the melancholic's withdrawal of interest from the external world, excessive self-interest, and self-reproach.

Bibring conceptualized depression as the emotional correlate of a specific state of the ego related to a fall in self-esteem. For Bibring, lowered self-esteem is the cardinal problem in depression. Self-esteem is the felt disparity between the ego ideal and the actual state as measured by the ego. Depression, like anxiety, is a primary experience, indivisible in nature. Other central features of depression include unfulfilled narcissistic aspirations and the painful awareness of ac-

tual or imaginary helplessness. Although many depressions have their roots in the oral phase of development, depressive roots beginning in later phases of development was proposed by Bibring.[7]

Like Bibring, Jacobson emphasized self-esteem as a central issue in depression. Jacobson believed that the mind develops by gradual formation of self and object representations. Roughly, self and object representations are the internalized images of oneself and others. Regulated by the superego, these self and object representations are invested (cathected) with libidinal, aggressive, or neutralized energy. Libidinal energy is sexual; aggressive energy is destructive. When sexual and aggressive cathexes are neutralized (altered) in favor of affectionate love relations and ego interests, the psychic energy is termed *neutralized energy*. The way a person feels about self and others depends on which representation is the recipient of the different types of energy. When aggressive or destructive psychic energy is concentrated on an internalized object, there is devaluation of the object.[24]

In infancy, the representation of self is fused or merged with the representation of others. Therefore, "a devaluation of others (an aggressive cathexis of the object representation) due to frustration is said to result also in a devaluation of the self, since the self is still fused with the representation of others."[5]

During growth and development in healthy persons, the superego develops into a depersonified agency. In pathology, the superego is not well developed and remains tied to people from the person's past and may be confused with external objects. This lack of development is a lack of differentiation. The lack of superego differentiation affects cathexis of self-representations.

In depression, when the ego is unable to

achieve gratification or pleasure, rage is aroused and there is an aggressive cathexis of self-image. In other words, aggression is turned upon the self-image. With aggressive cathexis, the self-representation is devalued. This devaluation of the self-representation results in a greater disparity between the self-image and the ideal self. Remember, in terms of ego psychology, *self-esteem* is the felt disparity between the ego ideal and the actual state as measured by the ego. In depression, then, the cardinal problem according to Jacobson is one of aggressive cathexis of self-representation that results in devaluation of the self-representation and lowered self-esteem. The lack of differentiation or the merging of worthless object representations with self-representation facilitates this process because, with fusion, aggressive cathexis of other representations also results in spontaneous devaluation of self.[25]

Drawing on the work of Freud and Jacobson, Leiderman presented three case studies on which he formulated the dynamics of loneliness and attempted to differentiate loneliness and depression. Depression is related more to aggressive drive components; loneliness, to libidinal drive components. In depression, there is cathexis of the self-representation with aggressive or destructive energy. In loneliness, there is an absence of hostility as the predominant affect. Depression probably derives from the earliest stages of development; loneliness, from later stages. The central issue in depression is loss. In loneliness, the central issue is the "uncompleted or undifferentiated self-object representations, or both, within the system ego."[31] In loneliness, the person feels incomplete and longs for another. Unlike grief and depression, loneliness is not dependent on the loss of a real object or an internalized object representation about which the person has ambivalent feelings.

The frequent occurrence of loneliness and depression together may be accounted for by the tendency of inadequate mothering and frequent separations to predispose the person to both loss and inadequate self-object differentiation. The infant normally creates an intrapsychic object representation of significant others in the environment. "The pathological process in self-object differentiation occurs when the appropriate individuals in the infant's environment are not available or are idiosyncratic, as in the case of identical twins."[31]

Interpersonal Theory

Interpersonal theory emphasizes relationships. People cannot grow up in a vacuum. Therefore, any consideration of the individual must also take into account others in the environment. Anxiety is another central concept in the theory. Motivation for behavior is avoidance of anxiety and the satisfaction of needs.[46]

Sullivan's writings on depression are highly descriptive and document the paucity of ideas, the repetitive tendency toward destructive situations, and the retardation of bodily processes.[45] Citing the hostility toward others that occurs during mania as evidence, Sullivan stated that "there is something other than loving kindness in the interpersonal relations of the depressed," as if others should suffer, too. He further commented on the person's almost protective attitude toward the depressive context.[47]

Developmentally, the future depressive receives total acceptance and care in infancy. In return, the child is very receptive to the significant other. Later, perhaps beginning in the second year of life, the child receives love and acceptance only when attempts are made to meet the expectations of significant others. The child learns early that that which is obtained should be deserved. Significant others subtly exhibit hostility toward the child by continually increasing expectations that are just beyond the child's capabilities. To obtain love, the child tries to meet expectations that tend to dangle forever beyond reach. Gratification remains in the future.[2] This process partially explains the depressive person's inability to feel pleasure, his tendency to set unreachable goals, and his difficulty with interpersonal relationships.

Sullivan did not directly connect loneliness with depression, but he did relate both to the need for human relationships. *Loneliness* is defined as "the exceedingly unpleasant and driving experience connected with inadequate discharge of the need for human intimacy."[46] An uncanny experience, loneliness defies description and baffles recall. Loneliness is so unpleasant and so feared that people will often confront anxiety-producing situations to obtain some relief from loneliness. Clinicians can describe loneliness only in terms of people's defenses against it. Fromm–Reichman noted that an individual, in suffering the most intense and freezing form of loneliness, is unable to remember what it was like to have relationships in the past or imagine future relationships.[17]

The roots of loneliness lie in the need for relatedness. The infant is born with a need for human relationships (*i.e.*, a need for tenderness). This need extends into childhood, a time when components that will ultimately appear as loneliness develop. These components are later expressed in the child's need for participation in activities. In the juvenile era, these components are visible in the need for peers and the need for acceptance. Many children experience a fear of ostracism at this stage because of difficult experiences with peers. In preadolescence, loneliness attains its final component—"the need for intimate exchange" with a chum,

friend, or loved one.[46] According to Sullivan, loneliness at this point has reached its full significance and will go on relatively unchanged throughout the life cycle. Weiss supported this position and proposed that the loneliness of emotional isolation is probably not experienced until early adolescence, when "parents are relinquished as attachment figures."[50]

Cognitive Theory

A key assumption of cognitive theory is that the way a person thinks and feels is significantly related to the way an individual cognitively structures experience. Beck believes a thinking disorder is the primary link in the chain of events resulting in depression. Other predominant and stressful symptoms of depression may be explained by an analysis of the cognitive distortion. Key concepts in the theory are the cognitive triad, schemas, and cognitive errors.[4]

The cognitive triad consists of three major cognitive patterns: 1) a negative view of self, 2) a tendency to interpret ongoing experience negatively, and 3) a negative view of the future. All other signs and symptoms of depression are a consequence of the negative thinking patterns. For example, excessive dependency is understood in terms of the person's view of self as inept and helpless, the overestimation of task difficulty, and the expectation that undertakings will turn out badly.

People constantly are confronted with stimuli. The concept schema designates stable cognitive patterns that are the bases for screening out, differentiating, and coding stimuli. Experiences are categorized and evaluated through a matrix of schemata. Specific environmental input may energize a previously inactive schema. In depression, "... patients' conceptualizations of specific situations are distorted to fit the prepotent dysfunctional schemas."[4] These overactive, idiosyncratic schemata override the normal, orderly matching of schemata. As the idiosyncratic schemata become more active, they are more easily evoked by a wider range of stimuli. In other words, as the depression worsens, the person's thinking becomes increasingly dominated by negative ideas and less related to the actual situation. Schemata explain the maintenance of painful, self-defeating attitudes in depression, even in the face of objective evidence to the contrary.

Faulty information processing is visible in the depressed person's tendency to structure experience primitively. Depressed persons are prone to make global judgments based on absolutist standards. They are more likely to attribute experiences to personal character defects and to consider experiences as fixed and irreversible.

Developmentally, the theory postulates that dysfunctional schemata are formed in early experience. Later in life, these schemata are activated by a particular kind of stress to which the person's cognitive organization is sensitive. The nature of the triggering stress (psychological, biochemical, physiological, or any other) depends on the person's sensitivity.

Drawing on the work of Beck and colleagues, and on attribution theory and behavioral theory, Young proposed a cognitive–behavioral theory of loneliness. *Loneliness* is defined as "the absence or perceived absence of satisfying social relationships, accompanied by symptoms of psychological distress which are related to the actual or perceived absence."[52] Key concepts are social reinforcement, attribution, assumptions, and automatic thoughts.

For Young, social relationships compose a particular class of behavioral reinforcement. For example, a person learns that confiding in a friend is pleasant and enjoyable.

Disruption of such a relationship creates a state of deprivation. Loneliness may result, but there is no cognitive discrepancy. Conversely, if a person perceives a relationship deficit, even when no such deficit exists, loneliness also may be experienced.

Negative affects compose the psychological distress of loneliness. Negative affects include depression, anxiety, anger, and bitterness. The particular affect experienced results from the person's explanation of the cause of loneliness, or *attribution*. For example, when a person attributes the social deficiencies to unchangeable personal defects (*internal stable attribution*), the feeling is likely to be one of depression and loneliness. When others are blamed for the social deficiencies (*external attribution*), a person is prone to feel angry or bitter. Changing attributions about the cause of loneliness can change the negative affect experienced.

Young also believes that lonely people hold maladaptive assumptions that are characteristic of loneliness. One example is the assumption, "There must be something wrong with me if I'm alone." Typical automatic thoughts (e.g., "I can't stand being alone") accompany assumptions.[51]

Finally, Young differentiates chronic, situational, and transient loneliness. *Chronic* loneliness (existing for a minimum of 2 consecutive years) involves long-term cognitive and behavioral deficits in relating. *Situational* loneliness occurs in crisis or loss situations. *Transient* loneliness describes the brief and perhaps daily feelings of loneliness.

Family Systems Theory

People are part of a family system extending from the present backward into time. As in any system, one part is interdependent on the other. The nuclear family consists of parents and their children and is part of the extended family, which comprises all other relatives. In Bowen's theory, depression is not viewed as an individual symptom, but rather as a reflection of dysfunction within the family system.[8] Depression is partially a learned response to anxiety and is determined by anxiety in the family system and one's basic level of differentiation.[10]

Differentiation of self, a key concept in Bowen's theory, refers to a person's ability to separate the intellectual processes (thinking) from the emotional processes (feeling). As the degree of differentiation of self decreases, the person is more prone to fusion. *Fusion is* the blending of self with others, thus creating a common self. As with nuclear particles that repel each other on becoming too close, individuals who become too close in fusion seek distance. Depressive dysfunction is one way of creating distance.

Bowen's differentiation-of-self scale describes human functioning along a continuum. The scale ranges from 0 to 100, with a few highly differentiated persons falling around 75 or 80. These rare people function at a high level of independence and are more flexible and adaptive. Their intellectual functioning can retain relative control in periods of stress. In contrast, people at the lower end of the continuum (0 to 25) are more emotionally dependent on others, less adaptive and flexible, function primarily, on a "feeling" level, and are easily stressed into dysfunction.[8]

Within this theory, *pseudoself* means beliefs, principles, and knowledge adopted from others, all of which are readily negotiable, depending upon the emotional environment. Less differentiated people have more pseudoself. Those who fall in the moderate range (25 to 50) of the differentiation scale are more likely to experience depression because of the large amount of pseudoself available for loss in fusion, and conse-

quently, depressive dysfunction. Deep and chronic depressions reflective of a lifelong automatic response to anxiety would be expected in persons functioning at the lowest levels of differentiation. People exhibiting higher levels of differentiation would be expected to experience fewer depressions of shorter duration.[10]

Developmentally, an individual born into a family becomes an automatic part of an ongoing emotional system. Emotional differentiation is largely dependent on the differentiation of parents. People marry others of a similar level of differentiation. Each person brings to marriage a piece of the undifferentiated ego mass from past generations. Through the multigenerational process, emotional problems are passed down from generation to generation. One way of handling an unresolved emotional attachment is through Bowen's concept of emotional cut off.[8] *Emotional cut off* is emotional distancing that may be achieved by an internal mechanism, such as depression, or an external mechanism, such as running away from home and cutting off contact with family members. Cut off is a way of handling the unresolved emotional attachment to parents. When cut off is used, a person carries the unresolved emotional attachment (need for closeness) into the current nuclear family, increasing the chance for fusion in the nuclear family. (Remember that fusion automatically results in distancing.) Withdrawal into self and emotional isolation (distancing) is the primary mechanism for handling anxiety and stress in depression. A family cut off nurtures this process, thus perpetuating depression.[10]

Further, with increased fusion in a marriage, one self may become dominant (drawing upon the common ego mass), whereas the other partner may become submissive or adaptive (losing self in the fusion). The adaptive position is represented by the depressed, underfunctioning person. The more fixed these positions become, the more difficult it is to evoke change in the family system. The fusion blocks opportunity for growth.

Bowen did not address loneliness; however, the concepts of differentiation and emotion cut off apply logically to loneliness. As with depression, less differentiated individuals, functioning primarily on a feeling level, would probably be most susceptible to chronic, intense states of loneliness. Rogers pointed out that individual separateness is essential for a strong union.[39] If differentiation enhances intimacy, then it probably also protects the person from loneliness. Further, Weiss proposed that loneliness results from *emotional* isolation (defined as a lack of intimate relationships), and *social* isolation (defined as a lack of socially supportive relationships). The family cut off imposes isolation, thus increasing the likelihood of loneliness.[50]

Biochemical Theory

In the past decade, nurtured by the scientific revolution, interest and research into the biochemical nature of depression have flourished. Although not necessarily negating psychodynamic theory, the framework favors a conceptualization of depression as a basic emotion, with both psychological and physiological correlates.[5] Presently, the three leading biochemical theories are the biogenic amine, the electrolyte, and the endocrine theories.

The biogenic amine theory arose out of serendipitous clinical observations and research endeavors. Many amines are under investigation, but those most frequently discussed are norepinephrine and serotonin. Both of these brain amines carry neuron messages across the synaptic gap. The theory proposes that an excess of one or both may lead to mania, whereas a depletion may lead to depression.[5] The observation that drugs like reserpine can induce depression in certain people, and that other drugs (the monoamine oxidase inhibitors and tricyclic antidepressants), can relieve depression in many other patients, supports this theory. Electroconvulsive therapy, extremely effective in the treatment of some severe depressions, has been shown in animal studies to increase the levels of norepinephrine and serotonin in the brain.[6]

The electrolyte theory emphasizes disturbances in brain electrolytes, particularly sodium and potassium. Normally, there is a higher concentration of sodium outside the nerve cell and a higher concentration of potassium inside. The cell's electrical behavior is determined by the interaction of these charged particles (sodium and potassium) through the cell membrane. If physical disorder or chemical imbalance upsets this electrical balance, the result is either in an abnormality in the cell's electrical behavior or in the transmission of a message along the nerve fiber. In depression, the balance may be upset, resulting in increases in residual sodium inside the cell.[11] Lithium, a drug found to be effective in the treatment of both clinical depressions and mania, is a simple ion. The positive response of patients to lithium (an ion much like chloride) provides support for this theory.[6]

The endocrine theory proposes that depression may be related to the adrenal cortex or to the sex hormones. First, endocrine disorders (such as hyperthyroidism, hypothyroidism, Addison's disease, and Cushing's syndrome) are frequently accompanied by affective disturbances that usually remit as the endocrine disorder is controlled. Second, the higher incidence of depression in women and the correlation of mood with hormone levels have been cited as further support of the endocrine theory. However, complex factors accompany the status of being female, and the psychological stresses often accompanying the periods of hormonal fluctuation (e.g., postpartum) must be considered.[18]

EVALUATION OF THE THEORIES

Because no single theory offers a completely satisfying explanation of depression or loneliness, a few of the predominant theories have been presented. The merit of any theory may be judged best by the application of evaluative criteria. Criteria provide a basis for judging the quality of a theory statement.[44] Key criteria for the evaluation of scientific theory to be briefly considered in this chapter are pragmatic adequacy, scope, and testability. *Pragmatic adequacy* is the usefulness of a theory in the real world. For health professionals, theory needs to be useful in a practice setting.[13] *Scope* is the amount and breadth of information as well as the completeness with which data are subsumed. *Testability* means that the theory can be or at least has the potential to be verified empirically.[19]

Each of the theories presented in this section has a variety of followers who attest to the usefulness of the theory in clinical practice. In practice, a theory is useful if it helps the nurse to understand the patient and the presenting symptoms better. For example, if, based on an awareness of psychoanalytic theory, the nurse encounters a depressed person who is turning anger or aggression inward, then the nurse may choose to help the person express the anger externally in physical activity.

With the exception of Kübler–Ross' theory of grief, all the theories have been derived from clinical work with severely depressed and lonely patients.[28] In applying the theories to mild and moderate depression and loneliness, the scope is arbitrarily expanded and the assumption is made that the psychodynamics of the phenomena are, in at least some respect, similar along the continuum. Another consideration of scope is the completeness with which data are subsumed. None of the theories account for all the data related to depression and loneliness. Each of the theories presents a specific perspective and accounts most thoroughly for data related to that particular perspective.

Beck's cognitive theory is probably the most well-tested of the theories.[4] Using the Beck depression inventory, Beck and his followers have worked persistently to gain empirical verification. In general, the other psychodynamic theories all present barriers to testing because the concepts are not easily operationalized. Research methods do not lend themselves readily to the measurement of such abstract concepts as ego and fusion. For example, Bowen cautions that the therapist should work with the patient over time before assessing level of differentiation.[8] The biochemical theories also present a serious impediment to empirical verification. The brain cannot be readily examined in a live subject. It is not possible to administer amines directly and measure their effect on depression because the blood–brain barrier blocks the amines. Brain substances are difficult to measure. Research on cerebrospinal fluid (CSF) holds promise, but this measurement is highly invasive. Although depression often accompanies thyroid dysfunction, in general depressed people do not show thyroid abnormalities.[18] However, some concepts from all the theories are testable by present-day methods. For example, the study of lowered self-esteem in depression and loneliness holds promise for increasing understanding of the phenomena and its relation to depression.

In summary, while no theory offers a panacea for the understanding of depression, theory does provide a base for explaining aspects of depression. Theory provides us with the best thinking of generations of scientists who have studied the complex phenomenon of depression in people. Drawing upon theoretical explanations of depression, the nurse may hope to better assess and manage care of the depressed and lonely patient.

NURSING ASSESSMENT

Subjective data compose the largest part of assessment for depression. Such an assessment requires that the nurse remain continually aware of self and alert to subtle as well as obvious cues. Refined listening skills are essential. Subjective assessment includes description of symptoms, family history, patient and family history, and suicidal potential. Objective assessment includes the physical examination and patient appearance.

SUBJECTIVE ASSESSMENT

Characteristics of Depression

Emotional Symptoms One of the most obvious symptoms of depression is sadness. The feeling may range from a mild, easily relieved response, to a more stable, severe state, perceived as unbearable. The sadness may be visible in the mere absence of humor or a forlorn expression. Eyes may fill with tears, the patient may shake with heaving sobs, or the pain may be so deep as to be beyond tears. The pain and sadness may actually seem to radiate outward, touching others. Sadness is the primary emotion of depression, but many other emotions play within the depressed person and may mask sadness.

Anxiety, which is often present, is a reaction to a nonspecific threat.[23] Signals of depressive anxiety include tension, worry, a foreboding feeling that something ominous is about to happen. The patient may be fearful of usual activities, for example, driving the car. The anxiety often relates to feelings of guilt and possibly to unconscious destructive wishes.

Guilt is a mixture of shame and anxiety.[46] The person often judges himself harshly against rigid standards. Unhappy with himself, the person feels responsible for wrongdoing and deserving of punishment. Automatic verbal whipping of self is one manifestation of self-inflicted punishment. Illness or even depression is sometimes perceived as a punishment. Guilt feelings may appear as the willingness to accept blame for a multitude of problems or as a giving up to illness or depression as one's just due.

Giving up is one sign of helplessness. The roots of helplessness may be traced to early infantile experience, when the person was truly incapable of meeting needs and was dependent on others in the environment. The person may feel inept at accomplishing work demands or even simple tasks like finishing a flower arrangement. Feelings of helplessness often result in excessive demands upon others in the environment. Demands are often accompanied by anger. Feelings of helplessness and anger may shift between patient and nurse.

Anger is a learned means of neutralizing the anxiety of interpersonal threat.[46] Anger counteracts feelings of helplessness. The depressed person may exhibit outbursts of anger or, more commonly, may have difficulty expressing anger. Anger that is unacceptable may be turned inward, toward the self. An absence of overt anger is often noted in loneliness.

Loneliness is an exceedingly unpleasant experience—feared, not chosen, and for which escape usually is sought. The lonely person may complain of feeling disliked, separate, misunderstood, and fearful of others' rejection or being alone.

Intellectual Symptoms Generally, a slowing in thought processes characterizes depression. The nurse may notice a hesitancy in responses, slowed nonrhythmic speech, limited concentration, or a paucity of thought content and verbalization. Difficulty in decision-making reflects ambivalence and self-doubt.

Negative content colors thought. The person focuses on his faults and gloom, selectively inattending to positive attributes and environmental stimuli. As the depression deepens, negative thoughts may become repetitive and ruminative.

In loneliness, the person may experience a cognitive disconnectedness with others. There may be an inner longing to communicate with someone on a particular area of interest or at a particular level of cognitive understanding. To quote Joseph Hartog, "The cognitive imperative to understand and be understood pervades interpersonal relationships."[21]

Physical Symptoms In depression, bodily processes tend to slow down. There is a lack of visible energy or enthusiasm. Activity often decreases, and tiredness may be a problem. The person may forget to drink or eat or may experience nausea at the thought of food. Weight loss and constipation are common. In women, menstruation may be altered. Diminished interest and participation in sexual activity are further reflective of withdrawal. A sensation of physical cold may mirror inner freezing feelings of isolation. Depressed and lonely people may wear excessive clothing, request extra covering at night, or set thermostats well about 70° F. Other somatic complaints (such as headache, pain, discomfort) are reported frequently, as if the person's body is screaming with mental anguish. Sleep disturbance is another classi-

cal and early sign of depression. Types of disturbance include insomnia, restlessness, early morning wakening, and excessive sleep. Key factors in diagnosis are whether sleep is experienced as refreshing, the actual number of hours slept per day, and variation from usual sleep patterns.

While bodily slowing is the primary physical pattern, many people react paradoxically. For example, if excessive anxiety accompanies the depression, the person may pace restlessly and exhibit other signs of anxiety. In an effort to fill up inner emptiness, a person may overeat drastically. Especially with loneliness, a person may ache for touching and try to substitute sexual acting out for longed-for caring.

Social Symptoms Social withdrawal is a hallmark of depression. Seeking comfort, the person protectively pulls into self. The withdrawal varies in intensity. As the depression worsens, other people are excluded more emphatically. The person may physically avoid people or remain quiet and withdrawn in their presence. New relationships are avoided. The longer a person stays inside the inner protective shell, the more difficult it becomes to rejoin the world of others. In loneliness, the withdrawal may be perceived as imposed, rather than chosen. When communicating, some lonely people may over-disclose or underdisclose.

Spiritual Symptoms In depression, the person's spirit is deflated. Motivation diminishes, and apathy and hopelessness may prevail. With loneliness, persons may experience a lack of meaning or a feeling of unrelatedness with the universe. Suicidal ideation may dominate awareness.

Family History Clinical depression and manic depression tend to run in families. The psychiatric diagnosis of a "major affective disorder" includes either a manic episode or a major depressive episode. According to the American Psychiatric Association (APA):

> Major Affective Disorders are more common among family members than in the general population. This is particularly true for family members of individuals with Bipolar Disorder.

Further, Bowen's multigenerational transmission process signals the nurse to assess not only for diagnosed clinical depression, but also for milder forms that have been passed through the generations.[8]

Patient History   The patient's history provides the nurse with a wealth of information. Was there an early childhood loss? Is there a personal history of lingering depression? Is the patient taking or has the patient ever taken any form of psychotropic medication? If so, what, when, and with what results? Is there a history of substance abuse? (Many people drink alcoholic beverages or use other drugs as a means of coping with depression.) All present medications should be assessed for possible side-effects to determine if the depression might be secondary to medication.

The nurse should try to identify any precipitating event that may have preceded the onset of depressive symptoms. Any event can serve as a depressive trigger. For example, a death, marital breakup, failure at work, promotion, financial distress, surgery, significant birthday, birth of a child, graduation of self or family member, diagnosis of illness, or the anniversary response to any such events could precipitate a depression. The key is the patient's perception of such events and the meaning attached to them. A description of the actual progression into depression is also useful.

Usual patterns of coping are extremely significant. How does the patient usually function? How has the patient coped with depression or loss in the past? What behav-iors have given the patient pleasure in the past? Are those pleasure-giving behaviors available to the patient now? If so, are they being used? What support system is currently available? The answers to these assessment questions can assist the nurse in establishing accurate diagnoses and are essential to planning effective nursing care. Information obtained from significant others completes the subjective assessment. People who know the patient intimately are the first to detect changes in mood and behavior.

Suicidal Potential   The nurse assisting patients suffering from depression and severe loneliness also confronts the possibility of patient suicide. Suicide does not occur at the deepest levels of depression, but rather in the midrange levels of depression, where energy is available for action. Because of personal anxiety related to self-destruction and the common American denial of death, the nurse may be selectively inattentive to suicidal clues.

Some indirect clues of suicidal intent include giving away valued possessions, morbid preoccupation with death, statements like, "I won't be seeing you anymore," suicide notes, or a struggling depression followed by a sudden calm and elevated mood (indicating perhaps that the struggle is over and the final decision has been made). Other clues include recent loss, absence of close ties, hopelessness, psychosis, or the presence of a progressively degenerative disease. Key risk factors related to lethality of suicidal attempts are age, sex, plan, and availability of means.[14] Mortality data indicate that adolescents, people over 50 years of age, and men tend to succeed at suicide more frequently. However, the incidence of attempted suicide is greater among women. If suicidal ideation is present, one must ask whether the person has developed a plausible plan. For example, has the means been identified? Does the person plan to shoot himself in the head with a gun or take an overdose of aspirin? Even more significantly, is the means readily available for carrying out the plan? For example, does the person have a loaded gun by the bed? If the person plans to take pills, has a bottle of lethal medication (like one of the tricyclic antidepressants) been hidden away at home?

In assessing suicide potential, all information should be considered together rather than in bits and pieces. However, any cues to suicidal intent, no matter how minor, should be shared with the team and with a mental health specialist. The nurse has the responsibility to the patient and to self to share such information and opinions. Failure to share such information could result in death for the patient and in the nurse having to live with the fact that personal failure to act may have contributed to a patient's death. If suicidal ideation is suspected, the patient should be asked directly, "Are you thinking about killing yourself?" The question will *not* plant the idea in the patient's thoughts; rather, the question will convey that the nurse is willing to help the patient with the problem if it exists. When such feelings are expressed openly, they are less likely to be acted on impulsively. Once the possibility has been identified, the treatment team may work together in assessment. With the help of specialists, a diagnosis may be reached and effective management planned.

OBJECTIVE ASSESSMENT

Because depression is often secondary to medical illness, the physical state of a person should be assessed thoroughly. For example, depression may be secondary to hypothyroidism or central nervous system (CNS) disorders. Depression may be a signal of physical illness or indirectly may precipitate illness due to neglect and emotional stress.

With regard to general appearance, the depressed person may look unkempt because of personal neglect. Posture is often slumped, with the spine curved as if the person carries an invisible and massive burden. Movement may be slowed, and eye contact limited or nonexistent because of the desire to retreat into self. Dark or drab-colored clothing may reflect the inner darkness of experience.

NURSING DIAGNOSIS

Nursing diagnosis may include specific statements related to behaviors outlined in the subjective assessment section. Generally, intensity and duration of a problem are indicators as to whether nursing interventions are warranted and whether referral to a mental health specialist is indicated. If the nurse and patient determine that problems exist, then priorities must be set. If observed symptoms are not readily responsive to nursing interventions, or if suicidal ideation is present, consultation with a mental health specialist is indicated. If the patient has a history of clinical depression or any form of severe enduring depression, then physician consultation for possible psychopharmacological intervention is indicated.

MANAGEMENT

GOALS

Because human beings are unique, there are no standard goals or interventions that can be applied uniformly. Nursing science is not now and may never be at that level of sophistication. The establishment of goals with a depressed person requires careful thought about the assessment information. The depressed person may have a tendency to 1) strive for goals rather than enjoy the present and 2) assess self-performance inaccurately.

The nurse accepts responsibility for keeping joint goals attainable and for assisting the patient in accurate evaluation. Specific goals must be individualized and be determined with each patient. For example, if a person accustomed to jogging is hospitalized for a joint injury and starts to display a depressed affect and angry outbursts, the nurse would work with the person to set a realistic goal that would facilitate release of anger without hampering the joint rehabilitation.

FRAMEWORK FOR INTERVENTIONS

Successful work with the depressed patient demands a supportive counseling framework. The nurse must strive continually to understand the unique person and to consider the problem from the patient's frame of mind. Through genuine caring and intensive listening, the nurse conveys supportive acceptance. For the severely depressed patient frequent brief contact is the best beginning. For the moderately to mildly depressed patient frequency and length of optimal nursing contact will depend on the patient's need to talk and on environmental demands. The most important factors to remember are that 1) uninterrupted quality time with the patient conveys more interest and respect than time that is not given to the patient specifically, and 2) contact should not be rapidly reduced when improvement is noted. Rapid reduction of time based on improvement conveys the idea that the patient is accepted because of the depression. Rather, with improvement, the nurse should use the time to reinforce the progress and help the patient make sense out of the depressive experience.

Interventions are planned based on the established goals, the depth of depression, the person's patterns of coping, and environmental sources available. In this chapter, selected examples of interventions are proposed to stimulate thinking about the possibilities. The nurse selects or creates actions that may best serve the specific patient encountered.

INTERVENTION: EMOTIONAL REALM

Sadness and Loneliness

Sadness is a natural healing response. When a loss is experienced, grief work must be done; it cannot be avoided.[28] The nurse needs to acknowledge and allow some pain. Acceptance may be conveyed through spending quiet time with the patient, through verbal empathetic acknowledgement, or by a caring touch. Nothing lasts forever, and the patient may need reassurance that this sadness, too, will pass. Refer to previous episodes of depression and point out that they did end. Help the patient identify what actions were beneficial in the past. On the other hand, excessive sympathy should be avoided so as not to perpetuate the problem.

Behaviors that have given pleasure in the past may be initiated in the present. For example, if a leisurely, warm bath is generally helpful to the patient, the practice of taking such a bath on a daily basis might be prescribed. Many people find classical music or a backrub soothing. To be effective, comfort measures must be meaningful to the patient. Also, the nurse's contact with the patient may serve to decrease feelings of loneliness. True communication serves to decrease the sense of isolation so characteristic of loneliness.

Anger and Anxiety

To help an angry patient, the nurse must be personally comfortable with anger. The patient may be feeling threatened and fearful. Remember, unprovoked outbursts of anger directed randomly at the nurse are not personal. At such times, skilled listening aimed at hearing what the patient is saying must take precedence over emotional reacting. Acknowledgment of the patient's feeling conveys acceptance of the patient as a person. Initial acceptance is essential to therapeutic change.[39]

Acceptance may be conveyed through attentive listening and an open and permissive atmosphere. These nurse behaviors encourage the patient's expression of feeling. For the patient who has difficulty expressing anger, minor daily irritations should be acknowledged. A little later, when the patient can acknowledge irritations, labeling of the feeling may be useful. The patient may need permission to feel angry. To convey permission, the nurse may firmly and simply state: "It is OK to feel angry." Permission may decrease the patient's anxiety over the expression of anger.

When anger has been turned inward in depression, the patient often fears the destructive power of such feelings. An accepting caretaker who is not intimidated by angry feelings may be a great source of relief to the depressed patient.[41]

Physical activity is an excellent channel for anger and anxiety. For the patient in good physical health, running therapy may be an effective approach.[43] Research findings have suggested that many mildly or moderately depressed patients participating in physical activity programs such as running report reductions in anxiety and symptoms of depression.[9,20,33] For the less physically active, walking or occupational therapy activities such as pounding with a hammer might be appropriate.

Helplessness

To treat an adult as helpless is demeaning. It fosters dependency, not growth. Yet the well-meaning caregiver or family member may readily assume an overfunctioning role in misguided efforts to help another. Overfunctioning of others reinforces a person's feelings of helplessness and inadequacy. Overfunctioning works to hold a person in the helpless position.

The nurse should encourage the patient to do everything possible for himself. Such a position fosters the use and further development of ability. Irrational demands should be discussed and refused.[32,43]

The nurse may also assist significant others in identifying their behaviors that foster patient underfunctioning. An overfunctioner can tone down more easily than an underfunctioner can pull up. A change in the overfunctioner's behavior in the primary emotional system fosters the underfunctioner's assumption of power.[8]

Another means of nurturing autonomy is to give the patient power regarding care or scheduling requirements. Such a tactic increases individual control over environmental stress.[28] Of course, this technique should be used judiciously in depressed patients who are suffering from indecision. Minimal goal-setting and making small decisions are appropriate for this patient.

Guilt

To the nurse, lamentings of guilt and the eager willingness to accept blame may seem irrational. Acknowledgment of such feelings by the nurse as belonging to the patient, not to the nurse, may be useful.[48] Also, exploring specifics of the situation and helping the patient become aware of the multidimensional self may broaden his perspective.[4]

Further exploration may result in the patient's more realistic perception of the guilt-producing situation in which responsibility is shared by all involved. After all, people cocreate situations. By helping the patient focus on positive aspects of self as well as the guilt-producing behavior, the nurse may broaden the patient's perception to include positive, as well as negative, dimensions of self. As always, in efforts to help the patient experiencing guilt, avoid arguments.

INTERVENTIONS: INTELLECTUAL REALM

Slowed Thoughts and Cognitive Distance

Communication that is clear and brief is most easily understood by the depressed patient.[22] Concise, simple statements are helpful. Frequent interaction allows less time for uninterrupted withdrawal into self. To counteract distraction, the nurse may choose to initiate early interactions in a quiet area. A light touch on the patient's arm can direct attention. To convey respect, the patient should always be given ample time for response. With minimal slowing of thought, the nurse may be able to facilitate interaction by introducing topics of interest to the patient.

In problems of cognitive distance, listening may enhance understanding. Also, facilitating the attainment of materials (books, instruments, equipment) may assist patients in engaging in cognitive activities. Referrals to special groups or to persons known to share similar interests or problems may nurture a sense of relationship.

Difficulty in Decision-Making

At peak intensity, depressed patients may feel distraught over minor decisions. Ambivalent feelings pull at the person, resulting in a "stuck" or worried position. In such cases, a planned schedule may be necessary to relieve the patient's burden. For minor problems, the patient may benefit from a procedure like making a list. With this tactic, the separation of positive and negative attributes of a problem in written form may make alter-

natives clearer. Also, discussion of foreseeable consequences may increase awareness of the ramifications of choices. New alternatives often arise in the course of discussion.

In addition to logical reasoning, decisions are made on the basis of values and beliefs. As Bowen pointed out, many people are not aware of their beliefs.[8] By encouraging identification of beliefs, attitudes, and values, the nurse helps the patient decrease pseudoself and facilitates differentiation.[10] This helps to decrease fusion and lessen withdrawal, as well as helping the patient to make decisions.

Negative Content

Direct rebuttal of negative content may result in the patient's thinking that the nurse does not understand the patient's weaknesses.[4] Arguments are futile. The nurse may try introducing alternative views, while being careful to label them as such. For example, the nurse might comment: "Another way of looking at this issue is that if your mother-in-law moves in with you, she will be able to share child-rearing responsibilities." As the nurse gets to know the patient, strengths will surface. Honest comments of positive regard for patient strength may be helpful.

Everyone needs to experience success. Successful experiences may assist the patient in reevaluating self in a more favorable light. The nurse can plan tasks and goals with the patient so that successful achievement will be probable. The identification of long-term goals, coupled with a realistic plan for accomplishment, may elevate hope for the future.

INTERVENTIONS: PHYSICAL REALM

Sleep Disturbance, Tiredness, Somatic Complaints

With insomnia and other somatic complaints, the nurse may recommend comfort measures (e.g., a backrub, hot bath, or warm drink). Sometimes, a relaxing activity like reading facilitates sleep. If thought processes are active, progressive relaxation training is an excellent and powerful technique. The patient is taught to relax the body's muscles through concentration. With high tension, muscle flexion and relaxation may need to be coupled with concentration.[34,37] In the relaxed state, creative visualization of pleasant and soothing experiences may be introduced to enhance the effect further. The nurse may record sessions for the patient to replay at home later. Anxiety reduction associated with comfort measures and relaxation exercises may also decrease perceived pain. Further, regular physical exercises may improve sleep and decrease feelings of tiredness.

Diminished Interest in Sexual Activity, the Ache for Touching, and Excessive Eating

Assisting or encouraging attention to grooming sometimes helps to lift the spirit. A warm bath may be followed by wearing a favorite gown in a pretty color or a favorite sweater or pair of jeans. Lipstick for a woman or cologne for a man may help the person feel more attractive. The actions must be meaningful to the person if they are to be effective in helping the patient feel more attractive.

With significant others, nongenital touching and holding may be recommended. Gentle touching tends to increase feelings of security. In some cases, pets such as small dogs are a wonderful outlet for the needs of touching. Touching may catalyze pent-up feelings. For example, for many patients a well-timed touch on the arm may trigger the release of tears. Together, comfort and expression of feelings may decrease excessive eating.

Inadequate Intake or Nausea

If necessary, the patient should be reminded to drink adequate fluids. Beverages usually enjoyed should be made available. At meal-time, small servings of favorite foods should be served. The company of the nurse or a significant other is essential because eating is a social activity. A flower on the table, a lighted candle, soft music, or some other meaningful environmental stimulus may further encourage adequate intake.

INTERVENTIONS: SOCIAL REALM

Withdrawal

Withdrawal breeds more depression and more loneliness. In deeper levels of depression, energy may be so limited that even minimal contact is taxing. Further, most people automatically respond to the depressed and lonely person by withdrawal. Withdrawal threatens relationships with these patients. Limiting the number of staff involved, but not the quality of contact time, saves some energy for the patient. Repeated assignment of the same staff may encourage a relationship, but will probably be extremely stressful to the staff. Therefore, the nurse must consider the patient and staff in planning care. The caregiver who agrees to work intensely in a one-to-one relationship with the depressed and lonely patient must have the emotional strength to engage in this relationship, or it will be ineffective. Ideally, the nurse who works with this type of patient would have a decrease in other responsibilities.

The family should be encouraged to maintain contact with the depressed person. This contact limits the patient's withdrawal. Opening the system to include extended family members spreads the emotional intensity. Also, nurse interaction with significant others in the patient's presence may help to shift the focus to external rather the internal concerns.[10]

Loneliness, Overdisclosure, and Underdisclosure

Maintenance of satisfactory social relationships has been related to lower levels of loneliness in widows,[3] college students,[12] and adults who responded to a newspaper survey in New York and Massachusetts.[40] Continued relations with others decrease isolation. Friends should be encouraged to maintain contact with the patient. Telephone conversations or letters may be recommended.

Group therapy is useful in correcting maladaptive communication processes. Through group interactions, a patient may receive feedback on behavior or test out new behaviors.[52] Referral to a group may be indicated for some patients who express excessive shyness or dysfunctional interaction patterns.

INTERVENTION: SPIRITUAL REALM

Hopelessness, Lack of Meaning, and Unrelatedness

The belief that one is a unique being is a requisite for integrated functioning.[15] The nurse conveys faith in the patient's uniqueness through all respectful contact.

Existential *angst*, or an intense feeling of anxiety or dread, may be a part of reaching greater awareness. Through confrontation with meaninglessness, one may hope to discover meaning. The existential paradox holds that one is simultaneously 1) of absolutely no value in the cosmos, and 2) of absolute value, never to be replaced.[35]

Persons experience *angst* when facing personal mortality or loss. The *angst*, although painful, may be a gate to greater awareness of meaning. The nurse's responsibility is to communicate caring during *angst* and to decrease the sense of unrelatedness through contact. In other words, the nurse may help the patient regain hope, meaning, and relatedness by being with the patient during these painful moments. Referral to the patient's religious leader or agency chaplain may also be indicated.

CONCLUSION

Patients experiencing depression present a tremendous challenge to the practitioner. The nurse's primary resource is the use of self. Human caring, respect, and knowledgeable intervention can facilitate healing as no other potent known; yet, people who work closely with depressed patients often experience depression themselves. The pain of depression and loneliness touches places deep within the human psyche. Depression can be contagious. To help the depressed effectively, the nurse must care for herself effectively. The nurse should pamper herself, exercise regularly, vent emotions, or apply any self-intervention necessary to maintain a high level of functioning. Clinical supervision or the team conference provides excellent opportunities for the nurse to obtain feedback and nurture objectively. Nursing practice with depressed patients necessitates the nurse maintaining intellectual control.

The challenge to nursing does not stop with interventions. To provide the best possible care requires that care be based on established knowledge. The clinical setting, not the laboratory, holds promise for the development of nursing knowledge about depression. Clinicians, researchers, and educators must work together in an unending search for increased knowledge in nursing practice with depressed patients. Descriptive and experimental studies based on practice are desperately needed if nurses hope to deliver optimal care to depressed and lonely patients and their loved ones.

REFERENCES

1. American Psychiatric Assn: Diagnostic and Statistical Manual of Mental Disorders, 3rd ed. Washington, DC, American Psychiatric Assn, 1980
2. Arieti S: Affective disorders: Manic-depressive psy-

chosis and psychotic depression. In Arieti S, Brody EB (eds): American Handbook of Psychiatry, 2nd ed, Vol 3. New York, Basic Books, 1974

3. Bahr HM, Harvey CD: Correlates of loneliness among widows bereaved in a mining disaster. Psychol Rep 44:367, 1979

4. Beck AT, Rush AJ, Shaw BF et al: Cognitive Therapy of Depression. New York, Guilford Press, 1979

5. Bemporad J: Critical review of the major concepts of depression. In Arieti S. Bemporad J (eds): Severe and Mild Depression. New York, Basic Books, 1978

6. Bernstein JG: Clinical Psychopharmacology. Littleton, Mass, PSG Publishing, 1978

7. Bibring E: The mechanism of depression. In Greenacre P (ed): Affective Disorders. New York, International Universities Press, 1953

8. Bowen M: Family Therapy in Clinical Practice. New York, Jason Aronson, 1978

9. Brown RS, Ramirez DE, Taub JM: The prescription of exercise for depression. Physician Sports Med 6:34, 1978

10. Cain AO: Assisting depressed clients and their families. In Collected Papers of the Second Southeastern Regional Conference of Psychiatric/Mental Health Clinical Specialists. Columbia, South Carolina Specialists in Psychiatric–Mental Health Nursing, 1981

11. Coppen A: The biochemistry of affective disorders. Br J Psychiatry 113:1237, 1967

12. Cutrona CE: Transition to college: Loneliness and the process of social adjustment. In Peplau LA, Perlman D (eds): Loneliness: A Sourcebook of Current Theory, Research, and Therapy, New York, Wiley-Interscience, 1982

13. Ellis R: Characteristics of significant theories. Nurs Res 17:217, 1968

14. Farberow NL, Heilig SM, Litman R: Techniques in Crisis Intervention: A Training Manual. Los Angeles, Suicide Prevention Inc, 1968

15. Frankl V: Man's Search for Meaning. New York, Beacon Press, 1959

16. Freud S: Mourning and melancholia (1917). In Jones E (ed), Riviere J (trans): Collected Papers, Vol 4. London, Hogarth Press, 1949

17. Fromm–Reichman F: Loneliness. Psychiatry 22:1, 1959

18. Futcher J, Howell A, Jackson–Keilin M: Depression. Irvine, CA, Concept Media, 1980

19. Goodson F, Morgan G: Evaluation of theory. In Marx M, Goodson F (eds): Theories in Contemporary Psychology, 2nd ed. New York, MacMillan, 1976

20. Griest JH, Klein MH, Eischens RR et al: Running through your mind. J Psychosom Res 22:259, 1978

21. Hartog J: Introduction: The anatomization. In Hartog J, Audy JR, Cohen YA (eds): The Anatomy of Loneliness. New York, International Universities Press, 1980

22. Hein EC: Communication in Nursing Practice, 2nd ed. Boston, Little, Brown & Co, 1980

23. Hinsie LE, Campbell RJ: Psychiatric Dictionary, 4th ed. New York, Oxford University Press, 1974

24. Jacobson E: The self and the object world: Vicissitudes of their infantile cathexes and their influence on ideational and affective development. Psychoanal Study Child 9:75, 1954

25. Jacobson E: Depression: Comparative Studies of Normal, Neurotic and Psychotic Conditions. New York, International Universities Press, 1971

26. Kerlinger F: Foundations of Behavioral Research, 2nd ed. New York, Holt, Rinehart & Winston, 1973

27. Kidd KK, Weissman MM: Why we do not yet understand the genetics of affective disorders. In Cole J, Schatzberg AF, Frazier SH (eds): Depression: Biology, Dynamics, Treatment. New York, Plenum Publishing, 1978

28. Kübler–Ross E: On Death and Dying. New York, MacMillan, 1969

29. Kübler–Ross E: Questions and Answers on Death and Dying. New York, MacMillan, 1974

30. Kübler–Ross E: Living with Death and Dying. New York, MacMillan, 1981

31. Leiderman PH: Pathological loneliness; A psychodynamic interpretation. In Hartog J, Audy JR, Cohen YA (eds): The Anatomy of Loneliness. New York, International Universities Press, 1980

32. Mendelson M: Psychoanalytic Concepts of Depression, 2nd ed. New York, Spectrum, 1974

33. Morgan WP, Roberts JA, Feinerman AD: Psychological effect of acute physical activity. Arch Phys Med Rehabil 52:422, 1971

34. Morris C: Relaxation therapy in a clinic. Am J Nurs 79:1958, 1979

35. Morris VC: Existentialism in Education. New York, Harper & Row, 1966

36. Moustakas CE: Loneliness. Englewood Cliffs, NJ, Prentice–Hall, 1961

37. Paul GL: Insight vs. Desensitization in Psychotherapy. Stanford, Stanford University Press, 1966

38. Peplau HE: Interpersonal Relations in Nursing. New York, Putnam, 1952

39. Rogers C: Becoming Partners: Marriage and Its Alternatives. New York, Dell Publishing, 1972

40. Rubenstein CM, Shaver P: The experience of loneliness. In Peplau LA, Perlman D (eds): Loneliness: A Sourcebook of Current Theory, Research, and Therapy. New York, Wiley-Interscience, 1982

41. Ruesch J: Disturbed Communication. New York, WW Norton & Co., 1959

42. Sachs ML: Running therapy for the depressed client. Top Clin Nurs 3:77, 1981

43. Steiner CM: Scripts People Live. New York, Bantam, 1974

44. Stevens B: Nursing Theory. Boston, Little, Brown & Co, 1979

45. Sullivan HS: Conceptions of Modern Psychiatry. New York, WW Norton, 1940

46. Sullivan HS: The Interpersonal Theory of Psychiatry. New York, WW Norton & Co, 1953

47. Sullivan HS: Clinical Studies in Psychiatry. New York, WW Norton & Co, 1956

48. Swanson AR: The client who generates depression. In Haber J, Leach AM, Schudy SM et al (eds): Comprehensive Psychiatric Nursing. New York, McGraw–Hill, 1978

49. Tillich P: The Eternal Now. New York, Scribner's & Sons, 1963

50. Weiss RS: Loneliness: The Experience of Emotional and Social Isolation. Cambridge, MIT Press, 1973

51. Yalom ID: The Theory and Practice of Group Psychotherapy. New York, Basic Books, 1975

52. Young JE: Loneliness, depression, and cognitive therapy: Theory and application. In Peplau LA, Perlman D (eds): Loneliness: A Sourcebook of Current Theory, Research, and Therapy. New York, Wiley-Interscience, 1982

3

Anxiety

Barbara Kersten Campbell

Anxiety is basic to our existence, varying with the experiences and circumstances of life. Anxiety may occur as a result of an underlying illness or may be independent of an organic etiology. It may present itself disguised by a variety of confusing signs and symptoms and go undetected by the unwary clinician. As nurses, we often are confronted with patients experiencing levels of anxiety that are destructive or disabling. To provide relief to these patients the nurse must have a solid understanding of the subject. This understanding leads to the ability to assess the patient's level of anxiety accurately, develop and implement a management plan, and to evaluate the outcome.

ANXIETY, STRESS, AND FEAR

Anxiety can be defined as an emotional response within a person to anything, either real or imagined, that may threaten that person's security. The threat may be to physical life (threat of death) or to psychological existence (the loss of freedom, meaninglessness). The threat may be to some other value identified with one's existence, for example, patri-

otism, the loss of another person, or success.[10]

Anxiety is a feeling of dread, an objectless fear that distracts one's mind. It is an unpleasant feeling of which a person wants to rid himself at any expense. The special characteristics of anxiety are the feelings of uncertainty and helplessness in the face of danger. Not all anxiety, however, is destructive or disabling. When anxiety exists in a mild degree it can be a motivating or stimulating force that influences and enhances development.[10] Anxiety produces energy that can be used in constructive ways. Most of us have, for example, experienced the feeling of being anxious prior to an important examination. As the test date nears, anxiety levels rise and the motivation to study harder occurs. If anxiety levels stay slightly elevated, performance is enhanced and higher levels of achievement are attained. DeRosis, in a particularly clear example, describes how the anxiety of frustration, anger, and helplessness has motivated women to break away from their image as dependent, subordinate persons, and make conscious and deliberate changes toward liberation.[4] Mild anxiety can also be viewed as a positive force serving to increase alertness and effort. For example, a patient may be motivated, because of anxiety about illness, to more positive health care habits.

Although the terms often are used interchangeably, anxiety is *not* synonymous with stress or fear. According to Selye, *stress,* is a "biochemical phenomenon, and it is not only independent of anxiety or other mental reactions, but it also doesn't have to be unpleasant. A great joy can be as stressful as a great pain."[5] Thus, stress is seen as more of a physiologic or biochemical response to a problem, while anxiety, according to May, "is how we relate to stress" (i.e., the emotional response to a stressful situation).[10] There is evidence to support the theory that the intensity of anxiety and consequent symptomatology is directly related to the degrees of stress, and that this interpretation may be grossly different from person to person. Stress may be a result of job loss, bereavement, marital difficulties or anything that significantly alters the person's support systems. Fear differs from anxiety in that fear is an emotional response to a consciously recognized and usually external threat or danger, whereas anxiety is not as well focused. The person experiencing anxiety is often unaware of what makes him anxious. Fear is usually short-lived, with few long-term manifestations, whereas anxiety usually lasts longer and may have a number of important effects on health.

NEUROTIC ANXIETY VERSUS NORMAL ANXIETY

There is an important distinction to be made between neurotic anxiety and normal anxiety. *Neurotic anxiety* refers to a state in which the response to anxious feelings is out of proportion to the perceived threat. *Normal anxiety* is in good approximation to the degree of perceived threat. Neurotic anxiety is the result of psychic conflict that is managed by varied and diverse neurotic defense mechanisms. These defense mechanisms are often so strong as to be inhibiting on an intrapersonal level, so that constructive and creative activity is limited. This type of problem often requires intensive psychotherapy. In contrast, normal anxiety, while also the result of intrapsychic conflict, results in less limiting adaptation that in no way inhibits successful intrapersonal relations.[12,13] The nurse is often confronted with both conditions. This chapter will, however, concentrate only on normal anxiety.

MECHANISM OF ANXIETY

CAUSES OF ANXIETY

Intrapersonal Conflicts

One common belief regarding the etiology of anxiety is that it results from the constant clash between man's instinctual drives and society's frustrating demands. To gain society's acceptance and parental approval, the individual's basic impulses must be controlled, modified, or sublimated. The individual is constantly fighting a battle between what he would like to do and what society mandates. (One may not, for example, tear limb from limb a policeman writing a parking ticket, although there may be an instinctual urge to do so.)

Psychosocial Threat

Conflict may also arise from the attempt to meet the demands of an overly strict superego. Horney described the rules and regulations imposed by the superego as a network of "shoulds" that are derived from our cultural, social, and familial heritage.[4] A person that has an extensive network of "shoulds" and a strong conscience finds it extremely difficult or impossible to live up to the demands he has placed on himself and, as a result, his anxiety flourishes. For example, many women believe they should be able to meet the demands placed on them by both family and career at the same time. This is often difficult or impossible to do. Anxiety flourishes when the network of "shoulds" is not being satisfied. Consider the following example. Mary was a 22-year-old who was certain that she had mononucleosis. The examining nurse noted that Mary was quite tense, and began a careful inquiry into the patient's social history. During the conversation Mary revealed that she had recently had her second child, and had been routinely up with the child at night so that her husband, a student, could have adequate rest. Because the patient was highly motivated toward her own goals of being an architect, she was resentful of this situation and felt that her own career goals had been derailed by the unexpected pregnancy. Mary believed that she should be able to carry out her mother and wife responsibilities as well as continue with her education. In light of this information, and after a thorough physical examination, the initial complaints of restlessness, muscle aches, headache and anorexia took on new meaning. Rather than having an infectious etiology, most of the symptomatology was the result of anxiety that could be attributed to Mary's intrapersonal conflict and a stressful home situation. Counseling the patient and her husband about their problems ultimately brought about resolution of the conflict and Mary's symptoms.

Physical Threats

Whatever the psychosocial etiology of anxiety, there are a number of environmental situations that are particularly apt to produce anxious feelings.[14] Anxiety may, for example, be produced by threats to the physical being. The threat of bodily injury, mutilation, or death is obviously stress-producing, leading to high levels of anxiety. Any situation that would threaten the person's fulfillment of biological needs causes anxiety. For example, the bedridden patient who is unable to walk to the bathroom and must rely on the nursing staff to assist him may fear embarrassment at this state of dependency. For the patient who has always been self-sufficient, this dependency is extremely stressful and the result may be high levels of anxiety.

Being in an unfamiliar or uncomfortable environment may cause anxiety levels to rise. The elderly patient who is exposed to monitoring equipment, alarms, and other loud noises, will certainly become anxious. Young children who are separated from family and placed in the seemingly sterile, unfamiliar environment of the hospital room or clinic will be likely to show manifestations of anxiety. Interrupted sleep and altered routines, often a result of hospitalization, can be very anxiety-producing.

Transference

Anxiety can be transferred from one person to another. Consider the situation in which the person who you are with is extremely anxious (i.e., wringing his hands, talking loudly and rapidly, and pacing). As you observe this person you will likely become increasingly uncomfortable and agitated yourself.

Unmet Needs

One way to view the etiology of anxiety is to recall Maslow's hierarchy of basic human needs. Maslow described a hierarchy of needs with primary or physiological needs at the base, and secondary or nonphysiological needs at the higher levels.[9] Only after the needs at the base of the pyramid have been relatively well gratified will the person focus on those needs higher up. The needs described by Maslow are, in ascending order:

- Survival needs (e.g., food, water, air, temperature, elimination, rest, pain avoidance)
- Stimulation needs (e.g., sex, activity, exploration, manipulation, novelty)
- Safety and security needs (e.g., safety, security, protection)
- Love needs (e.g., love, belonging, closeness, intimacy)
- Esteem needs (e.g., value and respect from others, value and respect of self [self-esteem])
- Self-actualization needs (e.g., the process of making maximum use of one's abilities)
- Cognitive needs (e.g., seeking knowledge, discovering things, working with ideas, knowing and understanding)
- Aesthetic needs (e.g., the desire for beauty)

The importance of this hierarchy of needs is that anything that threatens fulfill-ment of the needs may be a source of anxiety for the patient. The patient may be experiencing high levels of anxiety as a result of one or more than one of these causes (Fig. 3-1).

PATHOPHYSIOLOGY

The signs and symptoms created by anxiety have their origins in the autonomic nervous system (ANS). When a danger exists, either real or imaginary, physical or psychological, an anxiety response is triggered. The body's response to anxiety and fear is similar and is the result of activation of the sympathetic branch of the ANS. This produces a phenomenon known as the "fight-or-flight" response. Epinephrine, a hormone produced from the adrenal glands during the sympathetic response, prepares the body to defend itself against stress. The release of epinephrine stimulates the heart to beat faster, allowing for increased blood flow to vital organs and muscles. Epinephrine also stimulates glycogenolysis creating energy for cells. The energy that is created by the ANS response to

FIG. 3-1 *Causes of anxiety.*

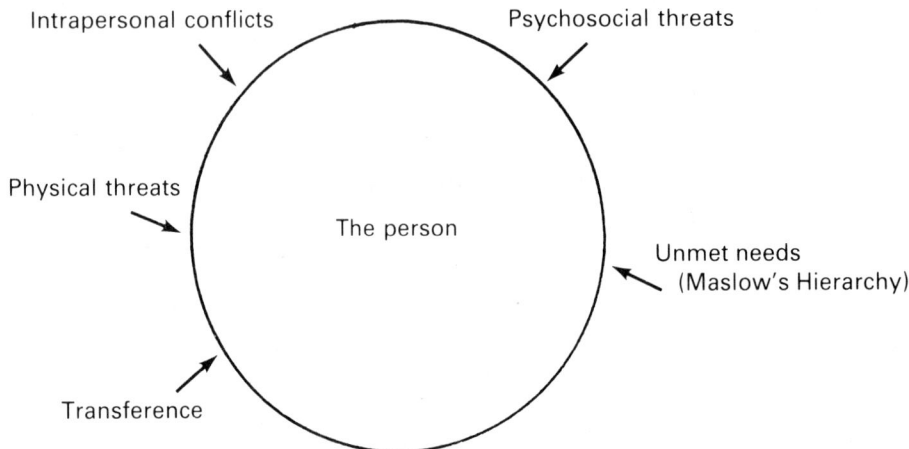

Intrapersonal conflicts

Psychosocial threats

Physical threats

The person

Unmet needs
(Maslow's Hierarchy)

Transference

anxiety primes the muscles for action. When no physical action is taken, the muscles are left in a state of excitement leading to muscle tension and spasm. Muscle tension seems to be a great source of discomfort for the patient creating a number of painful symptoms. Responses to anxiety caused by the sympathetic branch of the ANS are listed below.

In an anxiety reaction, as opposed to the fear reaction, the parasympathetic branch of the ANS is also prominently involved. In the anxiety reaction, there are noted increased frequency of urination, emptying of the rectum and occasionally decreased heart rate and lowered blood pressure (see the list). The parasympathetic influence may increase the amount of gastric acid produced with resultant gastric and duodenal ulcers.

Many disease states are believed to be caused in part by chronic levels of excessive anxiety. Conditions such as obesity, hyper-

tension, colitis, asthma, pseudo-seizures, ulcers, stuttering, immunological deficiencies, and sexual inadequacies may result from the body's inability continually to respond by means of the neuroendocrine system and make the necessary adaptations. The patient's physical health can be then directly related to mental health. Selye describes this phenomenon as the general adaptation syndrome.[8]

Since the list of signs and symptoms of anxiety is long and nonspecific, the nurse must assess the patient carefully in his milieu to make an accurate nursing diagnosis. She must consider not only the specific signs and symptoms but the circumstances under which they are occurring.

LEVELS OF ANXIETY

A person's level of anxiety is constantly changing depending upon circumstances of

Responses to Anxiety

SYMPATHETIC RESPONSES TO ANXIETY

Constriction of blood vessels
Increased heart rate, increased contractility, and premature contractions
Increased blood pressure
Dilated pupils
Dryness of mouth
Sweating (particularly of palms of the hands and the forehead)
Increased blood glucose
Increased free fatty acid level
Decreased motility of digestive tract
  Constipation
  Indigestion
  Cramping pain
  Distention
  Nausea without vomiting
  Change in appetite (anorexia or compulsive eating)
Bronchodilation
Chest pain (aware of palpitations at night)

Tingling of hands or feet
Cold, clammy hands
Increased muscle tension (headaches, bilateral frontal or occipital and gradually increasing during the day)
Tremors, twitching, trembling, restlessness, aching muscles, constant backache

PARASYMPATHETIC RESPONSES TO ANXIETY

Increased motility of digestive tract (diarrhea, mild cramping, no tenesmus, no blood or mucus)
Change in appetite
Increased micturation (no dysuria, pyuria, or hematuria)
Increased production of gastric secretions
Decreased heart rate and blood pressure

ADDITIONAL RESPONSE

Sleep onset disorder (taking more than 45–60 min to fall asleep)

daily life. Anxiety levels include relaxation, mild anxiety, moderate anxiety, and severe anxiety, and are characterized according to the following scheme.[14]

During level I or periods of relaxation, anxiety levels are lowest. For example, when a person is asleep or in comfortable surroundings, with all or most of his needs met, he will have minimal anxiety. The person thinking joyful thoughts, performing enjoyable activities or engaging in a happy social exchange is likely to be very relaxed. The person at this level will not be at his peak performance ability.

As events occur and decisions need to be made the anxiety level will rise. Level II is described as mild anxiety such as experienced when one must end the period of relaxation and begin work. At this level, the person will be alert, oriented to the people and happenings surrounding him, and motivated to perform. Learning abilities are enhanced by the increased alertness. This is the optimal state at which to function, since we are motivated to progress but not to the extent that learning would be inhibited.

Level III anxiety is characterized by feelings of discomfort or uneasiness. The person has an excessive amount of anxiety, evidenced by physical or emotional manifestations. The person's ability to function decreases. Creativity, learning, problem-solving, and attention span all are diminished. A patient who is ill-prepared for surgery scheduled to occur the following morning may exhibit level III anxiety. Fearing the possibility of pain, disfigurement, or death, the patient commonly experiences agitation, insomnia, palpitations, diarrhea, headaches, and muscle spasms. He frequently has displays of anger or hostility at the nursing staff and may become withdrawn. Subjectively the patient may complain of nervousness, of being short of breath, or of feeling dizzy. The person experiencing high levels of anxiety is preoccupied with the future, and shows an inability to experience fully the here and now. Recognizing signs and symptoms of anxiety, as in the situation above, is more easily done when examining the situation surrounding the patient.

Level IV is characterized by severe anxiety. The patient with severe anxiety cannot focus on what is really happening. There is a distortion of the environment. The person will behave in an irrational manner, thrashing and striking out, which leads to exhaustion or debilitation. Objective findings may include cool, clammy skin, dilated pupils, and hyperventilation. A family member shocked by the sudden, unexpected death of a loved one may experience such a reaction. This anxiety reaction is generally short-lived because the amount of energy expenditure rapidly results in exhaustion. The nurse working the emergency room or intensive care unit will be familiar with the person experiencing severe anxiety since the precipitating stress is often catastrophic in nature. Table 3-1 lists the signs and symptoms common during each level of anxiety.

NURSING ASSESSMENT

Assessing the level of anxiety in a patient or family member is an ongoing process. Ideally, the nurse will have a number of contacts with the patient and significant others, which will allow a relationship conducive to accurate assessment to be established. The nurse–patient relationship established during the initial assessment phase will continue to develop during the management and evaluation phase.

TABLE 3-1
LEVELS OF ANXIETY

LEVEL	SUBJECTIVE	OBJECTIVE
I *Relaxation*	Feels comfortable Learning, problem-solving not optimal	HR, BP, and R normal Resting comfortably Sleeping Relaxed appearance
II *Mild*	Enhanced ability to learn Awareness of surroundings Enhanced ability to problem solve Enhanced ability to make decisions Able to focus on what is happening	HR, BP, and R normal Alert, attentive
III *Moderate*	Decreased ability to solve problems Limited ability to focus on what is really happening Difficulty making decisions (simple tasks can seem a chore) Loss of confidence (feels timid, unassertive, and withdrawn) Sense of danger and perpetual dread Preoccupied with future Nervousness or dizziness Inappropriate anger and hostility Forgetfulness	Restless Excessive talkativeness Urinary frequency Altered motility of digestive tract: Diarrhea, indigestion, weight loss or gain, nausea Signs of muscle tension Headache, backache, tics Strained voice Increased or possibly decreased BP and HR Increased respiration
IV *Severe*	Disoriented, unaware of environment Bizarre perceptions, cannot focus on what is really happening Sense of doom No problem-solving or learning	Increased or possibly decreased HR and BP Increased respiration Dilated pupils Labored breathing Excessive sweating, pacing about Excessive talking, with rambling conversation Repetitive movement of hands and feet Altered digestive tract Sleep disorder

SUBJECTIVE ASSESSMENT

Even though the assessment process is ongoing, much information regarding the patient's level of anxiety will be evident during the first encounter. When given the opportunity, most patients will confide to the nurse about their concerns. The patient should be encouraged to talk about his physical and emotional health problems and related concerns. Much information can be obtained not only from the patient, but from family members and the interactions between family members. Whereas the patient may discuss the most overt causes of anxiety, that is, hospitalization, fear of surgery, or fear of pain, others close to him may uncover other, more covert, stresses such as financial concerns or marital discord.

Patients may have a myriad of subjective complaints that are a result of anxiety but often the patient does not recognize them as such. The nurse must be able to identify complaints that are indicative of anxiety. The symptoms will vary according to the level of anxiety experienced by the patient. Because of the unspent energy created by anxiety, the patient may have symptoms of muscle tension. The patient may complain of headache, pain in the neck, pain between the shoulders, and low back pain. Other symptoms include abdominal discomfort, dyspareunia, pruritus, premature ejaculation, fatigability, restlessness, and insomnia (Table 3-1).

Subjective complaints are interpreted only after examining the patient's physical and psychosocial status. Each patient and situation must be considered individually. Many patients complain of being dizzy, a symptom of anxiety, but not all of these patients have high levels of anxiety. The nurse needs to evaluate the symptom based on physical findings, history of illnesses, medication being taken, and stresses. Dizziness as a result of drug therapy or vascular disease must be differentiated from dizziness as a result of hyperventilation. Asking the patient if similar symptoms have occurred previously, and, if so, under what circumstances, may avoid guessing and assumptions by the staff.

After allowing the patient an opportunity to discuss his concerns, the nurse should determine how the patient has reacted to and coped with stresses in the past. Recognizing the patient's personality pattern will allow for greater understanding in planning care. For example, Mr. Leonard had always dealt with fear or stress by withdrawal and isolation. He had used these mechanisms unsuccessfully for years to decrease the discomfort of anxious periods. Prior to surgery for a vagotomy and pyloroplasty, Mr. Leonard became very restless, withdrawn, and hostile to the nursing staff. His nurse recognized additional symptoms of anxiety including insomnia, increased heart rate, and anorexia. Because the nurse was aware of his coping mechanisms, she was able to understand the basis of his behavior more fully and to take measures to dissipate the anxiety.

For some the symptoms of anxiety may become accepted as a personality characteristic. A woman may say, "I guess I'm just a born worrier," indicating that her symptoms are inherent in her personality structure. These attitudes have deep social roots nurtured through feelings of inadequacy and low self-esteem. Assisting patients to work through these feelings of inferiority and helplessness requires investigation of specific conflicts or concerns and an appropriate management plan.

Consider particular underlying medical disorders that may be contributing to the patient's anxiety. These disorders include both illness and effects of drug therapy. For example, side-effects of aminophylline and sympathomimetic drugs include increased heart rate and blood pressure, with resultant agitation. The hypertensive patient who is taking antihypertensive medication may experience impotence or loss of libido resulting in anxiety. The person may be consuming large amount of caffeine, tobacco, or alcohol, all of which contribute to feelings of anxiousness.

Anxiety often can coincide with alcoholism and drug abuse. An accurate history of the patient's use of alcohol or other drugs is necessary to avoid misdiagnosis and mismanagement. Anxiety and drug-related problems have many similar signs and symptoms but management is not necessarily the same for both. Each is a unique problem and should be treated as such.

PHYSICAL EXAMINATION

Making the diagnosis of anxiety as the etiology of the patient's complaints requires that no other organic cause can be found as well as identifying signs and symptoms indicative of anxiety. This is done by completing a thorough physical examination.

Before the physical examination, make the anxious patient feel as comfortable as possible. Give explanations about the procedures of the examination and an opportunity for the patient to ask questions regarding the examination. During the exam, drape the patient for comfort and to avoid embarrassment. As the exam progresses the nurse should keep the patient informed of what is being done and encourage the patient to talk of any discomfort or concerns. The nurse may uncover a source of anxiety for the patient during the exam. For example, Mrs. Jones made an appointment in the outpatient clinic for complaints of nervousness and inability to carry out her household responsibilities. During the interview the nurse identified Mrs. Jones as being highly anxious, but was unable to determine the cause of this problem. Mrs. Jones insisted that she was in perfect health, however, on examining the patient, the nurse found a breast lump that Mrs. Jones then admitted she had found previously. Without alarming Mrs. Jones, the nurse stated the significance of this finding and proceeded to outline a reasonable series of diagnostic tests. Although the patient had never admitted to being concerned about the breast lump, the nurse noticed that the patient's symptoms of anxiety were markedly reduced following the diagnosis of a benign breast cyst.

Several physical findings of anxiety may be observed during the interviewing process. The anxious patient may appear pale and be diaphoretic. Speech patterns are often altered. Patients may experience a strained voice, stuttering, rambling speech, or excessive talkativeness. They do not seem to be able to get comfortable and often pace or make repetitive movements of the hands and feet. The person's pupils may be dilated and breathing may be labored.

During the physical examination additional findings will support the diagnosis of anxiety (see "Responses to Anxiety"). Muscle tension has been noted to be a common physical finding of anxiety; however, the recognition of such muscle tension on physical examination often is difficult. Muscle tension frequently is manifested in the neck and shoulder area, in the lower back, and in facial muscles. Other physical findings may include tachycardia, abdominal distention, and diaphoresis. As mentioned previously, perform the physical examination coincident with a detailed history to make an accurate diagnosis. At each visit with the patient the nurse will gather new information about the patient's state of well-being and a complete physical examination need not be repeated. Abnormal physical findings will of course need to be monitored and evaluated at regular intervals.

PARACLINICAL DATA

There are tests that are helpful in classification and diagnosis that allow for increased objectivity. One such test is the Minnesota Multiphasic Personality Inventory (MMPI), which is an easy, inexpensive, and quick patient evaluation method. Additional tests used to evaluate the level of anxiety are the Hamilton Anxiety Scale (HAS) and the Anxiety Status Inventory (ASI). These are semiobjective rating scales in which specific cues for ratings of signs and symptoms are given, as well as instructions on how to rate quantitatively.[16]

NURSING DIAGNOSIS

LEVEL OF ANXIETY

Following the initial and each subsequent visit with the patient, the nurse will want to use her findings to form a conclusion about the patient's level of anxiety. Determining a person's level of anxiety is not easily done. There are qualitative and quantitative differences in traits or characteristics that do not lend themselves to strict classification. The nurse's own experience, judgment, and common sense must be relied on, as well as objective data.

Knowledge of the signs and symptoms related to the four levels of anxiety will assist the nurse in diagnosing the patient's anxiety level correctly and will allow her to implement appropriate interventions.

Accurate diagnosis may be facilitated by identification of the possible sources of the patient's signs and symptoms. As we discussed previously, the causes of anxiety may include intrapersonal conflicts, psychosocial threats, physical threats, transference, and unmet physical and emotional needs.

DIFFERENTIAL DIAGNOSIS

The diagnosis of anxiety as a cause of a patient's symptoms can be made only after it has been established that there are no organic illnesses present that could cause similar symptomatology. Often, this is done in collaboration with the physician. Diagnosis is often difficult because the symptoms of anxiety are rather vague and could be produced by a number of other disorders. The following sections describe a number of common presentations characteristic of anxiety states but that could also be caused by other disorders.

Dyspnea

A very common presentation of the anxious patient is the complaint of dyspnea. Typically patients complain that "I can't get enough air." They describe long dramatic "sighs" or yawning-type respiration that does not produce a satisfying feeling that enough air has been obtained. It is quite important, however, to distinguish this anxiety-related problem from asthma, which would also present as dyspnea. On physical examination, prominent expiratory wheezes would be heard in asthmatics, whereas these would not be heard in the anxious patient. In both cases tachycardia probably would be present. An anxiety state can be differentiated from emphysema primarily by consideration of the patient's history (smoking history, occupational exposure) and physical examination, in which prominent accessory muscles of respiration, increased anteroposterior diameter, and distant breath sounds suggest the diagnosis of emphysema. Although it would be far less common than anxiety state, spontaneous pneumothorax might also present as unexplained dyspnea and should not be overlooked. This diagnosis could be made by physical examination (absent breath sounds) or chest x-ray. It should be emphasized that in each case (asthma, emphysema, and spontaneous pneumothorax), the patients, sensing grave danger, would be expected to generate much ANS activity, and thus mimic the classic anxiety state.

Chest Pain

A number of anxious patients present with complaints of chest pain. Writing off a patient as "anxious" might be a critical mistake in the presence of underlying ischemic heart disease or pericarditis. For this reason the usual history and physical examination are undertaken. An electrocardiogram (ECG) may also be obtained under appropriate circumstances and compared with previous examinations. Patients with myocardial ischemia often have tachycardia and diaphoresis. They may also present with an extremely restless, anxious appearance. The diagnosis of anxiety reaction can be made in these circumstances only when myocardial ischemia or other serious heart disease has been excluded.

Nervousness

Nervousness, a common symptom of anxiety, is also a symptom of such endocrine disorders as hyperthyroidism, hypoglycemia and pheochromocytoma. Hyperthyroidism may cause weight loss, intolerance to heat, sinus tachycardia, atrial fibrillation, tremors, lid lag, and exophthalmos. When hyperthyroidism is suspected on the basis of history and physical examination, thyroid function tests (including T_4 bound, T_3 uptake, and the T_7 calculation) serve to confirm the diagnosis.

Hypoglycemia produces shakiness, tremor, sweating, weakness, and dizziness. The diabetic patient or the patient with a relative carbohydrate intolerance, who presents with nervousness accompanied by any of the above signs and symptoms, should have a blood sugar sample drawn and then be given candy or orange juice. When hypoglycemia or diabetes is suspected in the patient, a 2- or 3-hour glucose tolerance test generally can verify these conditions if they are present.

Pheochromocytoma produces marked hypertension, hypermetabolism, and hyperglycemia as the result of an oversecretion of epinephrine and norepinephrine. The sympathetic overactivity causes the patient to feel nervous and to present signs and symptoms similar to anxiety. When pheochromocytoma is suspected, a 24-hour urine collection for metanephrines and vanilla–mandellic acid (VMA) is useful to confirm the diagnosis.

Questioning the patient about dietary habits and drug usage may reveal the source of nervousness for many patients. Excessive ingestion of caffeine, cigarette smoking, cocaine, amphetamines, hallucinogens, high dose steroids, and alcohol can produce nervousness. Drug withdrawal may also produce anxietylike symptoms. Serum drug levels may be useful when drugs are considered as a possible etiology.

MANAGEMENT

Managing anxiety requires considerable imagination, time, effort, knowledge, and caring on the part of the nurse. One cannot rid oneself completely of anxiety, but the anxiety may be kept at a comfortable level so that the energy it produces can be used in a positive manner. Nurses cannot expect to accomplish this for patients. They can only expect to assist the patients in making certain changes for themselves. The nurse may be the crucial motivating force in this change process. Management may be solely the responsibility of the nurse, but will most likely involve the physician and other professionals. The physician may need to be consulted when the patient's anxiety level is severe enough to require sedation. To facilitate the best outcome, communication should be ongoing between the nurse and the physician regarding the patient's level of anxiety.

Depending on the situation, the management plan may range from quite straightforward to one that is more complex. For example, John was a 16-year-old adolescent who was admitted for an appendectomy. He had always been healthy, with no major mental or physical problems, and he was very upset about the possible effects of surgery, that is, pain, mutilation, and deformity. He was diagnosed as having level III anxiety. The nurse quickly implemented a plan consisting of comfort measures and education, and was available to offer reassurance and answer questions. In this situation, the high level of anxiety was directly related to the pending surgery, and the management plan was designed to reduce preoperative stress.

In comparison, Mrs. Prey was a 45-year-old housewife and retail clerk who made an appointment with the nurse practitioner for symptoms of headache, inability to make decisions, and nervousness. After an extensive history and complete physical examination, the nurse made the diagnosis of level III anxiety. The nurse discussed her findings with Mrs. Prey and then suggested that they work together to develop a management plan. The plan consisted of exploring the causes of Mrs. Prey's anxiety, focusing on a particular area of conflict, and identifying possible solutions. Mrs. Prey had to be willing to make necessary changes in her lifestyle to decrease her anxiety level.

In this situation, where the cause(s) of anxiety and the treatment are not as obvious, the management plan would require greater collaboration between the patient and nurse. Whatever the circumstance, it is important to keep the plan as simple as possible. A plan that is unrealistic or too complex will increase the possibility of failure and frustration.

COUNSELING

The person's anxiety level must first be minimized so that the patient is capable of learning, problem-solving, and reasoning. The patient must also be alert and motivated to make a change. People with high levels of anxiety generate energy that needs to be dissipated. The nurse can facilitate this release of energy by encouraging the patient to talk or to cry, or by encouraging physical activity. The nursing skills of talking to and listening to a patient must be developed and consistently included in patient care. Nurses often have difficulty justifying to themselves or other staff members time spent talking with patients. In a study done by Stockwell, nurses were found to hold the following views about talking with patients:[15]

- They felt guilty about talking with patients because other staff members would think that they were slacking.
- They felt uncomfortable during quiet periods but did not feel that talking with patients constituted work.
- Patients talked to most often were those that were liked by the staff.

However, verbalizing concerns are often anxiolytic for the patient since once fears are stated they often seem more manageable. A nurse can be of much help to the patient by encouraging him to talk and by being a good listener. The nurse should attempt to be respectful, nonjudgmental, and noncritical while listening to the patient. Interruptions by the nurse should be limited to providing direction when a patient begins to ramble or to prompt the patient to continue talking. Allowing patients to cry is often uncomfortable for the staff. Recognition of this response is important so that the nurses do not subconsciously prevent the distraught patient from this release. The nurse needs to be aware of the tendency to sedate the crying patient "for his own good." Some patients may rid themselves of anxiety by chewing gum or doing work with their hands. Anything that allows for the utilization of energy may help rid the patient of anxiety.

EMOTIONAL WELL-BEING

Increasing the patient's sense of well-being is particularly important in reducing anxiety. Creating an environment that is not overly stimulating, that is, without bright lights, monitoring devices, and loud or annoying noises, will increase the patient's sense of well-being. Personal belongings or familiar objects may be kept by the patient to increase his sense of security. Maintaining a calm, reassuring approach will help to control the anxiety.

PATIENT EDUCATION

Much anxiety can be eliminated through careful explanations of hospital or clinical procedures and diagnostic tests. The patient deserves accurate and appropriate information, in nontechnical, understandable language, regarding his illness. Repeated explanations may be necessary to avoid confusion because the anxious person may have altered cognitive functioning. Careless conversations between staff members should be avoided as they are easily misinterpreted by the patient.

PHYSICAL WELL-BEING

Keeping the patient as comfortable as possible may help to decrease anxiety. In instances in which nutrition has been poor, personal hygiene neglected, elimination patterns disturbed, or sleeping patterns altered,

the patient may benefit from a plan that attempts to correct these problems.

CONTINUITY

Providing constancy in the staff also promotes a sense of security in the patient. Once a satisfactory relationship has been established between the patient and nurse, it is usually beneficial to continue the relationship throughout the hospitalization or treatment program. If the nurse does have to stop caring for a patient, she should prepare the patient in advance to avoid feelings of abandonment.

MAINTENANCE OF CULTURAL VALUES AND RELIGIOUS BELIEFS

Exploring the patient's cultural practices and identifying areas of conflict may provide relief of anxiety. For example, Mr. Razka, a 76-year-old Lithuanian was admitted to the hospital because of uncontrolled diabetes mellitus and an ulcerated left foot. He had refused to eat his 2000-calorie ADA diet and in addition was not sleeping well. When the nurse sat down to talk with Mr. and Mrs. Razka, she learned that certain herbs and spices routinely were added to his diet at home, the absence of which made the hospital food unpalatable. The nurse also discovered that his nightly ritual before sleep was disturbed by the routine of the hospital staff. Consultation with the dietitian and simple reorganization of the staff's routine made Mr. Razka much more comfortable.

Religious beliefs and practices are important to the person's well-being and should not be neglected or ignored. The patient should be allowed to practice his religious beliefs as he wishes during hospitalization. Religious beliefs can be a very strong system of support for the patient and family members. It is important that opportunity be given for the patient or family to use the hospital chapel or visit with the hospital clergy. Allowing time for prayer or meditation can enhance relaxation.

ACKNOWLEDGMENT OF THE EXISTENCE OF ANXIETY

The next step in the management of anxiety is acknowledgment of its existence by the patient. Patients often object to being described as *anxious*. Adopting an alternative term ("nervous," "upset") is often justified as long as the management plan is not compromised. The nurse then assists the patient in learning about feelings, behavior, and possible causes of anxiety. This can be a time-consuming process; however, the patient often can explore these areas on his own after receiving the proper direction.

It is important to help the patient focus on the issue that is causing him to be anxious. Starting with only one issue keeps the problem manageable. One then determines how this particular issue is causing the patient to suffer. Has the patient been trying to find a solution to the problem or ignoring it?[4] According to Aquilera and Messick, people may be experiencing one or more of the following difficulties in managing anxiety:[1]

- Perceptions of the issues may be unrealistic.
- Coping mechanisms may be inadequate.
- Situational support may be insufficient.
- Complications resulting from discontinuation of psychotropic drug therapy may be involved.

If one of these difficulties seems to be present then the nurse should concentrate over a period of time on this issue. Once the solution has been identified and the ways in which the patient has responded recognized, the nurse can help the patient to examine which efforts have been ineffective. In attempting to find solutions, it is important not to become frustrated. If one solution does not work, the patient is encouraged to try another. Solutions should be kept realistic, and goals attainable.

SEVERE ANXIETY

Through all the nursing measures mentioned above, the goal is to decrease anxiety and prevent the occurrence of severe anxiety. Anxiety tends to escalate if not dealt with adequately in the early stages. When the patient experiences severe anxiety, the nurse will need to take control of the situation and provide direction for the patient. The patient may be disoriented and unable to focus on what really is happening. The nurse must remain calm and provide a calm, safe environment for the patient. She may walk with the patient or provide some simple activity to dissipate the energy created. Allowing the patient to cry or grieve provides an emotional release that need not be prevented by sedation. The patient who is likely to hurt himself or others may benefit from sedation. The patient who is severely anxious should not be left alone.

OTHER RESOURCES

The nurse is able to respond to many of the needs of anxious patients; however, there may be times when she will wish to refer the patient to other professionals for specialized therapy. Nurses need to familiarize themselves with individuals and agencies within the hospital and the community that may be beneficial in resolving the patient's anxiety. The new mother who has anxiety about breast-feeding may find support, reassurance, and helpful information from the La Leche League. A recent mastectomy patient may benefit from the empathy and advice offered by Reach for Recovery. The patient or couple with marital problems may be referred to a marital counselor, and the person with financial concerns often receives valuable information from the social worker.

Many patients find relief from the discomforts of muscle tension through physical therapy. Relaxation methods can be explored with the patient, as well as meditation, biofeedback, and various exercise programs.[3] Bioenergetics is a mode of therapy that combines emotional expression with physical expression and may be useful for persons who have difficulty talking about their feelings.

ANXIOLYTICS

As a result of the ambiguities surrounding the proper use of anti-anxiety drugs, these drugs have been widely prescribed and often abused. In 1979, over 60 million prescriptions were filled in the United States for benzodiazepines.[11] In trying to provide guidelines for distribution of anti-anxiety medication, Rosenbaum suggests that the following questions be considered:

Is the patient experiencing an illness or syndrome other than generalized anxiety, that could account for the patient's distress?

If not, is there an available nonpharmacologic intervention that is likely to effect symptomatic relief?

Is symptomatic treatment with an anxiolytic agent indicated, considering the potential benefits and risks, drug selection, and alternatives?

Anti-anxiety drugs are rarely necessary for the patient with varying degrees of normal anxiety. Most appropriately they are reserved for those patients with severe anxiety, or with neurotic anxiety that impairs functioning. Even then, drug therapy is used only in conjunction with other non-drug therapies.

The benzodiazepines are generally considered the mainstay of anti-anxiety pharmacotherapy. Various benzodiazepines differ in the rate of absorption, the formation of active metabolites, and the duration of activity, and they are chosen with these characteristics in mind. Elderly patients and patients with hepatic insufficiency are susceptible to excessive plasma accumulation of drug metabolites. Benzodiazepines with a shorter half-life of drug and active metabolites (e.g., lorazepam and oxazepam) are more appropriate for this group of patients.

Short-term clinical trials with the benzodiazepines indicate that they are relatively safe when compared to barbiturates, antihistamines, and propanediols.[2] The benzodiazepines are more selectively anxiolytic and have less addiction potential for short-term use at therapeutic doses. Anti-anxiety drugs should not be used over a long term, since they are expected only to diminish anxiety, not eradicate it. Problems of abuse occur when drugs are used in place of a more direct solution to personal conflicts. Even though genuine physiological addiction appears uncommon, evidence for psychological dependence is abundant. Critical clinical assessment at weekly intervals to evaluate the effectiveness of drug therapy is essential.

Drowsiness (especially when combined with alcohol) and impaired coordination are potential concerns for the patients taking benzodiazepines. Teratogenic effects include cleft lip and palate.[6] Withdrawal from certain drugs such as amitriptyline and imipramine may create high levels of anxiety in patients.[7]

CONCLUSION

The basic causes for anxiety are complex and poorly understood. Anxiety is, however, universal; elevation in the cost of health care delivery because of anxiety-related problems surely must be enormous.

The nurse has a unique opportunity to help patients suffering from anxiety-related problems. This help should be in the form of recognition of the anxious state, accurate differentiation from other non-anxiety–related problems, and management. An outline of this process is provided in the accompanying basic care plan. Critical to the implementation of these steps is the realization that the patient is suffering and needs help.

That the steps outlined here will be helpful is intuitively obvious but needs stricter documentation. Future research by nurses in this area should include an assessment of the effectiveness of nursing measures done to reduce anxiety levels. Sound research in this area is critically needed to ensure high levels of patient care and to add validity to nursing measures. Another area for research involves assessment of the effec-

tiveness of anxiolytic drugs in the management of normal anxiety. The nurse is in a strategic position that allows for a more thorough evaluation of the many aspects of this problem.

REFERENCES

1. Aguilera DC, Messick JM: Crisis Intervention Theory and Methodology. St. Louis, CV Mosby, 1978
2. Barsky AJ: Psychiatric and behavioral problems: Approach to the patient with anxiety. In Goroll AH et al (eds); Primary Care Medicine. Philadelphia, JB Lippincott, 1981
3. Benson H: The Relaxation Response. New York, Avon Books, 1975
4. DeRosis HA: Women and Anxiety. New York, Delacorte Press, 1979
5. Gray M: Neuroses, p 95. New York, Van Nostrand & Reinhold, 1978
6. Goldberg HL, DiMascio A: Psychotropic drugs in pregnancy. In Lipton MA et al (eds). Psychopharmacology: A Generation of Progress. New York, Raven Press 1978 1047–1055
7. Katerndahl D: Panic. Am Fam Physician 26, No. 1: 125–129 1982
8. Martin LL: Health Care of Women. Philadelphia, JB Lippincott, 1978
9. Maslow AH: Motivation and Personality. New York, Harper & Row, 1954
10. May R: The Meaning of Anxiety, rev ed. New York, WW Norton & Co, 1977
11. Rosenbaum JF: Current concepts in psychiatry: The drug treatment of anxiety. New Engl J Med 306, No. 7:401–404 1982
12. Rouhani GC: Neurotic anxiety is the result of unrealistic threats. Nurs Mirror 146:25–30 1978
13. Schweitzer L, Adams G: The diagnosis and management of anxiety for primary care physicians. In WE Fann et al (eds): Phenomenology and Treatment of Anxiety. New York, Spectrum, 1979
14. Smitherman C: Nursing Actions for Health Promotion. Philadelphia, FA Davis, 1981
15. Stockwell F: The unpopular patient. Research Project Series No. 2. London, Royal College of Nursing, 1972
16. Zung W: Assessment of anxiety disorder: Qualitative and quantitative approaches. In WE Fann et al (eds); Phenomenology and Treatment of Anxiety. New York, Spectrum, 1979

Basic Care Plan for Reducing Level of Anxiety

1. Show kindness.
2. Allow the patient to express his feelings.
3. Obtain complete history and physical examination; be honest about findings. Rule out organic problems.
4. Make assessment of the patient's level of anxiety.
5. Provide reassurance, perspective, explanations; suggest reasonable approaches to identified problems.
6. Provide an avenue for emotional release.
7. Reduce extraneous stimuli as much as possible.

BIBLIOGRAPHY

Ack M et al: Clues to the diagnosis of anxiety. Patient Care 12:158–186, 1978

Basic System: Anxiety: Recognition and intervention (a programmed instruction). Am J Nurs 65, No. 9:129–152

Cohn L: Coping with anxiety: A step by step guide. Nurs 79 9:34–37 December 1979

Dolan BP: A study of similarities and the differences in the concept of anxiety as found in the writings of selected contemporary psychoanalytic authors and in selected authors in professional nursing literature. Master's thesis, Catholic University of America, 1967

Greenblatt DS, Shader RI: Benzodiazepines in Clinical Practice. New York, Raven Press, 1974

Greenhill MH: Psychiatric perspectives in Medicine. Psychosomatics vol. 2, No. 6, 1961; Vol 3, Nos. 1 and 2, 1962

Hardin CH: Aspects of anxiety. 2nd and enlarged ed. Philadelphia, JB Lippincott, 1968

Jenkins RL: The medical significance of anxiety. Washington DC, The Biological Sciences Foundation, 1955

Keane B: The management of the anxious patient in the general hospital ward. Aust Nurses J: 7, No. 9:47–49

Kelly D: Anxiety and Emotions: Psychological Basis and Treatment. Springfield, IL, Charles C Thomas, 1980

Lesse S: Anxiety: Its Components, Developments and Treatments. New York, Grune & Stratton, 1970

Levitt EE: The Psychology of Anxiety. Indianapolis, Bobbs–Merrill, 1967

Marcinek MB: Stress in the surgical patient. Am J Nurs 77, No. 11:1809–1811, 1977

Rickles NK: Management of Anxiety for the General Practitioner. Springfield, IL, Charles C Thomas, 1963

Selye H: Stress: Anxiety's breeding ground. In Hollister LE (ed): The Ubiquitous Symptoms. New York, Medcom, 1972

Smith MJ, Selye H: Reducing the negative effects of stress. Am J Nurs 79, No. 11:1953–1964, 1979

Stephenson CA: Stress in critically ill patients. Am J Nurs 77, No. 11:1806–1808, 1977

4

Impairment of Body Image

Cynthia S. Darling-Fisher

Any person faced with illness or a change in normal body state will undergo an alteration of body image, even if it is only a transient alteration. Although such an alteration may in theory be perceived as either positive or negative, it is most often a negative change that calls for the involvement of health professionals. Impairment of body image can occur in persons going through normal maturational changes, as well as in persons subjected to major trauma. The main factors that determine how body image change will be handled are the person's perception of the degree of change that has occurred and the meaning it holds for him. Family, social, and cultural factors play important roles in the development of these perceptions and the consequent response to threatened or actual body image change. Because nurses and other health professionals are frequently in a position to influence patient perceptions of body state changes, they have opportunities to help people adjust to body image disturbances. However, to be most effective in doing this, it is essential for nurses to understand the concept of body image, its development, and its role in the person's definition of self and reaction to others.

The particular cause and extent of body

image change will dictate the interventions required in patient care. Specific problems such as obesity, ostomy care, or burn care all involve management issues that are to some extent unique. Nevertheless, there are broad principles that are central to the health care management of patients undergoing body image changes and that transcend the details of particular conditions. This chapter focuses on these principles. It addresses the definition of body image, the development of body image and body image disturbances, ways to assess the patient with a body image disturbance, and possible interventions for persons undergoing body image alteration. The information presented should be applicable to people undergoing a broad range of body image disturbances.

BODY IMAGE DEFINED

Body image has been described by many disciplines, each modifying the definition according to the perspective of the specific field. Nursing has taken a holistic view, in keeping with its approach to health care. Mattheis describes *body image* as a mental representation of one's body, which develops from internal sensations, emotions, fantasies, posture, and experience of and with outside objects and people. It is a perception of one's body that is determined largely by how one thinks that others view it. It includes a spatial idea of one's own body that changes according to both internal and external sensory information.[19] Norris adds that it is a "social creation...basic to identity and has been referred to as the somatic ego."[21] Body image is the picture one has of one's self. Although it is often thought of as a matter of conscious perception, it may have an unconscious dimension as well. It may or may not be consistent with one's actual body structure or with the way others view one. One's body image develops gradually through interactions with others. It is generally consolidated as one completes adolescence, although it is continuously modified throughout one's lifetime. It plays an important role in determining the person's sense of self-esteem and security and is an important aspect of one's self-concept.

When a change in body state occurs, there is often a lag in the person's awareness of this change and thus a delay in the alteration of body image. It is not unusual for an extremely obese person to see himself as the slender young man of several years before. He has not incorporated the 60-lb weight gain so obvious to others into his picture of his body. Acceptance of a change in body image is important for the person's adjustment to the body state change and to his ability to grow beyond it. Impairment occurs when the person is unable to cope with or adjust to a change in body image, and this inability interferes with his optimal functioning.

HISTORICAL PERSPECTIVE

The concept of body image evolved from observations of patients experiencing the *phantom limb phenomenon*, or the feeling that an amputated limb is still present and functional. This phenomenon, although undoubtedly recognized earlier, was first documented by Paré, a physician in the late sixteenth century. In the early twentieth century, neurologists carried out studies that further supported the concept of body image and substantiated the fact that one's body image is not necessarily consistent with one's anatomical appearance.[10,13,17]

One of the most important works for the development of the present concept of body image is Schilder's work *The Image and Appearance of the Human Body*. Schilder extended earlier models of body image (that had focused on postural and sensory perceptions of the body) to include interpersonal, environmental, and temporal factors. In this expanded concept, the attitudes and opinions of others assume particular importance in the formation of the person's body image. Schilder felt that the body image developed from birth through input from all sensations, with vision having the dominant influence. This developing image has a great deal of stability, or resistance to rapid change, and yet may eventually incorporate a variety of body state changes that occur over the course of person's lifetime. Schilder also believed that body image and ego were strongly intertwined. He emphasized the role of the ego in the development of body image and in the person's response to body image disruption.[24]

Subsequent research has expanded this view by exploring the person's attitude toward his body and his feeling about himself. Studies by Secord and Jourard and others show a strong relationship between *body cathexis*, the degree of satisfaction or dissatisfaction with various parts or processes of the body, and one's self concept during either sickness or health.[10,23] In this way, body image can be related to the organization and functioning of a person's personality, especially his perceived degree of security or insecurity, and his feelings of self-value.

Fisher and Cleveland, both psychologists, proposed an additional dimension to body image, the concept of body boundary. The *body boundary* is the perceived line of separation between one's body and the outside world. Body boundary becomes more distinct as the person matures. In early infancy the distinction between self and the environment is unclear. As the child grows these boundaries become more clearly demarcated. Physical and psychological changes occurring throughout the life span, such as normal maturational changes of adolescence, pregnancy, or old age, require frequent revisions of the body boundary. Definiteness of body boundary varies greatly among normal persons and will be influenced by cultural and social factors. Individual differences cannot be classified as normal or abnormal.[4]

The concept of body boundary is particularly appropriate for health providers since so many medical procedures and therapies assault the person's sense of boundary or separateness from the outside world.[5] Fisher and Cleveland developed a method for measuring definiteness of body boundary using the Rorschach and other projective tests. They found that people experienced different symptoms depending on the firmness of body boundary. People with definite body boundaries were more likely to develop "external" symptoms such as musculoskeletal disorders (arthritis, joint pain) and skin rashes. People with less definite boundaries were more likely to experience "internal" symptoms such as diarrhea, constipation, stomach pains, and ulcers. Body boundary distortions were also frequently noted in

people with psychological disturbances like schizophrenia.[10]

In summary, the concept of body image has evolved from the primarily physiological study of the phantom phenomenon, to an integration of physiological, psychological, and sociological factors. Further research has added the concept of body boundary and explored the application of body image concerns to individuals with routine health problems as well as those with psychopathology. Body image is recognized as an aspect of normal personality development. It is flexible and strongly influenced by the attitudes of others. The establishment of a well-defined body image is felt to be an important and necessary aspect of healthy development.[17,19] A person's attitude about his body image is also felt to reflect his sense of self-esteem and security.[23] Understanding the concept of body image and its development is important when dealing with people facing actual or potential threats to their body integrity. This knowledge will help in assessing body image disturbances when they occur, and in planning appropriate interventions to prevent disturbances or to help the person adjust to them.

MECHANISMS OF ALTERATIONS IN BODY IMAGE

NORMAL DEVELOPMENT OF BODY IMAGE

Body image development is an ongoing process occurring throughout the life span. It is the result of the integration of multiple perceptions of both internal and external environmental factors. It begins in the perinatal stage with the development of the embryonic and infantile nervous system.[17] The newborn acquires knowledge of his body from tactile impressions. Initially there may be no physical image or differentiation from the outside world. Sucking and feeding are among the earliest experiences, and it is usually assumed that the mouth is the first area to be stimulated and to become part of the infant's awareness of self. As the infant begins to use both hands, further exploration of his body and others begins. The infant's exploration of self, others, and objects provides the primary tactile and kinesthetic sensations that contribute to body image. Kolb states that these are the processes upon which the beginnings of self-awareness, individuality, and the sense of ego are founded.[17] Other sensations such as optic, olfactory, auditory, thermal, and pain play a secondary but important role in this initial development. As the infant grows and increases his capacity for intricate motor activities, the body image is modified continuously. In addition, interactions with family members and significant others impart an indelible impression on the child's concept of himself, his body, and its functions.[4,17]

As the infant develops, he begins to differentiate himself from his mother. His physical, cognitive, and motor skills develop at a rapid rate and with this development comes mastery over specific tasks, his body, and his environment. From his interactions with others, he learns that specific body parts are good and to be shared and that others are to be hidden.[21] Schilder states that there is an active connection between one's own body image and the body image of significant others. The closer the others are emotionally and spatially, the more influence they have on the person's identification and body image modification.[24] This can be seen in early development of parent–child relationships and becomes particularly evident in the ado-lescent period, when peer-group identification is important to the person. With resolution of the identity tasks in the adolescent period, body image becomes more firmly defined, though it still incorporates significant experiences and changes over time. Norris states that "once established, body image defines and places demands and limitations on what a person is capable of in life. Interpersonally, it expresses an individual's personality in many ways and with vivid representation."[21]

NURSING MODEL OF BODY IMAGE

Brown proposes a nursing model for the understanding of body image, based on a holistic view of the person in mutual interaction with the environment (Fig. 4-1).[4] This model includes three levels of bodily experience that may effect the person and six environmental variables that interact to develop and modify the body image. The person's developmental stage will mediate the impact of these variables at a given point in time.

The first level involves innermost somatic bodily experiences. These are derived from physiologic processes that influence the development of the core of the body image. Examples include endocrine and metabolic changes that occur during normal maturation periods (e.g., toddlerhood, adolescence, and old age). Alcohol and certain medications produce somatic changes at this level. Physiologic responses to fear and anxiety also act at the innermost level. These basic bodily experiences occur even in infants.[4,19]

Behavioral bodily experiences compose the second level. These experiences are derived from data acquired and processed by the perceptual system. Movement, touch, hearing, and thinking contribute to body im-

The elderly years
Middle age
Youth
Adolescence
School age
Preschool age
Toddlerhood
Infancy
Fetal life

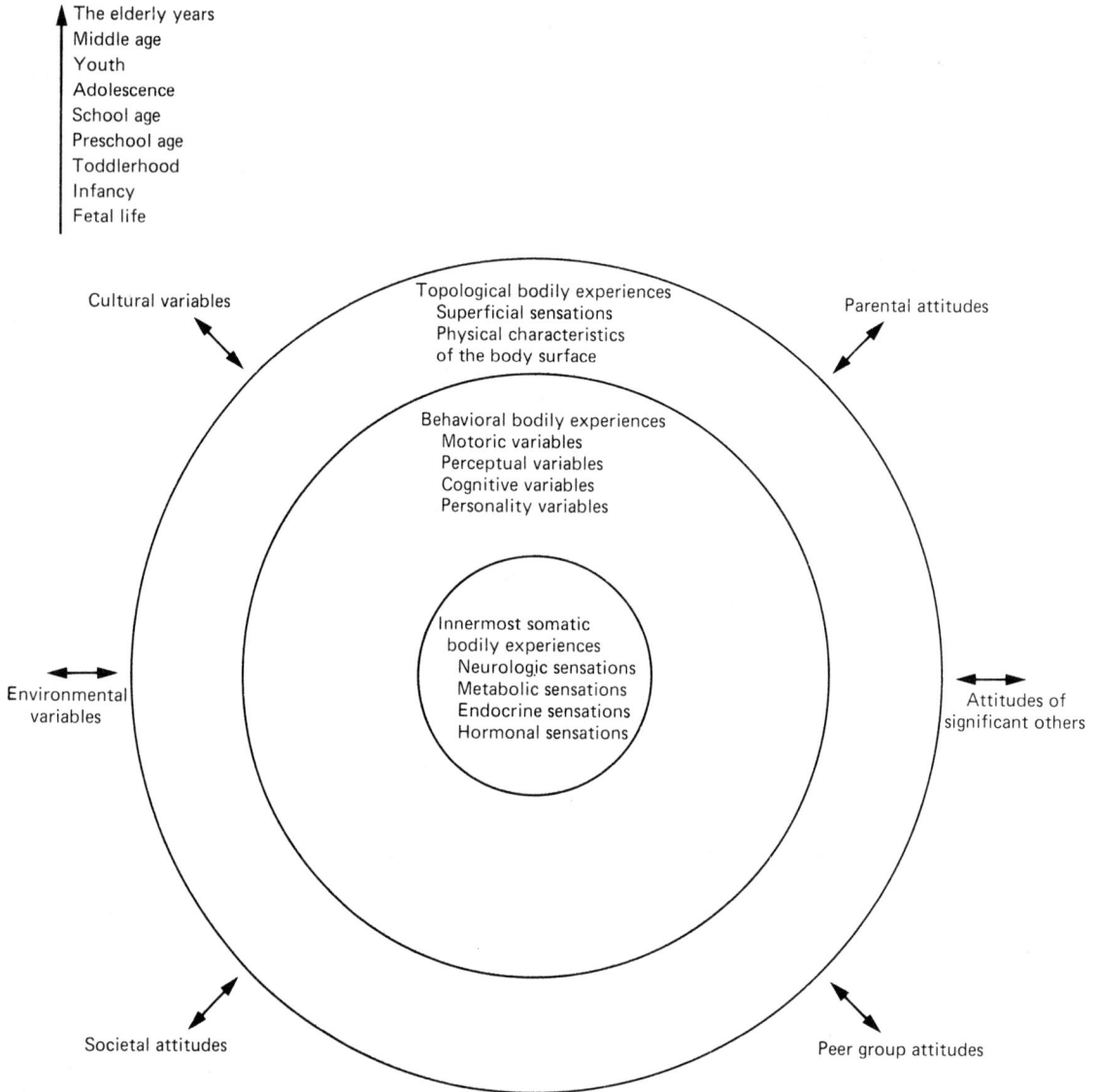

Cultural variables

Topological bodily experiences
Superficial sensations
Physical characteristics
of the body surface

Parental attitudes

Behavioral bodily experiences
Motoric variables
Perceptual variables
Cognitive variables
Personality variables

Innermost somatic
bodily experiences
Neurologic sensations
Metabolic sensations
Endocrine sensations
Hormonal sensations

Environmental
variables

Attitudes of
significant others

Societal attitudes

Peer group attitudes

FIG. 4-1　*Nursing model of body image. (Brown MS: Introduction to the concept of body image. In Bower FL (ed): Normal Development of Body Image, p 8. New York, John Wiley & Sons, 1977)*

age development at this level. Sensory stimulation is particularly important in the initial development of body image during infancy. Personality characteristics such as aggressiveness or docility mediate the person's experiences and thus influence body image development.[4]

The third level is the topological level of bodily experiences, including those sensations that emanate from the surface features.

The senses of pain, taste, hearing, and vision are included here. Physical characteristics often are experienced during interactions with others and are thus culturally and socially defined. The concept of body boundary falls in this area. As mentioned earlier, definiteness of the person's body boundary will have an impact on the person's responses to others and perhaps even in the types of symptoms he experiences. The body boundary will grow and change throughout the life span. Disease entities and therapies also will have an impact on it. The degree of definiteness of a person's body boundary may give clues to his ability to cope with stress and change.[4,19]

Brown identifies six external factors that influence body image development and the person's response to the body image change. These factors include parent, significant others, and peer group attitudes; cultural and societal influences; and general environmental concerns such as nutrition, financial resources, housing, and occupation.[4] The person's stage in life cycle development will mediate how various bodily levels and environmental factors interact. A person may experience conflicting responses from these different factors. A child's looks may be admired within his family and cultural group, yet when he attends school he may find that these same features are considered unusual or even undesirable. Studies have shown that a person's evaluation of an unclearly defined trait is based largely on evaluation of that trait by significant others. When a body defect or deformity occurs, the attitude of family and culture is a greater influence on a person's adaptation than is the defect itself.[17]

Because developmental stage plays such an important role in the formation of body image, it will be helpful to review normal developmental patterns. Erikson theorized that psychosocial development is achieved through negotiating a series of tasks that represent eight stages.[9] The tasks take into consideration the physical, cognitive, emotional, and social levels of the individual. One's success in negotiating a stage will influence one's ability to deal with the next stage. Tasks are negotiated not in an either/or manner but rather on a continuum. During the first stage of development, the sensory oral stage, the task of trust versus mistrust is met. This occurs during the first year of life when the infant is totally dependent on others. The infant's experiences with the nurturing person lay the foundation for his level of trust.[9]

The next task is autonomy versus shame and doubt. This is the muscular–anal stage, occurring at ages 1 to 3. During this period, there is great musculomotor development. The child learns to eat, talk, and control anal sphincter muscles. Parental figures become extremely important, and their opinions and attitudes carry great weight.[9] The body image is changing continuously due to rapid motor development, and the child experiences uncertainties concerning body boundaries.[18] During this period the child learns to relate to work or the performance of tasks. Failure to achieve mastery leads to feelings of shame, doubt, and inadequacy.

The third stage of development is the locomotor–genital stage, ages 3 to 6, encompassing the tasks of initiative versus guilt. During this period the child begins to develop a sense of sex role identity. Through identification with parent models, the child develops a sense of gender-appropriate behaviors.[9] With increased psychomotor and cognitive skills, the child becomes more curious about his body, particularly the genital area. At this time some form of masturbation may occur. Parental attitudes and responses towards the child's masturbation are felt to be an important determinant of the child's later sexual attitudes.[18]

During the latency stage, ages 6 to 11, the child strives for industry versus inferiority.[9] The child is learning technical skills, and school and peers become important features in the child's development. This may be the first time the child realizes that he cannot perform as well as others or that he is different from others.[18] The presence of a physical alteration such as the need to wear glasses or obesity may play an important role in the child's body image. If the child does not receive recognition for his efforts or achievements, inferiority or a sense of inadequacy may develop. During the end of this stage, the child may begin to experience the pubertal growth spurt. These normal changes make the child more self-conscious and concerned about appearance, especially in comparison with others. This heralds the beginning of the fifth stage of puberty and adolescence.

Erikson calls the tasks of this period identity versus role confusion, and it encompasses the ages of 11 to 18 years.[9] This is a transition period between childhood and adulthood and covers many important developmental changes. The adolescent is attempting to integrate his life experiences to form a sense of self. He is struggling with the dependency–independency conflict with his parents. One means of coping with this is to develop strong attachments to a peer group. Adolescent peer groups are very sensitive to similarities and differences. Therefore, an adolescent who does not or is not able to conform to the group norms may have difficulty being accepted. Problems may be related to normal developmental occurrences as well as to physical handicaps. The late maturer, the tall girl, the obese boy, or the hearing-impaired child all may face similar difficulties with peer groups due to their differentness. Towards the end of this period the adolescent begins to consolidate his own

identity and the standards of the peer group become less important.[18]

During the young adulthood period, ages 18 to 45, biologic change is completed but psychosocial development continues. Erikson calls the tasks of this period intimacy versus isolation.[9] The young adult is concerned with development of intimacy with another person. The person is secure enough in his identity that he is able to share himself with others, both in friendship and in a mutually satisfying sexual relationship. The person who fears losing his sense of identity develops a sense of isolation. The person who has been able to negotiate previous tasks and accept his body image is better able to develop meaningful and satisfying interpersonal relationships.[18]

The adulthood period addresses the tasks of generativity versus stagnation.[9] This stage spans the middle years of life, ages 45 to 65. During this period the adult is concerned with establishing and guiding future generations with a hope of bettering society. However, the adult may review his achievements and find that he has failed to accomplish what he had planned. He may feel incapable of generativity, which may precipitate a midlife crisis. The adult may see this period as his last chance to achieve in life and may become engrossed in satisfying personal needs. The result may be self-absorption and stagnation. Another concern may be the fear of old age. Regression to inappropriately youthful behavior may result as the adult attempts to deny his aging body. Conversely, the middle-aged adult may prematurely take on attributes of older adults. He may view every physical change as an indication of his aging, resulting in depression and isolation.[18]

Erikson's final stage is maturity, from age 65 onward, involving the task of integrity versus despair.[9] During this period, the adult comes to grips with his life. Thoughts about death are common, as is concern about not being capable of caring for an ailing significant other. Despair may develop. A mature adult who has developed a strong sense of self-worth and is able to place a value on past life experiences may be able to overcome these feelings. Otherwise, feelings of despair and disgust predominate, decreasing the person's sense of self-worth. Strength comes from an overall sense of satisfaction with one's life experiences and an acceptance of one's disappointments and triumphs. Many physical changes occur as this period progresses. These physiological changes may lead to alterations in body image boundaries, causing the person to focus on more internal sites.[10,18] These changes parallel the concerns of the middle-aged adult but are perhaps more extreme. Factors such as retirement, reduced income, and the death of significant others and friends are of particular concern.

The development of body image goes through many changes as the person grows and meets the challenges of specific developmental tasks. The infant starts with a hazy body boundary, focusing primarily on his mouth. The child progresses in his awareness of body image, but ambiguities concerning body boundaries may persist for some time. He then focuses on the genital region and develops a sense of gender identity. During adolescence he begins to consolidate his image of himself, and in adulthood he develops a realistic image of himself without unnecessary preoccupation with his body functions. The elderly person may tend to retreat toward the interior of the body structure, becoming once again preoccupied with body functions and losing some of the distinctness of the body boundary.[18]

It is helpful for the nurse to understand these concepts in order to plan individualized care. The person experiencing a body image change will be coping not only with the alteration itself but also with the demands of that particular stage. In addition, knowledge of the person's developmental stage at the time of a previous change in body image can give insight into his subsequent development and present day responses.

BODY IMAGE DISTURBANCE

Kolb describes five broad classifications of human condition that may lead to body image disturbance.[17] The first group is that of neurologic disorders affecting any part of the sensory or motor system. Stroke and spinal cord injuries are examples of this type of disturbance. Depersonalization or dissociation from the affected part is a common symptom of body image disturbance in persons with neurologic disorders. There are numerous reports of a stroke patient complaining that there is a strange body in his bed, when in fact it is his own affected limb.[13,16] Patients with neurologic problems like spinal cord injuries must adjust to loss of function in several body parts, resulting in loss of mobility, bowel and bladder control, and sexual function. Neurologic disorders have a primary impact at the behavioral level of bodily experience, although the other levels also may be affected.

The second group includes acquired or induced metabolic disorders that result in changes in body structure. Diabetes mellitus is an example of this. The person with diabetes may experience little or no outward change depending on the severity of the illness. However, injection of insulin may represent an invasion of the person's body boundary. The possibility of long-term complications such as vascular changes leading to lower extremity amputations, presents a significant threat to one's body image. With diabetes the innermost level of bodily experience is primarily affected, although other levels may be more severely affected as additional changes occur. Obesity also may be classified in this grouping and serves as an example of the importance of the cultural context in determining the nature of the body image change. In our present middle-class culture, obesity usually has negative connotations. However, some cultural groups equate obesity with signs of prosperity, beauty, and health. Disparity occurs when the two cultural viewpoints meet. It is not uncommon to hear an elderly woman bemoan the loss of her fine full figure and weight of 200 lbs while the young health provider praises her for her weight loss and trim figure. Although this type of disparity poses problems for communication, the real threat to body image comes from disparities between a person's perception of self and his perception of the ideal state encouraged by his immediate social and cultural environment. The critical role of perceptions is demonstrated forcefully by considering anorexia nervosa, in which it is clearly the person's perceived, rather than actual, body state that fails to match the perceived ideal. In this and other areas, unbalanced perceptions may create problems, even where they have little basis in reality.

A third group consists of somatic disorders leading to progressive deformity either early or late in life. Examples include cancer and rheumatoid arthritis. The cancer patient who has a progressive disease will become thinner, weaker, and have changes in skin color and texture throughout the course of the illness. The physical changes that occur may have many connotations to the patient and his family. They may represent loss of attractiveness and youth, causing the person to isolate himself from others, fearing their reaction. The changes may also represent the ravages of disease and death, causing grief and mourning. The person with rheumatoid arthritis experiences the progressive physical changes caused by contractures and other deformities, as well as decreased mobility. The person may equate these changes with old age and an inability to meet the expected task of guiding future generations, as in Erikson's generativity stage. This belief may lead in turn to self-pity; the person may stagnate, denying himself the opportunity to share and feel productive.[18]

The category most commonly associated with body image disturbances is that of acute dismemberment. Dismemberment can be the result of trauma or surgical procedure and can be a planned or emergency event. With the increased sophistication of trauma and burn care, the survival rate for people who suffer such injuries has increased. Specific details of the dismemberment will affect the person's response. The phantom phenomenon, or experiencing the lost body part though it is no longer present, is a normal adaptive response to acute dismemberment. (This phenomenon will be discussed in greater detail in the section on adaptation to body image change.)

The final group consists of disorders of personality development. This includes psychoneuroses, psychoses, and psychopathic states. Loss of body image boundaries and an inability to delineate clearly between one's self and the outside world is commonly seen in schizophrenic patients.[10,23] People demonstrating body image disturbances related to personality disorders usually require management by mental health specialists. The following discussion will focus primarily on people whose body image problems are related to the first four groupings presented.

FACTORS INFLUENCING THE PERSON'S RESPONSE TO BODY IMAGE CHANGES

How a person responds to a change in his body image is a function of many factors. In general, the intactness of the body image at the time of the alteration will have a significant role in the effectiveness of the person's adaptation and the eventual outcome.[16] People whose body image is well-defined before the change seem to cope better than those whose body image is still in the formative stages. Body image impairment is felt to be most traumatic during the adolescent period, when there is normally much concern about physical appearance and when the response of the peer group to the person is most influential. In general, adults in the later years have more stable self-images and are thought to cope better with such changes.

According to Brown, the patient's response to alterations in body image is greatly influenced by the following factors:

- The functional significance of the body part(s)
- The importance of physical appearance and pride to the person
- The visibility of the part involved
- The feasibility and availability of rehabilitation
- The speed with which the change occurred
- Previous coping patterns and their effectiveness.

These factors also apply to the family's response to a person's change in body image.[5]

The functional significance of specific body parts refers to both the physical and symbolic importance of the altered part to the person's sense of self and his interactions with others. Specific body parts may be highly invested with emotional significance, totally unrelated to actual physical function.

This may be apparent in situations in which the person's distress seems out of proportion to the body state change.

The cultural dimension of the significance of body parts is illustrated by a survey of the opinions of healthy Americans about their satisfaction with specific parts of their bodies. This showed that a person's satisfaction with his face was highly correlated with a positive sense of self-esteem.[3] This was true of men and women. For men, the body part that had the second most important image of self-esteem was the chest. For women, the second most important factor was the midtorso area, which the researchers interpreted as indicative of a concern about weight. Given this data, Americans experiencing facial disfigurement may be at higher risk for difficulties than would limb amputees. However, individual differences must always be considered.

Reaction to a distortion of the body image is also related to how much of the person's identity is invested in the involved part.[16] A surgeon may react more severely to loss of sensation in his fingers than to a comparable loss in his toes. A dancer, on the other hand, may have the reverse reaction.

The importance of physical appearance and pride is another significant factor in the person's adjustment to physical change.[5,16] Our culture places a great deal of emphasis on health, youth, and good looks. We are reared to take pride in the attractive aspects of physical appearance and to camouflage or hide the others. Nevertheless, there is variation in the amount of pride people place in their physical appearance. Some choose to focus pride on their intellectual abilities, their talents, or their careers; others may place their pride in their children. These attitudes, like most others, are influenced strongly by the person's view of himself, and values of family, significant others, and society as a whole. Such societal attitudes are not necessarily immune to change, as witnessed by increasing acceptance of the rights of the handicapped in this country. However, from the point of view of an individual, the cultural context may appear to show little or no flexibility.

The degree of visibility of the part involved also will influence the person's response to a body alteration. Obesity or facial deformities are examples of conditions that are difficult to hide. Colostomies, on the other hand, are generally visible only to the person and his intimate relations. However, there is always the risk of exposure if there is leakage or odor. Some feel that people with more obvious conditions respond better than those whose body image change is less obvious.[2] Even though those with more severe or obvious defects have to deal with the reactions of others and their own feelings, they may be forced to have more realistic expectations and therefore may respond more positively to surgery and rehabilitation. People with less visible deformities may place much energy in concealment of the alteration. This may in turn lead to anxiety and stress.

The feasibility and availability of rehabilitation is another influence on the person's response to body state change. New rehabilitative techniques and reconstructive procedures are continuously being developed. Mastectomy patients may now undergo reconstructive surgery to repair the deformity. However, the availability of reconstructive surgery is limited by the resources of a particular area. The type of body alteration experienced will also affect rehabilitation potential. Highly sophisticated limb prostheses have been developed to aid the amputee in his adjustment. Corrective surgery for severe burns, however, has sophisticated techniques but is less able to produce cosmetically satisfactory results. The person may not have the financial resources or geographical access to the most updated rehabilitative services. Awareness of this limitation may lead to frustration and despair.

The speed with which the change has occurred also influences the patient's response to a change in body state. In general, there is a lag between the occurrence of the body alteration, the person's awareness of the extent of the change, and his revision of his body image.[10] People undergoing progressive body changes often have time to acknowledge gradually the losses that are occurring and begin to work through the grieving process.

On the other hand, persons undergoing a sudden change of body image may have a traumatic response to the alteration. Acceptance of the change may be more difficult to achieve, and the manifestations of the grieving process may be more extreme. The phantom phenomenon is one example of a normal psychophysiological mechanism for helping the person cope with this change. Denial, anger, and depression are other normal behaviors.

Finally, the person's coping patterns and their effectiveness exert an important influence on the response to body state change. Coping patterns are the person's characteristic ways of protecting his self-esteem and reducing tension and anxiety.[8] They are problem-solving methods that the person has developed over time and that are effective in maintaining emotional stability. Coping patterns are highly individualized and are influenced by family, environment, culture, and level of maturity, as well as specific personality traits.[8,11] All people use coping or defense mechanisms, regardless of their level of adjustment. What form these mechanisms take depends on the person's situation and his social skill development. The healthy person uses many techniques to cope with anxiety whereas the emotionally troubled person uses only a few.[8,16] The importance of the past effectiveness of particular coping strategies is that this influences a person's tendency to rely on the same, or related, strategies in the future.

Common defense mechanisms used by people with a physical disability or body image change, defined by Freud, include: withdrawal, depression, denial and repression, projection, displacement, and rationalization.[8] Other commonly used coping strategies include: seeking information, turning to others for support, following orders, having faith in professionals, finding meaning for the disease and making the most of life, preparing for death, returning to employment, and a variety of tension-reducing strategies such as smoking, drinking, overeating, focusing on physical symptoms, or blaming oneself, someone, or something else.[11]

ADAPTATION TO BODY IMAGE CHANGE

Adaptive responses to body image change may take many forms. In addition to the coping behaviors discussed above, certain behaviors are commonly seen in persons adjusting to such a change. These include an experience of the phantom phenomenon, and an initial period of crisis followed by the normal grieving process.

The Phantom Phenomenon

The phantom phenomenon is an indication of normal adjustment to the sudden loss of a body part. It occurs in 98% of patients with limb amputations, and in 20% of patients having a mastectomy.[16,17] It has also been noted in cases involving traumatic or surgical loss of the nose, eyes, teeth, penis, nip-

ples, fingers, and toes. Both psychological and neurophysiological factors combine to produce the phenomenon.[17] In some cases the perception that the body part is still present and functional may be so vivid that the patient forgets the loss and attempts to use the missing part. The psychoanalytical interpretation of this phenomenon is that denial of the loss is the primary motivation for the behavior.[16] The sudden loss of the part is too rapid to accept. However, neurophysiological factors also play an important role in this response. Severed nerves have been shown to extend sensations to the point of amputation. Studies cited by Kolb show that the amputee is most aware of the distal portions of the phantom. Immediately following amputation, the person perceives the phantom as consisting of the entire extremity, but this perception gradually diminishes and resolves over time. The person may experience many different types of sensations. Most are annoying rather than agonizing and occur on an intermittent basis. The phantom sensation in a limb may be elicited by stimuli such as touch, changes in the weather, or emotionally disturbing incidents.[17]

The ability to experience the phantom phenomenon has been related in part to early sensory experience, to the mobility of the lost body part in relation to its place in space, and to its role in providing cues for establishing body position.[16] Children with congenital defects resulting in a missing body part or who experience amputations in infancy and early childhood (before 2 years of age) do not experience the phantom phenomenon. It is thought that due to a lack of early sensory experience, the part was not incorporated into the body image and therefore adjustment to the loss in the form of a phantom is not required.[24] Failure to report or experience a phantom phenomenon after the loss of a body part may occur following loss of internal organs, after gradual losses such as in leprosy, or may be because of psychological denial.[17] Phantoms of facial parts, breast, and genitalia are noted less frequently than those of the limbs but do occur. A facial phantom may present as a sensation of scratching or itching of the eye or nose, blinking of the eye, or a desire to palpate the nose. Breast phantom sensations may involve the whole breast, a portion of it, or just the nipple. Patients indicate sensations of itching, scratching, and heaviness such as being full of milk.[17] These perceptions are less vivid than those of the limbs and may occur more often with weather changes and menstruation. The phantom breast phenomenon occurs more frequently in younger women but does not appear to be related to the patient's attitude toward her breast, breast size, or concern over the loss.[16,17]

The phantom phenomenon commonly disappears after 2 years, although it has been reported to persist anywhere from a few months to 20 years. Only gradually does the new pattern of body sensations become assimilated into the body image.[17]

The presence of the phantom is an expected, healthy response to the amputation of a limb or body part occurring after early childhood. Lack of the phantom experience, particularly in a patient with a limb amputation, is a cause for concern. It may be an indication of massive denial of the loss, which in turn could prevent the person from adjusting to the situation.[16,17]

The Grieving Process

Grieving for the lost body part is also an adaptive response to a major body state change. *Grief* has been defined as "a complex combination of numerous emotions felt at the time of loss...These include anxiety, indifference, guilt, hope, hopelessness, helplessness, despair, ambivalence, anger."[6] The

grieving process has been described by Reed as the inner process of working through, managing, growing through, acknowledging, and making peace with a major loss or bereavement.[6] Most of the research on grieving has looked at adjustment to the death of a loved one. The grieving process for the person mourning a lost body part, feature, or capability is similar, yet it has its own unique qualities. Werner–Beland states that the loss experienced when a loved one dies is separate from one's self. One can learn eventually to live without another person. However, loss of one's own functioning is an ever-present reminder of what once existed. Although feelings diminish over time, events occur that remind the person of his loss. Grief returns each time the illness or disability becomes apparent or when it interferes with a hoped-for achievement.[25] Grieving behaviors have been described in terms of phases or stages. It is important to note that these are not necessarily sequential. Individuals and families will not necessarily experience each phase of the process, nor will they necessarily follow any prescribed order.[6] The phases describe adaptive reactions to loss and are helpful to the understanding of specific behaviors at specific times. They are not predictive of upcoming behaviors. Understanding of the person's response is essential in developing appropriate interventions. The person in the shock or denial phase may not be receptive to, or even capable of, understanding teaching about his prosthesis. However, in the acceptance phase, detailed instruction has great potential effectiveness.

Carlson presents an excellent summary of the major descriptions of the behavioral stages or phases that arise in response to life-threatening or life-changing events.[6] These include: Kübler–Ross' stages following diagnosis of a terminal illness (denial, anger, bargaining, depression, and acceptance); Fink's stages following a crisis (shock, defensive retreat, acknowledgment, and adaptation); Engle's stages in adaptation to a major loss (shock and disbelief, developing awareness, restitution, and resolution of loss); and Bowlby's identification of protest, despair, and denial. There is considerable overlap in these various descriptions, and Carlson has highlighted the similarities in her discussion of grief, grouping them into the precrisis, impact, retreat, acknowledgment, and acceptance phases.

The precrisis phase will occur if there is sufficient warning. This may be precipitated by an event such as a breast biopsy or a diagnosis of a progressively debilitating disease. The patient and family have a glimpse of possible future losses and may begin to prepare to cope with these changes.

In the impact phase, the person may be in a state of shock. "The reality of any catastrophic loss is generally too overwhelming for the individual to perceive accurately and integrate fully...the full reality of what has happened does not penetrate consciousness."[6] Initially, the patient and family may act euphoric or totally indifferent. Persons at this phase may require guidance and direction in terms of what needs to be done.

When awareness of the extent of the loss comes, severe anxiety generally occurs. This may reach panic proportions. Feelings of helplessness and devastation are not unusual.[6] Sensations of somatic distress, weakness, and despair are common. The person may experience a fight-or-flight type of reaction.[19] They may scream, attack, mourn, sigh, or cry. Attention to personal appearance may be lost, and there may be a pining for lost function.[6]

During the retreat phase, denial becomes the most common defense mechanism employed. The initial awareness of the significance of the loss may be so intolerable that avoidance mechanisms may become essential to maintain functioning.[6] Denial allows relief from the reality of the situation. Dreams, illusions, or hallucinations help maintain the impression that the loved one or lost object is still near.[17] Other methods of avoiding the pain of realization include involvement in many activities to avoid thinking about the loss and avoidance of people or activities that remind one of the loss. During the retreat phase the person may avoid discussion of the problem. He may refuse to look at the wound areas and may refuse treatment because he expects complete recovery. When his distorted perception of the situation is challenged, he may experience anxiety and anger. The length of time spent in this phase will vary according to type of loss, personality, and situational factors. Loss of a limb may be difficult to deny when its absence is so apparent. However, with injuries such as spinal cord damage or stroke, where the extent of permanent damage is unknown, persisting denial may continue for much longer periods.[22]

Defense mechanisms like denial are important in that they allow the person to regulate the amount of potentially disabling information that must be processed at one time. Over time the person allows more and more information to be assimilated, until he is able to acknowledge the loss.[6,20]

During the acknowledgment phase the person confronts the daily reminders of his loss. The person may experience an often "obsessional" review of events leading up the loss. This review may be conducted alone or with others and appears necessary for both emotional and cognitive integration of the loss event. This is a period of many emotions. The individual and his family may feel guilt or self-reproach at not being able to do something to prevent the event. They (the family and patient) may feel angry and blame others for what has happened. The anger may be turned inward, resulting in depression. There may be feelings of intense sadness. The person may vacillate between feelings of anger, depression, and bitterness. If suicide is contemplated it is most likely to occur during this period. Bargaining may occur; this may be with God or with others.[20]

Later in this period, the person may start to take an interest in his care. However, he may not be able to cope with future-oriented teaching. Managing the day-to-day realities may be all the individual and his family can deal with. This phase may last longer than the others, not uncommonly for several months. Gradually the person moves from predominant feelings of helplessness and hopelessness to feelings of hope. The focus begins to turn from what has been lost to what may be achieved.[25]

It is impossible to predict when this occurs or why. Patients indicate their readiness through verbal and nonverbal means. The patient's asking questions about his progress and seeking involvement in his care are indications of this transition. The ability to look at the scar or wound is another sign of progress.[22] Reconciliation of the past with the present is necessary for grief resolution. The person who belittles every achievement and refuses to let his old self die tends to remain unrehabilitated.[25]

During the final stage of acceptance and adaptation, the person organizes his life to integrate the realities of his loss. He may develop new meaningful goals or seek new methods to achieve goals that were important prior to his loss.[6] Healthy adaptation to the change can be measured by the patient's willingness to discuss the alteration in body image and his acceptance of help in the form of reconstructive and rehabilitative counseling and services.[17] The person is then ready to begin the adjustments that will allow him to return to a normal, if somewhat modified, life.

The family and significant others must work through the phases of grieving as well. While the patient is grieving his loss and trying to understand its implications for his life roles, the family also experiences the loss in terms of their entire system of role relationships.[25] Family members may become so involved in their own grief that they are unaware of or oblivious to the patient's experiences. Also, family members may pass more quickly through the grieving process and have difficulty understanding the patient's slower progress. The family may require support and encouragement from health professionals to understand the grief process and to maintain open communication with the patient and each other.

MALADAPTIVE RESPONSES TO BODY IMAGE CHANGE

Not all people are able to confront and accept a change in body image and the limitations that may accompany it. Exaggeration of normal defense mechanisms and generalization of the disability are common. These include massive denial, pervasive anxiety, severe depression, rebelliousness, and pervasive anger.[7,17]

Massive denial occurs when the denial mechanism, which allows for gradual acknowledgment and acceptance of the changes imposed by the disease or disfigurement, is exaggerated. This can be seen as a wish fulfilling mechanism to maintain the preexisting body image.[17] Extreme denial can result in: a failure to report the phantom phenomenon after a limb amputation; noncompliance with treatment regimens; nonparticipation in treatment planning; refusal of rehabilitation or assistive devices; and an unwillingness to modify living arrangements.[7] People experiencing extreme denial are unable to accept permanent disability or any change in previous patterns.

Pervasive free-floating anxiety also may occur. This is described as a feeling of dread that the person cannot assign to a specific cause. Somatic manifestations (e.g., irritability, hypersensitivity to light and sound, cardiac palpitations) may result. Coping mechanisms are weakened or ineffectual. Demanding behavior may be excessive and hysterical. The patient may become overly dependent on health providers and family.[7]

Severe depression is another maladaptive response. Depression is not an uncommon response to body image impairment. However, in severe depression there may be total apathy and social withdrawal from family, friends, and caregivers. Expressions of helplessness, hopelessness, and worthlessness are common. Kolb states that these reactions represent not only mourning for loss of the part but are also related to overexpectation of rejection and fear of separation from those upon whom the patient is dependent.[17] Repression of hostile feelings towards significant others may also be a part of this reaction. The depression may extend to all aspects of the person's life including his identity, roles, and relationships. He may become totally involved in his symptoms and exaggerate the severity of minor problems.[7]

Rebelliousness may result from the person's attempts to cope with the dependence–independence struggle precipitated by physical limitations. The feelings of lack of control and dependence on others may be so frightening or distasteful that the person will act to dispel them regardless of the consequences. Acting out behavior, refusal to accept medications, treatments, or to participate in planning care may occur not out of anger or denial but as an exaggerated expression of independence, derived from a need to resist dependency.[7,25]

Pervasive anger also may occur. This may be exhibited in diffuse and indiscriminately displaced anger, acting out toward objects and people, and physical and verbal abuse of family members or caregivers. Communication may become bitter and hostile. The patient may refuse to comply with treatment regimens or rehabilitative plans.

Some people may generalize the disability. Here the patient limits activities in such a way that he does not even attempt those that are possible. Invalidism becomes a way of seeking secondary gains from the chronic disease or disability.[7]

Psychotic reactions also may occur in response to body image impairment due to acute trauma or prolonged somatic disorders. Researchers have described psychotic reactions in patients suffering from acromegaly, Paget's disease, osteogenesis imperfecta, and dwarfism.[17]

People who develop maladaptive responses to their body image alteration generally will require referral to a mental health nurse or other specialist. Early identification of adjustment difficulties and referral can result in more rapid and effective treatment.[6]

NURSING ASSESSMENT

There are many means of obtaining the information necessary for an assessment of the person undergoing a change in body image. The assessment process is ongoing and will not be completed during one visit or interview. The nurse should make use of personal observations as well as standardized assessment formats (e.g., the health history). Patient encounters provide opportunities for observing the patient's verbal and nonverbal responses to his situation and the environment. The nurse's day-to-day interactions with the patient allow her to view and participate in the patient's adjustment process. Observation of the patient's interactions with family, significant others, and others in his environment, be they other patients, neighbors, or strangers, also provides insight into the patient's response to his illness. Home visits help the nurse assess the patient's environment and observe his adjustment in his own territory. Discussions with the patient and family help the nurse clarify some of these observations and ultimately include the patient and family in the management process. Questionnaires and care-plan formats have been devised by several authors to help the nurse organize the assessment and plan.[1,12] These tools tend to be oriented to specific disease entities or disabilities and can be a useful adjunct to the nurse's armamentarium (see sample assessment guide).

Although a complete assessment is ideal, it is not always possible. The nurse must be flexible in determining what information is essential at a given time and place. A patient and family who are in the midst of a severe crisis period may not be willing or able to give information about their attitudes toward the body image change. The primary information needed by the intensive care unit (ICU) nursing staff will have a different emphasis from that of the staff of the rehabilitation unit. Much of the information needed will be gathered over time while the patient, family, and health care providers develop a supportive and trusting relationship.

The assessment format for the person undergoing body image change includes information concerning the patient's identified concerns, his health history, and specific areas that have been identified unique to patient's undergoing a body image change.[5] These areas include the point in the life span when the disease or change occurred, the body levels affected by the alteration, the in-

teraction of the alteration with environmental variables, the patient and family's stage in the grieving process, the capability of the family to provide support and to accept the body image change, and the six specific factors that influence the patient's adaptation to the change.

THE PATIENT'S IDENTIFIED PROBLEM

Determine the patient's perception of the situation. The patient may have specific concerns that may appear nonrelated to the "obvious" problem. If the patient's concerns are not addressed, he may be unable or unwilling to accept the health provider's input or become involved in the management plan. Questions aimed at identifying the patient's concerns will vary according to each situation. Some general questions may be:

What concerns you most about the way you look?
How can we help you with this concern?
What do you think can be done? What would you like done?
What does this (change, procedure, loss) mean to you?

PAST PERSONAL HISTORY

General information about the patient's health history is necessary. This includes basic demographic data such as age, sex, race, marital status, employment, educational and economic status, information about past and present health, and psychosocial status. Much of this information already may be in the patient's chart. In addition, information about the patient's usual patterns of adaptation, daily activities, and view of himself will provide insights into his response to the body image change. Possible questions include:

Assessment Guide for the Individual with Plegia

Name _____   Location and type of injury/illness _____

Age _____   Occupation _____

ASSESSMENT FACTOR   **DATA**

1. What is the meaning of this illness/disability to this individual?
2. What was this individual's personality before the onset of this illness/disability?
3. Will this individual be able to return to his/her previous employment?
4. What is this individual's prognosis?
5. How dependent is this individual upon health care practitioners and significant others in meeting the activities of daily living (ADL's)?
6. How dependent is this individual upon the environment in meeting his/her needs?
7. Who are this individual's significant others?
8. How does this individual interact with his/her significant others?
9. Does the individual attempt to take an active role in meeting ADL's?
10. How much attention does this individual pay to personal appearance?
11. How much bowel and bladder control does this individual have?
12. Is this individual experiencing denial? depression? anger?
13. How much exhibitionism is the individual exposed to in meeting ADL's?
14. How much sexual functioning will this individual have?
15. Does this individual attempt to move his/her affected extremity(ies) with unaffected extremity(ies) independently?
16. Does this individual talk about his/her affected extremity(ies)?
17. Does this individual look at his/her affected extremity(ies)?
18. What does this individual say about the position of his/her affected extremity(ies) in space?
19. What does this individual say about his/her posture when sitting? lying?
20. What does this individual say about (abnormal) movements of his/her affected extremity(ies)?
21. What does this individual say about the size of his/her affected extremity(ies)?
22. What does this individual say about feelings/sensations in his/her extremity(ies)?
23. Is this individual able to judge the distance between his/her affected extremity(ies) and the environment? other unaffected parts of his/her body?

(From Beeken JE: Body Image Changes in Plegia. J Neurosurg Nurs, 10, No. 1:22, 1978)

How does he describe himself?

What is his typical day like?

How does he feel about himself and about the way he looks?

What does he like best about himself and about his looks?

What does he like the least?

What makes him feel good?

What is important to him?

Does he identify himself as disabled or limited in any way?

HISTORY OF BODY IMAGE ALTERATION

The following discussion is based on Brown's Nursing Model, presented earlier in this chapter. (See Fig. 4-1 and text pertaining to it.)

The Point in the Life Span at Which the Alteration Occurred

The impact of the alteration on the person will be influenced by the developmental tasks he is dealing with at the time of the change and at present. Knowledge of developmental status provides insights into the types of support that may be effective. Questions helpful to assess developmental status include:

How does the patient see himself as a person?

What are his life goals?

What specific developmental issues, such as sexual identity, peer, family, significant other relationships, and career goals is he dealing with?

Is he in the process of building a career?

Is he preparing for retirement?

How does he think the body image change will affect his present and future life situations?

The Level of Bodily Experience Affected by the Body State Change and by the Therapeutic Measures Employed

Consideration of the specific levels affected will emphasize the complexity of changes occurring and clarify the impact that the body state change may have on the person. At the innermost level, many of the changes may have a highly generalized physical manifestation (e.g., certain responses to medications or hormonal imbalances). These types of changes can be frightening simply because they may be very difficult for a patient to understand.[16] Changes at the behavioral level are more minimally apparent, as with muscle twitching or flaccidity, and yet their cause may be obscure to many patients. Topological changes, arising from the body surface, are the most obvious cause of body image disturbance. To assess the level(s) of bodily experiences affected, the nurse must have information concerning the nature of the body image alteration and any treatments or medications being used. Discussion with the patient about how he is experiencing the body image change will be helpful. Questions concerning the patient's perceptions of the change, what it feels like, any side-effects of medication, and any feelings about medications or treatments will also be of assistance.

The Interaction of the Body Image Change with Other Variables

Changes in the body state may affect the person's relationship with parents, significant others, peers, cultural group, society, and the physical environment. People may have strong ties to particular religious, cultural, and ethnic groups that influence their responses to health and illness and that may or may not be apparent from their appearance or surname. Questions concerning family, peer, and cultural relationships may include:

How does he describe his family?
What is the home like?
To whom is he closest?
Does he feel he belongs to any particular cultural group?
Are there any particular cultural beliefs he has about health and illness?
How does he feel the body state change will affect or has affected his relationships with parents, significant others, friends, and others?
How does he think others will react to him?
What does he worry about most?
How would he like others to react to him?
Does he know anyone else who has experienced a similar body state change? How did he react? How did his friends react?
How has this change altered his home environment, his relationships with family?

How detailed the assessment will be in each area depends on the importance placed on it and the patient's reaction to his body image change.

The Patient's and Family's Stage in the Grieving Process

Individuals and their families will experience a variety of expected behaviors in response to mourning over the body state change. Often they may be experiencing conflicting emotions that will influence their responses to each other and to interventions.

Identify the presence of responses such as denial, shock, hopelessness, helplessness, anger, bargaining, depression, acknowledgment, or acceptance of the altered body state. Questions helpful for assessing the patient's grieving process include:[7]

What was the patient's emotional response to information about the diagnosis and long-term implications?
Has he verbalized sad feelings about the situation?
Has he been able to cry in response to discussion of the losses and changes imposed by the disease process or disability?
Has he been able to discuss the meanings of the body image change to his life?
Has he been able to discuss what his life was like before the present situation, particularly in relation to those aspects that will be or have been drastically changed by the chronic disease or disability?
How does he handle the depression, anxiety, anger, and frustrations related to the losses?
Does he have an accurate perception of the situation and still retain either expectations or hope?
What efforts does the patient make to remain maximally functional and active?
How is he making decisions regarding the choice and timing of treatment?

Evaluate culturally prescribed responses toward grieving as well. Cultural norms may dictate the behaviors expressed and how the process is carried out.

The Availability and Capability of Family and Significant Others to Provide Support and Accept the Body Change

The influence of the family on the patient's rehabilitation has been documented repeatedly.[2,5,16,17] The family's ability to enhance the patient's adjustment depends on the other family members and the family's functioning as a whole. Determine whom the patient defines as "family" or "significant others." It is not uncommon for those persons most significant to the patient to be other than identified family members. Family and significant others play a significant role in helping the patient recapture his self-esteem and in maximizing positive input to minimize the enormity of the body assault.[16] Questions may include:

Whom does he find most supportive when he has problems?
Does he have any close friends or family?
How would he describe his family?
To whom does he feel closest?
Is the patient able to share his feelings with other family members? If so, with whom? If not, why not?

To assess the family system, determine the following:[7]

The patient's role in the family
The family's usual way of responding to the patient
The family's tolerance of expressions of both positive and painful feelings
The family's willingness and ability to act as a support for the patient and for each other
The family environment, personal resources, and ability to provide home care
The degree to which the patient and his partner can discuss and work through change in sexual functioning caused by the body state change
The family decision-making process.

Family members or significant others are not always able to cope with the changes resulting from the person's illness or disfigurement. Providing support or referral for family members and significant others will be a major goal in management of the patient's care. Therefore, understanding of their needs is essential for a thorough assessment of the patient with a body image impairment.

Factors Influential in the Patient's Adaptation to the Change

Much of the data necessary to assess the six factors identified by Brown as influential to adaptation may be obtained in questions presented in preceding sections.[5] However, there are instances in which it is helpful to focus on particular factors. The following section addresses these specific factors and proposes more detailed questions which can be used in their assessment.

- *Functional significance of the part involved*

  Determine what significance the patient places on the part. What does this impairment mean to the patient? Does it affect his self-identify? Is it necessary for the type of employment in which he is involved? Does it interfere with his recreational interests? Does it have an impact on his sexuality? How does his culture evaluate this type of impairment? How does it affect his marital relationship, peer relationships? How does society view this type of impairment? What importance does the patient place on the opinions of others? Whose opinions are important? Does the impairment interfere with his ability to communicate with others? Is this important to him?

  The patient's perception of the significance of the change and its impact on his life is a major concern. Whether this concurs with the reality of the situation is a secondary matter.

- *Importance of physical appearance to the person*

  Physical attractiveness is culturally defined, as is the importance placed on physical appearance. The person's value system is formed to a large extent by those around him: parents, peers, culture, and society.

  Determine the patient's and family's attitudes about physical attractiveness. What meaning does the physical change have for him? How important are good looks to his sense of self: What role did or do they play in his interactions with others, family, friends, employers, or clients? Is his livelihood based on appearance? Are his recreational activities based on appearance? Does physical appearance hold any cultural or religious significance to him? For example, whereas the prevailing middle-class American attitude places a high value on good looks, religious groups such as the Hutterites feel that physical beauty distracts from more valuable aspects of human life.[5]

- *Visibility of the part involved*

  Possible areas to explore include the following: How visible does the patient feel the alteration is? How comfortable is he with it? Has it affected his interactions with others? How have others reacted to it? Does he invest a great deal of energy in trying to hide the deformity? Does he spend much time worrying about other's reactions to it? What does he fear most about others' reactions to the body state change? How has he tried to cope with it? How does he react to others' reactions? How do his family, significant others, peers, and work acquaintances react to the body image change or distortion? How do these reactions make him feel?

- *The feasibility and availability of rehabilitation*

  The patient may have a more positive outlook if he is aware that rehabilitation is available. Evaluate the patient's level of understanding of rehabilitative services. It is also necessary to be aware of his expectations. What results does he expect from the treatment, therapy, or surgery? How does he think he will feel about his body after the attempted rehabilitation?[14] Evaluate the patient's resources and the services available. The patient who has neither funds nor access to rehabilitation services may feel great frustration and hopelessness over his situation.

- *The speed with which the change occurred*

  A patient who has experienced a relatively rapid or traumatic change in body state may perceive himself as being in a different situation from a person who has experienced a more prolonged deterioration of body state. Neither condition is necessarily easier for patients to adapt to, but a patient may perceive the difference as significant. Data in this area may be obtained from the chart, from observations of the patient, or from the patient's description of how the change occurred.

- *Past and present coping patterns*

  In times of crisis people will first attempt to use those coping patterns or defense mechanisms that they have used in the past.[8] Understanding the person's response to past stresses or similar situations (e.g., previous surgery) will give some clues as to how the person may respond initially to this particular stressful event. This awareness may also explain responses that may otherwise seem inappropriate or bizarre. Ask the patient or family members how the patient usually responds to everyday stresses, to crises or previous surgical procedures. Also ask how successful these responses have been in resolution of previous crises. The patient may have particular supportive techniques or support systems that he has found helpful. These may not necessarily be healthful or advisable but to be aware of them is important. Identify strengths, such as a sense of humor or an ability to work with others. Possible questions to assess coping ability include: Has anything like this ever happened to him before? How has he handled other stresses in his life? What stresses cause body responses? What parts of his body are affected when stressed? How does he usually deal with tension and anxiety (e.g., exercise, verbalization, smoking, consumption of alcohol, or drugs)? What methods usually work? Who is able to help him when he is under a great deal of stress?

NURSING DIAGNOSIS

The nursing diagnosis for the patient with a body image impairment will vary depending on the patient and his particular situation. Four general areas are important to consider in the development of the nursing diagnosis.

DETERMINE THE PRESENCE OF A BODY IMAGE CHANGE OR DISTURBANCE

One's body image is based on many factors. The person's perception of the completeness or intactness of his body image is the prime identifier of body image disturbance. Either the person's own sense of body image disturbance or his exhibition of behaviors that indicate disturbance may form the basis for the diagnosis.

DETERMINE ADAPTATION TO BODY IMAGE CHANGE

When there is a change in body state, all behavior is directed at helping the person cope with this change. To develop an effective management plan, the nurse must determine whether the patient's response is adaptive or maladaptive. *Adaptive behaviors* will help the patient work through the grieving process, ideally reaching a point of acceptance of a change in body state and integration of this change in the formation of a new body

image. These behaviors primarily require supportive counseling, although in some instances referral is necessary. A *maladaptive response* will prevent the patient from reaching a state of equilibrium and acknowledgment of the body image change. Patients experiencing this type of response will most often require referral for further psychological intervention. Early identification of patients in need of referral will assist the rehabilitation process greatly.

DETERMINE THE DISEASE-SPECIFIC FACTORS THAT AFFECT THE PERSON'S RESPONSE TO BODY IMAGE CHANGE

There are many causes of body image impairment. While all share some commonalities, each will place specific demands on the individual and his family. In developing a nursing diagnosis, these demands should be identified. The concerns experienced by the person with a colostomy and the skills that need to be learned for management of this disorder will be different from those required of the newly diagnosed diabetic patient.

DETERMINE THE FAMILY'S OR SIGNIFICANT OTHER'S LEVEL OF ADAPTATION

Much of the person's response and progress will be dependent on the adaptation and acceptance of those people whose opinions and support are important to him. To achieve optimal rehabilitation, the family's or significant other's level of adaptation must be identified and supported as well as that of the patient. Again, as with the patient's response, families may require supportive counseling or referral for more indepth therapy depending on their level of adaptation.

MANAGEMENT

The overall goal of the management process is acceptance of the changed body structure, with eventual establishment of a new body image and resumption of a fulfilling life-style.[16,17] This does not mean that the person prefers the new image to the old but that he has acknowledged the reality of the situation and is able to continue with the growth process. Interventions are primarily interactive in the sense that the nurse uses herself as a teacher, facilitator, helper, and source of support to the patient and family.[14]

The primary nursing modalities used include: supportive counseling in the form of active listening and interpretation of verbal and nonverbal cues; assisting the patient to use his own resources and encouraging problem-solving skills; patient and family teaching aimed at present and future needs; and direct nursing care specifically related to the type and extent of body image change and impairment.

Henker has divided interventions for persons undergoing body image changes into three phases: the preparation phase, the encounter phase, and the follow-up phase.[15]

THE PREPARATION PHASE

The preparation phase occurs in situations in which potential body image disturbance can be predicted, such as scheduled surgery or therapy that causes hair loss, weight gain, or other physical changes. Henker identifies two primary management goals for this phase: 1) establishment of a supportive and trusting relationship with the patient and family, and 2) preparation of the patient and family for the changes that are to occur.[15]

To develop a supportive relationship, one member of the health care team should be identified as the primary person with whom the patient and family relate, whereas other members provide additional support and reinforcement.[2,15] Selection of the primary person will depend on the specific situation and personalities involved. The family may informally choose the person they feel most comfortable with, or a primary nurse or physician may be assigned to the patient. It is important that someone assume this role to assure continuity and coordination of care.

The primary caregiver is often the most effective person to prepare the patient and family for the changes that are about to occur. Preparation involves both education and supportive counseling. The teaching plan should be based on assessment of the patient's level of comprehension, the type of procedure, and the patient's level of fear and anxiety. Verbal descriptions, specific literature, and visits from people who have recovered from the procedure may be useful. The patient and family should be informed of specific reactions that are expected to occur with the change, such as the phantom phenomenon. In conjunction with this, supportive counseling focuses on encouraging the patient to express his feelings, fears, and anxieties about the procedure. Reassurance, when appropriate, as to the normality of feelings may reduce anxiety. Family members also should be encouraged to share their feelings. Early development of open communication between the patient and family members and significant others should be facilitated, for family support is a key factor in the person's adjustment to the impairment.

THE ENCOUNTER PHASE

During the encounter phase, the person experiences the bodily change and adapts to it by working through the grief reaction. Patients dealing with loss may experience a variety of emotional responses. It is important to recognize that the patient's response is a form of coping, even though his method may appear to be inappropriate or inadequate. The defenses used by the patient help to soften the impact of the loss, so that feelings can be faced and worked through.[7]

Henker identifies the aims of intervention in the encounter phase as: helping the patient to understand his crisis; helping him express his present feelings; identifying the patient's coping mechanisms, encouraging those that are constructive; and reopening the social world to the person.[15] The patient's responses during this phase will vary according to his place in the grieving process. It is important to remember that these response patterns are descriptive for each stage but not necessarily predictive of preceding or subsequent behaviors. The patient may skip a stage or return to an earlier one; there are many individual differences in response. Therefore, nursing interventions need to be directed at the presenting behaviors exhibited by the patient or family member(s).[20]

Acceptance of and support for the patient's and family's feelings provide the foundation for the management process. Interventions focus on helping the person regain his sense of acceptance and self-esteem. In the earlier phases of the grieving process, when the patient and family are trying to cope with the reality of the situation, supportive counseling and direct care interventions predominate. However, as the person becomes able to acknowledge and accept the change that has occurred, patient teaching and anticipatory guidance assume greater importance. Interventions that help the patient to achieve or maintain control of his functions should be encouraged. However, these must be tailored to the patient's readiness to assume an active role in his care. In the earlier phases of the grieving process, the patient may need clear directions. Involvement may involve asking the patient to perform specific tasks. As the patient becomes better able to make decisions or assume control, his involvement can be encouraged by following patient suggestions about personal care routines or sequencing of care, and by allowing the patient to assume an active role in the management plan. More detailed interventions for patients undergoing disruptions in body image will be presented in terms of the common behaviors manifested in the different stages of the grieving process (discussed in the Mechanisms section).

Impact

Individuals in the impact or shock phase of the grieving process may need interventions that help to orient them to their situation. Reminders of where they are and what has happened are helpful. Simple and direct answers are required, because the patient and family may be too overwhelmed to cope with many details.[22] The patient may need guidance to carry out the most routine activities and therapies.[6] It may be necessary to enlist the aid of supportive friends or relatives or write simple directions for those involved.

Retreat

Persons in the retreat phase primarily exhibit denial, either verbally or through their behavior. Nursing interventions should allow the patient to deny his loss to the extent necessary without reinforcing the denial. Treatments should be explained in clear, concise terms. Teaching regarding future abilities may be ineffective at this time. The patient is denying long-term disability; therefore, long-term means for coping with disability have little meaning to him. Exploration of feelings, encouragement of verbalization, and emotional support may be the most effective approach.

When the patient verbally expresses his denial, confrontation is not necessary; however, acknowledgment of the feeling expressed will allow the patient to verbalize further and to explore his fears and anxieties. For example, a patient who denies the loss of his leg might be encouraged to discuss his feelings with the comment, "It must be hard for you to believe this has happened to you."

The patient may also use symbolism to seek reassurance or validation of his loss. In a casual discussion the patient may jokingly add, "At least I can get a job in a freak show." The nurse may choose to laugh at the humorous way in which this is said, but a more effective approach might be to help the patient verbalize his concern about being unacceptable, or a "freak," and then focus on the positive aspects of his changed body image.[22]

Anger may be expressed during this phase, as well as at other times. The anger may be justified or may be the projection of feelings of inadequacy onto others. Anger is a normal response to the grieving process, and the patient must learn to express his anger without fear of abandonment. If the criticisms are unjustified, it is best simply to listen and not take the remarks personally or become caught up in defending one's colleagues or oneself. A constructive approach would be to help the patient to dispel the anger by not becoming upset and by encouraging the patient to ventilate feelings and to become self-sufficient to the degree that the conditions and his motivation allow.[20]

Acknowledgment

During the acknowledgment phase the nurse has the opportunity to gather more information about the patient's needs. In this period the patient and family begin to express their feelings and fears. The patient experiences daily reminders of his loss. He begins to question who he is. He is experiencing strange bodily sensations, loss of feeling or contact, detachment, or depersonalization.[22] The patient may experience a variety of emotions. He also may become obsessed with a review of the events that led up to the change. He may become angry and blame others or feel guilt and self-reproach. Profound sadness and depression are common.[6] Because emotions may be changing frequently and abruptly, nursing interventions need to be flexible. As in the retreat phase, anger and blame may be aimed at the health providers. It is important to recognize this as normal, although difficult to deal with, behavior.[6,20] Allowing the patient to express his feelings without defensiveness may be the nurse's most effective approach. At this stage, advice is counterproductive.

The depressed patient will need help to feel better about himself. His self-esteem is regained gradually. Compliments and assistance often add further to the patient's sense of guilt and low self-worth. Allowing the patient to perform simple tasks for which he can feel achievement is a more effective way to raise self-esteem. He may have difficulty coping with complex ideas, planning, or decision-making. The nurse should encourage the patient to express his feelings and then communicate acceptance of them to him. Referral will be necessary if the depression persists and hinders further adjustment.[7] The nurse should be alert to potential suicidal behavior, such as withdrawal, loss of interest in everything, or verbal references to planning suicide or "giving up."

Patients who express suicidal thoughts or behaviors should be encouraged to discuss them, and therapeutic follow-up should be arranged. Direct questions about suicidal feelings are not harmful, and generally those

who have considered suicide will feel relieved to discuss it.[6] Reassurance that feelings of anger, depression, bitterness, guilt,
and shame are to be expected during this
phase is important. Both verbal and nonverbal support is required.

During the acknowledgment phase, the
patient will exhibit behaviors that demonstrate his adaptation and should be encouraged.[20] A patient may frequently review what
has happened. This is a common way of resolving feelings about the changes that have
occurred. The patient may ask questions repeatedly about what happened and what is
happening, what to anticipate in terms of his
healing, family relationships, work, and recreational activities. He may peek at the
changed area or feel it. He will watch others
to learn their feelings about the change. The
response of others will reinforce or negate
his sense of worth as a person.[14,20] The nurse
should respond to the change as a matter of
fact, and be positive in acceptance of it. The
person who is anxious to show others his
wound or scar is also looking for acceptance
and approval of the changed body part. Emphasize the patient's abilities while at the
same time allowing the patient to accept his
limitations. Involving the patient in his care
will help him regain a sense of control over
the situation. Family members also should be
included in the patient's care, particularly if
their help will be needed on the patient's
return home.[20]

Another means of encouraging realistic
acknowledgment of the patient's altered
body image is to arrange interactions with
other patients who have similar problems.
This could be in the form of one-to-one interactions or as group support sessions. The approach will depend on individual preference. Reentry into the social world should be
encouraged as soon as possible.

Depending on the type of change, the
patient may need to learn new communication skills. Anticipatory guidance may be
planned to help the patient deal with the responses of others, family and friends as well
as strangers. This may be accomplished by
encouraging the patient to discuss his fears
about others' reactions by role-playing encounters and the patient's reaction to them,
or by actually attempting interactions with
others. The patient may begin by visiting
other patients or by interacting with visitors
and family. However, it is essential to provide opportunities for the patient to discuss
his feelings about these encounters, what he
liked about them, what problems arose, and
how he dealt with them or could deal with
them at another time. Learning effective
communication skills is particularly important in the patient's interactions with family
and friends. Open communication and sharing of feelings should be supported and encouraged. If extreme difficulties arise or can
be anticipated, referral to a mental health
specialist should be considered.

Acceptance

During the acceptance or adaptation stage,
the patient begins to reorganize his life. He
develops new goals or new methods for
achieving prior goals. He views health providers in a positive light and seeks out ways
to improve himself and his situation. The patient and family are mobilizing their internal
and external resources and seek encouragement and reassurance.

During this phase, the patient becomes
most receptive to teaching. He needs detailed
instructions about his care and may follow
them literally. General instructions should
be avoided, since the patient and family may
not be able to translate abstract goals to specific details.[22,25] For instance, rather than tell-
ing the patient to increase his activities grad-

ually, provide specific recommendations. Nursing interventions may involve a variety of teaching modalities, such as provision of information, written materials, problem-solving techniques, and role-playing.[6] The approach will vary according to the individual situation. Reinforcement and encouragement is necessary, especially when the patient is learning new procedures.

Family supports are particularly important during this phase because most of the actual reconstruction occurs between the patient and his family.[22] The nurse should meet with the whole family to discuss patient education issues, concerns about patient progress, and patient and family adjustment. Individual meetings with key family members such as a spouse, parent, or grandparent are also effective ways to provide additional reinforcement for patient care.[2]

The patient and family may need to restructure their relationships depending on the extent and impact of the change. There may be role reversal between parent and child. Sexual difficulties may occur between the patient and his partner. Such difficulties will need to be addressed to facilitate the adjustment process. In many instances, problems may be alleviated by helping the patient and family members to share their concerns and problem-solve jointly. For example, a father may feel frustrated by the overprotectiveness of his family. However, through sharing his feelings with them, he may learn that they were only trying to show concern for him by their assistance. A compromise may then be worked out so that the patient has more responsibility and the family can be more constructive in their caring.

Sexual concerns are common between patients and their partners following a body image alteration. It is important to provide an opportunity for the patient to discuss his concerns and clarify any misconceptions that he or his partner may have. This is another situation in which open communication can alleviate or prevent problems. The nurse should treat the issue in a matter-of-fact manner, sensitive to the patient's values, attitudes, and preferences. It may be enough to inform the patient that sexual concerns are common for people experiencing a change in body structure or a specific illness, and that the nurse or a specific staff member will be available to discuss any questions or concerns that he or his partner may have. This lets the patient know that his concerns are normal and that there are resources available to him should he desire them. It is important for the nurse to feel comfortable discussing sexual issues if she is going to offer counseling. Otherwise, her discomfort will be communicated to the patient and will hinder open discussion. If the nurse is not secure in raising these issues, she should refer the patient to another provider. In some instances, patients and their partners may need or desire specific counseling by a sex therapist.

Family members may benefit from group meetings for relatives of persons undergoing body image alterations. Family support groups allow families to share and work through their feelings about loss, grief, and helplessness. They can share their struggles and successes in coping with the impaired person. In these groups, family members can express feelings of hostility toward the patient or toward those who make it difficult for the patient to adapt. In addition, group members can teach each other new ways of coping with the situation. They can make suggestions about ways to deal with school, work, and social groups. They may also be able to deal directly with confrontation or acting out among members. These groups may be hospital- or community-based. Both are extremely effective ways of helping families cope.[2]

THE FOLLOW-UP PHASE

Rehabilitation is a long-term process that requires evaluation and monitoring. Henker labels this third phase of intervention the follow-up phase.[15] The grieving process for the person with a chronic disability or deformity may never reach total resolution. It is modified over time but may recur with reminders of the loss.[25] Monitoring the adjustment process is important. Henker recommends occasional reinforcement sessions to help the person discuss his progress and express concerns that have developed.[15] Follow-up care is also important to keep the patient informed of the latest improvements in treatment, medication, and rehabilitative devices.

The frequency of follow-up care needs to be individualized to the patient's particular situation. Selection of the caregiver responsible for the follow-up will depend on the patient's wishes, the health care system, and the resources available. In many situations, a nurse is the person most appropriate and capable of providing follow-up.[15] This could be a community health nurse, a clinical nurse specialist in charge of the patient's particular clinic or clinical area (such as ostomy care or oncology), a primary care nurse clinician, or a mental health nurse specialist. The main concern is that someone assume this responsibility.

The goals or limitations of individual settings will also determine if referral is necessary for ongoing care and evaluation. The specialized nature of present hospital settings requires referral from one group of providers to another. When the patient's condition is stabilized, he is transferred from the ICU to a general floor. Referrals are made as the patient's progress or lack of progress is evaluated. Often a patient will adapt well to his body alteration in the hospital setting but have great difficulty on his return home. The

patient returning home faces many challenges. The hospital may have become a protective haven for him. He now has to deal with different activities and an environment that may remind him constantly of his former capacities. The family, too, may have many needs and concerns to discuss. New routines and patterns will need to be developed and new frustrations may also arise.

The community health nurse can be most effective in helping the patient and family cope with the challenges of returning to the home environment. She may provide anticipatory guidance to the family in preparation for the patient's return home. Helping the family problem-solve and maintain open communications will be another task for the nurse. Patient and family education will involve reinforcement of previously learned care, as well as modification of plans to suit the patient's and family's needs in the home. The nurse often will act as a facilitator for the patient in negotiating the health care system. She will provide ongoing communication with other health team members as well. The community health nurse also can provide an excellent understanding of the community services and resources available to support the patient and family.

Community support groups and societies geared to the needs of persons with specific problems are also helpful in assisting the patient and family to work through the adjustment process. Agencies such as the American Heart Association, American Cancer Society, or the American Arthritis Association often provide educational materials, equipment, and support groups for patients and families. Community mental health services are available for those who would like or appear to need more in-depth help in adjusting to their body image alteration. Bernstein emphasizes that exchange of information is necessary to plan care for the disfigured person in the community.[2] People need to know the resources available to them and what to expect from them. In turn, those working with the disfigured need to have an understanding of the family system, the job situation, the public and community attitudes, and the educational system to develop realistic plans.

CONCLUSION

The concept of body image is an essential part of a person's self-concept and plays a strong role in his sense of self-esteem. Impairment of body image is determined primarily by the person's perception of the change, the meaning that it holds for him, and the reactions of those significant to him. Impairment of body image may occur with what appears to be a relatively minor scratch, with the invisible changes caused by a chronic disease, or with obvious disfigurement. How severely a person responds will be the result of many factors. People experiencing a loss caused by a modification of body image will experience the grief reaction. Specific disease entities or injuries will also add to the tasks required of the patient in his adjustment to body image change. The nurse can be extremely effective in helping the patient and his family work through the grieving process and adjust to the body image change. Interventions are aimed at helping the patient and family to regain a sense of acceptance and self-esteem and may combine supportive counseling and health teaching, along with provision of direct personal care.

Many research questions concerning body image remain unanswered. The role of the family is acknowledged as important but not well documented in the body image literature. Ways to improve family involvement in care and ways to help families cope need further investigation. The impact of maturational changes on the person's body image needs exploration, particularly in the adult years. Prevention of body image disturbance should be a major concern for nursing. This has begun with preoperative teaching but deserves further exploration. Accident victims compose a large number of those people who experience body image alterations. Accident prevention and determination of effective means to carry this out is greatly needed.

Nurses are in a prime situation to help patients adjust to body image change. Their impact can be felt in wellness and illness care. Continual awareness of the impact of a body image alteration on a patient's health and well-being is essential for optimal health care management.

REFERENCES

1. Beeken JE: Body image changes in plegia. J Neurosurg Nurs 10, No. 1:20–23, 1978
2. Bernstein NR: Emotional Care of the Facially Burned and Disfigured. Boston, Little, Brown & Co, 1976
3. Berscheid E, Walters E, Bohrnstedt G: The happy American body: A survey report. Psychol Today 1, No. 6:119–131. 1973
4. Brown MS: In Bower FL (ed): Normal Development of Body Image, pp 1–106. New York, John Wiley & Sons, 1977
5. Brown MS: The nursing process and distortions or changes in body image. In FL Bower (ed): Distortions in Body Image in Illness and Disability, pp 1–19. New York, John Wiley & Sons, 1977
6. Carlson CE: Grief. In Carlson CE, Blackwell B (eds): Behavioral Concepts and Nursing Intervention, 2nd ed, pp 87–112. Philadelphia, JB Lippincott, 1978
7. D'Aflitti JG: Disability and chronic illnes. In Haber J, Leach AM, Schudy SM et al (eds): Comprehensive Psychiatric Nursing, 2nd ed., pp 759–789. New York, McGraw–Hill, 1982
8. Eisenberg MG: Psychological Aspects of Physical Disability. New York, NLN Publication, 1977
9. Erikson E: Childhood and Society, 2nd ed. New York, WW Norton & Co, 1963

10. Fisher S, Cleveland SE: Body Image and Personality, 2nd ed. New York, Dover Publications, 1968

11. Friedman BD: Coping with cancer: A guide for health professionals. Cancer Nurs 3, No. 2:105–110, 1980

12. Gallagher AM: Body image changes in the patient with a colostomy. Nurs Clin North Am 7, No. 4:669–676, 1972

13. Gorman W: Body Image and the Image of the Brain, pp 9–57. St. Louis, Warren H. Green, 1969

14. Gruendemann BJ: The impact of surgery on body image. Nurs Clin North Am 10, No. 4:635–643, 1975

15. Henker FO: Body-image conflict following trauma and surgery. Psychosomatics 20, No. 12:812–820, 1979

16. Kleeman K: Distortions in body image in adulthood. In Bower FL (ed): Distortions in Body Image in Illness and Disability, pp 73–96. New York, John Wiley & Sons, 1977

17. Kolb LC: Disturbances of the body-image. In Arieti S (ed): American Handbook of Psychiatry, Vol IV, 2nd ed, pp 810–837. Organic Disorders and Psychosomatic Medicine. New York, Basic Books, 1975

18. Lambert VA, and Lambert CE: The Impact of Physical Illness and Related Mental Health Concepts. Englewood Cliffs, NJ, Prentice–Hall, 1979

19. Mattheis RF: Holistic health concepts. In Haber J et al (eds): Comprehensive Psychiatric Nursing, 2nd ed, pp 79–135, New York, McGraw–Hill, 1982

20. Murray RL: Principles of nursing intervention for the adult patient with body image changes. Nurs Clin North Am 7, No. 4:697–707, 1972

21. Norris CM: Body image: Its relevance to professional nursing. In Carlson CE, Blackwell B (eds): Behavioral Concepts and Nursing Intervention, 2nd ed, pp 5–36. Philadelphia, JB Lippincott, 1978

22. Roberts SL: Behavioral Concepts and the Critically Ill Patient, pp 75–96. Englewood Cliffs NJ, Prentice–Hall, 1976

23. Secord P, Jourard S: The appraisal of body cathexis: Body cathexis and the self. J Consult Psychol 17, No. 5:343–347, 1953

24. Schilder P: The Image and Appearance of the Human Body. New York, International University Press, 1950

25. Werner–Beland JA: Grief Responses to Long-term Illness and Disability. Reston, Va, Reston Publishing, 1980

5

Fatigue

Marilyn Doerman Kellum

Fatigue is a common symptom that everyone experiences at some time in life. It occurs at the end of a busy day, after exertion, with an illness, or accompanying psychologic stress. Fatigue can be a normal and expected response, or it can be a disproportionate and limiting response for which the person seeks care. Although fatigue is a common experience and is understood to mean that the person is tired and unable to continue, helping the person with fatigue can be complicated and difficult.

Fatigue is a complex symptom because potential causes can arise from every body system, for example, endocrine, cardiovascular, and musculoskeletal. Fatigue can also be a symptom that reflects a combination of causes. It is an important symptom because it affects a person's sense of well-being and ability to function. When a person experiences fatigue, he is unable to continue activities, may fear an underlying illness, or may be very dissatisfied with his inability to perform or to achieve a desired goal. Although fatigue is a single symptom, it can have widespread effects.

It is generally acknowledged that, as a symptom, fatigue requires thorough evalu-

ation and management because it can be a nonspecific symptom of underlying physiologic or psychologic pathology.[1,7,9,12] Nurses often deal with fatigue in patients and are in a position to help the patient manage the symptom. Nurses must be able to identify the causes of fatigue and recognize areas of need for possible intervention. This chapter develops an approach for assessing the causes of fatigue and providing management strategies to assist the patient with fatigue.

For the purposes of this chapter, *fatigue* is defined as the perception of tiredness, lack of energy, and an inability to continue. Fatigue involves more than a tired muscle, physiologic processes (e.g., accumulation of metabolic wastes), or a decrease in work output. All of these are part of a process that leads to fatigue, but they are incomplete without the person's evaluation of his feelings in relation to these events. Fatigue is a person's *total* response to physiologic, psychological, and situational factors. It integrates physiologic and psychological variables and is a person's evaluation of his status in relation to the task at hand. It may result in a feeling of inadequacy and a loss of the sense of well-being. It is a total response that, if inappropriate and extreme, will impede the person in daily activities and detract from the overall satisfaction with life.

MECHANISMS OF FATIGUE

PROCESS OF FATIGUE

An understanding of the process of fatigue helps the nurse to clarify causative factors and their interactions. The result is the same, but what causes the symptom may be quite different. Fatigue due to overexertion is managed in a different way than is fatigue from extreme stress.

The development of fatigue is an interactive process that involves the physical environment, physiologic processes, the patient's psychological state, and the situation. S. H. Bartley, a psychologist who has written extensively on fatigue, has developed an explanation of its pathophysiology that includes physiologic and psychological components, their interactions, and effects (see Fig. 5-1).[4]

He describes a series of phenomena that lead to fatigue: impairment, disorganization, discomfort, and decrease in activity. Each occurs at a particular level of function: cellular, systemic, subjective, objective, and evaluative. The initial disturbance can occur at any level, but eventually all levels become involved. Fatigue is the final, generalized response.

Impairment occurs at the cellular level. *Impairment* is the decreased ability of cells to function, which results from a depletion of energy stores (e.g., oxygen, adenosine triphosphate, glycogen), and an accumulation of metabolic waste products (e.g., lactic acid, pyruvate). Repeated contractions of a skeletal muscle result in impairment; the fibers contract less effectively and recovery time is delayed. Impairment produces physiological and secondary psychological changes.

Disorganization occurs at the systemic level of function and can result in fatigue. Body systems integrate the functions of cells, tissues, and organs to achieve a task. The car-

FIG. 5-1   *The process of fatigue. (Data partially from Bartley SH: Fatigue: Mechanism and Management. Charles C Thomas, Springfield, IL 1965)*

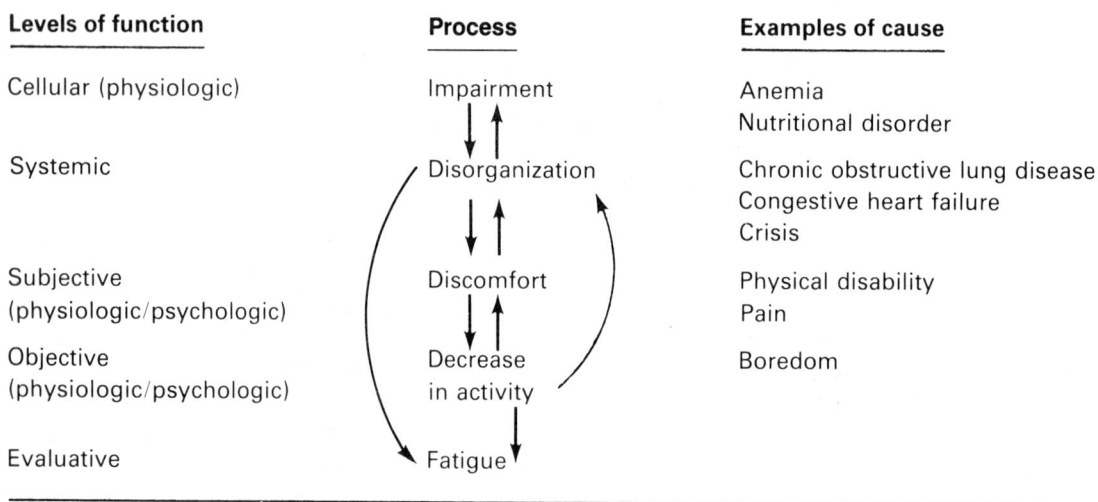

Levels of function	Process	Examples of cause
Cellular (physiologic)	Impairment	Anemia Nutritional disorder
Systemic	Disorganization	Chronic obstructive lung disease Congestive heart failure Crisis
Subjective (physiologic/psychologic)	Discomfort	Physical disability Pain
Objective (physiologic/psychologic)	Decrease in activity	Boredom
Evaluative	Fatigue	

diovascular system, for example, is responsible for the delivery of nutrients and oxygen to the cells and also for the removal of metabolic waste products. *Disorganization* is the failure of a system to act in an integrated and effective manner. It is a crucial step in the process of fatigue.

Disorganization can be a result of cellular impairment, as in the example of muscle contractions. A muscle, after repeated contractions, becomes weak and tremulous.[1] Chronic obstructive lung disease alters the respiratory system's ability to oxygenate blood adequately. Disorganization occurs when the body attempts to compensate for this derangement. Difficulty in breathing, decreased oxygen, and increased carbon dioxide lead to a decreased exercise capacity, anxiety, and respiratory acidosis.

Disorganization can also be a psychological phenomenon without impairment as its cause. The nervous system analyzes sensory information from internal and external sources in an attempt to arrive at an appropriate response.[7] Disorganization occurs when this fails. Anxiety can cause disorganization in thought processes that result in the person's being unable to think and act effectively. Anxiety can also cause palpitations, fast movements, and disturbed gastrointestinal function, leading to impairment.

Discomfort is the subjective experience of fatigue. For example, muscles will ache after repeated use. The sense of being unable to meet a demand or live up to a self-expectation also leads to the feeling of discomfort. Whether sensory or cognitive, discomfort can lead the person to stop a task before his physiological limit is reached.

A *decrease in activity* is the objective result of this process. The person becomes less effective and work output decreases. If a muscle contraction has become weak, the muscle can no longer accomplish the same amount of work. Mental as well as physical activities are affected. Thought processes can slow or become less effective. Depression is an example of slowing thought processes and a decrease in physical activities.

The feeling of fatigue is the net response to the process. It is based on the evaluation of body feelings and sensations, the realization that effectiveness has diminished, and the urge to withdraw or discontinue an activity. Fatigue can be a response that is normal or expected, protective, or pathologic. The person can view fatigue as a normal or abnormal response, and that view will affect his reactions, self-expectations, and expectations of the health care provider.

In summary, fatigue can be caused by both physiological and psychological processes, either separately or in combination. Although many studies have looked at the biochemical and work output parameters of fatigue, there are few data to document clinically relevant aspects of the symptom. Allan reviewed 300 cases in which fatigue or weakness was the chief complaint.[3] He found that 20% of these were caused by a physical disorder, whereas 80% were caused by psychologic factors. A more recent study found that approximately one third of patients reporting fatigue had a physical etiology.[12] These studies do give an estimate of the proportional representation of physiological and psychological causes of fatigue.

THE TYPES OF FATIGUE IN CLINICAL PRACTICE

To analyze the symptom, it is useful to have an idea of the common etiologic factors that lead to fatigue and a set of diagnostic categories into which they fall. Because fatigue can stem from so many varying causes, an organized approach is necessary to assess a patient's fatigue effectively. The accompanying

The Basic Types of Fatigue

NORMAL

Prolonged or unusual physical exertion
Inadequate rest
Unusually hectic schedule
Stress
Boredom or unstimulating daily routine

PATHOPHYSIOLOGIC

Acute infection: Prodrome or sequela
  Viral infection
  Mononucleosis
  Hepatitis
Chronic infection
  Endocarditis
  Tuberculosis
Endocrine or metabolic disorders
  Diabetes mellitus
  Hypothyroidism
  Pituitary disorders

Addison's disease
Chronic renal failure
  Hepatocellular failure
Malignancies
Anemias
Nutritional disorders
Congestive heart failures
Chronic obstructive lung diseases

SITUATIONAL

Extreme stress
Crisis: Personal or developmental, career, family, financial
Problem with a close relationship

PSYCHOLOGICAL

Anxiety
Depression

(Note: Fatigue may result from a combination of these causes.)

box outlines and gives examples of the four categories of fatigue: 1) normal, 2) pathophysiologic, 3) situational, and 4) psychological.

Normal fatigue is an expected response to any exertion, change in daily activities, added stress, or a decrease in physiologic reserve. For example, a hectic schedule, prolonged physical exertion (especially without adequate conditioning), or an inadequate amount of sleep (because of an unusually busy schedule or a transient stress reaction) all are apt to lead to normal fatigue. To some extent, fatigue will always occur after physical exercise, but often the patient's condition and endurance can be improved. Impairment probably occurs first with a depletion of oxygen and a build-up of metabolic wastes. Stress, physiologic or psychological, has been found to lead to a generalized physiologic response.[14] It can interfere with clear

thinking and effective action. Stress can easily lead to impairment, discomfort, and decreased work. Normal fatigue resolves quickly and predictably with rest and a moderate change in life-style. The person's restorative ability is an important factor in diagnosing this type of fatigue.

Fatigue can also be a symptom of disease or the result of a *pathophysiologic* process. Acute illnesses, especially viral infections, can be preceded and followed by periods of fatigue. Chronic disease, for example, anemia and chronic obstructive lung diseases, can result in continual impairment of physiological reserve, predisposing the patient to fatigue. Nutritional disorders such as obesity or an inadequate diet (nutrients or calories) are also pathophysiologic causes of fatigue. Ordinarily, the person with pathophysiologic fatigue cannot expect to overcome the problem simply by resting and adopting a change in life-style; the person's restorative ability is diminished.

Situational fatigue is a variant of normal fatigue. It occurs in unusual, fairly transient circumstances that produce periods of extreme stress, during which normal coping mechanisms are inadequate. Crises occur when a person is confronted with a problem he is unable to resolve by using the usual repertoire of actions and resources.[2,6] If the crisis continues without successful resolution, tension and discomfort build. Tension and discomfort, if prolonged or severe, lead to anxiety, a sense of helplessness, and finally to disorganization. Fatigue is the response to the increase in energy that a crisis requires, and to the disorganization and anxiety that an unresolved crisis creates. Career crises or job change, death in the family, problems in a close relationship, and developmental crises are examples of fairly common situations that require an unusual amount of energy and resources to resolve, all of which can lead to fatigue.

Finally, fatigue may be a symptom of significant *psychological* disorders, depression and anxiety being the most common causes.[7,9] Depression causes a decrease in activity, for example, a low voice, psychomotor slowing, and loss of interest in previous activities. Fatigue is the evaluative response to these changes. Anxiety is a systemic response and an energy utilizer. If prolonged, it leads to disorganization and exhaustion. These disorders are more chronic than the problems of situational fatigue, and may require long-term counseling by a mental health practitioner.

NURSING ASSESSMENT

When fatigue is an unexpected or disproportionate response to exertion and begins to interfere with daily activities, it becomes a concern to the patient. He will report fatigue as a symptom and seek care. Often, the patient suspects physical illness as the cause and may wonder if he might be anemic, have a vitamin deficiency, or some underlying and as yet undiagnosed physical illness. A thorough assessment is necessary to determine the pattern of fatigue, associated physiological and psychological manifestations, and the significance that the symptom has for the patient.

SUBJECTIVE DATA

It is necessary first to clarify exactly what the patient means by fatigue. Specifically, what changes have occurred? Activity patterns may have changed and the patient may be unable to maintain the previous level of activity. Responsibilities and circumstances may have changed, resulting in increased demands upon the patient or unrealistically high self-expectations. This increase in activity resulting from a job change, a new family member, or financial pressure, can lead to fatigue. Sleep and rest patterns may be altered. The patient may require a marked increase in sleeping time, such as naps, more hours per night, or report problems with sleep that result in an inadequate amount of sleep. One important differentiation to make is between *fatigue* and *weakness*. Weakness involves muscular strength and function.[1] A complaint of weakness implies a neuromuscular problem that requires a different evaluation. Clarifying the symptom and its effects provides the nurse with the basis for further assessment and areas of focus for subsequent management.

Pattern

The pattern of fatigue is important and is helpful in establishing the cause of fatigue.

Normal fatigue is alleviated predictably with adequate rest and relaxation. Fatigue from a physical cause improves with rest and worsens with activity. The pattern of psychologic fatigue seems to be the opposite; the patient is tired in the morning and may improve during the day.[7] The onset and duration of fatigue should be assessed. Fatigue that has been present for greater than 4 months has been found to be more commonly associated with psychologic problems.[12] Fatigue that is transient, in which the person is exhausted at one moment and full of energy the next, is apt to be from psychological or situational causes.

Associated Signs and Symptoms

The patient should be asked about any other signs or symptoms that have occurred. Fever and general malaise, for example, accompany fatigue that is secondary to an acute or chronic infection. Weight changes can be associated with nutritional disorders, hypothyroidism, or neoplasms. Dyspnea can be present with congestive heart failure, anemia, or chronic obstructive lung disease. Fatigue that is accompanied with difficulty falling asleep, palpitations, and gastrointestinal disorders may indicate anxiety. Early morning wakening and functional complaints associated with fatigue may lead to the diagnosis of depression.[9] The associated signs and symptoms cover a wide range of possibilities, but as specific ones are elicited, the nurse can begin to narrow potential causes of a patient's fatigue.

Psychosocial Factors

Situational factors can play a major role in fatigue, being the sole cause or exacerbating a preexisting condition that has left the patient with limited reserves, for example, chronic physical or psychological illness. Stressors must be identified. They can stem from a recent change or can be chronic in nature, such as long-term job dissatisfaction, a disabled household member, chronic marital problems, or financial worries. Fatigue is also a major symptom in depression and during periods of grief.[7]

Nutrition History

An assessment of fatigue should include a diet history. Insufficient calories or inadequate nutrients can be a cause of fatigue. Asking the patient about routine diet habits, that is, what is eaten for meals and snacks during a normal day, provides the nurse with an idea of the balance and appropriateness of the patient's diet. Weight gains or losses are an indicator of a change in diet or metabolism and should be noted. Alcohol, a depressant, and caffeine, a stimulant, are commonly consumed substances that affect performance and energy levels. Use of these substances should be noted.

Medications

Fatigue is a side-effect of many drugs, including over-the-counter medications. The dosage and purpose of all medications used by the patient should be recorded. Antihypertensives, minor tranquilizers, hypnotics, antidepressants, and antihistamines all have sedation as a side-effect.

Family History

Baseline data about close family members' health should be obtained. A family history of diabetes, anemia, endocrine disorders, or depression may be significant. A family history also may elicit information about a serious health problem of a close family member that is affecting the patient (i.e., causing concern and worry, or requiring the patient's time and energy in providing care to that person).

Past Medical History and Review of Systems

The review of systems will elicit any additional signs and symptoms that may be related to fatigue. A checklist or form that the patient fills out is a thorough and efficient way to obtain these data. The patient's past medical history also should be noted. A diagnosed chronic disease, for example, is significant since medications, a change in physiological status, or a change in situational factors can be possible sources of fatigue.

The focus of the review of systems should be on determining the presence of signs and symptoms that are commonly associated with fatigue. Fevers and lymphadenopathy are present in acute and chronic infections. Weight loss often is associated with diabetes mellitus or cancer. Skin changes can indicate an endocrine disorder. Nausea and jaundice are associated with hepatitis. Nervousness and difficulty falling asleep may indicate anxiety.

The review of systems can be quite extensive and may not be appropriate in every situation. The nurse must use judgment in determining the time and energy to invest in this part of the history. Awareness of the common physiologic and psychological causes of fatigue can help the nurse to focus the examination on the appropriate areas.

OBJECTIVE DATA

The physical examination is based on the preceding history. Signs and symptoms reported by the patient should be investigated and verified by a physical examination. A complete physical examination is appropriate when the patient fears an underlying disease, has reported a wide range of signs and symptoms, or when obtaining baseline data for providing primary health care. Necessary objective data also can be found in hospital records (e.g., an admitting history and physical examination, progress notes). Those data can be reviewed and used as necessary.

General Appearance

Observe the patient's general appearance. An unkempt appearance and a flat affect may be a sign of depression. An increased or decreased activity level may be obvious and a sign of agitation or depression. Begin to evaluate the patient's nutritional status by observing the general appearance. Does the patient's weight seem to be appropriate for his height? Ill-fitting clothes may indicate a recent weight change.

Vital Signs

Note heart rate, respiratory rate, blood pressure, and temperature. Tachycardia or palpitations can mean that the patient is anxious or has cardiovascular pathology. An increased or altered respiratory rate can be present in chronic lung disease. To monitor for a fever, the patient can be asked to check his own temperature at home.

Integument

Observe the skin for color, turgor, and lesions. Jaundiced skin is present in hepatitis and liver disease: pale skin may indicate an anemia: cyanosis can be present with chronic obstructive lung disease and worsening congestive heart failure. Hypothyroidism and poor nutrition lead to dry skin. Rashes can be present in viral illnesses.

Examine hair and nails also. Hair can become dry and brittle with inadequate nutrition. Circulatory insufficiency can cause a hair loss (most commonly seen on the lower extremities). Clubbing occurs when there is inadequate oxygenation present and is a symptom of anemia, congestive heart failure, and chronic lung disease. Check capillary refill.

Head, Ears, Eyes, Nose, and Throat (HEENT)

Examination of the eyes can reveal signs of a neurologic disorder, damage to blood vessels secondary to diabetes mellitus, and liver failure. Examining the pupils for reactivity and eye movements for extraocular movements are basic neurologic tests that should be done. A fundoscopic examination is important to evaluate the extent of vascular damage that occurs secondary to diabetes mellitus. Scleral icterus is a sign of liver disease and can be present in hepatitis before jaundice appears.

Examine the throat. Tonsillitis is a sign of infectious mononucleosis. Posterior cervical lymphadenopathy also is present in infectious mononucleosis. Palpate the neck for lymphadenopathy and an enlarged or irregular thyroid gland.

Respiratory

Note respiratory rate and character. Labored breathing or exertional dyspnea can be a sign of congestive heart failure or chronic lung disease. A barrel chest and purse-lipped breathing are present in emphysema. Adventitious lung sounds, (i.e., rales, rhonchi, wheezing) are present with underlying respiratory diseases that can range from bronchitis to pneumonia to chronic lung disease.

Circulatory

Assess the heart and peripheral vascular system. Auscultate the heart for rate, rhythm, and extra sounds. A murmur may be a sign of endocarditis or vascular disease. Heart failure often results in a third heart sound. Check peripheral pulses for strength and symmetry. Note edema, if present.

Gastrointestinal

Obtain a baseline weight and record recent changes. Bowel function is significant. Tarry stools may indicate a blood loss in the gastrointestinal tract. Hard, infrequent stools are a sign of constipation that may mean an inadequate diet or hypothyroidism. Diarrhea may be functional or a sign of an illness. The abdomen should be examined for tenderness and organomegaly.

Neuromuscular

Evaluate the neuromuscular system for muscular weakness, tremors, paralysis, and range of motion. Diseases such as myasthenia gravis, Parkinson's disease and arthritis cause weakness and loss of function that can be a cause of fatigue.

Any type of neuromuscular disability resulting from the above diseases, an injury, or a stroke can result in an increased difficulty in performing necessary daily activities. An evaluation of the patient's ability to be mobile, to dress and feed oneself, and to perform other required daily functions can be significant. A daily routine that is complicated by a neuromuscular disability can lead to fatigue.

Paraclinical Data

Laboratory studies are used to confirm a clinical diagnosis or to rule out certain, specific diseases. Testing should be selective. A complete blood count with a differential is useful to diagnose anemias and infections. A urinalysis and fasting blood suger level can detect abnormalities in glucose metabolism. Other studies, again dependent upon the preceding assessment, may include: a monospot, liver functions, thyroid evaluation, serum electrolytes, and blood urea nitrogen.

NURSING DIAGNOSIS

The nursing diagnosis includes determing the type of fatigue, the processes involved, and the effects on the patient. This enables the nurse to plan appropriate care that is aimed at correcting the underlying cause and helping the patient to cope with changed abilities. Understanding the probable causes and changes that have occurred as a result of the symptom is necessary for effective intervention.

NORMAL FATIGUE

Normal fatigue is identified primarily through the history. Rest is restorative, and fatigue develops as the day progresses. The physical examination and laboratory tests are normal. This is reassuring to the patient if illness is feared as the cause of fatigue. Often, the patient has identified the problem already or pinpoints the cause while the nurse is collecting data.

PATHOPHYSIOLOGIC FATIGUE

If the nurse suspects an illness based on the assessment data, a physician should be consulted for diagnosis of the illness and medical treatment. Acute and chronic disease can cause fatigue. The history will reveal associated signs and symptoms. Abnormalities may be present on physical examination and on laboratory data. Table 5-1 summarizes associated signs and symptoms that occur with illness-related fatigue. Decreased activity tolerance and improvement with rest are a common pattern for pathophysiologic fatigue.

SITUATIONAL FATIGUE

A history of recent crisis or an accumulation of stressful events is critical to the diagnosis of situational fatigue. The patient may report associated symptoms, (e.g., palpitations, sleep disturbances, gastrointestinal upsets) with this. Rest is not necessarily restorative and the patient may start the day feeling fa-

tigued. The physical examination is usually normal, although tachycardia, increased bowel sounds, or other signs of stress may be present.

PSYCHOLOGICAL FATIGUE

Psychological disorders, most commonly anxiety and depression, cause fatigue. Early morning awakening, crying spells, and functional complaints may be associated with depression. Anxiety may be accompanied by nervousness or uneasiness and sleeping problems. Medications used to treat psychological problems can have fatigue as a side-effect.

Fatigue can be a combination of the four types from a variety of causes. Fatigue can be an additive response, for example, a person with stable congestive heart failure who must care for a sick spouse in the home. A psychological stress can exacerbate an illness, and fatigue results from both the physiologic and psychological changes. This obviously complicates diagnosis and management of fatigue.

MANAGEMENT

The management of fatigue involves a wide range of nursing interventions, such as physical nursing care, monitoring medical regimens, counseling, teaching, and referral. These interventions can be directed at any level of the fatigue process. In some instances, the nurse may choose to treat the basic impairment, for example, preventing overexertion in a patient with inadequate oxygenation. In normal fatigue that results from a demanding schedule, the nurse may counsel the patient about setting priorities. This intervention is at a systems level. With some

TABLE 5-1
ASSOCIATED SIGNS AND SYMPTOMS IN PATHOPHYSIOLOGIC FATIGUE

	SIGNS	SYMPTOMS (IN ADDITION TO FATIGUE)
Addison's disease	Hyperpigmentation Decreased weight Postural hypotension	Nausea, vomiting Weakness
Anemia	Decreased hemoglobin Decreased hematocrit Pallor	Shortness of breath History of blood loss Dyspnea on exertion
Chronic obstructive lung disease	Barrel chest Labored or shallow breathing Purse-lipped breathing	History of smoking Decreased activity tolerance Chronic cough Sputum production
Congestive heart failure	Third heart sound Edema, rales Jugular venous distention	Shortness of breath Paroxysmal nocturnal dyspnea
Diabetes mellitus	Glycosuria Decreased weight Ketoacidosis Elevated blood sugar	Polyphagia Polyuria Polydipsia
Hepatitis	Jaundice Elevated liver function test Hepatomegaly Liver tenderness Dark orange urine Clay-colored stools	Nausea Decreased appetite
Hypothyroidism	Increased weight Dry skin	Intolerance to cold Constipation
Infectious mononucleosis	Exudative tonsillitis Fever Enlarged posterior cervical nodes	Headache Nausea Sore throat Malaise
Viral infections	Fever	Recent upper respiratory infection symptoms Nausea Headache Myalgia

patients, certain limitations are unalterable and interventions that assist at another level must be planned. Knowledge of the type of fatigue and an understanding of the basic underlying processes enable the nurse to plan appropriate systematic strategies.

The patient–nurse relationship is important when dealing with fatigue. A trusting relationship must be built and maintained. The patient should be able to discuss feelings freely with the nurse, since fatigue is primarily a perception. The nurse, in turn, must be able to share observations about the patient's fatigue and to suggest ways of intervening that the patient accepts. A sound nurse–patient relationship enables the patient to be open about the feeling of fatigue and gives the nurse credibility when suggesting strategies.

NURSING MANAGEMENT OF NORMAL FATIGUE

Developing a reasonable, healthful daily routine is basic to the management of all types of fatigue. Routines and habits free a person from many nonessential decisions and actions that can consume time and energy.[13] Any change in routine, such as illness or added stress, requires reorganization and energy expenditure. A balanced diet, regular exercise, and adequate rest are sound health habits and provide necessary physiologic requirements. These provide optimum conditions for functioning and enhance the body's restorative ability, both of which are important in managing fatigue or preventing its development.

Exercise

Aerobic exercise (e.g., jogging, walking, swimming) improves cardiovascular and respiratory efficiency. During aerobic exercise, the heart rate should be maintained at the patient's training heart rate (approximately $220 - age \times 80\%$). An exercise session includes a warm-up (5–10 min stretching or slow walking), 30 min of aerobic activity, and then a 5-min cool-down period of slow walking.[10] The patient should exercise three to four times per week. Exercise programs are quite often available in the community, and patients may be referred to these. There also are many books on setting up a personal exercise plan. Medical conditions like heart disease or chronic obstructive lung disease may be a contraindication to exercise or require a modified exercise program after consultation with a physician.

Sleep

Disturbance in the patient's sleep routine can lead to fatigue. Transient sleeping problems such as difficulty falling asleep, frequent awakenings, and early awakening, can occur as a result of stress or situational variables. An interruption in normal circadian rhythms (e.g., rotating shifts or jet lag,) can cause sleeping problems. Misuse of sleeping medications and caffeine a few hours before sleep can cause sleep disturbances. Insomnia can become a chronic problem and may require referral for treatment of an underlying psychological problem. Sleep habits and needs vary among individuals, but each person has definite requirements. A decrease in the number of hours of sleep required occurs with aging. The patient should be assisted to develop a sleep routine that allows for adequate rest. A comfortable sleeping environment (noise, light, bed), regular hours, and exercise promote relaxation and sleep.* A bedtime routine, use of relaxation techniques, and consistent rising time each morning are a few examples of ways to facilitate sleep.

Stress

Fatigue can occur in response to stress. Mediated by the endocrine and nervous system, the response to stress has demonstrated a link between psychological stress and disease (e.g., hypertension, peptic ulcer disease). Stress can give rise to many symptoms,

*Carse C; Alteration in the Sleep/Wake Cycle: A Nursing Protocol for Sleep as a Component of Health Promotion and the Nursing Management of Insomnias, 1979 (unpublished)

such as muscle tightness, gastrointestinal disturbances, and a sense of anxiety. The patient who is experiencing stress may need help in identifying its causes, that is, job or family demands. Once identified, the nurse, with the patient, can explore different ways to respond to stressful situations. Deep muscle relaxation, meditation techniques, exercise, and pursuing activities that the patient enjoys are common interventions in stress management.[8] (Chapter 6 delineates specific relaxation and meditation techniques.)

Planning Priorities

Unrealistic self-expectations, an inability to set priorites, and increasing demands on one's time and energy lead to an actual or, in some cases, a perceived loss of effectiveness and control. Self-expectations that are incongruent with actual abilities and available resources lead to fatigue. Fatigue occurs from overwork or the feeling that one is unable to meet a demand. Inability to set priorities decreases a person's effectiveness and ability to accomplish tasks.

Fatigue can occur from actual overwork. The patient may not realize his expectations or goals require an increase in energy expenditures. A change in circumstances, for example, a job change or a new baby in the family, can result in increased responsibilities.

In all of these cases, fatigue is the result of the patient's being unable to set expectations at a level consistent with the existing internal and external conditions. The nurse can provide the patient with an objective evaluation of these conditions, assist the patient in setting priorities, and help the patient formulate reasonable self-expectations.

One method of setting priorities is to make a list of those activities that the patient feels need to be done. Then the patient categorizes the activities into things that must be done that day, that week, and that month. The activities within each group are ranked from first to last. Thus the patient avoids expending energy each day deciding what must be done and when.

Motivation

Motivation plays an important role in fatigue. An individual's motivation affects his view towards a task and also his performance. A lack of motivation can cause fatigue before a physiologic limit has been reached. This has been noted by psychologists in industrial settings.[1] Working with the patient to establish goals and to be able to anticipate long-term rewards and outcomes can provide a motivating force. Goals should be both short-term, leading to a sense of accomplishment, and long-term, providing direction and meaning for the patient.

An unchanging routine provides little stimulation or satisfaction. A sense of fatigue often accompanies boredom. Interventions are aimed at providing varied experiences and should include identification of ways to alter daily routines. Lunch with a friend, pursuing a favorite activity or hobby, or participating in a group activity all add interest to the day's routines. The nurse can help the patient plan a schedule to include enjoyable tasks. A break in routine such as a short vacation provides new and different experiences.

The management of normal fatigue involves helping the patient: 1) develop healthful practices (e.g., exercise); 2) achieve insight into the cause(s) of the fatigue and develop realistic self-expectations; and 3) plan a reasonable daily routine that provides direction and stimulation. These are basic principles of fatigue management and are useful areas that should be examined for possible intervention in all types of fatigue.

NURSING MANAGEMENT OF PATHOPHYSIOLOGIC FATIGUE

Pathophysiologic fatigue is associated with illness. The treatment of this type of fatigue involves identifying the underlying cause, the medical treatment to stabilize the condition, and specific nursing care. Nursing care includes interventions at all levels, for example, monitoring physiologic response to a medical regimen, assisting the patient to develop energy-saving routines, providing for basic comfort, and helping the patient to cope with the effects of illness. With pathophysiologic fatigue, the nurse must have an understanding of the physiologic processes and their potential effects on fatigue development. Interventions must be planned at levels at which it is possible to make a change. Impairment may be unalterable, like a decreased cardiac output in congestive heart failure, but organizing daily routines to provide for rest periods helps minimize further impairment, disorganization, and discomfort.

At the cellular level, the treatment of pathophysiologic fatigue includes: 1) diagnosing and treating the underlying disorder; 2) monitoring response to therapy; and 3) preventing further impairment. Collaboration with a physician usually is necessary. The physician makes the medical diagnosis, stabilizes the condition, and implements a medical regimen. The nurse works closely with the physician to monitor therapies and prevent further impairment.

Congestive heart failure, for example, occurs when the heart becomes an ineffective pump. The cells are unable to obtain oxygen and nutrients. Medical treatment includes digitalis, vasodilators, diuretics, and a sodium-restricted diet to improve the heart's efficiency. In monitoring the patient's response to therapy, the nurse observes for signs of digitalis toxicity and worsening failure (e.g., increased edema or decreased activity tolerance). Helping the patient to obtain adequate physical and emotional rest decreases the cells' oxygen requirement by decreasing the heart's workload, therefore decreasing tissue demands and promoting diuresis.[11] This helps prevent further impairment.

An alteration in daily routines often occurs as a result of illness. The patient may have limited physiologic reserves, be unable to perform some activities unassisted, or may have increased responsibilities as part of a treatment (e.g., insulin injection, physical therapy program, a new diet). The nurse can assist the patient to develop a reasonable daily routine that prevents disorganization and augments limited physical capacity.

The nurse can also help the patient to determine what activities need to be done and how best to do them. The patient may be able to do some things unassisted, such as a partial bath or preparing meals, but may require assistance with other activities. Pacing activities to allow for ample rest prevents fatigue and still enables the patient to accomplish certain tasks. Often, the nurse caring for a hospitalized patient will plan activities, that is, bath, meals, and bed change, all with intervals of rest between them. However, the ambulatory patient also may need assistance in pacing daily activities.

Illness can cause considerable discomfort, both physical and psychological. Physical discomfort, such as pain or fever, interferes with rest. Other symptoms that are associated with illness may cause discomfort that can interfere with basic functions. Nausea and anorexia that occur with hepatitis or as a side-effect of chemotherapy can lead to inadequate nutrition and result in a feeling of fatigue. Interventions should include provision for the patient's comfort. Position changes, a comfortable environment, maintaining a balanced diet, and preventing overexertion, are all basic areas that should be included in the management of pathophysiologic fatigue.

Nurses working in a hospital setting should counsel patients with an acute illness or anticipating surgery to expect some degree of fatigue, which may be a lingering symptom during recovery. Knowing this, the patient may not be alarmed or discouraged when he is home and experiences easy fatigability. The patient with a chronic disease may need to alter his responsibilities and self-expectations. This may be a difficult process and require the support of the patient's family. The nurse can provide guidance by acknowledging the patient's changes and feelings about it, assisting in planning daily routines, and helping the patient to set realistic goals.

The nurse must be aware of resources available from the patient, family, or the community, that could provide the patient with needed assistance. A community nurse referral may be necessary to ease the transition from the hospital to home. The management of pathophysiologic fatigue involves consideration of the total individual, that is, the illness, response to illness, physiologic and psychological reserves, situational factors, and environment.

NURSING MANAGEMENT OF SITUATIONAL FATIGUE

A problem or crisis requires an increased expenditure of time and energy and can lead to situational fatigue. The nurse can assist patients to cope with and to resolve crises through a problem-solving process developed by Aguilera and Messick.[2] Understanding the crisis is the first step. In talking with the patient, the nurse must assess the problem and find out:

1. The patient's perception of the event(s)
2. What supports are available to the patient
3. The patient's past means of coping.

Not only does this define the problem for the nurse, it can help clarify the problem for the patient. Crises can be additive, and coping strategies may have been tried without their usual results. The resultant confusion and disorganization may have obscured the basic issues.

The next step is to plan appropriate interventions. The nurse and patient must consider possible actions and evaluate the different alternatives in terms of past experiences, how well they have worked in the past, and the reasons.

Actions and strategies are planned that begin to alleviate the symptoms produced by the crisis and that begin to resolve the crisis itself. Helping the patient to understand the crisis and providing an opportunity to ventilate feelings can be beneficial side-effects of the problem-solving process. Crisis causes tension and anxiety to develop. Exercise, a short break in routine such as a weekend trip, or planning an activity that the patient enjoys and considers to be a reward, are useful suggestions. Interventions that lead to resolution also are considered by the patient and nurse. Specific actions are planned and possible consequences are anticipated.

There are several types of crises.[6] Developmental crises are a normal and predictable part of growth and maturation. The young adult must establish independence. Parenthood is another example of a developmental crisis of the adult. Anticipated life events, such as school, marriage, or seeking employment, are other types of crisis. Failure, personal disaster, losses, and other unexpected life events can result in crisis. Often, a combination of these is the final precipitating factor. One problem could be handled and resolved, but a combination of events (*e.g.*, loss of a job and a new baby) results in crisis.

Enabling the patient to define the crisis, to use coping mechanisms, and to develop a potential solution helps him mobilize energies and resources into effective actions. This process can prevent or resolve symptoms brought on by crisis, one of which is fatigue.

NURSING MANAGEMENT OF PSYCHOLOGICAL FATIGUE

Psychological fatigue results from more complex psychological disturbances and may be a long-term or chronic problem. Fatigue often is associated with depression and anxiety. The patient with a psychological disorder requires counseling and assistance in identifying the underlying conflicts and losses he is experiencing. This counseling may be done by the nurse, if qualified. (Helpful techniques in counseling depressed or anxious patients are discussed in Chaps. 2 and 3.) Other helpful strategies are the same as for situational and normal fatigue. Referral to a mental health practitioner is indicated if the disorder is severe (more than minimal interference with functioning in job, school, other activities, or relationships). Consultation with a physician is indicated if the nurse feels that pharmacologic intervention is required. Psychological disorders may require long-term therapy. The nurse must be able to make a reasonable judgment that a psychologic process exists, begin to discuss this with the patient, and initiate appropriate referrals.

COMMON THREADS OF MANAGEMENT

The management of fatigue reflects the complexities of the symptom. Fatigue is a symptom that has integrated a person's physiological capabilities and psychological state. The causative factor may be from either or both. Basic to managing and preventing fatigue is promotion of a healthful, balanced life-style. This includes exercise, a balanced diet, adequate rest, and dealing effectively with stress. The nurse is in a position to make observations, recommend change, and teach patients basic health principles.

Helping the patient to retain or regain control over his situation and affairs is an important part of fatigue management. People function more effectively, with less discouragement or disorganization, when they are able to do things at their own pace, minimize interruptions, and can vary activities. The hospitalized patient has relinquished control over his environment. The nurse should be sensitive to this and include the patient as much as possible in developing the plan of care.

Helping the patient to develop realistic self-expectations gives the patient sound guidelines for planning activities. Expectations determine a person's goals and are the basis of self-evaluation (*i.e.*, did he perform or achieve as expected?). Discouragement and fatigue can occur if the person does not meet self-expectations. Motivation is another important behavioral factor when considering fatigue because it has a definite impact on performance. Long-term goals and potential rewards affect motivation. The patient may need help clarifying his goals and expectations.

CONCLUSION

Some degree of fatigue is a frequently encountered symptom. Everyone has experienced it at the end of a long day, during crises, or when ill. It can be a distressing symptom that affects both performance and image of one's self as a capable, functioning person. The nurse must be able to identify the problem and deal with it systematically. A complaint of fatigue requires clarification as to cause, type, and potential areas of intervention. The nurse also must be alert for the patient who is experiencing fatigue, but has not complained about it. A denial of fatigue and decreasing activity tolerance is more apt to be a sign of underlying pathophysiology.[7] Counseling the patient to expect a degree of fatigue following illness, surgery, or during times of stress may prevent discouragement and alarm.

Because many people look to health care providers for an explanation of their fatigue and ways to handle it, it is necessary that nurses have a thorough understanding of the symptom. Research needs to be done to clarify fatigue, the types, degree, effects, and effectiveness of interventions. Fatigue is a complex symptom with many different causes. It requires a diverse approach: developing a credible and therapeutic relationship with the patient, integrating physical and psychological problems, and being able to intervene at many levels.

REFERENCES

1. Adams RD: Lassitude and asthenia. In Isselbacher KJ, Adams RD, Braunwald E, Petersdorf RG et al (eds): Harrison's Principles of Internal Medicine, 9th ed. New York, McGraw–Hill, 1980
2. Aguilear DC, Messick JM: Crisis Intervention; Theory and Methodology, 2nd ed. St. Louis, CV Mosby, 1974
3. Allan FM: The differential diagnosis of fatigue. N Engl J Med 231:414, 1944
4. Bartley SH: Fatigue: Mechanism and Management. Springfield IL, Charles C Thomas, 1965
5. Bartley SH, Chute E: Fatigue and Impairment in Man. New York, McGraw–Hill, 1947
6. Burgess AW, Lazare A: Psychiatric Nursing in the Hospital and the Community, 2nd ed. New Jersey, Prentice–Hall, 1976
7. Engle GL: Nervousness and fatigue. In MacBryde CM, Blacklow M (eds): Signs and Symptoms; Applied Pathologic Physiology and Clinical Interpretation. Philadelphia, JB Lippincott, 1970
8. Farquhar JW: The American Way of Life Need Not Be Hazardous to Your Health. New York, WW Norton, 1978
9. Goroll AH, May LA, Mulley AG (eds): Primary Care Medicine. Philadelphia, JB Lippincott, 1981
10. Hanson PG, Giese MD, Corliss RJ: Clinical guidelines for exercise training. Postgrad Med 67:120, 1980
11. Luckman J, Sorensen KJ: Medical–Surgical Nursing: A Pathophysiologic Approach, 2nd ed. Philadelphia, WB Saunders, 1980
12. Morrison JB: Fatigue as a presenting complaint in family practice. J Fam Pract 10:795, 1980
13. Ryden MB: Energy: A crucial consideration in the nursing process. Nurs Forum 16:71, 1977
14. Selye H: The Stress of Life. New York, McGraw–Hill, 1956

6

Chronic Pain

Terry Vandenbosch

Pain is a complex phenomenon. It has been described as a response to noxious stimulation, a threat, an experience that is partly perception, partly reaction, an emotional state, and a product of consciousness.[5] Theories about pain include physiological, psychological, behavioral, sociological, and anthropological viewpoints. Any definition of pain is limited, because each person's pain experience is unique.

A useful definition of pain is proposed by McCaffery: "Pain is whatever the experiencing person says it is, existing whenever he says it does".[37] The definition acknowledges the subjectivity of the pain experience. It also "legitimizes" the person's pain. However, McCaffery's definition assumes the person's pain perceptions and responses are in the conscious mind and can be described. A more comprehensive definition based on the gate control theory of pain states that *pain is a complex experience in which painful sensory input is altered by a distinctive and interactive neural system before the input evokes pain perception and response.*[45]

Any discussion of pain should distinguish between acute and chronic pain. Acute pain is short-term (< 6 mo) and has a known, treatable cause or a defined course of illness. Anxiety is the dominant emotion associated with acute pain. Chronic pain is of longer duration (> 6 mo) and the pathology of the pain cannot usually be removed or altered. Depression and anger are the most common emotions associated with chronic pain. Behavioral literature defines chronic pain on the basis of pain behaviors.[20] The person suffering from chronic pain learns and uses consistent behaviors that often are maladaptive for dealing with his environment. Some clinicians divide chronic pain into long-term pain (e.g., from arthritis), and progressive pain (e.g., cancer pain). *Benign pain* is a term used to define chronic pain that is long-term but nonprogressive.

Chronic pain is a devastating problem. LeShan describes the person with chronic pain as living in the cosmos of a nightmare. His sense of being is blurred, and the pain seems to obliterate the rest of the body. He is conscious only of the area that is providing the overwhelming sensation.[33] As a result of chronic pain, the person often has problems of unemployment, restricted social activities, altered family roles and relationships, depression, anger, and substance abuse.

The problem of chronic pain in our society is increasing. People are living longer with chronic diseases and disabilities that are associated with chronic pain. To assist these persons to lead productive, satisfying lives, we need to help them learn to use strategies for coping with pain.

DEFINITION OF TERMS

Pain Threshold and Pain Tolerance

Pain threshold is the point at which a noxious stimulus is perceived as pain. It is assumed to be primarily physiological. It depends on the person's having an intact peripheral and sensory nervous system.[52] *Pain tolerance* is the duration of time and the intensity of pain that a person accepts before making a verbal or overt pain response.[52] Pain tolerance is influenced by psychological and sociocultural factors.

Pain Perception and Pain Reaction

Early researchers and clinicians divided pain experiences into two parts: pain perception or sensation, and pain reaction.[62] The terms *pain sensation* and *pain threshold* are similar: *pain sensation* is the point when the person is conscious of a painful sensation; *pain reaction* refers to motor, emotional, and cognitive responses that occur after the pain is consciously perceived. Pain reaction is assumed to be mediated by psychological factors, such as the meaning of pain to the individual and sociocultural factors.[62]

The introduction of the "gate control" theory of pain has added a new perspective to the terms *pain threshold, pain sensation,* and *pain reaction.* The *gate control theory of pain* proposes that psychological and sociocultural factors significantly influence and alter pain sensations *before* they are perceived.[43] The terms are useful for clinicians if they are interpreted with the understanding that pain threshold and pain sensation measure more than physiological sensation.

Pain Experience

The term *pain experience* is used extensively throughout this chapter. The term was first suggested by Hardy, Wolff, and Goodell and is the individual's integration of all aspects of pain.[25]

Psychogenic and Somatic Pain

In the past, pain has been classified as psychogenic or somatic; *psychogenic pain* being pain whose causes are psychological, and *somatic pain* being pain whose causes are physical. As one learns about the complexities of pain experiences, it becomes more difficult to make a distinction between psychogenic and somatic pain. The person with pain of primarily psychological origin can feel as much physical pain as the person with pain of physical origin. Conversely, the person's emotions affect the physical sensation he experiences. It is appropriate to assess the pain sensation and the person' emotional state no matter what the cause of the pain. A person with a strong emotional component to the pain may need psychological interventions. However, these need not be done at the exclusion of other types of interventions.

MECHANISMS OF PAIN

ENDORPHINS

In 1975 researchers discovered naturally occurring substances, *endorphins,* in the human brain that have effects similar to morphine. Endorphins act by inhibiting the transmission of painful stimuli to the central nervous system (CNS). Researchers now believe that endorphins are hormones and neuromodulators that play a role in pain, sleep, stress, shock, drug intoxication (e.g., alcohol and Valium), depression, schizophrenia, and sexual behavior.[7, 24]

One study on endorphins reported

higher pain tolerances in persons with above average levels of endorphins in their cerebrospinal fluid (CSF).[58] In another study the narcotic antagonist, naloxone, actually reversed the effects of acupuncture, suggesting that endorphin release mediates the effectiveness of acupuncture.[13] Another recent study reported increased endorphin levels in women who increased their exercise levels to 45 min a day.[10] It may be that many interventions alter pain by increasing the level of endorphins.[59] Because of the increasing research in this area, many people believe that experts may soon be able to develop an effective, nonaddicting treatment for pain relief, and begin to understand how pain affects the whole person.[61]

CHARACTERISTICS OF PAIN

The characteristics of pain are important aspects of pain. The type of sensation a person describes is related to the area of the body where the pain originates. *Cutaneous pain is* pain that originates in skin or subcutaneous tissue. Somatic pain originates in bone, nerve, muscle, and other tissues that support these structures. Visceral pain originates in body organs located in the trunk. Table 6-1 summarizes the different characteristics of pain according to origin. However, because pain is a subjective experience, the table should be used only as a general guide in understanding characteristics of pain sensation.

GATE CONTROL THEORY*

A widely accepted theory of pain is termed the *gate control theory of pain.* The gate control theory proposes that incoming painful

*Adapted from Lindberg JB, Hunter JL, Kruszewski AZ: Person-Centered Nursing Care: Introduction to Professional Practice, Philadelphia: JB Lippincott, 1983.

sensations are altered and modulated at differing levels in the CNS *before the person perceives the pain.* The intensity and quality of perceived pain is affected by competing factors in the CNS. There is some controversy and conflicting evidence about the gate control theory; some of the details may need revision. However, the evidence for *gating,* or modulation of painful sensory input, in the spinal cord is strong.[43] The gate control theory differs from the older specificity theory of pain in that the specificity theory proposed a *single* pain pathway in the CNS. The amount of pain perceived was assumed to be directly proportional to the amount of painful stimulation. This concept is not true for the gate control theory.

The discussion of the gate control theory focuses on factors that modulate incoming pain sensations, how the factors interact at the "gate" in the spinal cord, and neurotransmission to the higher CNS.

The gate control theory proposes that the substantia gelatinosa (SG), an area of specialized cells in the dorsal horn of the spinal cord, acts as a gating mechanism (see Fig. 6-1). This gating mechanism alters and modifies the arriving pain sensations before they reach the cerebral cortex and evoke the perception of pain. Three major factors interact at the gate: 1) pain receptors and pain fibers, and their interaction at the gate; 2) the effect on the gate of cognitive and emotional elements that are also called higher CNS functions; and 3) the descending neural input from the brain stem.

Pain Fibers

Two major types of fibers that carry sensations important for pain perception are small diameter and large diameter receptor fibers. *Small-diameter fibers* transmit high threshold, or more intense, pain sensations. Some small-diameter fibers rapidly transmit intense, highly localized pain sensations,

TABLE 6-1
CHARACTERISTICS OF PAIN AS COMMONLY RELATED TO SOURCE OF PAIN

SOURCE	LOCATION	INTENSITY	QUALITY	CHRONOLOGY
Cutaneous	Well-localized	Correlates with intensity of stimulus	Bimodal sensation may occur Sharp, tingling, stinging Abnormal surface sensations may occur	Correlates with stimulus changes, tissue damage May be steady or throbbing in inflamed tissues
Deep Somatic	Poorly localized May localize with tendon, periosteum, ligament pain May be referred to body surface	Correlates with intensity of stimulus and with movement of involved area	Vague, aching, boring, dull Cutaneous tenderness may accompany	May be steady or change in character with stimulus change or movement Correlates with stimulus changes
Visceral	Poorly localized May localize as duration extends May be referred to body surface	May be severe with colic May increase if not relieved Correlates with intensity of stimulus	Vague, dull, aching, burning If continues may become sharper If due to obstruction may be gripping, cramping, twisting	Obstructive pain generally occurs in cycles Untreated pain may mount Correlates with stimulus changes

(Johnson M: Assessment of clinical pain. In Jacox A [ed]: Pain: A Source Book for Nurses and Other Health Professionals, p 152. Boston, Little, Brown & Co, 1977)

whereas others slowly transmit vague, dull, or crushing pain that is more generalized, making it difficult to locate the exact area of pain. *Receptors* for the small-diameter fibers are free nerve endings located in the skin and deeper body structures such as tendons, muscles, and internal organs. These receptors send out pain impulses when they are stimulated by chemical, thermal, or mechanical agents.

There are many chemical agents in the body that can cause pain. Bradykinin and potassium, which are released when a cell is destroyed, can stimulate pain sensation. Buildup of lactic acid in muscles is another chemical that can cause pain. Thermal agents include fire or hot water. Examples of mechanical agents might be a strong blow to the body or changing the dressing on an open wound.

Large-diameter fibers transmit the sensations of touch, vibration, warmth, and light

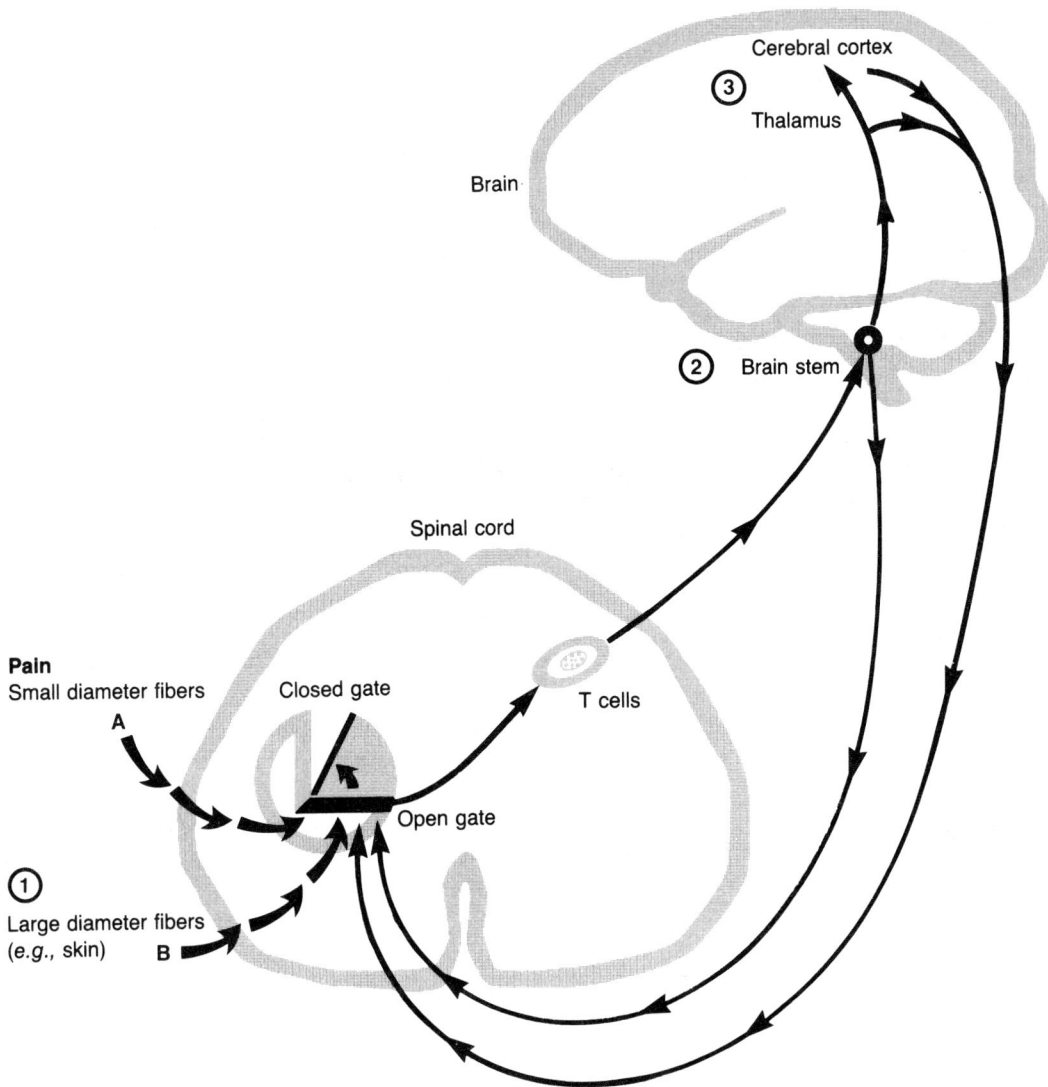

FIG. 6-1 *Gate control theory of pain. One influence on the gating mechanisms is the ratio of large to small fibers activated (A) impulses traveling on small-diameter nerve fibers cause the gate to be held open; (B) impulses traveling on large-diameter fibers generate feedback to the gate, almost closing it. Transmission of pain impulses through gates in the spinal cord is affected by the following: 1) activity in large and small sensory nerve fibers; 2) projections from the brain stem reticular formation; and 3) projections from the cerebral cortex and thalamus. (Hassid P: Textbook for Childbirth Educators. New York, Harper & Row, 1978)*

pressure. Receptors for the large-diameter fibers are located mainly in superficial structures. Large-diameter fibers are myelinated and conduct impulses rapidly. However,

they adapt to stimuli whereas small-diameter fibers do not. *Adaptation* means that the large diameter fibers do not continue sending impulses to the gate with long-term, continuous stimulation. An example of adaptation of these fibers is the diminished sensation and awareness experienced with the long-term wearing of wristwatches or rings. Impulses that are created by stimulation of the receptors of large- and small-diameter fibers are conducted along the fibers to the cell bodies in the dorsal root ganglia. The cell fibers then synapse at the SG. The interaction of the large- and small-diameter fibers at the gate is one cause of the alteration or modulation in the pain sensation. Stimulation of the large-diameter fibers that synapse at the SG inhibits and modifies the pain sensations arriving on the small diameter fibers.[45] For example, a pregnant woman is taught to modify the pain sensation by rubbing her abdomen during labor contractions.

Cognitive and Emotional Factors

Within the CNS is a pathway for constant input from the brain down to the gate in the spinal cord. Normally this input is inhibitory and keeps the gate or SG partially closed to painful, small-diameter fiber sensations. Emotional changes, such as a high anxiety level, decrease the inhibitory input and allow the pain sensation to pass through the gate unchecked. Depression also alters the inhibitory input.

Brain Stem Activity

Areas in the brain stem receive input about somatic, visceral, and autonomic activity, and proprioception, and relay the information to other areas of the brain. The brain stem has a pathway for constant *inhibitory* input to the gate. Changes in somatic, visceral, and autonomic activity can affect the amount of pain impulse inhibition that occurs at the gate. An example of this might be the person who finds his pain is minimized by an increased activity level.

The Gate

The pain sensations arriving at the gate can be modulated by the large-diameter fibers and one's emotional state, before one has actually perceived the pain. Three features help to determine how much pain a person will perceive. The first is the ongoing cognitive and emotional input that precedes and occurs with the pain stimulus. The second is the intensity of the pain stimulus in terms of *numbers* of fibers stimulated and the *frequency* of impulses. For example, a small burn to the finger would not stimulate as many receptors as a burn to the hand. The third is the relative balance of activity in large versus small fibers.[45]

Some neurophysiologists maintain that the gate or SG is also a storehouse for pain memory. Pain impulses are recorded in the SG similarly to photographic film registering visual events. If the memory of the original injury is not reactivated, the pain images gradually fade. However, the memory traces of the pain can be revived by a different irritant and the same type of pain can be reestablished.[41] This, in part, could account for some chronic pains that have no obvious physical cause. A commonly occurring example of this phenomenon is low back pain. The cause of the pain may be removed by surgery, yet the pain often returns for no apparent reason.

Neurotransmission After the Gate

After being altered at the gate, the pain impulses go to the transmission cells (T cells) which, like the SG, are located in the dorsal horn of the spinal cord. The T cells transmit the impulses along spinal cord pathways to the thalamus, reticular formation, limbic system, and the cerebral cortex. The reticular formation and limbic system are responsible in part for emotions and sympathetic responses to the pain sensation. The cerebral cortex helps us to interpret and evaluate the pain. Thus, the pain sensation evokes emotions and thoughts, as well as physical reactions. There are several key points to remember about the gate control theory:

- Because modulation of the pain sensation occurs at the gate, there is no direct relationship between the amount of tissue damage and the amount of pain a person experiences.
- Emotions and thoughts about pain affect the amount and quality of pain a person perceives.
- A person can perceive a physical pain from emotional causes.
- Because there are many factors that interact to modulate the pain sensation, multiple interventions are appropriate for pain relief.
- The gate control theory can help to predict the kinds of interventions that might be appropriate.

FACTORS THAT AFFECT PAIN

The gate control theory of pain provides the basis for identifying factors that affect pain. The following factors are described in more detail to understand better their relationships to chronic pain.

Sociocultural Factors

Socialization about pain begins at an early age. In families that place a great deal of attention on pain, the child learns early that pain-related behaviors get attention and other behaviors do not. Not only does this begin to set a lifelong pattern of focusing on pain, it may also encourage the person to interpret as painful, stimuli that others may term uncomfortable. Pain-prone behavior also develops when parents hold unrealistically high expectations of their children. The children develop a low level of self-esteem, and feelings of guilt and hostility. Pain may serve as a ''punishment,'' or way of atoning for not being a perfect child.

Some researchers report familial tendencies for developing problems with pain. This could be because of an interplay between genetics, constitutional factors, and socialization. Significant past experiences with others suffering from acute and chronic pain have been implicated as determinants of the manner in which a person copes with a present pain.

The person in chronic pain does not function in isolation from the rest of the family. Family members' roles are altered when a member has pain. The person with chronic pain tends to restrict socialization, which can alter family socialization and support systems. It may also become necessary for other family members to find or change jobs. In addition, maladaptive family coping patterns develop, such as hostility and guilt towards the family member in pain, resulting in angry flare-ups and overcompliance with the needs of the person in pain.

Persons with complaints of pain are more likely to come from a lower socioeconomic class.[54] This is probably because of poorer housing, nutrition, and medical care.[28] Persons from a lower socioeconomic background may not have access to treatment programs for prevention of problems and assistance with adaptation to chronic illnesses. Sternbach suggests that people from the working class are more likely to express emotional stress and conflict in somatic difficulties, including pain.[54]

Occupations that cause high amounts of stress may predispose the person to illness and pain. Pain such as low back pain is related to occupations in which weightlifting and bending are common.

The health care practices of different ethnic, racial, and religious groups also can affect the development of pain and the person's ongoing pain experience. For example, black Americans generally have less access to quality health care than whites, which may predispose them to more problems with pain.[28] Baptists, who believe in predestination, may respond passively to efforts to involve them in a pain program because they do not believe they can change their situation.[49] There are numerous articles that report differences in pain expression and pain tolerance, depending on race and culture.[5, 16, 29] Research results on the effects of age and sex on pain tolerance are contradictory; hence, it is not possible to make generalizations that have a research base about pain tolerance.[5, 16, 28, 30]

Emotional Factors

A person's emotions play a role in the development of chronic pain and in the person's ongoing pain experience. There is some controversy over whether emotional difficulties result in pain or develop because of the pain. Nevertheless, persons with chronic pain invariably have emotional difficulties. Well-documented research reports the existence of emotional difficulties before the development of many chronic pains (e.g., migraine, low back pain, and phantom limb pain). Hostility, guilt, resentment, anxiety, and preoccupation with bodily functions (hypochondriasis) all have been reported as pre-disposing to chronic pain development. Persons with high expectations for themselves and rigid guidelines that are difficult to meet, may develop hostility, a chronic sense of guilt, and low self-esteem. For them, chronic pain becomes an acceptable way to discharge hostile feelings toward relatives. The pain neutralizes the guilt and results in less tension.[48] Parkes reported two significant personality variables in amputees who had phantom limb pain: rigidity and compulsive self-reliance.[47] These persons were unable to accept the need to be dependent on others. A hostile ambivalence toward dependency often is seen in persons with chronic pain.[47] Furmanski, in his study of persons with migraine, reported that attacks of migraine began when hostilities accumulated beyond the person's capacity for tolerance of frustration.[21] The person transformed his emotional distress into physical symptoms. Increased muscle tension from high anxiety levels may predispose persons to development of pain and increase the intensity of that pain.

Continued coping with chronic pain over time leads to loss of hope about the future and to depression. The person's main focus becomes the pain. As a result, depression, despair, and hypochondriasis commonly occur with chronic pain.

Evidence is accumulating that the daydreams and thoughts people have about their pain affect their pain experience.[9, 38, 51] There is also evidence that self-statements people make affect their pain experience.[12] For example, a person who continually focuses on his pain and thinks to himself, "This is the worst thing that can happen to me," is probably more depressed and has more problems with pain than the person who believes he has the ability to cope.

Other Factors

Other factors that affect the person's pain experience are rest, sleep, and dietary habits. Adequate sleep and nutrition help the person maintain the energy to cope with pain.

PAIN VALUES

One's familial and cultural background and life experiences influence one's view of pain.

Nurses often assess a person's pain based on their own values about pain. A recent study reports that nurses tended to infer differing amounts of physical pain and psychological distress based on their patient's socioeconomic status, age, sex, ethnic background, and on the nature and extent of the illness. In addition, nurses who have a history of a significant experience with pain tend to infer more pain in their patients.[16]

An important aspect of pain management is examining one's values about pain. Nurses' and health care professionals' attitudes and actions can affect their patients. Part of the patient's self-image relates to how significant others view him. Recent research shows that the social environment can alter a person's pain perception and pain tolerance.[14] The staffing patterns, attitudes, and knowledge of nurses caring for the person in pain also has an effect on the person in pain. For example, many different people in one day having close contact with a patient could detrimentally affect his ability to form trusting therapeutic relationships. Confusion and conflict in the patient's treatment can occur if nurses hold differing views on pain management.

Another aspect of pain to consider is the priority and accountability given to pain management in the health care setting. In most settings, nurses are accountable for recording and reporting vital signs and managing physical care, yet they are not usually accountable for developing consistent pain management philosophies and treatments.[56]

The information in the chart, Examining Pain Values, can be used by health professionals to make themselves more aware of their own values regarding pain and the effect these attitudes have on patients. This information can be used as a guide to change those attitudes.

QUANTITATIVE MEASUREMENT OF PAIN

Measurement of chronic pain is complex. There is no measure that accurately quantifies the pain experience. However, by assessing pain sensation, the quality of pain, and psychological aspects of pain, one can gain an understanding of the person's pain experience.

The best measure of a person's pain is what he says about the pain. Observation of a patient's behavior as a means of quantifying the amount of pain he experiences is extremely unreliable. Increases in blood pressure and changes in autonomic responses are also unreliable.[55] People with chronic pain adapt to pain physiologically and socially. In addition, behavioral and autonomic signs of pain are influenced by one's cultural background.[57]

Pain sensation can be measured by using a scale. Clinical data that may be used for future research is best quantified using a numeric scale of 0 to 100. The patient is asked to rate the pain *intensity* rather than the qualities of pain or the emotions associated with the pain. Estimate the present pain and pain at other times. Use words to help define the endpoints of the scale (see Fig. 6-2A). Zero is described as no pain and 100 is pain so intense a person could not bear it for more than two min. If people have difficulty assigning a number to the pain, a pain-rating scale can be used. Although the pain-rating scale, using descriptive words, is more open to interpretation than the numerical scale, it is easy for patients to use (see Fig. 6-2B).

A simple scale developed by researcher Ronald Melzack that helps to measure the emotional aspect of chronic pain is listed in Figure 6-2C.

Another way to measure pain is to review the words people use to describe their

Examining Pain Values

PERSONAL PAIN VALUES

1. How did important people (mother, father, grandparents) in your life respond to their own pain? to your pain?
2. Are there childhood experiences with pain that affect your response to pain?
3. Did you ever get extra privileges or attention because you had pain?
4. Do you ever feel as if pain is given to people to make them strong?
5. Do you talk a great deal about pain when you have it? How do you feel about people who talk a great deal about their pain?
6. What do you think about when you have pain that is uncomfortable?
7. What do you do when you have pain that is uncomfortable?
8. Are there times a person should endure more pain?
9. Are certain pains more legitimate than others? Does it depend on the severity of illness?

SOCIOCULTURAL PAIN VALUES

What do you think about some of the ideas concerning pain in our American culture? For example:

Men are tough and do not cry when they are hurt.
Men tolerate pain better than women.
Adults can endure more pain than children.
Older persons experience less pain.
If no physical reason for pain can be found, then you must have emotional problems.
People in pain should be pampered.
All pain should be avoided.
Pain should be relieved.
Nurses and doctors are experts on pain.
Doctors and nurses will take away the pain.

ORGANIZATIONAL PAIN VALUES

1. Is there an organizing philosophy concerning the patient's responsibility in assessing, preventing, relieving, and minimizing his own pain?
2. What information about pain coping measures and their limitations should nurses be held accountable for?
3. What information concerning pain is charted and passed on in the nursing report?
4. What are the responsibilities of RNs, LPNs, aides, doctors, psychologists, technicians, and therapists in helping patients to manage pain?

(Data partially from Ingersoll B, Chenoweth B: Coping with Aches and Pains: An Education/Support Group Model. Booklet published by Turner Geriatric Clinic, University of Michigan Hospitals, Ann Arbor MI, October 1981 and from Fagerhaugh SY, Strauss A: How to manage your patient's pain...and how not to. Nurs 80 10:44, 1980)

pain. Melzack and Torgerson categorized the words people use to describe their pain into three categories (see Table 6-2). The categories are

1. Sensory (words that describe the sensory qualities of pain)
2. Affective (words that describe emotion and autonomic responses)
3. Evaluative (words that describe the overall subjective intensity of pain).

Under each of the three categories are subcategories containing words that are rank ordered. For example, under the category "Sensory" and the subcategory "Temporal," a flickering pain is assumed to be less than a quivering pain. To administer the tool, the nurse should read the adjectives aloud to the person and check the words that the person chooses. One way to derive a score is simply to count the total number of words checked. A more complex way of scoring in each cate-

0-100 NUMERIC SCALE

A

| 0 10 20 30 40 50 60 70 80 90 100 |

No pain   Moderate pain   Unbearable pain

SIMPLE DESCRIPTIVE SCALE

B

| 0 | 1 | 2 | 3 | 4 | 5 |

None   Mild   Moderate amount of pain   Quite a lot of pain   Very bad pain   Unbearable pain

MELZACK'S SCALE

C

Mild   Discomforting   Distressing   Horrible   Excruciating

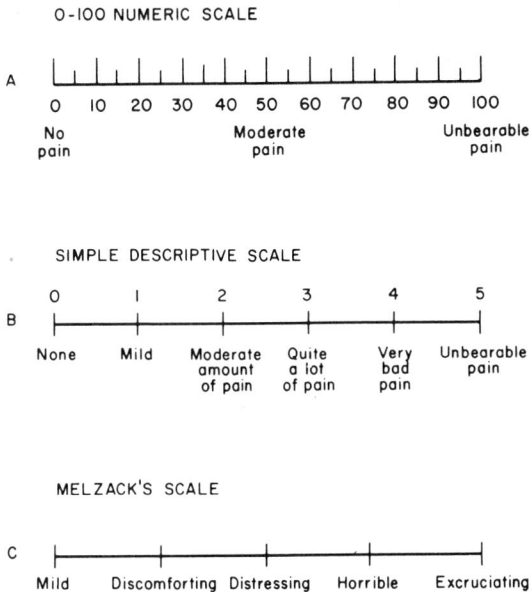

FIG. 6-2 *Pain scales. (Stewart ML: Measurement of clinical pain. In Jacox AK (ed): Pain: A Source Book for Nurses and Other Health Professionals, 1st ed, p 111. Boston, Little, Brown & Co, 1977)*

gory can be found by rating information on the McGill Pain Questionnaire, from which this chart is derived.[42]

NURSING ASSESSMENT

Assessment data should be collected from both the person in pain and a minimum of one family member.[55] An assessment guide can be used to explore factors contributing to the person's pain experience. If the data collected in the initial assessment are to be used as baseline data for future comparisons of progress, they must be recorded carefully and must be specific. For example, not only is the patient's perception of the degree of his social restriction important, but also the number of times per day or week that he socializes with people outside of the immediate family. Early in the interview, the per-

son's expectations for pain relief and what he would like from the nurse should be explored. This information will help the nurse to focus on collecting data in the area of the patient's concerns. It may not be appropriate to collect all of this information in the initial interview. Because chronic pain is a complex problem, the nurse continues to assess factors that contribute to the person's pain experience throughout the initial stages of building a relationship.

SUBJECTIVE DATA

Demographic Variables

Demographic variables include age, sex, ethnic identification, race, economic status, employment status, educational level, and current medical diagnosis and prognosis.

Pain Sensation

The pain sensation describes the location of the pain; quality of the painful sensation (e.g., burning, aching, stabbing quality); when the pain began; factors that precipitate or increase pain, variations in pain intensity over days, weeks, and months. Ask the patient to estimate pain sensation on a scale from 0 to 100 (see Fig. 6-2A) to rate the pain at its worst, at its best, the current pain level, and alleviating factors.

Quality of Pain

Ask the person to describe the quality of pain in his own words or use the word adjective checklist adapted from the McGill Pain Questionnaire (see Table 6-2).

Psychosocial, Cognitive, and Cultural Factors

Review affective and evaluative adjectives chosen from the McGill word adjective checklist, or ask the patient to assess pain on

TABLE 6-2

CLASSES AND SUBCLASSES OF PAIN DESCRIPTORS AS RATED BY PATIENTS

CATEGORY	DESCRIPTORS	CATEGORY	DESCRIPTORS
SENSORY			
Temporal	Flickering		Hurting
	Quivering		Aching
	Pulsing		Drawing
	Thumping		Blurred
	Throbbing		Steady
	Beating		Heavy
	Pounding	**AFFECTIVE**	
Spatial	Jumping	Autonomic	Nauseating
	Flashing		Sickening
	Spreading		Suffocating
	Radiating		Choking
	Shooting		
		Sensory	Tender
Punctate pressure	Pricking	(miscellaneous)	Taut
	Boring		Rasping
	Drilling		Splitting
	Stabbing		Tearing
	Lancinating		
	Penetrating	Tension	Nagging
	Piercing		Fatiguing
			Tiring
Incisive pressure	Sharp		Exhausting
	Cutting		Dragging
	Lacerating		
		Punishment	Racking
Constrictive pressure	Pinching		Punishing
	Nipping		Grueling
	Tight		Cruel
	Squeezing		Vicious

5-point scale developed by Melzack (see Fig. 6-2C). Assess the emotional state, both current and past. Assess the level of anger, hostility, and depression. Assess the level of dependence/independence and inquire about past actions in seeking pain relief, expectations concerning pain relief or pain minimization, past history of dealing with other types of pain, and roles played by family members in dealing with the person's pain. Explore the person's background for significant experiences of observing or relating to persons with similar problems with pain; explore religious beliefs and cultural values, and assess mental "pictures" of pain and self-statements about pain.

TABLE 6-2
CLASSES AND SUBCLASSES OF PAIN DESCRIPTORS AS RATED BY PATIENTS (Continued)

CATEGORY	DESCRIPTORS	CATEGORY	DESCRIPTORS
	Pressing		Killing
	Binding		Torturing
	Gnawing		
	Biting	*EVALUATIVE*	Annoying
	Cramping		Bearable
	Gripping		Troublesome
	Crushing		Miserable
			Distracting
Traction pressure	Tugging		Agonizing
	Pulling		Ugly
	Wrenching		Intense
			Intolerable
Thermal	Hot		Unbearable
	Burning		Savage
	Scalding		Violent
	Searing		
		Fear	Fearful
Brightness	Tickling		Frightful
	Tingling		Terrifying
	Itchy		Dreadful
	Smarting		
	Sticking	Affective–	Grinding
		evaluative–	Wretched
Dullness	Dull	sensory	Awful
	Sore	(miscellaneous)	Blinding
	Numbing		Wicked

(Johnson M: Assessment of clinical pain. In Jacox A [ed]: Pain: A Source Book for Nurses and Other Health Professionals, p 150. Boston, Little, Brown & Co, 1977. Adapted from Melzack R, Torgerson WW: On the language of pain. Anesthesiology 34:54, 1971)

Effects of Pain on Life-style

Assess the activity level in detail; for example, list the number of times per day spent sitting up and the amount of time in a chair. Assess changes in the activity level related to pain, degree of restriction of social activities, effects of pain on employment, amount of disruption of family life, and type of planning for the future.

Associated Manifestations

Associated manifestations, such as nausea and dizziness, should be noted.

Past and Current Medical History

Medications

Names and doses of medications, including prescription and over-the-counter medications, amounts and times taken, type of pain relief experienced with pain medications, and side-effects of pain medications should be assessed.

Other Factors

Assess degree of fatigue and quality of sleep, nutritional intake, other pain-coping strategies such as warm baths and menthol rubs, distraction, and other current and potential stressors for the patient or family.

OBJECTIVE DATA

A complete physical examination should be done. Pay particular attention to weight, physical appearance (neat vs disheveled), guarding of painful areas, alterations in gait or mobility, and emotional affect.

NURSING DIAGNOSIS

After collecting data, the nurse analyzes it to arrive at a nursing diagnosis. Because the diagnosis reflects problem areas with which the patient wants assistance, the problem list should be developed with the patient. An initial problem list can be made with the assumption that it will change as the treatment program progresses.

When writing the actual diagnosis, consider whether the person's problem is the pain itself or difficulties as a result of the pain. With chronic pain, the nurse often is assisting the person to adapt to a different life-style. Examples of problem statements are as follows: 1) pain related to poor body mechanics, 2) restricted socialization related to decreased self-esteem and pain.

An area that frequently is neglected is assessment of the person's strengths. Persons with chronic pain are accustomed to receiving health care when they have problems.

Assisting them to maintain and develop strengths helps them to begin to consciously learn their own coping skills and to develop self-reliance. In addition, strengths often may be used to help with other problem areas. (An example of a strength that can be used for assisting with other problems might be: patient maintains positive relationship with close and extended family.)

Another aspect to consider is whether or not the patient's problem is within the realm of the nurse to treat. Assisting persons with adaptations to their chronic pain *is* within the expertise of nurses. Information on referrals is in the treatment section of this chapter.

MANAGEMENT

GENERAL CONSIDERATIONS

Working with persons in chronic pain is not easy. Restricted socialization, maladaptive family coping patterns, narcotic abuse, over or underweight, decreased physical endurance, economic and occupational problems, and emotional difficulties are common problems.

The person with chronic pain usually has sought many different health care providers to help with the pain. It may take a great deal of time to build trust in the relationship because the person has had a history of "failures" with other health care providers. People with chronic pain may not be motivated to try new approaches to pain management. They may believe that trying psychological approaches to pain management is an admission that the pain is not physical in origin. They need to be helped to see pain as a problem with *both* psychological and physical components. Learning to cope with and minimize pain takes a great deal of work and practice on the part of the person in pain. The rewards come slowly, and patients can become discouraged and despondent. In addition, the person in pain often expects a solution to the pain problem. When no easy solution is available, anger may be directed toward the nurse or others.

Management of chronic pain includes psychological, sociocultural, and physiological interventions. Sternbach says psychological approaches of pain management seldom abolish pain, but frequently reduce it, and results are longer lasting than with many surgical procedures in which the pain often returns within 6 to 18 months.[54]

The systematic study of chronic pain is relatively recent. Many interventions have not been thoroughly researched. Areas requiring research include timing of interventions, types of techniques, and characteristics of persons with pain. Reliable data on the long-term results of current pain management programs is sparse.[36]

Chronic pain programs with a strong behavioral component define the success of a pain management program in terms of decreased pain behaviors, increased physical and social activities, decreased use of health care resources, increased occupational activity, and increased ability to manage emotional distress. Pain sensation is relieved significantly for some patients, minimized for some, unchanged for a substantial number, and in a few cases, worse. Different behavioral programs report long-term, follow-up success rates ranging from 37% to 50% for decreasing pain sensation.[36]

Evaluation of the effectiveness of pain management programs is essential. Evaluation and revision is a continuous process. Clear, measurable goals and reliable pain measurement tools help to ensure adequate evaluation. There is a critical need for nurses to publish effective pain management programs and techniques to build a solid base for management of pain.

The setting in which the nurse practices and her expertise will help to determine the specific pain program that the nurse develops with the patient. In addition, the nurse offers a unique service when she develops a pain management program based on the person's perceptions of his need. Five broad areas that help to define the nurse's role in assisting the person to achieve an optimal state of wellness can be defined:

- Build trust
- Promote positive orientation
- Promote patient's control
- Promote strengths
- Set achievable health-directed goals.[18]

GOALS

One of the most important steps in working with patients with chronic pain is to assist them to set incremental, achievable goals. Goals that address activities that the person would like to accomplish and that improve or maintain the quality of life are most appropriate. Goals of complete pain relief are usually not realistic. Goal-setting confirms that the nurse can help the person with his problems. Referrals to other health care providers also may be considered at this step.

Sternbach suggests that persons set goals in three areas of their life: occupational, recreational, and social.[53] A time frame for meeting these goals helps keep them realistic. Ninety days or less is suggested for nonprogressive chronic pain.[9] If the patient sets the goals, they will reflect what the patient wants. Goals also will be more measurable if they are defined in two steps. The patient first identifies the goals. The second step is defining the measurement so that it is clear when a goal has been met (Fig. 6-3). Some

Sample	
	Date: _Feb. 7_
	Time: _12 noon_

I want to	I've reached my goal when
1 Return to work	I'm well enough to begin working at least 3 days a week
2 Make love with Bill like we used to	I'm able to enjoy sex without pain
3 Sleep more soundly	I sleep 8 consecutive hours without awakening
4 Stop taking pain pills	I can throw all my medications away
5 Drive a car	I can drive by myself to Don's school
6 Go to a movie	I can sit in a crowded theater comfortably for 2 straight hours
7 Go to a nightclub and dance	I can stand the loud noises and dance without pain
8 Not have to depend on doctors	I can stop seeing Dr. Carlton
9 Travel to see my sister	I can visit Martha in Oregon at Christmas
10 Climb stairs more quickly	I can climb 20 stairs, one right after the other

FIG. 6-3 Goal setting. (Reprinted with permission from Bresler DE, Trubo R: Free Yourself from Pain, 1st ed, p 40. New York, Simon & Schuster, 1979)

patients may need more ideas and help than others in phrasing realistic measurable goals.

Difficulties can occur in goal-setting if the patient's pain is not stabilized. A person with a rapidly progressive cancer may set day-to-day goals, whereas a person with chronic low back pain may be able to set goals for the next 90 days. If the patient avoids setting realistic goals, consider other life issues that affect his ability to set goals.

Common issues are lack of acceptance of the chronic nature of the pain, and a belief that the nurse or health care provider has the responsibility to provide pain relief. Other issues could be overwhelming stresses in the patient's life at that particular time, or secondary gain from the pain. Sternbach analyzes pain behavior from a transactional analysis viewpoint. He discusses a number of maladaptive "pain games" played by persons with chronic pain. Some persons avoid honest interactions by playing "games." Sternbach estimates approximately 10% of persons with chronic pain engage in pain games to a significant extent. (Refer to Sternbach's book for an extensive discussion of pain games.[52]) It is appropriate to assess the issues that are affecting the patient's ability to set goals and work through some of those issues. In most cases, some type of meaningful, short-term goal is possible.

Setting short-term goals and working to meet them are important interventions. The patient sees the progress he is making in relation to the problem. It creates positive expectations about the future that help to counteract helpless or hopeless feelings. Many goals also help to distract the person from preoccupation with pain. In addition, occupational goals may bring about greater economic stability for the person.

INITIAL INTERVENTIONS

Management begins with the first interaction between the patient and the nurse through development of a relationship that establishes trust. Listening and empathy promote trust and help the person to view the nurse as someone who is interested in his welfare. Data gathering also becomes an intervention because it is one of the beginning steps in assisting the person to gain insight into factors that affect pain experiences.

Education about ways of coping with pain are described throughout the chapter. Education about factors that alter pain experiences is important. An approach to this education would be to include a description and drawing of the gate control theory of pain. The gate control theory helps patients to see the importance of emotions and pain, legitimizes the pain experience, and assists them to see the nurse as someone who understands pain and can be helpful.*

Other considerations when planning care include making interventions that are additive, use of the placebo effect, reviewing current coping methods, and adapting interventions for the person. Interventions are more effective when more than one is used. Not only is the effect additive, but it helps the person to look at a range of alternatives for assistance with pain. A placebo effect can result from the influence one person has on another and can enhance the effect of interventions. Interventions need to be adapted to the patient in light of the current coping methods the person uses.

A recent trend reported in the literature is to screen persons with acute pain for their potential to develop chronic pain. Persons with acute pain who have many of the characteristics of persons with chronic pain are susceptible to developing chronic pain. It is suggested that interventions such as prescribing pain medications on a regular schedule (not p.r.n.), asking the patient to keep charts about activity levels, exploring family behavior, and assisting with occupational alternatives are helpful in preventing problems of chronic pain. Regularly scheduled return visits and promotion of positive coping strategies help to change the pattern of seeking nursing and medical attention

*VanMeter M: Personal communication. Ann Arbor, Michigan, 1981

and reinforcement for pain and illness behaviors.[15]

EMOTIONAL AND COGNITIVE INTERVENTIONS

Behavior Modification

Principles of behavior modification are used extensively in most inpatient pain clinics. Behavioral assessment focuses on identification of pain behaviors and reinforcers for pain behaviors. Treatment focuses on removal of reinforcers for pain behaviors and positive reinforcement of alternate behaviors that are incompatible with pain behaviors and that help to develop a positive adaptation. Pain behaviors are observable behaviors such as activity level in a 2-hour time period. Cognitive behavior modification views thoughts and images as behaviors. Thoughts and images are not observable for quantification; however, a log or journal can be used to have the person record thoughts, feelings, and activities. As the person records pain behaviors, he should also record the pain rating. Bresler has devised a pain rating scale for what he terms a "daily comfort log" that has a gauge of a minus 10 to a plus 10. This scale can be particularly useful because it not only helps the person focus on thoughts and activities that affect pain, but also on behaviors that have a positive effect (see Fig. 6-4). Minus 10 represents the person's pain when it is at its worst. Minus 1 represents minimal discomfort. The plus ratings quantify pleasure. Journal entries should be made a minimum of once an hour, and more if possible. Patients should keep a journal for approximately 1 week. Hourly logs of activity and socialization that record types of activities and amount of time spent on each are also helpful. Interventions to assist persons with socializing and activity are described in other sections of this chapter.

Reinforcers for pain behaviors can be identified when reviewing the journal and analyzing the person's relationships with his family. As discussed earlier in this chapter, reinforcement for pain-prone behavior often occurs in childhood. The family and spouse relationships often continue to reinforce pain behaviors. Interventions that assist persons to identify reinforcers and to work on altering them are needed. Interventions to assist persons to alter thoughts and feelings are included in the sections on relaxation and guided imagery.

Handling Anger and Depression

Within the framework of a therapeutic relationship, the nurse can assist the person to cope with depression and anger, both of which are common problems with chronic pain.[46] Ways of dealing with depression include helping the person to gain insight into factors that affect emotional states, and helping the person to find and use his "inner guide" (described in the section on mental imagery). Promoting positive expectations and hope about the future is also necessary. Just as Kübler–Ross says that not taking away hope is essential for dying persons, the same concept can be applied to persons with chronic pain.[32]

Nurses can help people to handle anger by helping them to acknowledge and express their anger, direct it appropriately, understand that anger is a common experience for persons in pain, and then assist them to use anger as a motivating force. Anger can be expressed in physical and emotional ways. It may be helpful for the person to hit pillows or other objects. Anger also can be expressed in a letter or in a tape recording. Some persons have learned from childhood not to express anger. They may turn their anger inward and instead of anger, experience guilt and depression. Acknowledgment that it is

					Sample

Record on a scale of −10 to +10
  −10 to 0 = pain
  0 to +10 = pleasure

Date: ___Feb. 3___

Time	Activity	Feeling	Duration	Rating	Comments
8:30 am	Shower	Weak	10 min	−1	Still trying to wake up; feeling very "average."
8:50 am	Eat breakfast	Relaxed	15 min	0	
9 am	Watch TV	Amused	1 hour	+1	Takes my mind off my problems
10:15 am	Read the mail	Angry	10 min	−5	Doctor bill arrived, his fee is more than expected
10:40 am	Balance checkbook	Anxious	20 min	−3	We're spending too much money
11:30 am	Housework	Depressed	45 min	−2	Can't do the things I used to
12:30 am	Phone call from my daughter	Elated	15 min	+5	During the entire call I was barely aware of discomfort
1 pm	Planning for summer vacation	Hopeful	40 min	+2	Maybe there still is room for pleasure in my life
3 pm	Call from women's club	Frustrated	5 min	−1	Had to turn down request to help at charity lunch
5:40 pm	Cooking dinner	Bored	35 min	−3	It's so monotonous
6:25 pm	Bill comes home from work	Relieved	5 min	−1	He showed me a lot of affection, made me feel better
6:30 pm	Eat dinner	Stimulated	20 min	+1	Good conversation about taking our vacation soon
8 pm	Watch TV	Lethargic	2 hours	−2	My mind wanders; thinking about future
11 pm	Get ready for bed	Fatigued	10 min	−4	Very weary, really need to sleep

Notes:

FIG. 6-4   Daily comfort log. (Reprinted with permission from Bresler DE, Trubo R: Free Yourself from Pain, 1st ed, p 34. New York, Simon & Schuster, 1979)

all right to be angry and that there are reasons to be angry may help to alter depression and assist them to begin to handle angry feelings. As a result of childhood experiences and current relationships, persons in pain often direct their anger towards others, especially the health care provider, who may be a physician, nurse, or other person. The patient needs assistance to see that there are reasons for his anger, such as the grieving process and current situations. Anger can become a productive emotion if it is channeled. Sternbach describes an active, well-adapted housewife with chronic pain who expressed both anger and resentment that she used constructively as motivating forces to cope with the pain. She refused to "roll over and die."[53]

SOCIOCULTURAL INTERVENTIONS

Family involvement is important when working with persons in chronic pain. Family relationships often promote and maintain painful life-styles by positively reinforcing maladaptive pain behaviors. A spouse who finds that his needs are attended to by the significant other only when he is having physical difficulties promotes a pain-prone type of pattern. It can also perpetuate pain behaviors such as bed rest. Maladaptive patterns develop over time and can be difficult to change. The family dynamics are often complex. Many clinicians find a behavioral approach useful in assisting families to maintain and establish adaptive, positive interactions. Analysis of the "reinforcers" for pain behaviors is essential. The nurse works together with the person and family to set goals for family behaviors. At times, a contract between husband and wife or the person and the family may be helpful. If a measurable behavior change can be identified by the person in pain and the family, a simple contract that states, "I will ——— in return

for ———," can be developed. Families and persons in pain can be assisted to identify non-pain behaviors and then provide reinforcement for them.

Education of the family concerning the person's pain program and their potential involvement in the program is essential. After meeting with the person in pain it is often helpful to meet with a close family member to help understand the person's familial environment. Meetings with the family, the person in pain, the nurse, and other health care providers can help to increase the likelihood of a successful program by ensuring consistent follow-through.

Structured groups also can be helpful for persons with chronic pain. Groups are a good forum for finding out about common concerns and sharing them. Most importantly, people can share coping strategies and develop support systems. Sternbach states that groups are often successful because persons in pain are more likely to accept constructive analysis of their behavior from other persons in pain, rather than from one of the health care providers.[52] Groups also can be used to help educate persons about chronic pain.

Assisting the person in pain to develop an extended social support network is also important. Because persons in pain tend to withdraw, they may lose socializing skills that they once had. Assistance in setting goals for increasing socialization will help reestablish self-esteem.

OCCUPATIONAL INTERVENTIONS

Persons in pain often need referral to a job-training skills center or a therapist who assists them to find other occupational and vocational work. Economically, our system of reimbursement tends to promote painful life-styles. Health care reimbursement often covers physical interventions, but may not be as liberal in coverage of social and psychological treatments. Because persons in pain often come from "laboring" occupations, their only way of maintaining an income may be to receive some type of disability payment. Helping these persons to find a satisfactory alternative is a challenge.

HOLISTIC INTERVENTIONS

Holistic interventions are interventions that involve every aspect of the person and the environment in which he moves. These interventions can be used to mobilize coping strategies and to assist in evaluation of life goals and values. Many of the interventions in the other sections include actions that are also holistic; however, the following interventions are commonly associated with holistic health.

Supporting Adaptive Responses

Nutrition and sleep problems are closely linked to pain. An adequate, balanced nutrition helps to maintain maximum energy resources to cope with pain. Sufficient sleep also helps to restore and maintain energy. Persons with pain are particularly vulnerable to difficulties with nutrition and sleep. Persons may be overweight because of inactivity from pain. They also may prepare poorly balanced meals due to difficulties with meal preparation. The pain also contributes to sleepless nights. Assistance with nutritional and sleep difficulties is essential in pain management.

Relaxation Techniques

Relaxation techniques can have numerous positive outcomes for the person with pain. According to McCaffery, relaxation can have the following effects: reduction in the effects of stress, decrease in anxiety, distraction from pain, and decrease in muscle tension and muscle contraction. It also can combat fatigue, produce a state of increased suggestibility, facilitate sleep, and enhance the effectiveness of many different types of pain interventions such as the TENS (transcutaneous electrical nerve stimulator).[37]

A wide variety of relaxation techniques have been developed in recent years. The person gains maximum benefit from the use of relaxation techniques when they are individualized. Relaxation techniques are best if they are learned when the intensity of pain is lowest. It is also essential to identify past coping styles and to assist the person to find a comfortable technique. Techniques can be evaluated on mental or physical emphasis, or both.[22] Amount of active involvement or passivity is also important. Transcendental meditation has more of a mental emphasis, whereas Jacobson's progressive relaxation technique has a physical emphasis. The Jacobson technique requires active muscular contraction.[27] Benson's relaxation response involves more passivity and focusing on breathing.[6]

Relaxation techniques occasionally have the effect of increasing awareness of pain and other bodily discomforts. In these cases, using a more active technique, adding a mantra for distraction, or using the technique when the intensity of pain is lower may be helpful. Many excellent resources for learning relaxation therapy are available and are listed in Appendix D.

Guided Imagery

Imagery often is referred to as daydreaming or using one's imagination. Use of guided imagery means that the person is alert, concentrating intensely, and imagining sensory images.[37] Persons who are successful in altering their pain experience are helped not only because the pain is more manageable, but also because they learn that they can exert some control over their pain. They may begin to have more positive expectations and hope about their future. Many patients report decreased pain and, at times, dramatic reductions in pain with guided imagery techniques. However, there are very few controlled clinical studies that report a long-term follow-up of the effectiveness of imagery techniques.

This section on guided imagery discusses imagery in relationship to pain management. General guidelines on the use of guided imagery can be found in many sources (see Appendix D).

For persons in pain, *imagery* can be defined as "use of one's imagination in a special way to achieve a specific, desired (or therapeutic) goal."[37] The images may include one, or all of the senses of vision, hearing, movement, touch, smell, and taste. It is well established that vivid imagery can produce both emotional and physiologic reactions to the imagined event or situation. In fact, Klinger states that experiencing something in imagery is in many ways equivalent to experiencing it in actuality.[31]

The way in which the nurse helps the patient to use imagery depends on the individual circumstances. In most cases, imagery will be used to try to minimize pain. Imagery can also be used to create pleasant experiences and life-enhancing attitudes. Imagery used in the latter context may support and create adaptive responses; however, it probably will not directly affect the pain the person reports.

The way a person is able to imagine events or situations reflects the same method with which he approaches things in general. It is currently popular to determine whether a person uses primarily the right or left hemisphere of the brain for coping. People who predominantly use the right side of the brain are considered to have richer, more vivid imagination. People who predominantly use the left side of the brain are considered to be more verbal and thought-process oriented. Recent evidence suggests that a person needs both sides of the brain to use imagery effectively because imagery involves not only a production of image sensations, but also an evaluative component that processes and "makes sense" of the images.[2] Different types of imagery are discussed later.

The following guidelines may be helpful when assisting persons in pain with guided imagery:

1. Assess the person's current use of his imagination and the vividness of his imagery.
2. Begin guided imagery with a relaxation technique. This reduces muscle tension and helps the person become receptive to relaxation.[2]
3. Use one image at a time to achieve maximum effect (e.g., do not switch between glove anesthesia and symptom substitution).
4. Ask the person to practice guided imagery 3 times a day.
5. Have the person try the techniques for a week. Ability to use imagery for events and situations takes time to learn.
6. Help the person to learn techniques when the pain is at a lower level. This allows the person to concentrate on learning to achieve the desired response with less difficulty.[37]
7. Ask the person to purchase a tape or record the imagery technique and practice with it. Learning the technique is then reinforced.
8. Ask the person to keep a record in a journal of the level of pain before and after each guided imagery experience.

General precautions for the use of imagery also apply to using imagery for persons with chronic pain. In addition, McCaffery suggests that the person retain enough awareness of pain so that pain as a protective mechanism is preserved. One way to do this is to ask the person to agree to trust part of his mind to monitor the pain and inform him of potential or actual harm.[37]

Many therapists use the concept of an inner guide or inner adviser.[9,51] The person develops an image of another person, often a respected authority figure or an imaginary living creature (a playmate) who helps him to gain access to unconscious images and drives. This inner adviser keeps the person informed about his feelings, expectations, and progress in incorporating new beliefs. In addition, many people turn to their inner adviser for consultation about pain and pain-related behavior and feelings. This imagery technique helps the person use the "logical" or left hemisphere to get in touch with the right hemisphere. As with any learned behavior, it may take some time to identify and develop the inner adviser. It is appropriate to emphasize with patients that the inner guide is merely a symbol of their inner self with which they are generally out of touch (see Appendix A).

Bresler has elaborated on three other types of imagery useful for persons with chronic pain. These are symptom substitution, glove anesthesia, and mind-controlled anesthesia.[9] *Symptom substitution* involves "sending" the pain to another part of the body or changing the type of pain sensation. For example, a person might send low back pain to the knees or little toe where it might be more manageable. A stabbing pain might be transformed to a pricking pain. The person relaxes and is instructed to continue moving or transforming the pain with each breath. With *glove anesthesia*, the person imagines that the hand is numbed and then transfers the numbness to other painful parts

of the body (see Appendix B). *Mind-controlled anesthesia* involves asking the person to make three drawings of the pain, with the pictures representing the pain at its worst, at its best, and as it would appear at a pleasure level of +10 level (see Appendix C). A creative nurse can also assist the person to alter his images of pain.

Other Holistic Interventions

Other holistic techniques to assist persons with chronic pain are biofeedback, acupuncture and acupressure, touch therapy, and hypnosis. (These techniques are not detailed in this chapter.)

SENSORY INTERVENTIONS

Sensory interventions are interventions that alter the sensory input to the SG, the gate in the dorsal horn of the spinal cord. Sensory interventions include interventions such as rubbing, which stimulates the large-diameter fiber input and thereby decreases pain, and interventions that alter small-diameter fiber (painful) input. Another way sensory interventions may decrease pain is to provide physical sensations that compete with pain sensations at the level of the brain stem.

Interventions that stimulate large-diameter fibers and thus help to alter the pain sensations are rubbing or tapping an area with one's fingers, using hot water bottles or heating pads, and employing metholatum rubs and massage. These interventions are most effective when the surface area directly over the painful site or on the opposite side of the body is stimulated. Because large-diameter fibers adapt to continuous stimulation, sensory interventions such as massage and metholatum rubs may work for a limited period of time. Persons will need to experiment with the timing, duration, and method of rubbing and massage to determine what is most effective for them.

Recent articles have recommended the use of ice to help to decrease pain.[38, 40] It is assumed that ice is effective by slowing down the pain impulses transmitted to the gate. Guidelines for the frequency and duration of the use of ice are not well established. One institution reports moderate pain relief and improved joint function for persons with arthritis when ice packs are applied above and below the affected joint three times a day for 20 minutes.[38] Contraindications for the use of ice are decreased sensation or poor circulation to the area where ice is applied.

Use of the TENS is becoming common. The TENS is a small portable battery-operated unit that delivers low-voltage electricity to the person's skin. It is believed that the unit is effective in controlling pain through peripheral blockade of some small-diameter fiber activity and through stimulating the release of endorphins.[26] The units are available from many pharmacies on a physician's prescription. Results with the TENS unit are variable. Some persons report dramatic relief of pain, others find their pain minimized or unaltered. Pain minimization with the TENS unit is related to the person's motivation to use the unit and the skill of the person instructing the person in its use. Persons need assistance with learning how to use the control settings and electrode placement. Electrical voltage, pulse width, and pulse rate can be adjusted. It can take a great deal of adjustment to find settings that are effective. Electrode placement is variable. The following are areas of electrode placement that have been reported: above and below the painful area, over the course of the involved nerve, over dermatomes, or over acupuncture points.

PHYSICAL INTERVENTIONS

Physical interventions include pacing activities, using principles of energy conservation, correct use of body mechanics, working on increasing exercise, and working on correct posture and gait. These interventions decrease muscle strain, increase mobility, develop competing stimuli for pain impulses, conserve energy, and reduce fatigue. Exercise may increase endorphin levels, which would tend to decrease pain; however, the amount and quality of exercise needed to increase endorphins is not yet known.

Learning to pace activities is an important intervention for a person with chronic pain. Pacing activities means undertaking activities and then stopping them before pain begins to *increase*. Persons who become frustrated with their inactivity and then increase activities for 1 day are often then bedridden for 2 to 3 days afterwards. A schedule of regular work and rest periods allows much more activity to be accomplished. Baseline activity is recorded for a 1-week period, after which the person determines the average length of time that he can do activities. Sternbach suggests setting a timer with the average length of time for activities before the pain increases, and then planning a 15 to 30-minute rest break.[52] He says further that patients who follow a schedule may find that the first few weeks they work for 45 minutes and then take a 15-minute break. The next few weeks they may work for 50 minutes and take a 15-minute break. Over a period of weeks they can often reach 2, 3, or 4 hours of activity before needing a break. Persons with cancer may not be able to increase activity time; however, pacing activities will help them to conserve energy. Use of principles of energy conservation and work simplification also decreases fatigue.

Pain can also be caused by muscle tension due to immobility. People with arthritis or people who have difficulty moving independently (e.g., in hemiparesis) may find that their pain is minimized through active and passive range of motion. In her work with persons in a hospice program, Dolan reports that proper positioning and body alignment often help to decrease pain. She describes a woman who had hemiparesis from a brain metastasis and whose severe leg pain was relieved by using corrective measures for footdrop.[17]

Proper body mechanics and posture will also help to decrease muscle strain and decrease fatigue. This aspect of pain management is discussed in Chapter 7.

ENVIRONMENTAL INTERVENTIONS

The environment can have a significant impact on pain. Anderson describes a person with terminal cancer pain whose pain improved as soon as he was moved from a medical–surgical hospital to a hospice.[1] The nurse can assess the patient's home environment and help persons to organize it. This may help to prevent excessive fatigue and increase the person's feeling of social usefulness and self-esteem.

MEDICATIONS

Two major classes of medications are used for persons with chronic pain: analgesics and antidepressants. Other medications may be prescribed for pain from specific diseases, such as anti-inflammatory agents for arthritis. Tranquilizers are not usually prescribed for persons with chronic pain. However, for pain associated with muscle tension, mild tranquilizers and muscle relaxants may be beneficial. In addition, many persons use over-the-counter medications for pain and sleep. The potential for abuse of over-the-counter drugs is high.

For persons with terminal disease, narcotic analgesics are the drugs of choice. For many years Brompton's cocktail, an opiate mixture for oral use, was advocated for use for persons with cancer pain. Recently, however, controlled studies have demonstrated that neither Brompton's cocktail nor heroin has advantages over the use of morphine.[36] The regimen used in many hospices is a high initial dose of narcotics, followed by a lower dose that still helps the person to remain comfortable.

The timing of medications is crucial in managing pain. For persons with cancer pain, the aim of drug therapy is to anticipate and prevent pain in addition to treating pain. Medications should not be given p.r.n., but rather on a regular schedule.[1] This breaks the cycle of pain associated with the anticipation of pain. McCaffery believes there is a recent trend in the United States and Canada to undertreat cancer pain with narcotics. Narcotics are not usually recommended for stable, nonterminal, chronic pain.

People with chronic, nonprogressive pain should have their narcotics, analgesics, and other medications withdrawn over a specified time period. Initially, the person records his medication use for 1 week and then the average 24-hour drug consumption is computed. A pharmacist can prepare a "pain cocktail" that incorporates the person's medication into one single, flavored mixture. The pain cocktail is taken on a regularly scheduled basis, which avoids the pattern of using medications as the person's major coping strategy. Active ingredients in the pain cocktail are reduced by 10% every week or 10 days.[23] Many persons will be able to decrease the level of medication to zero. Others will decrease their consumption significantly. Persons with serious addiction problems should be in an inpatient setting, preferably a unit where staff are knowledgeable about chronic pain.

Antidepressants are beginning to come into wider use in the treatment of chronic pain. Because of the close relationship between chronic pain and depression, it is speculated that some of the same neurotransmitters are involved in both pain experiences and depression. Antidepressants help to increase levels of important neurotransmitters that mediate pain, sleep, and mood in the CNS. The tricyclic antidepressants, especially amitriptyline, are the most frequently used.[54] Imipramine may also be useful. Doses are usually less than doses used for depression alone. Fifty to one hundred mg once a day is a usual dose. However, in a recent study, 129 persons who did not have an identifiable organic cause for their pain were treated with the higher doses of antidepressants often prescribed for depression. They reported significant improvement in their pain.[8]

Many of these drugs have serious side-effects. Teaching persons to monitor and to manage common side-effects is essential.

MEDICAL–SURGICAL INTERVENTIONS

Numerous medical specialties are involved in working with persons with chronic pain. Family physicians may work with patients on an outpatient basis. Neurosurgeons, neurologists, anesthesiologists, and psychiatrists all contribute to the medical care of persons with pain. Persons with long-term, chronic pain have usually been seen by a number of these medical specialists.

Most surgical procedures are directed toward interruption or destruction of sensory pathways to the cerebrum.[39] Follow-up data on large numbers of persons electing surgery for pain relief indicate that very few techniques have long-term success rates.[60] For most persons, pain returns anywhere from 6 to 18 months after surgery.[54] Persons who elect surgical procedures often face the possibilities of operative complications, such as loss of all sensations or loss of motor control of certain parts of their bodies, and the even-

tual return of the pain. Persons with a terminal disease may elect a surgical intervention to ease their pain. Cancer pain is frequently treated with peripheral nerve blocks and intraspinal blocks. Surgery to correct the underlying pathophysiology of a chronic pain problem can be successful in relieving pain.

Another surgical procedure that was promising in the early 1970s was direct electrical stimulation of the spinal cord and parts of the brain. Electrodes were implanted surgically in either the brain or spinal cord. Habituation to the electrical stimulation developed in a large number of persons, so this procedure is not performed on a regular basis. Continuous, low level cutaneous electrical stimulation is superior to implanted electrodes.[54]

REFERRALS

Because the person with chronic pain often has complex problems, referrals are frequently necessary. Referrals will depend on the areas of expertise of the nurse and the individual problems of the patient. Referrals are commonly made to physical therapy for complex gait and mobility problems. Referrals to agencies that train people for different occupations are essential. In addition, referrals to a social worker, psychologist, or psychiatrist may be necessary. Referrals to a physician are made when there is a consistent change in the pain quality or pain sensation. A nurse should work closely with a physician when the person's chronic pain is not in a stable pattern.

The advantages of developing an interdisciplinary team to work with persons with chronic pain are numerous. However, an individual practitioner with a broad knowledge base will be able to assist the person with chronic pain.

People who are not making progress in

meeting realistic goals may need referral to an inpatient or outpatient pain program. A list of pain clinics in the United States can be obtained from the American Society of Anesthesiologists, 515 Busse Highway, Park Ridge, Illinois 60068. Careful examination of the treatment modalities and qualifications of the practitioners is important because currently an accreditation program for pain clinics does not exist.

SUMMARY

This chapter reflects an overall philosophy that the person in chronic pain must be helped to attain an adaptive coping state through the help of the nurse, other appropriate health care providers, and by using the person's own resources. A discussion of pathophysiology, commonly used terms, and factors that influence a person's pain helps set the basis for understanding the selection and effectiveness of interventions. Interventions are divided into ten categories that contain many practical ideas and ways to help the person experiencing chronic pain.

REFERENCES

1. Anderson JL: Nursing management of the cancer patient in pain: A review of the literature. Cancer Nurs 5:33, 1982
2. Bakan P: Imagery, raw and cooked: A hemispheric recipe. In Shorr JE, Sobel GE, Robin P et al (eds): Imagery: Its Many Dimensions and Applications. New York, American Association of Mental Imagery Proceedings, Plenum Press, 1980
3. Barber TX, Spanos NP, Chaves JF: Hypnosis, Imagination, and Human Potentialities. New York, Pergamon Press, 1974
4. Beecher HK: Measurement of Subjective Responses. New York, Oxford University Press, 1959
5. Benoliel JP, Crowley DM: The patient in pain: New concepts, Publication No. 3362-PE. New York,
6. American Cancer Society Professional Education Publications, 1974
6. Benson H: The Relaxation Response. New York, Avon Books, 1975
7. Berger PA, Akil H, Watson SJ et al: Behavioral pharmacology of the endorphins. In Creger WP, Coggins CH, Hancock EW (eds): Annual Review of Medicine: Selected Topics in the Clinical Sciences, Vol 33, Palo Alto, CA, Annual Reviews, 1981
8. Blumer DB, Heilbronn MH, Pedraza E et al: Systematic treatment of chronic pain with antidepressants. Henry Ford Hosp Med J 28:15, 1980
9. Bresler DE, Trubo R: Free Yourself from Pain. New York, Simon & Schuster, 1979
10. Carr DB, Bullen BA, Skrinar GS et al: Physical conditioning facilitates the exercise-induced secretion of beta-endorphin and beta-lipotropin in women. JAMA 305:560, 1981
11. Chapman RC: Pain: The perception of noxious events. In Sternbach RA (ed): The Psychology of Pain. New York, Raven Press, 1978
12. Chaves JF, Brown JM: Self-Generated Strategies for the Control of Pain and Stress. Presented at Annual Meeting of the American Psychological Association, Toronto, Canada, August 1978
13. Chung SH, Dickenson A: Pain, enkephalin and acupuncture. Nature 283:242, 1980
14. Craig KD: Social modeling influences on pain. In Sternbach RA (ed): The Psychology of Pain. New York, Raven Press, 1978
15. Cummings D: Stopping chronic pain before it starts. Nurs 81, 11:60, 1981
16. Davitz JR, Davitz LL: Inferences of Patients' Pain and Psychological Distress: Studies of Nursing Behaviors. New York, Springer Publishing, 1981
17. Dolan MB: Controlling pain in a personal way. Nurs 82, 12:144, 1982
18. Erickson H, Tomlin E, Swain MA: Modeling and Role Modeling: A Theory and Paradigm for Nursing. Englewood Cliffs, NJ, Prentice–Hall, 1983
19. Fagerhaugh SY, Strauss A: How to manage your patient's pain . . . and how not to. Nurs 80, 10:44, 1980
20. Fordyce WE: Behavioral Methods for Chronic Pain and Illness. St. Louis, CV Mosby, 1976
21. Furmanski AR: Dynamic concepts of migraine: A character study of one hundred patients. Archives of Neurology and Psychiatry 67:22, 1952
22. Gallard L: Easing stress: How to help patients learn to relax. Patient Care 14:138, 1980
23. Halpern L: Analgesic drugs in the management of pain. Arch Surg 112:861, 1977
24. Holaday JW, Loh HH: Endorphin–opiate interactions with neuroendocrine systems. In Neuro-

chemical Mechanisms of Opiates and Endorphins: Advances in Biochemical Psycho Pharmacology. Vol 20. New York, Raven Press, 1979

25. Hardy JD, Wolff HG, Goodell H: Pain—controlled and uncontrolled. Science 117:164, 1953

26. Ignelzi RJ, Sternbach RA, Callaghan M: Somatosensory changes during transcutaneous electrical analgesia. In Advances in Pain Research and Therapy, Vol 1, New York, Raven Press, 1976

27. Jacobson E: You Must Relax, 5th ed. New York, McGraw–Hill, 1978

28. Jacox AK: Sociocultural and psychological aspects of pain. In Jacox AK (ed): Pain: A Source Book for Nurses and Other Health Professionals. Boston, Little, Brown & Co, 1977

29. Johnson M: Assessment of clinical pain. In Jacox AK (ed): Pain: A Source Book for Nurses and Other Health Professionals. Boston, Little, Brown & Co, 1977

30. Kim S: Pain: Theory, research and nursing practice. Advances in Nursing Science 2:43, 1980

31. Klinger E: Therapy and the flow of thought. In Shorr JE, Sobel GE, Robin P et al (eds): Imagery: Its Many Dimensions and Applications. New York, American Association of Mental Imagery Proceedings, Plenum Press, 1980

32. Kübler–Ross E: On Death and Dying. London, Collier–MacMillan, 1969

33. LeShan L: The world of the patient in severe pain of long duration. J Chronic Dis 17:119, 1964

34. Lindberg JB, Hunter JL, Kruszewski AZ: Person-Centered Nursing Care: Introduction to Professional Practice. Philadelphia, JB Lippincott, 1983

35. Lipman AJ: Drug therapy in cancer pain. Cancer Nurs 3:39, 1980

36. Malec J, Cayner JJ, Harvey RF et al: Pain management: Long-term follow-up of an inpatient program. Arch Phys Med Rehabil 62:369, 1981

37. McCaffery M: Nursing Management of the Patient with Pain, 2nd ed. Philadelphia, JB Lippincott, 1979

38. McCaffery M: Relieving pain with noninvasive techniques. Nurs 80 10:55, 1980

39. McDonnell D: Surgical and electrical stimulation methods for relief of pain. In Jacox AK (ed): Pain: A Source Book for Nurses and Other Health Professionals. Boston, Little, Brown & Co, 1977

40. Medical News. JAMA 246:317, 1981

41. Mehta, J: Major Problems in Anesthesia, Vol 2, Philadelphia, WB Saunders, 1973

42. Melzack R: The McGill pain questionnaire: Major properties and scoring methods. Pain 1:277, 1975

43. Melzack R, Dennis SG: Neurophysiological founda-tions of pain. In Sternbach RA (ed): The Psychology of Pain. New York, Raven Press, 1978

44. Melzack R, Torgerson WW: On the language of pain. Anesthesiology 34:1, 1971

45. Melzack R, Wall PD: Pain mechanisms: A new theory. Science 150:971, 1965

46. Merskey H, Spear FG: Pain: Psychological and Psychiatric Aspects. London, Bailliere, Tindall & Cassell, 1967

47. Parkes CM: Factors determining the persistence of phantom pain in the amputee. J Psychosom Res 17:97, 1973

48. Pilowsky I: Psychodynamic aspects of the pain experience. In Sternbach RA (ed): The Psychology of Pain. New York, Raven Press, 1978

49. Pumphrey JB: Recognizing your patients' spiritual needs. Nurs 77 7:64, 1977

50. Siegele DS: The gate control theory. Am J Nurs 74:498, 1974

51. Simonton C, Matthews–Simonton S, Creighton JL: Getting Well Again. Toronto, Bantam Books, 1981

52. Sternbach RA: Pain: A Psychophysiological Analysis. New York, Academic Press, 1968

53. Sternbach RA: How Can I Learn to Live With Pain When It Hurts So Much? LaJolla, CA, Scripps Clinic Medical Institutions, 1977

54. Sternbach RA: Clinical aspects of pain. In Sternbach RA (ed): The Psychology of Pain. New York, Raven Press 1978

55. Stewart ML: Measurement of clinical pain. In Jacox AK (ed): Pain: A Source Book for Nurses and Other Health Professionals. Boston, Little, Brown & Co, 1977

56. Strauss A, Fagerhaugh SY, Glaser B: Pain: An organizational-work-interactional perspective. Nurs Outlook 22:250, 1974

57. Tursky B, Sternbach RA: Further physiological correlates of ethnic differences in responses to shock. In Weisenberg M (ed): Pain: Clinical and Experimental Perspectives. St. Louis, CV Mosby, 1975

58. Van Knorring L et al: Pain perception and endorphin levels in cerebrospinal fluid. Pain 3:359, 1978

59. West AB: Understanding endorphins: Our natural pain relief system. Nurs 81, 11:5, 1981

60. White JC, Sweet WH: Pain and the Neurosurgeon: A Forty Year Experience. Springfield, IL, Charles C Thomas, 1969

61. Wilson RW, Elmassian BJ: Endorphins. Am J Nurs 81:722, 1981

62. Wolff HG, Wolf S: PAIN. Springfield, IL, Charles C Thomas, 1958

Appendix A

THE INNER GUIDE MENTAL IMAGERY PROCESS*

The steps below are designed to help you establish initial contact with an Inner Guide, whatever form it takes. Once you have found it, you may call upon it whenever you wish during your regular, three-times-a-day mental imagery.

1. Sit in a comfortable chair, feet flat on the floor, eyes closed. Use a relaxation process to get very comfortable and relaxed.
2. In your mind's eye, see yourself in a natural setting that gives you a feeling of warmth, comfort, peace, and serenity. Select the spot from your memory or your fantasies. Concentrate on the details of the scene. Try to experience it with all your senses—as if you were really there.
3. Notice a path emerging near you, which winds toward the horizon. Sense yourself walking along this path. It is pleasant and light.
4. Notice that in the distance there is a radiant blue-white glow, which is moving slowly toward you. There is nothing threatening about the experience.
5. As the glow comes closer, you realize it is a living creature—a person (whom you do not know) or a friendly animal.
6. As the person or creature comes closer, be aware of the details of its appearance. Is the creature masculine or feminine? See its shape and form as clearly as you can. If your guide is a person, notice details of face, hair, eyes, bone structure, build.

7. If this person or creature makes you feel warm, comfortable, and safe, you know it is an Inner Guide.
8. Ask the guide's name, and then ask for help with your problems.
9. Engage the person or creature in a conversation, get acquainted, discuss your problems as you would with a very close friend.
10. Pay careful attention to any information you receive from your guide. It may come in the form of conversation or through symbolic gestures, such as the guide's pointing toward something or producing an object that represents its advice.
11. Establish an agreement with your guide about how to make contact for future discussions.
12. Then when you are ready, let your consciousness come back slowly into the room where you are sitting and open your eyes.

Appendix B

GLOVE ANESTHESIA*

Before beginning, take a moment to get comfortable and relax . . . Sit upright in a comfortable chair, feet flat on the floor, and loosen any tight clothing or jewelry or shoes that might distract you . . . Make sure you won't be interrupted for a few minutes . . . Take the telephone off the hook if necessary . . . Now take a few slow, deep abdominal breaths . . . inhale . . . exhale . . . inhale . . . exhale.

Focus your attention on your breathing

*Reprinted with permission from Simonton O.C., Matthews-Simonton S. and Creighton J.L.: Getting Well Again. Toronto, Bantam Books, 1978.

*Reprinted with permission from Bresler DE, Trubo R: Free Yourself from Pain pp 384–388. New York, Simon & Schuster, 1979 throughout this exercise, and recognize how easily slow, deep breathing alone can help to produce a nice state of deep, gentle relaxation...Let your body breathe itself, according to its own natural rhythm...Slowly... easily...and deeply...

Now close your eyes and begin the exercise with the signal breath, a special message that tells the body that you are ready to enter a state of deep relaxation...exhale... breathe in deeply through your nose...and blow out through your mouth...You may notice a kind of tingling sensation as you take the signal breath...Whatever you feel is your body's way of acknowledging the experience of relaxation, comfort, and peace of mind...

Remember your breathing...slowly and deeply...As you concentrate your attention on your breathing, give your body a few moments to relax deeply and fully...Feel all the tension, tightness, pain, or discomfort draining away, down your spine, down your legs, and into the ground...With each breath, you may be surprised to feel yourself becoming more and more deeply and fully relaxed... comfortable...and at ease...Enjoy this nice state of relaxation for a few minutes...

Now with your eyes remaining closed, imagine that a small table is being placed in front of you, on which sits a bucket filled with a sparkling clear, odorless fluid...Can you see it in your mind's eye?...Is the bucket a metal or plastic one? What color is it?...

The fluid is an extremely potent anesthetic, one so powerful that it easily penetrates any living tissue, quickly rendering it insensitive to all feeling. In a moment, at the count of three, you will be asked to lift your right or left hand, and dip it into the imaginary bucket up to the wrist level...If you proceed through these actions as if they are real, you may be surprised to discover that the relief you experience will also be real...

One...two...three...Raise your hand and slowly dip it into the bucket...Feel your fingertips tingle as the anesthetic is quickly absorbed...Slowly dip your hand deeper and feel the numbness move up to your knuckles...Across your palm and the back of your hand...To your wrist...

The skin on your hand may now feel constricted and "tingly," and as the anesthetic quickly penetrates deeper, you may notice a numb, woodenlike feeling in the muscles of your hand and fingers...As it seeps even deeper, the bones themselves may lose all feeling...

Gently swirl your hand around in the bucket to ensure the deepest possible penetration of the anesthetic solution...Sense any remaining feelings in your hand moving out the tips of your fingers, floating down softly to the bottom of the bucket...Continue to swirl your hand around for as long as it takes to achieve total anesthesia—a deep feeling of tingly numbness.

In a moment, at the count of three, I will ask you to remove your hand from the bucket and gently to place it directly on the part of your body that hurts...This will permit you to transfer the feeling of numbness from your hand into the area of your discomfort, and in exchange, any tension, tightness, pain, or discomfort will flow from this area back into your hand...You can then dip your hand into the bucket once again to repeat the exercise...

One...two...three...

Now remove your hand from the bucket and place it directly on the part of your body that hurts...Imagine all the deep feelings of numbness from your hand streaming into your body, and simultaneously, picture your hand beginning to absorb your body's discomfort...

Gradually, the same numbness that quickly developed in your hand is now permeating the affected part of your body...Can you sense the skin constricting?...And the muscles losing all feeling as the numbness penetrates even deeper?...Can you experience your hand becoming filled with the sensations you once experienced only in that affected area?...Slowly rub your hand around the once-painful area until you feel you have transferred as much anesthesia (and absorbed as much of the discomfort) as you can. Allow yourself to be surprised to notice what an immediate difference this has made...

Then, dip your hand once again into the bucket to repeat the exercise...Swirl your hand around in the anesthetic solution, and allow the transferred feelings of discomfort to move out through your fingertips, and float gently down to the bottom of the bucket...

At the same time, feel your hand once again react to the anesthetic, deeply absorbing it through the skin, into the muscles and bones...Fill your hand once more with the feeling of total numbness...It will probably take much less time to achieve this state than it did the last time, but continue to swirl your hand around for as long as it takes, whether that be a few seconds, or even a minute or more...Soak up as much numbness as your hand possibly can...

When you're ready, put your hand back on your area of discomfort...Once again, transfer the numb, relaxed feeling deeply into the area, and if there is any remaining discomfort, take away as much of it as you can...Gently rub your hand over the area until you are ready to dip it another time...

Repeat the transfer process as many times as you wish...For each time you repeat it, you will be able to experience an even greater amount of comfort and relief in the affected area...And each time you repeat it, it will become easier and easier...

When you are ready to end this exercise, simply shake your hand briskly to return quickly all the feeling to it that existed before the exercise began. After completing this session of Glove Anesthesia, you may be surprised to notice that you will feel not only relaxed and comfortable, but energized with such a powerful sense of well-being that you will easily be able to meet any demands that arise...

To complete the exercise, open your eyes and take the signal breath...Exhale...Inhale deeply through your nose...Blow out through your mouth...And be well...

© 1976 by David E. Bresler, Ph.D.

Appendix C

MIND-CONTROLLED ANALGESIA*

This tape contains a Mind-Controlled Analgesia technique that you can use to help transform your current pain experience into what you want it to be...

Before beginning, take a moment to get comfortable and relax...Sit upright in a comfortable chair, close your eyes, and loosen any tight clothing or jewelry or shoes that might distract you. Make sure you won't be interrupted for a few minutes...Take the telephone off the hook if necessary...Now take a few slow, deep abdominal breaths... inhale...exhale...inhale...exhale...

Focus your attention on your breathing throughout this exercise, and recognize how easily slow, deep breathing alone can help to produce a nice state of deep, gentle relaxation...Let your body breathe itself, according to its own natural rhythm...Slowly... easily...and deeply...

Now let's begin the exercise with the signal breath, a special message that tells the

*Reprinted with permission from Bresler DE, Trubo R: Free Yourself from Pain pp 372–373. New York, Simon & Schuster, 1979

body that you are ready to enter a state of deep relaxation...Exhale...Breathe in deeply through your nose...and blow out through your mouth...You may notice a kind of tingling sensation as you take the signal breath...Whatever you feel is your body's way of acknowledging the experience of relaxation, comfort, and peace of mind...

Remember your breathing...Slowly and deeply...As you concentrate your attention on your breathing, give your body a few moments to relax deeply and fully...Feel all the tension, tightness, pain, or discomfort draining away, down your spine, down your legs, and into the ground...With each breath, you may be surprised to feel yourself becoming more and more deeply and fully relaxed...comfortable...and at ease...Enjoy this nice state of relaxation for a few minutes...

Remember your breathing, slowly and deeply from the abdomen...Now take a brief inventory of your body, starting at the top of your head, working down to the tips of your toes...Is every part of your body totally relaxed and comfortable? If so, wonderful. Enjoy how good it feels...

However, if there is still any part of your body that is not yet relaxed and comfortable, simply inhale a deep breath, and send it into that region, bringing soothing, relaxing, nourishing, healing oxygen into every cell of that area, comforting it and relaxing it...As you exhale, imagine blowing out—right through your skin—any tension, tightness, pain, or discomfort from that area...Again, as you inhale, bring relaxing, healing oxygen into every cell of that region, and as you exhale, blow away—right through the skin and out into the air—any tension or discomfort that remains in that area...

In this way, you can dispatch your breath to relax any part of your body which is not yet as fully relaxed and comfortable as it can be...

Breathe slowly and deeply, and with each breath you may be surprised to find that you have become twice as relaxed as you were before...and that you are able to blow away twice as much tension and discomfort as you did with the previous breath...inhale...exhale...Twice as relaxed...Inhale...exhale...Twice as comfortable...

Now, paint a picture in your mind's eye of your discomfort at its very worst...Recall the symbolic picture you drew as fully and as clearly as you possibly can...(Try to remember this image, since it will soon become a thing of the past...) Can you vicariously experience the agony that was once associated with it?

Now...watch how quickly your discomfort passes as you transform this image to the one of your discomfort at its best...See how powerfully the mind's eye affects what you experience...As you carefully examine this second picture in your imagination, notice how different you feel...Fully sense the experience of your discomfort at its best, and allow this image to become strong, natural, and real...

An even more powerful way to stimulate the body's healing abilities is to transform the second picture to the third one...Unlock your creative potential, and dissolve any remaining pictures of discomfort into the image of how you most want to be...Use your imagination to see yourself exactly as you want to be...

You don't have to tell your body how to heal itself, for it already knows...All you need to do is to tell your body what you want it to do, how you want it to be...Then watch what happens through your mind's eye...

If a part of your body has been injured, for example, you may see and experience a rush of new blood to that area, carrying with each heartbeat the oxygen and vital nutrients essential to the healing process...In your imagination, you may see your body's immune system spring to life—the white blood cells racing to the injured area to metabolize and carry away any damaged tissue . . . Watch closely as the areas of irritation, inflammation, or infection are replaced by the formation of new, healthy tissue . . . See in your mind's eye what happens as the area of discomfort becomes healed and restored . . .

By focusing your attention on the experience of being as you want to be, you help your body make it a reality . . . You may continue to work with this image for as long as you like . . . Breathe slowly and deeply, and sense the healing process in action . . .

When you end this exercise, you may be surprised to notice that you feel not only relaxed and comfortable, but energized with such a powerful sense of well-being that you will easily be able to meet any demands that arise . . .

To complete the exercise, open your eyes and take the signal breath . . . Exhale . . . Inhale deeply through your nose . . . Blow out through your mouth . . . And be well . . .

© 1976 by David E. Bresler, Ph.D.

Appendix D

AIDS FOR LEARNING RELAXATION AND IMAGERY

Audiotapes

Relaxation

1. Budhzynski TH: Relaxation Training Program. BMA Audio Cassette Publications, 1974.
   200 Park Avenue South, New York, NY 10003
2. Carrington P: Clinically standardized meditation (CMS) Self-Regulated Course (audiotapes and manual). Pace Educational Systems, 1979.
   P.O. Box 113, Kendall Park, NJ 08824
3. Cotler SB, Guerra JJ: Self-Relaxation Training. Research Press, 1976.
   Box 3177, Champaign, IL 61820

4. Stroebel CG: Quieting Response Training. BMA Audio Cassette Publications, 1978.
   200 Park Avenue South, New York, NY 10003

Imagery

1. Cassetes available from:
   BMA Audio Cassettes Publications.
   200 Park Avenue South
   New York, NY 10003
   (212) 674–1900
2. Prerecorded tapes of D.E. Bresler's techniques available from:
   Center for Integral Medicine
   P.O. Box 967
   Pacific Palisades, CA 90272

Books

Relaxation

1. Benson H: The Relaxation Response. New York, William Morrow & Co, 1975
2. Carrington P: Freedom in Meditation. Garden City, NY, Doubleday & Co, 1978
3. Cautela JR, Groden J: Relaxation: A Comprehensive Manual for Adults, Children, and Children with Special Needs. Champaign, IL, Research Press, 1978
4. Davis M et al: The Relaxation and Stress Reduction Workbook. San Francisco, New Harbinger Publications, 1980
5. Jacobson E: You Must Relax. 5th ed. New York, McGraw–Hill, 1978
6. Mitchell L: Simple Relaxation. New York, Athenaeum Publishers, 1979
7. Rosen GR: The Relaxation Book: An Illustrated Self-Help Program. Englewood Cliffs, NJ, Prentice–Hall, 1978

Imagery

1. Bresler DE: Free Yourself from Pain. New York, Simon & Schuster, 1979
2. Kroger WS, Fezler WD: Hypnosis and Behavior Modification: Imagery Conditioning. Philadelphia, JB Lippincott, 1976
3. McCaffery M: Nursing Management of the Patient with Pain, 2nd ed. Philadelphia, JB Lippincott, 1979
4. Samuels M, Samuels N: Seeing With the Mind's Eye: The History, Techniques and Use of Visualization. New York, Random House, 1975
5. Simonton OC, Matthews–Simonton S, Creighton JL: Getting Well Again. Toronto, Canada, Bantam Books, 1978

7

Low
Back
Pain

Margaret M. Jacobs

Low back pain is a common health problem that most people experience at least once during their lifetime. It has been a problem recorded in cave drawings, managed by Hippocrates, and described in the Bible. The pain can range from a minor, annoying, self-limited episode; to an extremely painful, disabling condition that impairs a person's mobility and prevents an active life-style. Although there is an abundance of literature about low back pain, little of it is validated by research findings. Numerous factors contribute to the problem, and in most people the cause of the pain will not be found. Hence, low back pain is a complex problem both to evaluate and to manage. This complexity frequently produces frustration for the patient, the family, and also for the health care provider. Continuity of care and coordination of care is essential in addressing this frustration, restoring the patient's health to its highest level, and minimizing its impact on the family.

The nurse has a vital role in the care of these patients by providing direct care, continuity, and coordination of care given by other health providers. The purpose of this chapter is to provide a guide for the nurse in the interpretation and nursing management of low back pain. The chapter reviews pathophysiology and contributing factors involved in producing low back pain, and provides an assessment guide and management strategies for the nurse to use in caring for patients with low back pain.

INCIDENCE AND ECONOMIC IMPACT

Although the incidence of low back pain is high, the actual incidence can only be estimated because most people do not seek medical care for it, and most data are from hospitalized patients or those involved in specialty clinics. One estimate from the National Center for Health Statistics is that there are 18 million physician visits for low back pain each year.[7] Another study estimates that 2% of a general practitioner's patients have complaints of low back pain each year.[33] The Division of Health Care Statistics reports that in 1980 there were 96,000 hospital discharges with a diagnosis of lumbago and 21,000 with lumbago with sciatica.*

*Division of Health Care Statistics, National Hospital Discharge Survey, National Center for Health Statistics, 1980. Unpublished data

More females than males were hospitalized with these diagnoses, most patients were white, and most were between 15 and 65 years old.

Low back pain is the second most common reason (after upper respiratory infections) for sick time from work.[1,15,16,33] It is a major cause of loss of wages and long-term disability. The National Safety Council reports that 25% of all injuries are related to job injuries from overexertion, primarily from lifting, but including push-and-pull injuries. They estimate that 12 million people lost work days and over 1 billion dollars were spent in workman's compensation costs.[32] In 1976, approximately 38% of the compensation paid for all disabling injuries in the United States was for back injuries.[22,24] In another study of those disabled, one fifth were unable to work, two fifths made a job change, and two fifths were limited in the type of work they could perform.[33] Only 50% of those off work over 6 months return to work.[17] In summary, low back pain is a major health problem that has a large economic impact on society.

DEFINITIONS

The most common terms used in reference to low back pain include lumbago, sciatica, herniated disk, slipped disk, trigger points, and recurrence. Standard definitions are unavailable. For the purpose of this chapter, the terms are defined as follows:

Low back pain: Pain experienced in the lumbar area extending from the first lumbar vertebra to the first sacral vertebra. The pattern of low back pain can vary and is discussed in a separate section.

Lumbago: Lumbar back pain with an abnormal back examination (usually muscle spasm or pain on palpation of the back but no neurologic symptoms).

Sciatica: Pain radiating down the sciatic nerve, over the buttocks, posterior thigh, calf, and into the foot. Movements that cause stretching or pressure on the nerve produce pain. Neurologic deficits are commonly associated with it.

Trigger point: Focal area of hyperirritable muscle tissue that is painful with stimulation or palpation

Herniated disk: Displacement of an intervertebral disk that can be of several degrees of severity. Low back pain with sciatica and neurologic deficits usually are present.

Slipped disk: Lay term for a herniated disk

Recurrence: A second episode of symptoms following a symptom-free period

Lumbar lordosis: Concavity of lumbar spine

Swayback: Exaggerated lumbar lordosis

MECHANISMS OF LOW BACK PAIN

ANATOMY AND PHYSIOLOGY

The spine consists of thirty-three vertebrae, which are divided into five regions: seven cervical, twelve thoracic, five lumbar, five sacral (which are fused together) and four coccygeal vertebrae. Low back pain involves primarily the lumbar vertebrae and, to a minimal extent, the sacrum. Therefore, the following discussion is limited to the anatomy and physiology of the lumbar spine. The lumbar spine supports the weight of the body and its movement, and distributes that weight to the lower extremities.

To accomplish its support function, the lumbar spine has a complex structure. The lumbar vertebrae are aligned in a concave

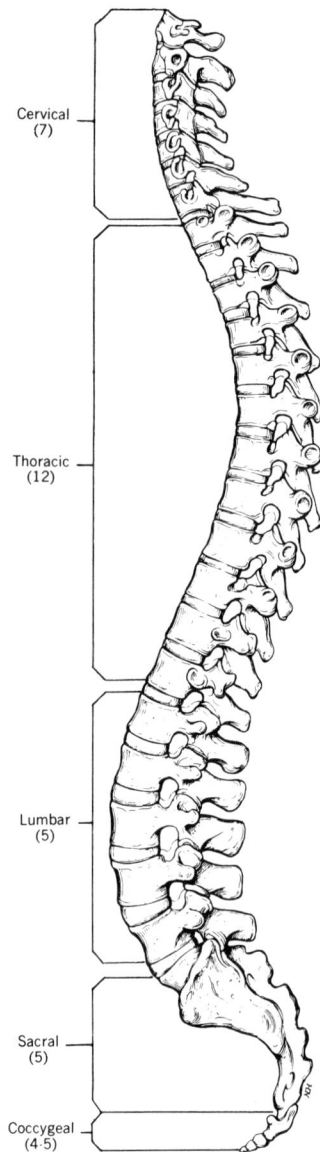

Cervical
(7)

Thoracic
(12)

Lumbar
(5)

Sacral
(5)

Coccygeal
(4-5)

FIG. 7-1 *Lateral view of the vertebral column.*

manner forming a lordotic curve (Fig. 7-1). There is a large degree of movement in three planes: flexion–extension, lateral bend, and axial rotation.

The anterior portion of the lumbar spine consists of large vertebral bodies and intervertebral disks (Fig. 7-2). A *disk* is an avascular, fibrocartilaginous structure located between two adjacent vertebral bodies. It acts as a shock absorber. It consists of the inner nucleus pulposus, which is a gelatinous substance, and the outer annulus fibrosus, which is a tough, fibrous material.

The posterior portion of the spine consists of the extensions from the vertebral bodies: the pedicles, laminae, spinous processes, and ligaments that together form the vertebral (spinal) canal. The lumbar spinal canal is triangular-shaped. The spinal cord terminates at the first lumbar vertebra and the spinal nerve roots run vertically as the *cauda equina* (Fig. 7-3). The spinal nerve roots exit above the disk through the intervertebral foramen, which are formed by the pedicles of two adjacent vertebrae. The superior articular process of one pedicle joins the inferior articular process of the adjacent pedicle at the *facet joint*. The disks, intervertebral foramen, and facet joints can be sites of pathology, contributing to low back pain.

Ligaments and muscles support the lumbar spine. The anterior and posterior longitudinal ligaments hold the vertebral bodies and disks together. In contrast to the posterior longitudinal ligament, the anterior longitudinal ligament is broad and strong. Transverse and spinous ligaments extend laterally and posteriorly, connecting the spinous processes. The ligamenta flava connect laminae and also the articular facets. Muscles involved in the support of the spine include the paraspinous muscles (in particular, the sacrospinal muscles), abdominal, gluteus maximus, iliopsoas, and hamstring muscles. They provide the spine with stability during movement.

The innervation of the lumbar spine is poorly understood, which makes localizing

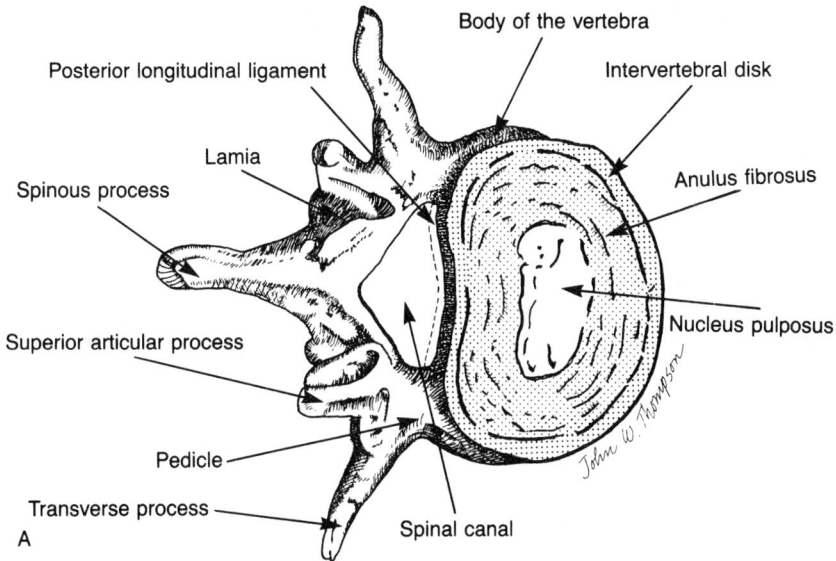

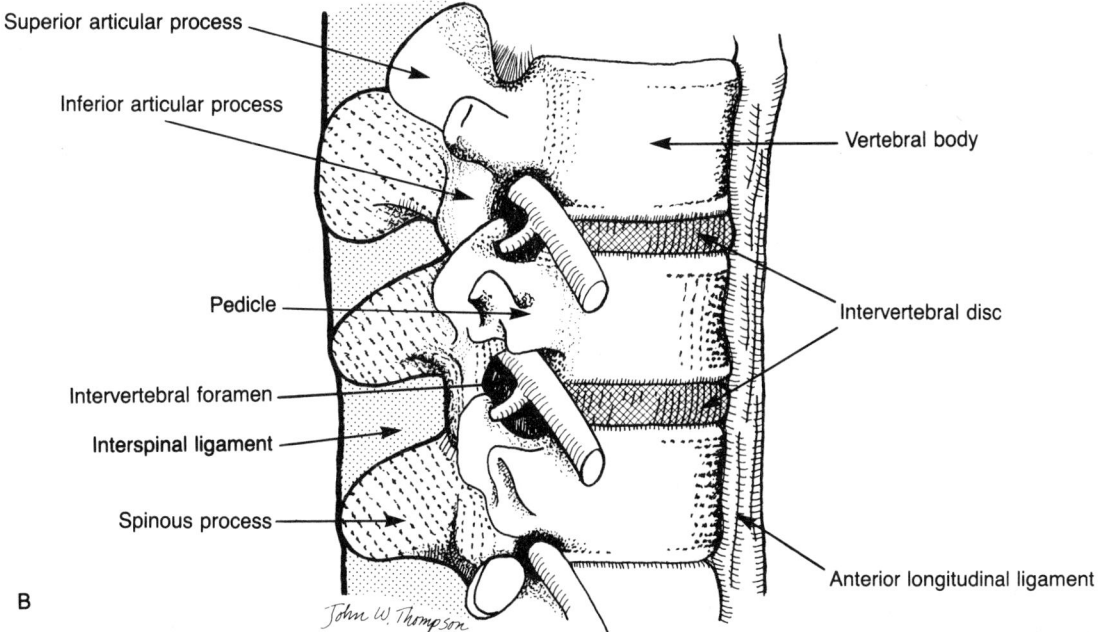

FIG. 7-2 *Cross section of the lumbar vertebrae. (A) Superior view; (B) lateral view of adjacent lumbar vertebrae.*

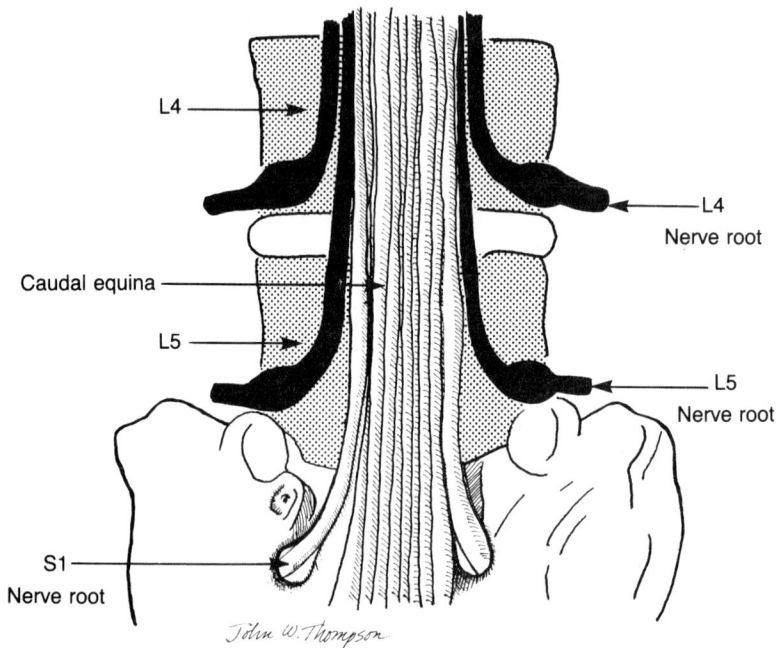

FIG. 7-3 *Posterior view of nerve root pathways from the vertebral column.*

low back pain to specific structures difficult. It is known that the vertebral bodies have no sensory nerve endings. There are pain nerve endings in the ligaments, muscles, periosteum of the bone, outer part of the annulus fibrosus, and synovium of the articular facets. The fibers join to form the sinovertebral nerves and enter the spinal column through the lumbar vertebrae and first sacral vertebra.[30] There appears to be sensory overlap between vertebral areas, which may contribute to the diffuse nature of low back pain.

Mechanical stress properties of compression, torsion, and shear affect the lumbar spine. *Compression* is a downward force on the spine that tends to squeeze vertebrae together. Compression on the lumbar spine is greatest in the sitting position, less in the standing position because the load is distributed to the legs, and least in the recumbent position. Abdominal compression, through good muscle tone, diminishes the compression stress on the lumbar spine. *Torsion* is a force that causes a twisting motion. *Shear* is a force causing sliding or slipping (opposite movement of two connecting parts in the same plane). The lordotic curve accentuates torsion and shear in the lumbar area. Torsion, shear and compression stress are modified by the strength of the supporting musculature (especially the abdominal muscles), posture, and the presence of underlying pathology of the spine. These forces, combined with the amount of movement of the lumbar area, make the low back susceptible to injury and, consequently, pain.

Pressure develops within the intervertebral disk when compression, torsion, and shear stress are placed on the lumbar spine. According to research by Nachemson, the intradiscal pressure varies according to the position of the spine, the type of stress applied, and the amount of support the lumbar spine receives (Fig. 7-4).[20, 21] The pressure varies in the same manner as compression loads and is lowest in the supine position and greatest in the sitting, bent-forward position. It is less with standing than sitting. Coughing, straining, and laughing increase intradiscal pressure, as does adding weight to the arms. Lifting objects while the legs are straight and back bent significantly increases the pressure, but if the back is kept straight and the knees and hips flexed, the pressure increases only slightly. The greater the distance between the load lifted and the body, the larger the rise in the intradiscal pressure. Supports, such as armrests (or inclining backrests in cars), decrease intradiscal pressure. Knowledge about the effect of body position and mechanical loads on the lumbar spine and the consequent effect on low back pain have implications for management recommendations that are discussed later in this chapter.

PATTERNS OF LOW BACK PAIN

The pathophysiology of low back pain is not well understood. Research has been unable to pinpoint the site of origin of the pain, partly because the innervation of the spine is not well understood, and because the spine is difficult to examine due to its location. Low back pain can be confined to the lumbar area, radiate from the lumbar spine outward into the lumbar sacral dermatones and into the hips or legs, or be referred from the pelvic and abdominal viscera into the low back itself.

The pattern of the pain is influenced by various factors. It can be produced by irritation, pressure, or injury of the nerve roots within the spinal canal or as they exit from

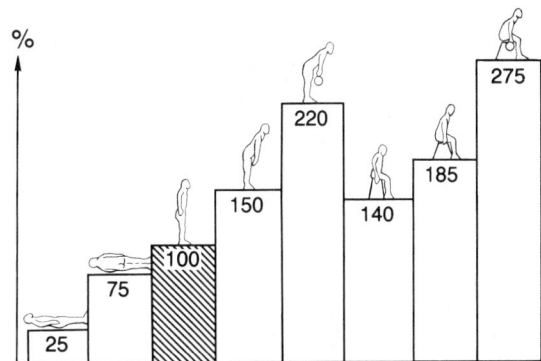

FIG. 7-4 Relative change in pressure (or load) in the third lumbar disc in living subjects in various positions. (Redrawn from Nachemson AL: The lumbar spine: An orthopaedic challenge. Spine 1:59, 1976)

the canal through the intervertebral foramen. The pain may arise from irritation or injury to the facet joints, ligaments, or muscles in the low back. Local pain occurs with any condition or injury involving lumbar pain nerve endings, and is felt near the affected part of the spine. The pain can be sharp or dull, and will vary in intensity with movement. It can be steady or intermittent. Pain referred to the lumbar sacral dermatones will vary in the same manner as local pain. Pain referred from the viscera to the low back will not be affected by movement.

Radicular pain is produced by compression or irritation of a spinal nerve root, usually proximal to the intervertebral foramen. However, the pain can be due to entrapment of the nerve root within the foramen. The sciatic nerve is involved most often because it consists of the fourth and fifth lumbar and first sacral nerve roots. The pain radiates down the posterior aspect of the thigh and into the foot. Either the posterior, lateral, or anterior aspect of the leg is involved, depending on which nerve root is affected. Coughing, sneezing, straining, and flexing the spine stretch the lumbar nerve roots and

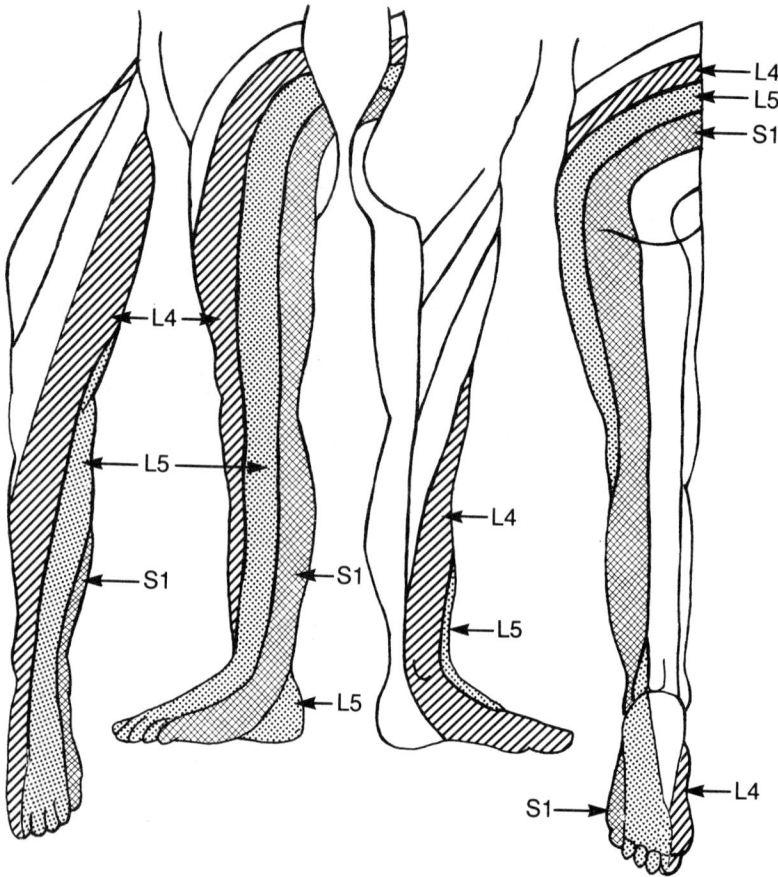

FIG. 7-5 *Dermatome chart of the lower extremity. (Redrawn from Keegan JJ: Diagnosis of herniation of lumbar intervertebral disks by neurological signs. JAMA 126:868, 1944. Copyright 1944, American Medical Association)*

aggravate radicular pain. Neurologic deficits (numbness, tingling, paresthesia, weakness, atrophy, deep tendon reflex loss) can accompany radicular pain. Findings depend on which spinal nerve is involved (Fig. 7-5).

Identified pathophysiology, such as osteoarthritis or degenerative disk disease, may or may not produce low back pain, and pain can be present without any specific abnormality identified in the spine. The pattern of pain exhibited also can vary both in its location, radiation, and intensity, given the

same anatomic abnormality. More than one factor can contribute to the pattern of pain experienced, making determination of the cause and the management approach difficult.

ETIOLOGY OF LOW BACK PAIN

The etiology of low back pain is controversial because the pathophysiology is not well understood. In most people, no cause will be found. However, many conditions appear to

Causes of Low Back Pain

Mechanical
    Lumbar muscle strain
    Intervertebral disc degeneration
    Fracture
    Spondylolysis and spondylolisthesis
Nerve root entrapment syndromes
Arthritis
    Osteoarthritis
    Ankylosing spondylosis
    Rheumatoid
Congenital abnormalities
Metabolic disorders
    Osteoporosis
    Osteomalacia
Tumors
Infection
Extraspinal
Psychosocial

cause or contribute to low back pain (see "Causes of Low Back Pain"). The most common group of causes is mechanical in nature and includes strains, fracture, intravertebral disk degeneration (including herniated disk), spondylolysis and spondylolisthesis. Injury or poor body mechanics frequently contribute to mechanical causes of low back pain.

Lumbar muscle strain often follows a specific movement, such as bending, lifting, twisting, or falling. Sudden motion, combined turning and lifting, repeated lifting, and prolonged unchanged positions also can cause strain. Poor physical conditioning prior to initiating athletic activities, sporadic participation in sports, weakened abdominal muscles, and obesity increase the probability of lumbar strain. Women who do not recondition their abdominal muscles postpartum often experience lumbar muscle strain.

Poor posture also contributes to lumbar muscle strain. Normal posture keeps a balance between the cervical and lumbar lordo-ses and the thoracic kyphosis. Poor posture accentuates lumbar lordosis: the head is thrust forward and the abdomen and buttocks protrude, creating swayback. Weak abdominal muscles and obesity aggravate poor posture. High heels accentuate poor posture by increasing lumbar lordosis. Postural changes from pregnancy can produce lumbar strain and pain. The added weight is centered anteriorly, which causes a compensatory, exaggerated lumbar lordosis to maintain balance. Patients without evidence of a specific etiology for their low back pain often are categorized as having muscular strain or lumbago, rather than having low back pain of unknown etiology.

Strained muscles or sprained ligaments are the most common types of mechanical injury causing low back pain, but compression fractures, which result from a fall or some other trauma, also cause low back pain. Fractures are more common in the elderly. If the trauma is minimal, underlying pathology such as osteoporosis, malignancy, or long-term steroid therapy, which predisposes the spine to fracture, frequently is present. Shear and torsion stress can produce fractures involving the transverse processes, whereas compression fractures usually involve the vertebral bodies. Partial dislocation of a lumbar facet joint from trauma also can produce pain.

Intervertebral disk degeneration is another cause of mechanical low back pain. The pain can be severe, chronic, or recurrent. Degenerative disk disease occurs more frequently in men and in the 30 to 60 year-old age group. The disks between the fourth and fifth lumbar vertebrae, and between the fifth lumbar vertebra and the first sacral vertebra, are involved most frequently.

Golub describes three stages of degenerative disk disease.[13] Stage I, nuclear degeneration, is characterized by instability due to softening and fragmentation of the disk. Repeated trauma may accelerate this process. Patients may have intermittent episodes of low back pain. Stage II, nuclear displacement, occurs after some type of injury (e.g., flexion or torsional stress), leading to retrodisplacement of the disk. The injury does not have to be severe. In older people, a sneeze or trivial movement can cause displacement. Vertebrae with degenerative changes withstand mechanical stress poorly. The displacement (herniation) is usually unilateral and can be of several degrees. The nucleus can bulge through the weakened posterior annulus (prolapse), rupture through the annulus but not through the posterior longitudinal ligament (protrusion), or rupture through both the annulus and posterior longitudinal ligament, with a fragment extruding beyond (extrusion). Occasionally the extruding fragment can break off into the spinal canal. Stage III, fibrosis and repair, is characterized by collagen formation, which acts to stabilize the disk. Repair takes a long time because disks are avascular.

Other causes of mechanical low back pain include spondylolysis and spondylolisthesis. Spondylolysis is a structural defect in the vertebral isthmus (pedicle) of the spine. Spondylolisthesis is a more progressive defect and is characterized by forward displacement of one vertebral body on another. These conditions may be asymptomatic or may produce low back pain. They can be congenital, but usually are acquired through trauma and are aggravated by tension and shear stress. Degenerative changes and arthritis of the facet joints may be associated with it.

Nerve Root Entrapment

Nerve root entrapment syndromes, which can cause low back pain and sciatica, are conditions that modify the normal configuration of the intervertebral foramen. Degenerative changes in this area involve the disk and facet joints and affect the specific spinal nerve that passes through the canal. The fourth and fifth lumbar vertebrae are most susceptible. Osteophyte formation may narrow the canal, causing pressure on a nerve. *Spinal stenosis* is narrowing of the lumbar spinal canal, which causes pressure on the spinal roots prior to their entering the intervertebral foramen. This condition is most commonly seen in the elderly with degenerative disk disease. The pain is intermittent and is partially relieved by stopping the activity that produced the pain.

Arthritis

Arthritic conditions can contribute to low back pain. Osteoarthritis of the lumbar spine, especially the facet joints, can produce a nerve root entrapment syndrome. Pain is worse in the morning and better after exercise. *Ankylosing spondylitis*, a progressive inflammatory arthritic condition, is more common in men, involves destruction of the sacroiliac joints as well as the vertebrae (including the lumbar vertebrae), and leads to immobilization of the spine. Rheumatoid arthritis can involve the lumbar spine but is not a common cause of low back pain.

Congenital Abnormalities

Congenital abnormalities of the spine are common but by themselves probably do not cause low back pain. They may, however, predispose the patient to mechanical causes previously mentioned. Congenital abnormalities found in the lumbar spine include *facet tropism* (asymmetry of the facet joints), spina bifida occulta, and transitional vertebrae, including lumbarization of the first sacral vertebra and sacralization of the fifth lumbar vertebra. Transitional vertebrae are seen on x-ray film. Lumbarization essentially is a sixth lumbar vertebra while sacralization occurs when the fifth lumbar vertebra is fixed to the sacrum. Neither of these conditions has been found to cause low back pain.

Other Causes

Less common causes of low back pain include metabolic disorders, tumors, and infection. Metabolic disorders, such as osteoporosis, osteomalacia, Paget's disease, and heavy metal poisoning can cause low back pain. Osteoporsis is the most common of this group of disorders as a source of low back pain. Osteoporosis is usually found in postmenopausal women and can be asymptomatic until a minor trauma precipitates an episode of pain. The pain is relieved with rest. Tumors of the lumbar spine producing low back pain are rare but include benign tumors (e.g., hemangioma and meningioma) and malignant tumors (multiple myeloma and metastatic cancer from the breast, lung, prostate, kidney, and gastrointestinal tract). Infection is another relatively rare cause of low back pain. Tuberculosis and osteomyelitis are included in this group.

Low back pain can be referred pain from extraspinal sources. Extrinsic sources include gynecologic disorders (dysmenorrhea, retroverted uterus, endometriosis, fibroids, ovarian cyst, and pelvic inflammatory disease), prostate disease, renal disease (calculi, infection, neoplasm), hip disease, idiopathic lumbar scoliosis not treated in adolescence, pregnancy, abdominal masses, abdominal aortic aneurysm, Leriche's syndrome and gastrointestinal disease (inflammatory bowel disease, cancer). Other visceral diseases, such as peptic ulcer, pancreatic disease, and cholecystitis refer pain to the middle or upper back rather than the low back.

Psychosocial factors predispose to, precipitate, and perpetuate low back pain, rather than act as a single cause.[4] Both psychosocial factors and organic disease often are present simultaneously. Predisposing psychosocial factors include personality, work, home, and demographic characteristics. Several studies in the literature relate high scores in the depression, hysteria, and hypochondriasis sections of the Minnesota Multiphasic Personality Inventory (MMPI) with patients having low back pain, regardless of whether organic causes are also identified.[6,23] These personality characteristics seem to contribute to a patient's perception of pain. People with hypochondriacal and hysterical characteristics are more anxious; anxiety produces muscle tension, which causes pain. Pain causes more anxiety and, hence, a positive feedback cycle evolves that perpetuates the pain. Emotions of frustration and helplessness aggravate this cycle. The source of the patient's anxiety is often not known; other coping mechanisms are not developed, and the outlet for the stress is somatic.

Work characteristics of heavy or repeated lifting, forward stooping, long periods of unchanged positions, sudden maximal physical efforts, and vibrational stresses are predisposing factors. Nachemson found that truck and tractor drivers have a higher incidence of low back pain, as do people who drive to work.[20,21] People with sedentary jobs have a greater incidence than those with jobs that involve standing and walking.

Other factors such as sporadic exercise, multiple pregnancies, and poor physical fitness increase one's risk for low back pain. Persons active in sports involving rotational movements, such as golf, tennis, baseball, gymnastics, and football have a higher risk. Fatigue, socioeconomic and emotional stress (e.g., job dissatisfaction, divorce, and alcohol abuse), education level, religion, age, a history of smoking, and chronic cough are risk factors. People who are more aware of their bodies also have a higher incidence. How often each risk factor is present before an episode of low back pain is not known, but more than one factor usually is present.

Precipitation of low back pain may at times be related to psychosocial stress, but this relationship has not been well studied. Significant life events before the onset of low back pain may be elicited during the history. Trauma or incorrect body mechanics during an activity often precipitate an acute episode of pain.

Psychosocial factors are associated with the duration of symptoms. Regardless of the presence of organic disease, the pain can be prolonged and result in invalidism and disability in the presence of depression, anxiety, hysteria, fear, or anger. However, chronic pain also can cause these emotions. A person's emotional makeup and life situation affect the perception of pain and the reaction to it. One's attitude can influence the outcome of the treatment program, frequently negatively. The patient may develop pain disability behaviors (e.g., moaning, wincing, and overcautious behavior) that may impede recovery. Subconscious secondary gains may result that perpetuate the pain and suffering by bringing rewards (attention, manipulation of significant others) or meeting dependency needs that the person is unable to obtain in other ways.

Another psychosocial factor that may perpetuate low back pain is malingering. This entity differs from secondary gain in that there is a conscious deception of the health care provider and others for the purpose of gaining some reward from the illness, often monetary compensation.

Psychosocial factors, the methods that the patient uses to cope with pain, and the chronicity of the problem affect family relationships and relationships with others. Relationships can be strained by the attention the person demands and role changes that occur. Chronic low back pain can force the person to relinquish functions such as earning income or doing household chores. Community involvement may decrease. Other family members may assume new roles (employment, cooking) that often create conflict within the family structure and result in resentment, frustration, and guilt in both the patient and family members.

CLINICAL MANIFESTATIONS OF LOW BACK PAIN

Low back pain can present as an acute episode, intermittent acute episode, or a chronic problem. An acute episode can progress into a chronic problem. Recurrences of acute low back pain are common, both as isolated episodes as well as exacerbations in patients with chronic low back pain. The recurrence rate can be as high as 50% in the first year following an acute episode.[31] The more frequent the recurrence, the poorer the prognosis. To evaluate the pain, the nurse needs to be aware of the clinical manifestations of low back pain based on its etiology.

Low back pain from lumbar strain and sprain usually follows an injury or a movement such as bending, twisting, or lifting. The patient may feel something "give" in his back. Cold weather or a draft may precipitate an episode. The onset of pain can be immediate or gradual, beginning with a dull ache or stiffness that increases in intensity over hours or days. The pain is limited to the low back and buttocks and rarely radiates down the legs. Motion of the spine produces pain but coughing or straining does not. The pain is worse at the end of the day. Lumbar strains are normally episodic occurrences but can occasionally be chronic if poor posture is an aggravating factor. Pain is relieved by rest.

TABLE 7-1
NERVE-ROOT–ASSOCIATED NEUROLOGIC DEFICITS

ROOT	DISC	NEUROLOGIC DEFICITS
L_4 root	L_3–L_4 herniation	Absent or decreased knee reflex Quadriceps atrophy and weakness
L_5 root	L_4–L_5 herniation	Extensor weakness of great toe Numbness and pain along L_5 dermatome (top of foot) Weak heel-walking
S_1 root	L_5–S_1 herniation	Absent or decreased ankle reflex Numbness, pain along S_1 dermatome (lateral foot and sole) Weak toe-walking Calf atrophy

Muscle spasm of the paraspinous and gluteal muscles usually is palpated on exam and will intensify the pain. No neurologic deficit is elicited.

A herniated disk presents as an episode of severe low back pain that usually follows trauma or sudden movement, in particular a flexion–rotation force. Making a bed is a common precipitating factor. In older people with degenerative disk disease, a sneeze or trivial movement can cause it. The pain radiates down the leg in a dermatome distribution and is caused by compression of the nerve root by the disk (see Fig. 7-5). The pain is aggravated by movement of the spine except in one direction, which relieves it. The exam shows flattening of the lordotic curve and a list away from the side of the herniated disk. Flexion is limited; it produces radicular pain. A herniated disk compresses the nerve root below it. For example, a herniated disk between the fourth and fifth lumbar vertebrae causes pressure on the fifth lumbar nerve root. Paresthesias, hyper or hyposensitivity, numbness, and weakness may be reported in the dermatone distribution of the nerve root (see Table 7-1). The fifth lumbar and first sacral roots are involved most frequently. Straight-leg raising stretches the nerve root and elicits pain. Clinical findings are usually unilateral. If the herniation is large and involves caudal compression with parasympathetic involvement, bowel, and bladder sphincter control may be compromised.

Nerve root entrapment syndromes also can result in neurologic deficits. However, the pain pattern will differ and specific sensory and motor loss will be absent. For example, pain from spinal stenosis is relieved with flexion and sitting.

Arthritis in the lumbar spine produces pain with motion and is relieved by rest. Range of motion is reduced. Morning stiffness may be present. The pain does not radiate, but the patient usually has pain in other joints as well.

The pain of a spinal tumor has a insidious onset, gradually increases in severity, is not relieved by rest, and occurs at night.

Pain from extraspinal sources is not related to movement.

NURSING ASSESSMENT

SUBJECTIVE DATA

Pain is difficult to describe, making a detailed history from the patient with low back pain difficult to obtain. If the back pain has been chronic, the patient may have difficulty recalling accurately when and how it began, any past examinations, and tests or types of medicine and treatment used in the past.

Demographic Variables

Identify age, sex, marital status, employment status, occupation, education level, religion. The elderly are more likely to have fractures or cancer; those under 25-years-old, muscle strain or ankylosing spondylitis; and ages 25 to 50 years, disk herniation.

Description of Complaint

Quality Is the pain sharp, dull, stiff, constant, or intermittent? Is it getting worse or better?

Severity The severity of the pain is determined by the amount of interference in activities (work, recreation). Does the pain confine the patient to bed? Does it interfere with sleep (*i.e.*, wake up at night, cannot fall asleep)?

Location Is the pain point tender or diffuse, bilateral or unilateral to spine? Does the pain radiate, and if so, where (extremities, buttocks)? Have patient point to the pain's pathway.

Onset What was the patient doing when it began? Inquire about bending, twisting, lifting, trauma, laughing, sneezing, coughing, or no precipitating factor. Was the onset immediate or gradual? Disk pain is usually immediate; muscle strain delayed until next day.

Duration Determine the duration of the current pain. Ask about previous epi-

sodes, length of time between episodes. If backaches occur intermittently over many years, malignancy or infection is unlikely.

Aggravating and Alleviating Factors Factors that affect the pain include activity, sports, rest, body positions (sitting, lying, walking), sleep positions, mattress quality, sneezing, coughing, laughing. Note effect of food.

Associated Manifestations Symptoms may include weakness, numbness or tingling, paresthesias in the extremities, loss of bowel or bladder control, burning and frequency of urination. Note a relationship to menstrual cycle, fever, concurrent illness, pregnancy. Inquire about other pain sites (joints, abdomen, neck).

Past Medical History

Establish any history of trauma, obesity, arthritis, recent lumbar puncture, chronic steroid use, cancer, past hospitalizations, and tests and procedures.

Psychosocial History

Daily Activities Ask about sleep, appetite, energy level, sexual activity, mood, and hobbies. Ask about regular exercise (and types), overall physical condition.

Occupation Is the patient employed—part-time, full-time, or on disability? Identify body positions involved in the job, feelings about the job and co-workers. Check for job stress (deadlines, supervisory responsibilities). Evaluate motivation and ambition level; ask about compensation or litigation.

Emotional Assessment Assess emotional stress, fatigue, anxiety, depression, and emotional makeup. Depression may be masked by physical symptoms. Identify recent life changes, recent significant events (divorce, death). Observe for feelings of helplessness and fear, denial of any emotional difficulties. Identify dependency needs.

Pain Perception Determine the patient's attitude and feelings about the pain and his locus of control. Is the disability emphasized? The patient's perception of his pain will affect his description of his symptoms.

Coping Mechanisms Identify past, present, positive or negative mechanisms. Identify self-care abilities.

Family and Interpersonal Relationships Evaluate family interactions, attitudes of family members regarding the patient's pain. Determine effect on family members. Determine supportiveness. Does the family encourage inappropriate pain behaviors?

Medications

Note past and current medications, with type and dosage. Note chronic corticosteroid use, analgesic's effectiveness, alcohol use, or illegal drug use. There is a high incidence of spinal infection among drug addicts.

Other Professionals Involved

Identify other physicians (check for doctor-shopping), lawyer, insurance company, employer, or chiropractor who may be involved.

OBJECTIVE DATA

The physical exam is necessary to determine the etiology of a patient's back pain, to determine the severity of the problem, and to monitor the patient's progress during treatment. The physical exam should be directed primarily to the muscular–skeletal and neurologic examinations of the low back and lower extremities. A general physical examination, including abdominal and rectal examinations, and a pelvic examination for women, is needed to evaluate possible extraspinal causes. The physical examination may be done by the nurse or physician, depending on the clinical skills and role of the nurse.

Particular aspects of the exam pertinent to the evaluation of low back pain follow.

General Appearance

Observe for inappropriate affect (i.e., smiling during painful movements), obesity, manner of dressing.

Muscular–Skeletal Examination

Gait Observe patient walking (limp), getting on and off exam table, lying down, and sitting. Does the patient support himself on the good side, place hand on area of discomfort, favor one side? Is there stiffness? Look for decreased arm swing on one or both sides (may indicate muscle spasm).

Evaluate toe walking; note inability or unilateral weakness (one heel lower than other), which may indicate a first sacral nerve (S_1) radiculopathy.

Evaluate heel walking; observe for inability or unilateral weakness (decreased dorsiflexion), which may indicate a fifth lumbar nerve (L_5) radiculopathy.

Stance Note posture and curvature of spine. Exaggerated lordosis indicates poor posture and possible weak abdominal muscles. Lack of lordosis of the lumbar spine may indicate muscle spasm. Observe for list (pelvic tilt), possibly due to muscle spasm or sciatica. A severely bent-forward posture may indicate psychosomatic overlays. Standing on one leg may indicate sciatica.

Range of Motion of Spine Observe for limitations in flexion, extension, side bend and rotation, and for movement causing pain. Muscle spasm usually limits motion. If range of motion is good in all directions, muscular–skeletal disease is unlikely.

Flexion: Normal flexion causes reversal of lordotic curve. Bending at hips and not reversing the curve results from muscle spasm or sciatic pain. Asymmetry indicates muscle spasm.

Side bend: Assess for pain on opposite side due to stretching of a pulled muscle, causing spasm. Degenerative arthritis, old fractures, or anklyosing spondylitis can cause pain with side bend.

Extension: Extension is limited with spasm and with inflammation or a fracture, may produce pain in leg or buttock due to sciatica, sacroiliac joint, or hip pain.

Sitting Posture Note if erect, leaning, sitting on hands, ability to lie flat. Severe muscle spasm causes the patient to flex the knees.

Muscle Tone and Strength Observe for symmetry; observe or measure circumference of thighs and calves for atrophy (greater than ½ inch difference between legs). Observe for atrophy of buttocks. Unilateral atrophy is from disuse or a neurologic deficit due to disk herniation. Bilateral atrophy could indicate spinal cord involvement. Atrophy can occur after a few days of disuse. Assess muscle strength for symmetry. Diminished strength of big toe extensor is indicative of fifth lumbar nerve root involvement.

Leg Length A short leg can cause back pain.

Range of Motion of Hip Note presence of pain, which may indicate hip disuse. Patrick's test (Faber's sign) is internal and external rotation of the hip with the knee flexed and, if positive for pain, usually indicates hip disease.

Back A helpful anatomical marker is that the level of the top of the iliac crests marks the fourth lumbar process. Observe curvature; check for scoliosis in an upright and a flexed position.

Palpate and percuss spinous processes and paraspinous muscles. Observe for a prominent L_5 process. A palpable step between two vertebrae is associated with spondylolisthesis. Note area(s) of tenderness and firmness (indicating muscle spasm). if severe pain is elicited, consider infection or another local pathologic process; percuss costovertebral angles for tenderness to evaluate kidney involvement. Palpate sacroiliac joint, for tenderness.

Straight-Leg Raising (Lasègue's sign): Indicative of sciatic pain. With patient in a supine position, raise each extended leg up until it approaches 90°. Note whether pain is elicited, at what angle the pain occurs, and the location of pain. Pain when the leg is between 0° and 60° is indicative of sciatica. Pain when the leg is extended beyond 60° may be due to other sources (tight hamstrings). Pain in the low back or pain radiating down the leg is a positive test. If findings are equivocal, dorsiflex the foot and repeat the test to confirm the presence of sciatica. The test can also be done in the sitting position. Note when the patient leans backwards (indicative of pain) as well as a verbal report of pain. Bent-leg raising does not produce sciatica.

Chest Expansion Ankylosing spondylitis is a cause of diminished chest expansion.

Lateral Pelvic Compression Apply pelvic compression while the patient is lying on one side to elicit sacroiliac joint pain.

Neurologic Examination

Patellar and Achilles Deep Tendon Reflexes Note unilateral absent or diminished reflexes.

Sensation of Lower Extremities Note decreased or absent sensation in a sensory dermatome distribution, using sharp versus dull, and light touch. Patients with hysterical characteristics may have a "stocking" distribution of decreased sensation.

Other Specific Exams

Abdominal Examination Palpate for a pulsatile mass and listen for a bruit over aorta.

Pulses   Palpate femoral, popliteal, posterior tibial, and dorsalis pedis pulses and note if absent.

Rectal Exam   Palpate for sciatic nerve or sacroiliac joint tenderness or for a mass.

Indicators to Help Differentiate Patients Felt to be Malingerers and Compensatory Patients

History   The patient has an inappropriate affect and answers questions grudgingly, is often uncooperative during exam and treatment and is often unpleasant. Patient also is inconsistent when recounting the history, with disability emphasized, not the pain. Pain is widespread.

Physical Exam   Gait shows marked lumbar lordosis. Patient walks very swiftly. Elevation of arms produces pain. Range of motion of spine is minimal but symmetrical. Pain is not unilateral.

Burns' Bench Test   Patient kneels on chair and bends over to touch floor. A patient with sciatica and organic disease can reach within 15 cm of the floor; a malingerer usually cannot. However, hip or knee disease can prevent a patient from doing this test. This test is only one indicator and should not be used as the sole basis for identifying a malingerer.

PARACLINICAL DATA

There are no strict guidelines as to what diagnostic tests to order. The helpfulness of each test depends on which etiology is suspected.

Back X-Rays

Back x-rays may include anterior–posterior view, right and left oblique views, sacroiliac joints, and hips. These have traditionally been done routinely to evaluate low back pain to rule out tumor, infection, and metabolic disease. However, x-ray films usually do not show pathology.[2,26,27] For example, disk pathology is not identifiable on x-ray films. Most pathology findings that are identified are insignificant and do not correlate with the patient's symptoms.[2,5,11,16,20,21,27] For example, degenerative findings are common in asymptomatic people. Back x-ray films are most useful to confirm suspected diagnoses rather than provide new information. The cost effectiveness and usefulness of routine x-rays are currently being questioned. The literature now recommends x-rays to confirm a suspected diagnosis, to evaluate persistent pain over 1 month duration, or if necessary, to reassure a patient.

Large companies have used x-rays as a pre-employment screening tool to identify people at risk for low back pain. By not hiring these people, disability compensation costs and sick time potentially are reduced. However, screening back x-rays have been consistently shown to have little predictive value.[11,16]

Blood Work

Usually none is necessary unless a specific etiology is suspected and blood work can confirm the diagnosis.

Electromyography

Electromyography (EMG) is a noninvasive procedure used to evaluate referred pain down the lower extremity (sciatica). It is helpful to document a neurologic deficit due to a disk herniation and to differentiate a compressive syndrome from a neuropathy.[15] EMG will show nerve irritation or damage. Most accurate results are obtained approximately 2 weeks after the onset of pain.

Myelogram

A myelogram is done if a tumor is suspected or immediately before surgery to identify the level of a disk herniation.

Discography

In the past, discography (injecting dye into a disk space) was done to evaluate a disk space. This procedure was felt not to be useful. It is still performed before injection of chymopapain into a disk for the treatment of disk disease.

Bone Scan

A bone scan may be ordered if a neoplasm is suspected.

Computerized Tomography (CT) Scan

The CT scan has been recently recommended to confirm spinal stenosis and foramenal nerve root entrapment syndrome. This technique is not widely used.

Psychological Testing

The MMPI test or Holmes and Rahe Schedule of Recent Life Experiences can be useful to help differentiate suffering and disability owing to psychological rather than organic factors.

A study by Sternbach showed patients with low back pain scored high in the hypochondriasis and hysteria scales on the MMPI.[6, 25] Patients involved in litigation elevate these scores and the depression score. However, one cannot determine an organic versus psychological etiology based on these scores; they merely identify areas to evaluate further.

NURSING DIAGNOSIS

Nursing diagnoses can be made relating to the following areas.

ETIOLOGY

The nurse should collaborate with the physician to determine the etiology if the assessment reveals indicators of a cause other than muscle spasm. A specific etiology may not be identified. The severity of the problem cannot be determined by the etiology alone. Although the etiology can determine potential use of specific therapeutic procedures (such as injection, surgery), the majority of the management program depends on whether the pain is acute or chronic.

DIFFERENTIATING ACUTE FROM CHRONIC LOW BACK PAIN

Acute low back pain is an isolated episode of recent onset, with duration of symptoms less than 3 months. Chronic low back pain has a duration of over 3 months, may be constant or may be frequent, intermittent episodes of acute pain. Psychosocial problems are strongly associated with chronic low back pain (discussed earlier in the chapter). The patient with chronic low back pain emphasizes his suffering. He often is unable to work, is supported by social security or disability benefits and is a frequent user of the health care system. Therefore, identifying potential chronic low back pain patients during the initial episode of acute pain and directing interventions to prevent chronicity is a priority.

IMPACT ON LIFE-STYLE

The impact of low back pain on a person's life-style can be enormous and results in long-term disability. Functional limitations, if present, should be monitored, and return to full activities recommended as early as possible.

PSYCHOSOCIAL IMPACT

Determine whether identified psychosocial factors have predisposed, precipitated, or prolonged the patient's pain. Negative behaviors expressing demanding, depressed, angry, or hopeless feelings can make the patient unwilling to participate fully in his care. Secondary gains, such as dependency needs, will also affect response to treatment negatively. Indications of a strong psychosocial component include persistent pain with no identified etiology, a vague description of the pain, multiple pain sites in addition to the low back, emphasis on the disability, and a normal physical exam.[2, 4, 14, 27]

IMPACT ON THE FAMILY

Chronic low back pain can disrupt family relationships, communication, and role structure. Family members need assistance with adjusting to changes within the family unit and in assisting the patient in his rehabilitation.

PRESENCE OF COMPENSATION OR LITIGATION

For legal purposes, the physician should be involved closely in the evaluation and management of patients involved in compensation or litigation. Malingering should be ruled out. Compensation depends on whether the etiology is work-related. A herniated disk usually is compensable, but a lumbar strain or sprain may not be, depending on whether a causal relationship between the job and injury is found. The physician's role in compensation or litigation issues is to determine the severity and nature of the complaint, not whether it was employment-related.[16]

MANAGEMENT

Comprehensive management of low back pain can be provided by an individual nurse or through a multidisciplinary approach involving a physician, physical therapist, social worker, psychologist, and vocational rehabilitation counselor. The approach is based on the setting (inpatient versus outpatient) and the specific needs of each patient. The extent to which the nurse provides the care or coordinates the care given by others will depend on the nurse's education and expertise and setting. The nurse should refer the patient to a physician if persistent pain does not improve with bed rest or if progressive neurologic deficits are noted. Medical therapy and procedures require collaboration or referral.

The management of low back pain is divided into two general approaches: management of *acute* low back pain and of *chronic* low back pain. The management section addresses mechanical low back pain, including muscle strain and degenerative disk disease (in particular disk herniation), nerve root entrapment syndromes, and psychosocial factors. It does not address infection, tumor, or extraspinal sources because of the significantly lower incidence of these causes, and the more minor role the nurse has in their management.

GOALS

The goals of management of low back pain are

1. To eliminate or decrease the pain as quickly as possible
2. To help the patient return to his full activity level as soon as possible
3. To teach the patient ways to help prevent recurrences

The patient must be included in developing a management program with which he feels comfortable because the strategies involved require patient participation. They cannot be done to or for the patient.

ACUTE LOW BACK PAIN

Management of acute low back pain is initially conservative, and nonsurgical. Ninety percent of patients are better after 1 month of treatment and ninety-eight percent are better within 2 months.[27,28] Acute low back pain usually is treated on an outpatient basis. Patients may be hospitalized for conservative management if they are unable to comply with restrictions while at home. Surgery and invasive procedures are done in the hospital. Initially, patients should be seen once a week to monitor their progress.

Bed Rest

Bed rest is the primary intervention for acute pain. However, if the pain is mild, avoiding activities that aggravate the pain (e.g., lifting and bending) may be all that is needed. The purpose of bed rest is to relieve the stress on the low back. It reduces compressive and torsional pressure on the nerve roots and on the disks. It minimizes the inflammatory response and helps decrease any edema present. It allows muscle spasm to subside. It also prevents further irritation while the area heals. Sitting does not rest the back. Bed rest is with bathroom privileges only. The patient should be horizontal or in a semi-Fowler's position with the lower back rounded (reversing the lordotic curve). The patient can lie on his back with pillows under the knees or on the side with both knees flexed. He should not lie on his back without knees and hips flexed or be in a prone position. These positions accentuate the lordotic curve, put pressure on the nerve roots, and aggravate muscle spasm. Prolonged immobilization can lead to muscle wasting and should be avoided. One to two weeks of bed rest is usually sufficient. The length of time can be as short as a few days depending on the patient's response and level of compliance.

Compliance is jeopardized by boredom resulting from strict bed rest. Diverting activities facilitate compliance and keep the patient's mind off the pain. The patient is prone to constipation due to inactivity and narcotics. Prevention through diet and fluid intake should be encouraged. If the pain continues after 3 weeks the patient should be referred to a physician. After activities have been resumed, frequent rest periods (two or three times daily) in bed are recommended.

Medication

Analgesics and muscle relaxants frequently are used alone or together for acute back pain. Narcotics are used for severe pain. Aspirin or acetaminophen with codeine is a frequent choice. Plain aspirin or acetaminophen every 4 hours is frequently used for mild pain. Nonsteroidal anti-inflammatory medicine may be used if arthritis is present. Use of muscle relaxants for spasm (also provides some mental ease) may reduce pain by increasing the patient's pain tolerance and also tolerance of prolonged bed rest. Diazepam is often the drug of choice. *Cyclobenzaprine HCl* (Flexeril) and *methocarbamol* (Robaxin) are also used. Initially, a fixed schedule for pain medicine can help prevent the pain–anxiety–pain cycle. Medication is appropriate for the acute episode and usually can be tapered or discontinued after the first week.

Exercise

Start back-stretching exercises early in the management program to help relieve muscle spasm while the patient is still on bed rest (Fig. 7-6, 7-7, 7-8). Exercises that increase strength and tone abdominal and lumbar musculature should be delayed until the pain has been relieved on bed rest (Fig. 7-6 to 7-12). Any exercise that causes pain needs to be discontinued. The patient gradually in-

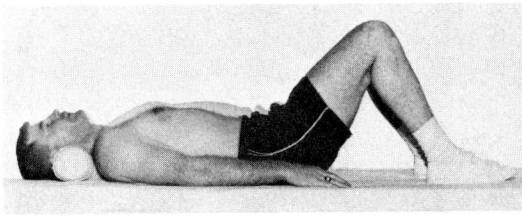

FIG. 7-6 Exercise 1. Take a deep breath, expanding the chest as much as possible, exhale slowly, allowing the chest to return to its normal position. Keep the back and neck flat. Repeat this deep breathing exercise very slowly 5 or 6 times. (Ishmael WK, Shorbe HB: Care of the Back, Industrial edition 2, p 20. Philadelphia, JB Lippincott, 1976)

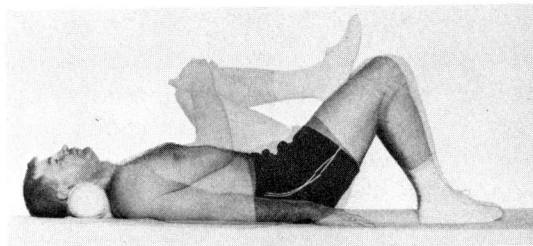

FIG. 7-8 Exercise 3. Draw both knees to the chest, then grasp the knees with the hands, drawing the knees as near to the chest as possible. This can be repeated 5 or 6 times. It is well to hold the knees pressed against the chest for 25 seconds each time. Before raising the knees, tighten the abdominal muscles and hold the back flat. (Ishmael WK, Shorbe HB: Care of the Back, Industrial ed 2, p 20. Philadelphia, JB Lippincott, 1976)

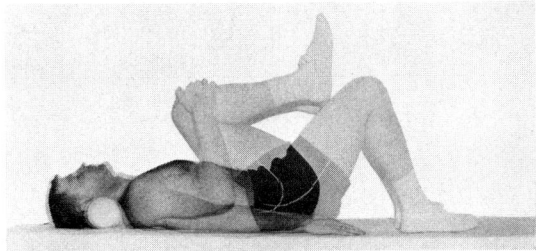

FIG. 7-7 Exercise 2. Draw one knee up to the chest, bring it up tight with the hand, then return it slowly to the original position. **Do not allow the knee to straighten out.** Next, draw the other knee up to the chest, then return it to the original position (keeping knee bent). Repeat with each leg from 10 to 20 times. (Ishmael WK, Shorbe HB: Care of the Back, Industrial edition 2, p 20. Philadelphia, JB Lippincott, 1976)

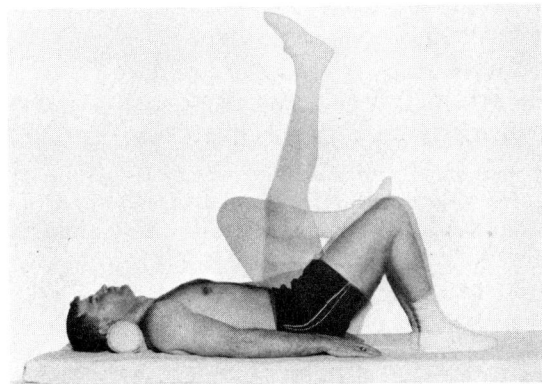

FIG. 7-9 Exercise 4. Draw one knee to the chest, then straighten that knee, pointing the leg upward as far as possible, bend knees and return to original position. Alternate with the opposite leg, repeating this cycle 4 or 5 times. (Ishmael WK, Shorbe HB: Care of the Back, Industrial ed 2, p 20. Philadelphia, JB Lippincott, 1976)

creases the number of times an exercise is done until he reaches the maximum number recommended. (Further discussion of exercise for patients with low back pain is found in the management of chronic low back pain section.)

Heat and Massage

Moist heat and massage may help relax paraspinal muscle spasm. Hot baths or showers, in addition to local heat, may help. Their effectiveness has not been validated.

Traction

Traction has not been found to be valuable in the treatment of low back pain. The only benefit is that it keeps the patient in bed, allowing the back to rest.

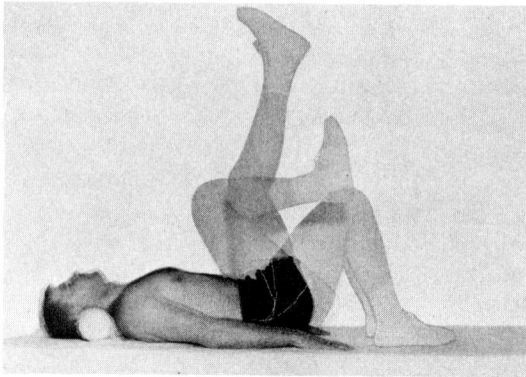

FIG. 7-10   Exercise 5. Do not start this exercise until the others have been done for 3 or 4 weeks. Draw both knees to the chest, then straighten both, pointing the feet upward; return to original position. This can be repeated 3 or 4 times. (Ishmael WK, Shorbe HB: Care of the Back, Industrial ed 2, p 21. Philadelphia, JB Lippincott, 1976)

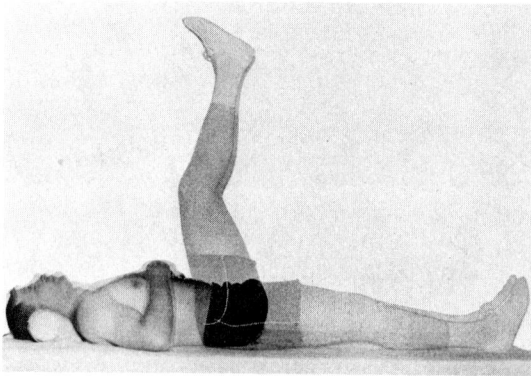

FIG. 7-11   Exercise 6. Raise both legs to vertical position and return, keeping legs straight throughout. It requires a strong back and abdominal musculature to accomplish this exercise. The back must be kept flat at all times or low back strain could occur. Do not attempt this exercise until all soreness has disappeared from the back. (Ishmael WK, Shorbe HB: Care of the Back, Industrial ed 2, p 21. Philadelphia, JB Lippincott, 1976).

Corsets and Back Braces

Corsets and back braces limit movement of the lumbar spine and increase the support of the abdominal wall. Use of these devices is

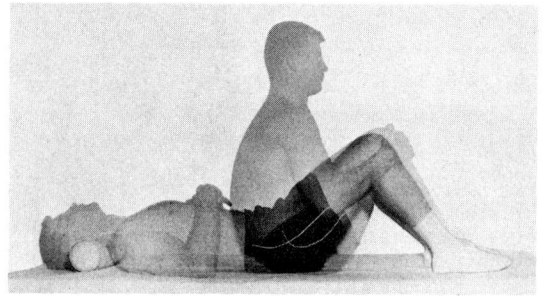

FIG. 7-12   Exercise 7. Pull up to the sitting position, keeping the knees flexed at all times. This exercise can be facilitated by having someone hold the feet to the floor or by hooking them under a piece of heavy furniture. (Ishmael WK, Shorbe HB: Care of the Back, Industrial ed 2, p 21. Philadelphia, JB Lippincott, 1976)

not encouraged because prolonged use decreases the strength of the abdominal muscles and will ultimately perpetuate the problem. At best, use a corset short-term for acute pain.

Surgery

Surgical treatment for disk herniation is rarely necessary. When surgery is indicated, simple diskectomy usually is performed. Fusion has been found not to have any significant advantage.[13, 21] Indications for surgery include: pain unrelieved with 6 to 12 weeks of strict bed rest and progression of neurologic deficits, including bladder or bowel dysfunction while maintaining bed rest, foot drop, and paraparesis. Surgery is occasionally performed for spondylolisthesis with marked instability and spinal stenosis. Surgery is preceded by a myelogram to locate the lesion; it is not done as an exploratory procedure. Surgery may eliminate severe leg pain, but it may not eliminate all of the low back pain. Patients with secondary gain or who are involved with compensation have a poor surgical success rate.[12, 20, 21] A 6-week postoperative recovery period follows the surgery and frequently patients do not resume normal activities for three to six months. Some patients never return to work and seek additional surgery to relieve pain.

Chemonucleolysis

Chymopapain is an enzyme that is injected under x-ray into a herniated disk. It causes lysis of the cartilage, which reduces intradiscal pressure and results in symptom relief. The use of this technique is controversial. The success rate is reported to be approximately 50% and, hence, is much less effective than bed rest.[20, 21, 30] Some authorities recommend it as an alternative to surgery.[19]

Progression of Activities

Activities are resumed as soon as possible, progressing as symptoms permit. After the patient is pain-free while on bed rest, short periods of walking around the house can begin. If an activity causes pain, the patient discontinues or decreases it by half and then gradually builds back up. If significant pain occurs, bed rest is reinstituted. Sitting for long periods should be avoided. The type of chair used should allow for ease in getting to a standing position. While sitting, the patient should keep his knees higher than his hips. A firm mattress or use of a bedboard can be helpful. Minor discomfort or stiffness should not interfere with increasing the patient's activities.

Recommendations for body mechanics, exercise, and prevention of recurrence are the same as those found in the management section for chronic low back pain.

CHRONIC LOW BACK PAIN

Chronic low back pain usually leads to changes in life-style. The pain interferes with personal, social, and work relationships and capabilities. The invalid role is readily assumed. Patients with chronic low back pain respond poorly to both conservative and surgical treatment. There frequently is no clear pathophysiology, which makes management difficult. These patients continue to seek out health care looking for an easy cure, often take little responsibility for their own care, and can undermine that care. However, the patient has a large role in the management of chronic low back pain. Management must include the psychosocial factors related to chronic pain, help the patient become more independent and less pain-centered, and relieve or diminish the pain. Management usually is done on an outpatient basis; however, there are a few comprehensive inpatient rehabilitation programs for patients with chronic low back pain. A multidisciplinary approach may be helpful in providing a comprehensive program. Continuity by the nurse is essential so that progress may be evaluated, strategies modified, and services coordinated. Patients should have scheduled visits at regular intervals for follow-up. Inappropriate tests, unnecessary medicine, and surgery should be avoided.

Patient Education

The patient needs to learn about low back pain; the cause, the anatomy and physiology of the spine, the management program, and how to prevent recurrences of the pain. This education can be done on an individual basis or in a group format.

Body Mechanics

Teach the patient proper use of the spine to minimize stress on the spine and surrounding muscles. Proper body mechanics can be taught by the nurse or a physical therapist.

Standing Suggest that the patient stand against a wall and flatten the back against it to learn proper posture. While standing still, the patient should have one foot on a footrest to diminish lumbar lordosis. Avoid hyperextension of the low back (swayback).

Sitting Knees should be higher than hips, and back flat without lumbar lordosis. The back is slightly curled. Squatting and sitting on the floor cross-legged also helps to diminish pain. The patient should avoid sitting for long periods, should move around, and should use arm rests whenever possible.

Sleeping The patient should sleep on one side with knees and hips bent or on the back with pillows under the knees, and avoid a prone position. Use of a firm mattress or a bedboard for added support is recommended.

Lifting There are no controlled studies to document which method is best. Some authorities feel that the position most comfortable is best. Specific recommendations vary, depending on the size and weight of the object, distance from the body, the frequency and duration of lifting, and the height of the lift. General recommendations include: keep the load close to the body, with feet shoulder-width apart for stability to prevent slips or falls. Bend knees and use legs to lift. A patient may need to strengthen the quadriceps before doing any lifting. The back may be slightly bent but do not lean forward. Avoid sudden movements and lifting and twisting simultaneously. Avoid lifting higher than the waist. Do not lift weights over 35% of one's own body weight. Avoid lifting over 20 lb. This limit may be less, depending on other aggravating factors.

Avoid Twisting Pivot on feet to avoid rotational stresses. Do not lean forward without bending the knees.

Driving Sit closer to the wheel so knees are flexed and higher than hips. Avoid driving a standard shift with a clutch. Avoid long car rides; stop at least every 2 hours.

Walking Encourage patients to walk independently without use of a cane or crutches. Patients need reassurance that walking is safe and desirable.

Other Suggestions High-heeled shoes should be avoided. Advise and assist overweight patients to reduce until they have reached their normal body weight.

Exercise

Exercise for chronic low back pain consists of exercises for the low back, including flexion exercises that tone and strengthen the abdominal and lumbar musculature and general conditioning exercises. Exercises can be taught by the nurse, physical therapist, or the physician. Treatment of the acute phase of low back pain with bed rest leads to unconditioned muscles. Chronic low back pain patients usually feel that they cannot do any general exercise.

Flexion Exercises Flexion exercises are done twice daily (see Fig. 7-6 to Fig. 7-12). If pain (not discomfort) is produced, stop that particular exercise for a week and then attempt again. An exercise can be done up until the point at which pain is produced, and then gradually built up until the complete exercise can be done. Exercises six and seven are not done until *all* pain has disappeared from the back. The back must be kept flat or lumbar muscle strain may occur. After 3 to 4 weeks, a bent-knee sit-up can be done, with the patient curling up to a sitting position and then uncurling.

General Conditioning Exercises General conditioning can help the patient to gain flexibility and strength to increase activities of daily living, as well as prevent future episodes of lumbar strain. Strengthening leg muscles is important to aid lifting. General exercise should not be started until all acute pain has disappeared, and the amount of exercise should be increased slowly. Walking and swimming are highly recommended. Bicycling is another good exercise; however, use of low handlebars can aggravate back pain. Sports that may aggravate low back pain include golf, tennis, and jogging. Back flexion exercises can be included as part of the warm-up. General exercise should be done a minimum of three times per week. Intermittent vigorous exercise (less than three times per week) can cause lumbar strain and create frustration for the patient. If the patient's back begins to feel tired, he should rest lying on his back with knees bent.

Medications

Analgesics and muscle relaxants are not helpful in managing chronic pain except for exacerbations. These agents can impair mental alertness and potentially lead to drug dependency. Medication should be tapered and discontinued whenever possible.

Activities of Daily Living

Patients with chronic low back pain need specific guidelines on how to increase activities. Bed rest is appropriate for exacerbations of pain (e.g., an episode of acute pain) only. If the patient has been on bed rest, he should begin walking for 5 to 10 minutes several times per day. The length of time out of bed can be increased quickly as long as the activity does not produce pain. If an activity causes pain, it should be stopped and strength built up before attempting it again. Minor discomfort should not eliminate activities. Sitting for extended periods should be avoided. Long car rides or plane rides aggravate lumbar pain. The patient should get up and move around every 1 to 2 hours. Vacuuming and making beds should be avoided until the patient has been pain-free with less strenuous activities for several weeks. Vibrating equipment can aggravate pain and should be avoided. Shoveling snow and other heavy lifting should be avoided.

Endurance can be increased by conserving energy and simplifying work. For exam-ple, long complex tasks can be broken down into smaller units. Rest periods are important. Overdoing activities or pushing oneself when tired can precipitate more back pain. Modification of the number of hours spent standing or sitting, minimizing lifting, and frequent short rest periods can help to prevent aggravation of pain. As patients realize that activities can be performed without pain, they are more willing to do other activities and become more independent.

Job change may be necessary if the present job involves activities or positions that aggravate low back pain. Vocational rehabilitation is an important resource to help retrain people and return them to the work force.

There is a wealth of patient literature to augment the patient's knowledge about his problem and its care. Lay literature includes pamphlets and books; (e.g., Rudinger, E: *The No More Back Trouble Book*).

Counseling

Chronic pain patients often have a heightened awareness of pain. Suffering responses can perpetuate the pain–disability cycle. Counseling helps the patient to cope and to take responsibility for being an active participant in the management program. Many patients will not achieve complete pain relief. Counseling is directed at helping the patient live as normal a life as possible with little or no pain medication. The patient needs to understand the relationship between emotions and symptoms. He may resist acknowledging this relationship initially. He needs to learn new coping strategies to deal with dependency needs, feelings of hopelessness, and frustration. Strategies like problem-solving and assertiveness training can be applied to work and home stress situations. A physical outlet such as walking or knitting helps. Socialization with others needs to be encouraged. Psychiatric counseling may be needed for the patient to deal with underlying depression or anxiety. Behaviors and changes should be reinforced. The patient needs to learn ways to control activities and situations that increase pain. Feeling some control over the pain can help to relieve the feeling of hopelessness and reduce the expectation of pain during activities.

Chronic pain can place a great deal of stress on family and marital relationships. The nurse should provide opportunities for family members to express feelings and concerns. They need to learn what the patient is capable of doing, and to ignore pain behaviors and reinforce productive behaviors. Flexibility regarding role function can assist the patient in becoming more independent.

Relaxation Techniques

Relaxation techniques are used to reduce muscle tension and spasm. Relaxation of tensed muscles breaks the pain/muscle tension/pain cycle. Relaxation techniques are also helpful to pace activities or cope with stressful situations. Lay literature on relaxation is available and includes Herbert Benson's *The Relaxation Response.* One simple relaxation technique is to alternately tighten and relax every muscle group of the body, starting at the toes and progressing to the head. Special attention is directed to the low back area. Imagery can be used simultaneously. A more detailed discussion of these techniques is found in the chapter on chronic pain.

Biofeedback

Biofeedback techniques help patients consciously reduce muscle tension and spasm. Referral is usually needed to enter a biofeedback-training program. Electromyographic biofeedback is considered an adjunct

therapeutic strategy when other measures have failed. Biofeedback and relaxation techniques can be used simultaneously.

Hypnosis

Hypnosis can be useful as an adjunct strategy to help the patient gain control over pain by blocking the perception of pain. The patient learns self-hypnosis and uses it on a regular basis. He is instructed not to eliminate all pain perception to ensure that pain from other sources is perceived. Counseling is needed simultaneously to address underlying emotional issues that are not helped by hypnosis. The patient should be referred to an expert if this technique is chosen.

Manipulation

The effectiveness of manipulation is controversial. There are different types of manipulation (rotational and sudden hyperextension) and the studies on manipulation do not always agree which is preferable. Nor do studies agree if manipulation is more effective than placebo.[8, 9, 10, 18, 29] Manipulation may cause herniation of a degenerated disk and should not be used if any neurologic deficits are noted on examination.

Lumbar Facet Joint Injection and Injection of Trigger Points

Lidocaine (Xylocaine) can be injected into trigger points of muscle pain. Lidocaine (Xylocaine) and corticosteroids can also be injected into the facet joint using fluoroscopy for treatment of lumbar facet arthropathy. Pain relief may last up to 6 months.[3] These two procedures are not widely used and have not been proven effective.

Other Procedures

Other procedures have been tried but are not commonly used in the treatment of chronic low back pain. These include sympathetic

nerve blocks, TENS, and dorsal column stimulation. These only provide short-term
symptom relief and are expensive.

Prevention

Preventive measures are appropriate for patients with acute or chronic low back pain.
Flexion exercises should be done daily. They
are helpful prior to strenuous exercise or
other activities. Aerobic exercise at least 3
days a week will help keep a person in general good physical condition, decreasing the
risk of injury. Weight should be maintained
in the normal range. Good posture and body
mechanics, as outlined in the chronic pain
management section, with the patient wearing low heels on shoes, and avoiding heavy
lifting or other activities that have caused
pain in the past will help prevent further episodes. Obtaining the proper rest and relaxation is important, since acute injuries frequently occur when the patient is tired.

SUMMARY

Low back pain is a common health problem
that can be an acute, self-limited episode or a
chronic debilitating problem. The pain can
be confined to the lumbar area, radiate into
the hip and leg, or be referred from the pelvic
or abdominal viscera. Multiple conditions
contribute to the incidence of low back pain
but in most people a cause will not be found.
Psychosocial factors have a strong role in predisposing, precipitating, and prolonging the
pain. After serious pathology has been ruled
out, the nurse can manage patients with low
back pain or coordinate a multidisciplinary
approach. Initially, frequent visits provide
support and guidance for the patient and
help to achieve fast resolution of the problem. Management differs depending on
whether the pain is acute or chronic; how-

ever, the goals are the same: to relieve the
pain as quickly as possible, to help the patient return to the highest activity level possible, and to teach the patient how to avoid
recurrences. Achieving these goals requires
the patient's full participation in the management program.

REFERENCES

1. Anderson JAD: Back pain in industry. In Jayson, M (ed): The Lumbar Spine and Back Pain. New York, Grune & Stratton, Inc. p. 29–46, 1976
2. Boy RJ: Evaluation of back pain. In Goroll AH et al: Primary Care Medicine: Office Evaluation and Management of the Adult Patient. Philadelphia, JB Lippincott, 1981
3. Carrera GF: Lumbar facet joint injection in low back pain and sciatica. Radiology 137:665–667, 1980
4. Crown S: Psychosocial factors in low back pain. Rheumatol Rehabil 17:77–92, 1978
5. Currey HLF et al: A prospective study of low back pain. Rheumatol Rehabil 18:94–104, 1979
6. Dennis MD et al: The Minnesota Multiphasic Personality Inventory: General guidelines to its use and interpretation in orthopedics. Clin Orthop 150:125–130, 1980
7. Donovan L: Low back pain: Where care is the key to recovery. RN 41:71–24, 1978
8. Doran DML, Newell DJ: Manipulation in treatment of low back pain: A multicentre study. Br Med J 2:161–164, 1975
9. Evans DP et al: Lumbar spinal manipulation on trial: Part I: Clinical assessment. Rheumatol Rehabil 17:46–53, 1978
10. Farfan HF: Mechanical disorders of the low back, pp 212–230. Philadelphia, Lea & Febiger, 1973
11. Frymoyer JW, Pope MH: The role of trauma in low back pain: A review. J Trauma 18, No. 9:628–634, 1978
12. Gainer JV, Nugent GR: The herniated disc. American Family Practice 10, No. 3:127–131, 1974
13. Golub BS et al: Cervical and lumbar disc disease: A review. Bull Rheum Dis 21:635–642, 1971
14. Gottlieb H et al: Comprehensive rehabilitation of patients having chronic low back pain. Arch Phys Med Rehabil 58:101–108, 1977
15. Grabias SL, Mankin HJ: Pain in the lower back. Bull Rheum Dis 30, No. 8:1040–1045, 1979–1980
16. Hadler NM: Legal ramifications of the medical defi-

nition of back disease. Ann Int Med 89:992–999, 1978

17. Hirsh T: The billion dollar backache. National Safety News 115:51, 1977
18. Hoehler FK et al: Spinal manipulation for low back pain. JAMA 245, No. 18:1835–1838, 1981
19. Leavitt F: A comparison of patients treated by chymopapain and laminectomy for low back pain using a multidimensional pain scale. Clin Orthop 146:136–143, 1980
20. Nachemson AL: A critical look at conservative treatment for low back pain. In Jayson M (ed): The Lumbar Spine and Back Pain, pp 355–365. New York, Grune & Stratton, 1976
21. Nachemson AL: The lumbar spine: An orthopaedic challenge. Spine 1, No. 1:59–71, 1976
22. National Safety Council: Accident Facts. Chicago, National Safety Council, 1975
23. Nehemkis AM: The predictive utility of the orthopedic examination in identifying the low back pain patient with hysterical features. Clin Orthop 145:158–162, 1979
24. Owen BD: How to avoid that aching back. Am J Nurs 80:894–897, 1980
25. Robinson GE: A combined approach to a medical problem. Can J Psychiatry 24:138–142, 1980
26. Sarno JO: Psychosomatic backache. J Fam Pract 5, No. 3:353–357, 1977
27. Schurman DJ, Nagel DA: Low back and leg pain. Primary Care 1, No. 4:549–563, 1974
28. Sims–Williams H et al: Controlled trial of mobilisation and manipulation for low back pain: Hospital patients. Br Med J 2:1318–1320, 1979
29. Thorn GW et al (eds): Harrison's Principles of Internal Medicine. New York, McGraw–Hill, 1977
30. Troup JDG et al: Back pain in industry: A prospective study. Spine 6, No. 1:61–69, 1981
31. US Dept. of Health and Human Services: Work practices guide for manual lifting. Cincinnati, Ohio, DHHS (National Institute for Occupational Safety and Health) Publication No. 81–122, 1981
32. Wood PHN: Epidemiology of back pain. In Jayson M (ed): The lumbar spine and back pain, pp 13–27. New York, Grune & Stratton, 1976

BIBLIOGRAPHY

Barras Sr A et al: Low back pain: Why we must get tough. Part 3. RN 41:78–81, 1978

Brown MD: Diagnosis of pain syndromes of the spine. Orthop Clin North Am 6, No. 1:233–248, 1975

Burton C et al: Treating low back pain in the elderly. Geriatrics 33:61–69, 1978

Crasilneck HB: Hypnosis in the control of chronic low back pain. Am J Clin Hypn 22, No. 2:71–78, 1979

Cummings D: Stopping chronic pain before it starts. Nurs 81 11:60–62, 1981

Evanski PM et al: The Burns' test in low back pain: Correlation with the hysterical personality. Clin Orthop 140:42–44, 1979

Fahrni WH: Conservative treatment of lumbar disc degeneration: our primary responsibility. Orthop Clin North Am 6, No. 1:93–103, 1975

Flower A et al: An occupational therapy program for chronic back pain. Am J Occup Ther 35:243–248, 1981

Friedmann LW, Cassvan A: Guide to evaluation of low back pain and sciatica. Hospital Medicine 16:9–20, 1980

Gilbertson B: Low back pain: What to look for . . . what to do, Part 2. RN 41:75–77, 1978

Gramse CA: For control of severe pain: Dorsal column stimulation. Am J Nurs 8:1022–1025, 1978

Greenfield S et al: Nurse-protocol management of low back pain. West J Med 123:350–359, 1975

Grimes D: Back school: Teaching patients to love their backs. Resident and Staff Physicians 26: 60–68, May 1980

Hastings DE: Back pain: A multifaceted syndrome. Postgrad Med 62:159–165, 1977

Iveson J: Prevention: How to stay healthy. Part 8: Back strain. Nurs Mirror 149:22 November 1, 1979

Keim HA: Diagnostic problems in the lumbar spine. Clin Neurosurg 25:184–192, 1978

Keim HA, Kirkaldy–Willis WH: Low back pain. New Jersey, Clinical Symposia (CIBA), 1980

Kelsey JL et al: The impact of musculoskeletal disorders on the population of the United States. J Bone Joint Surg 61A:959–964, 1979

Kester NC: Evaluation and medical management of low back pain. Med Clin North Am 53, No. 3:325–540, 1969

Leavitt F et al: Affective and sensory dimensions of back pain. Pain 4:273–281, 1978

Magora A, Schwartz A: Relation between the low back pain syndrome and x-ray findings: Part 2. Transitional vertebra (mainly sacralization). Scand J Rehabil Med 10:135–145, 1978

Millard L: Low back pain: Guide to evaluation. Hospital Medicine 14:79–90, 1978

Mooney V, Cairns D: Management in the patient with chronic low back pain. Orthop Clin North Am 9, No. 2, 1978

Mooney V, Robertson J: The facet syndrome. Clinical Orthop 115:149–156, 1978

Nachemson A: Lumbar intradiscal pressure. In Jayson M (ed): The Lumbar Spine and Back Pain, pp 257–269. New York, Grune & Stratton, 1976

Newman RI et al: Multidisciplinary treatment of chronic pain: Long-term follow-up of low back pain patients. Pain 4:283–292, 1978

Nigel AJ, Fischer–Williams M: Treatment of low back strain with electromyographic biofeedback and re-laxation training. Psychosomatics 21:495–499, 1980

Thomas LK et al: Physiological work performance in chronic low back disability. Phys Ther 60(4):407–411, 1980

Tucker LE: Diagnosis: Back pain of extraspinal origin. Hospital Medicine 17:52–64, 1981

Yates A: Treatment of back pain. In Jayson M (ed): The Lumbar Spine and Back Pain, pp 341–353, New York, Grune & Stratton, 1976

8

Headache

Margie Van Meter

Headache is one of the most common human discomforts. It is thought that 90% of the population have headaches at some time. It ranks with fatigue, hunger, and thirst in incidence. Although many people who suffer from headaches never seek assistance from health care professionals, some 30 million people do each year. The U.S. Department of Health and Human Services Vital and Health Statistics lists reasons for visiting the physician in a National Ambulatory and Medical Care Survey.[40] The following numbers were compiled: visits to private physicians' offices were 1,154,550,000, with 30,797,000 visits for headache as a symptom, and 18,342,000 visits for headache as the principal symptom. This discomfort affects women more than men, and although it occurs in people from infancy to old age, it occurs more commonly in the years between puberty and the climacteric. The affliction spans the continents and has spanned the centuries. Thousands of neolithic skulls have been found which have marks of trephination in them, indicating that surgical procedures to the head were done. This practice seems to have been fairly universal because trephined skulls have been found in almost every continent. Pain in the head was very likely the symptom that motivated the medieval surgeons to use a chisel and mallot to perform cranial surgery. Paintings from earlier centuries show various treatments for headache, including surgical procedures for the removal of what was believed to be a "head stone," and the use of herbs, compresses, and massage of the neck muscles to relieve wrenched necks.[26] An epic poem from 3,000 B.C. gives evidence of a description of migraine. The poet is talking about heaven.[3]

> The sick-eyed says not, I am sick-eyed.
> The sick-headed says not, I am sick-headed.

This may mean that the "sick-eyed" (referring perhaps to scintillating scotoma) was also "sick-headed." Because migraine could afflict a sensitive poet, the thought of heaven to him was a place where there would be no migraine headaches.

The simple definition for headache given by Dorland is "pain in the head, cephalgia."[11] The term *headache* is commonly restricted to an unpleasant sensation in the region of the cranial vault, the area from below the orbits, to over the scalp and back to the occipital region. Facial and pharyngeal neuralgias, cervical, eye, ear, and sinus pain are not classified as headaches.

Webster's definition of headache also includes "a vexacious situation, a baffling problem or source of trouble or worry."[42] This use of the term may stem from the human experience of many vexacious situations resulting in a person's having a headache. Newspaper headlines use the term *headache* in this way. Some examples from one newspaper include: "Clark's biggest headache: his defensive line," "Soviet hippies causing headaches," "US grain embargo causes headache."

The significance of a headache is often abstruse, since it may be a symptom either of disease or of tension. In most instances headaches are benign, that is, they do not threaten the survival of the sufferer. The dual significance of possible serious disease or minor discomfort necessitates the careful evaluation of the report of headache. The unpleasant sensations that occur around the cranium are not described adequately by the simple term *headache*. There are several types of headaches, each with its own probable mechanism, triggers, and treatments.

The mechanisms and treatment of chronic headache will be the major focus of this chapter. A broad range of nursing interventions are required to assist the patient with chronic headache to prevent the circumstances that result in headache. Nursing interventions for the symptom of acute headache are also included, using principles related to the headache mechanism; however, the various underlying diseases are not extensively described.

MECHANISMS OF HEADACHE

NORMAL ANATOMY AND PHYSIOLOGY

There are pain-sensitive and pain-insensitive structures in the head.[6,32] Pain-sensitive structures include the scalp and its under-lying muscles, parts of the periosteum, the dura at the base of the skull, the extracranial, dural, and intracerebral arteries, the extracranial and intracerebral veins and the venous sinuses, the pain fibers of trigeminal, glossopharyngeal, and vagus cranial nerves, and the upper cervical nerves. Pain-insensitive structures include the cranial bones, the diploic vein within the bones, most of the dura, pia, and arachnoid, all of the brain parenchyma, the ependymal lining of the ventricles, and the choroid plexus within the ventricles.

Traction, displacement, and inflammation of pain-sensitive venous structures, arteries, cranial nerves, and upper cervical nerves are chiefly responsible for headaches arising from intracranial structures.[6] Lesions stimulating pain-sensitive intracranial structures on or above the superior surface of the tentorium cerebellae result in pain in various regions in front of a line drawn vertically from the ears across the top of the head (Fig. 8-1). The pathways of this pain are contained in the fifth cranial nerve. Stimulation of the pain-sensitive intracranial structures on or below the inferior surface of the tentorium cerebellae result in pain in various regions behind the line described. The pathways for this pain are contained mainly in the ninth and tenth cranial nerves and the upper three cervical nerves.[6]

FOUR BASIC MECHANISMS OF HEADACHE PRODUCTION

The basic mechanisms resulting in headache are vascular, muscle contraction, traction, and inflammation.[6]

Vascular

The mechanisms producing a vascular headache are distention, traction, dilation, compression, or inflammation of blood vessels

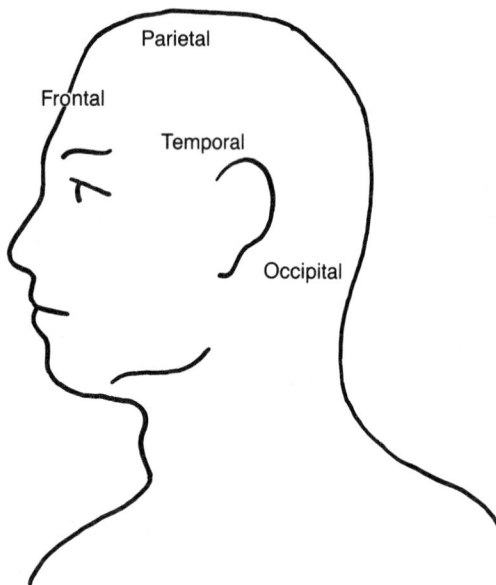

FIG. 8-1 *Divisions of the cranium.*

about the scalp and intracranium. Of the structures covering the cranium, the arteries are particularly sensitive to pain. The category of vascular headache, is a large hodgepodge of head pains ranging from the effects of a hangover or hunger, to severe, disabling migraine and cluster headaches.

A variety of conditions and substances such as febrile and toxic states, anoxemia, and vasodilating agents can cause a generalized dilation of the intracranial and extracranial arteries. The intracranial arteries are very sensitive to humoral influences.[16] Chemicals produced by inflammatory foci, fever, and migraine sensitize the pain-nerve endings in the perivascular area resulting in a lowered pain threshold in the inflamed tissues. The blood vessel dilation and the lowered pain threshold result in a diffuse, pulsating headache due to the painful distention of the dilated and inflamed blood vessels, which pulsate with each cardiac systole. Straining and jolting aggravate the pain.

A headache produced experimentally by histamine results principally from the stretch of the wall of the cerebral arteries rather than the extracranial arteries.[6] Although the data is fragmented, the distention of the intracranial arteries also is the likely mechanism of headache pain associated with acute infection and sepsis. The headaches associated with nitrites, anoxia, hunger, hypoglycemia, caffeine withdrawal, hangover, and postconvulsive states have a similar mechanism. The intensity of the headache produced by histamine is proportional to the degree of dilation and stretch of intracranial vessels and perivascular tissues. After histamine release, the vessels distend and the number of stretch impulses arising from their walls increases, accentuated with each pressure wave from the cardiac systole. Normally, the blood vessel walls absorb changes in pressure and thus the variation of pressure in the vessels is directly transmitted to sensory end-organs in and about their walls in the subarachnoid space. The resulting unusual flood of afferent impulses causes pain.

Muscle Contraction

Continually contracted musculature has a decreased blood supply because of reflex vasoconstriction. The pain of acute scalp muscle contraction headache has been attributed to contraction of muscles alone; however, ischemia of the muscles and accumulation of metabolites that cause pain are also probable factors.[6]

Sustained muscle activity as the cause of pain is only a partial explanation, especially for the person suffering chronic muscle contraction headache. A substantial group of muscle contraction headache sufferers has no appreciable increase in electromyographic (EMG) activity about the head and neck; nor do they have arterial abnormalities associated with their pain.[19,31] Hence, the psychological determinants or components of the pain, and the concept of chronic pain as a variant of a depressive state, must be considered in the mechanism producing a headache.[5]

Inconsistent EMG findings in persons with muscle contraction headache and successful pain reduction with tricyclic antidepressants suggest that chronic scalp muscle contraction and depression may result from cerebral norepinephrine and serotonin deficiencies; thus, there may be more than one mechanism to explain muscle contraction headache, that is, acute muscle contraction and a central neurotransmitter deficit. A third component may be an increasing autonomy of the underlying mechanisms. Repeated episodes of persistent muscle contraction from worry, depression, or traction on the muscle may result in the physiological mechanisms functioning independently of their original cause.[31]

Traction

Traction on intracranial pain-sensitive structures, such as large arteries, veins, venous sinuses, and cranial nerves that contain pain fibers, results in pain. There may be either direct traction upon pain-sensitive structures or traction by displacement from a distance. Intracranial mass lesions (e.g., a brain tumor, hematoma, abscess, or aneurysm) can cause headache only when they are in a position to exert pressure or traction on vessels or other pain-sensitive structures.[16,32] This may happen long before intracranial pressure (ICP) rises; therefore, headache can occur with or without increased ICP.

Inflammation

The headache associated with meningeal irritation has been attributed by some to increased ICP. However, dilatation and congestion of inflamed meningeal vessels are also involved. The pain probably is initiated by chemical irritation of nerve endings of the meninges.[32] A lowered pain threshold occurs in the inflamed tissues of structures within or adjacent to the coverings of the brain. These inflammatory changes usually are most marked in the dura, vessels, and nerves in the base of the brain. The headache is pulsatile because of distention of the vessels with each cardiac systole.

Scalp arteries also can become inflamed, particularly the temporal arteries. When inflammation occurs, the vessels dilate, the surrounding tissue becomes more sensitive to the pain, and there is a pattern of pulsatile pain.

Combinations of Basic Headache Mechanisms

More than one mechanism and more than one sensitive structure are involved in the headache of intracranial disease:

Traction and displacement of pain-sensitive vessels

Distention and dilation of intracranial arteries

Inflammation in or about any pain-sensitive structure

However, intracranial headaches eventually become vascular whether the initial intracranial mechanism is vascular, traction, or inflammation because the main consistent structures involved are blood vessels. Thus, traction, inflammatory, and vascular headaches can have the sensation of throbbing head pain.[14] All head pain has a reflex muscle contraction component to it. Just as pain in any part of the body results in reflex muscle contraction, any pain about the head causes scalp, neck, and shoulder muscle reflex contraction. If the muscle contraction is intense and sufficiently prolonged to cause

TABLE 8-1
ACUTE AND CHRONIC HEADACHES CLASSIFIED BY FOUR BASIC MECHANISMS

VASCULAR	MUSCLE CONTRACTION	TRACTION	INFLAMMATION
Migraine	Chronic scalp muscle contraction	Tumor	Meningitis
Cluster	Depressive equivalent	Cerebral edema	Subarachnoid
Fever	Cervical arthritis	Cerebral hematoma	hemorrhage
Toxins	Temporomandibular joint disease	Lumbar puncture	Temporal arteritis
Metabolic		Dural tear	Arachnoiditis
Hypertension			

pain, the headache then has a combination of mechanisms involved in its production.

PRIMARY AND SECONDARY HEADACHES

Headaches fall into two major classifications: 1) acute (secondary) headaches resulting from an organic or toxic vascular etiology with varying degrees of seriousness; and 2) chronic (primary) headaches that represent an overreactivity of physiologic mechanisms.[4,43] These latter headaches are benign but can have a troublesome impact on the person's comfort and life. Chronic headaches can have a pattern of constant, dull pain, recurrent episodes of acute pain, or a combination of both. One of the four basic mechanisms of headache is more prevalent in each type of acute or chronic headache. Table 8-1 shows this relationship.

Causes of Acute (Secondary) Headaches

Intracranial Mass Lesions Acute headaches include the intracranial mass lesions of brain tumors, hematomas, and brain abscesses.[14] In some people with brain tumors, headache may be an early symptom, but in others headaches are not prominent. Every patient with progressive or persistent headache should be suspected of having a brain tumor and the possibility should be explored. The headaches from a mass lesion tend to be progressive in their development and the location of the pain is influenced by the site of the lesion.

Hypertension A headache due to essential hypertension, although less common than is sometimes believed, may occur when the systolic pressure is higher than 170 mm Hg or the diastolic pressure is higher than 110 mm Hg.[39] The mechanism of the headache is uncertain; however, the pain is vascular and occurs when the extracranial and intracranial arteries dilate. Characteristics of a hypertensive headache include a daily dull to moderate occipital or frontal headache, which frequently occurs at night or in the early morning. It clears during the day, often after 1 hour of the patient's being out of bed. It is aggravated by effort, lifting, stooping, and jolts to the head. Patients with minimally increased blood pressure who report headaches need evaluation of the headache for other causes.

Ischemic Cerebrovascular Disease The incidence of headache from ischemic cerebrovascular disease ranges from 9% to 64% according to various study results. The headaches can involve any of the cerebral vessels and can result from thrombus, embolus, infarction, or transient ischemic attack.[12]

Various hypotheses have been suggested as to the mechanism of the production of the headache in ischemic cerebrovascular disease. The most current has to do with platelet response to the damaged endothelium. Platelets may release into the blood vessel lumen serotonin, prostaglandins, and other substances that react on the pain-sensitive vessel walls. This process has been identified in the production of migraine headaches, and it could be the cause of headache in thrombotic disease in which platelets are also involved.[12]

A headache may precede the clinical symptoms of a neurologic insult, although most often it occurs simultaneously with the actual evidence of the vascular event.[20] Usually the headaches are ipsilateral to the occluded vessel. When the carotid circulation is involved, the headache is anterior, and when the vertebrobasilar vessels are affected, the headache is posterior.[7]

The majority of the headaches are mild to moderate; however, they can range from barely noticeable to excruciating. The headaches seem to be vascular in nature, being described as throbbing or steady.[12]

Other symptoms associated with the vascular ischemia are visual disturbances similar to a migraine aura, or transient monocular blindness. Contralateral neurologic deficits may also be present.[7]

Meningeal Irritation   Meningitis, subarachnoid hemorrhage, and arachnoiditis cause meningeal irritation. Infection or blood in the cerebrospinal fluid (CSF) produces inflammation of structures within and adjacent to the coverings of the brain. Chemical substances are released that irritate and sensitize nerve endings to pain.[1] The inflammatory changes usually are most marked in the dura, vessels, and nerves at the base of the brain. The headache is throbbing because of the painful vascular distention, is very intense, usually occipital, and involves nuchal rigidity.

Fluid manipulation in the lumbar arachnoid space during diagnostic lumbar punctures traumatizes pain-sensitive intracranial structures.[1] It seems probable that in the upright position, a low intraspinal fluid pressure permits caudal displacement of intracranial structures, which exerts traction on the dural attachments. The headache disappears when the CSF leak stops, the CSF is replaced, and the pressure is restored.

Toxic Vascular Headaches   This classification includes conditions that produce a vascular headache as part of a symptom complex.[1] Fever is the most common cause of nonmigrainous vascular headaches. The intensity of the headache increases as the fever gets higher. Prostaglandins that are released by the pyrogen (the direct cause of fever) cause dilation of the cerebral vessels and thus produce a headache.[23] Vasodilation of the extracranial and intracranial arteries can also result from other conditions and toxins, and include pathologic conditions such as alcohol use, hypoglycemia, hypoxia, altitude, hypercapnia, or toxic substances that are pharmacologic (e.g., nitrites and vasodilators), and non-pharmacologic (e.g., carbon monoxide and industrial nitrates). Withdrawal from drugs such as caffeine or ergot can also result in a vascular headache.[18,35]

Alteration in cerebral blood concentrations of oxygen, carbon dioxide, and glucose can produce changes in the cerebral blood flow. A decrease in the cerebral arterial oxygen content or, to a greater extent, increased carbon dioxide tension, causes profound cerebrovascular dilation.[23]

The toxic vascular headache is usually a diffuse, pulsating headache that is moderate to severe and may be associated with malaise and anorexia. It may occur daily and be intermittent or constant, occipital or generalized.

Temporal Arteritis This disorder affects the pain-sensitive temporal artery. Inflammation produces throbbing, persistent pain. It occurs in the older person, is associated with tenderness of the temporal artery to palpation, and can result in loss of vision. Medical treatment should be sought immediately because it is essential to treat the condition at an early stage if permanent disturbances of sight are to be avoided.[15] Prednisone is the standard treatment.

Causes of Chronic (Primary) Headaches

Chronic primary headaches are divided into vascular and muscle contraction headaches. Migraine and cluster headaches are chronic vascular headaches.

Migraine The definition of *migraine headache* from the Ad Hoc Committee on Migraine is

> Recurrent attacks of headaches, widely varied in intensity, frequency, and duration. The migraine headaches are often familial, the attacks are commonly unilateral in onset, are usually associated with anorexia and sometimes with nausea and vomiting, and some are preceded by or associated with conspicuous sensory, motor, and mood disturbance.[2,8]

Migraine, which leads to vasodistention and inflammation, is primarily a neurochemical disorder with secondary vascular change. It is the result of a complex mechanism that involves vasoactive events and substances, including platelet aggregation, fluctuations in the level of amines (serotonin and norepinephrine), bradykinin release, prostaglandin biosynthesis, free fatty acid elevation, impaired monoamine oxidase function, histamine release, basophil and mast cell degranulation, and immunoglobulin and compliment activation.[7,25,33] Migraine attacks

result in not only head pain but altered functioning in most systems of the body (Table 8-2). Important factors in the production of the pain of a migraine are the dilated vessels and the perivascular accumulation of substances that sensitize the vessels to pain.

Although the vascular component of a migraine is well established, many pathophysiologic events are still unclear, and the sequence of events is not known. The vascular changes in migraine involve both intracranial and extracranial vessels. The initial biochemical changes involve the brain and produce symptoms of an aura. The aura or prodrome symptoms precede the onset of the headache phase, usually by 15 to 20 minutes. The symptoms may be irritability, exhaustion, visual disturbances, or sensory disturbances, for example, numbness and tingling, slurred speech, and confusion. Visual symptoms are the most common pre-headache disturbance in classic migraine. A secondary phase of vasodilation and inflammation of extracranial vessels produces the headache and residual tenderness in the post-headache phase.

A genetic predisposition to neurovascular instability is an important factor in migraine.[6,25] The condition is often inherited as a Mendelian dominant trait. The person's psychologic and biologic states, as well as environmental stimuli, interact with the genetic tendency that results in migraine headaches.

Change, either external or internal, can trigger a migraine headache. The external and the internal triggers can be either physiological or psychological. (See "Triggers for Vascular Headache"). The exact mechanism(s) by which light, odor and emotions, and so forth change the physiological functioning that results in pain is still not determined. Although it is accepted that emotional disturbances can cause headache, a

TABLE 8-2
ASSOCIATED SYMPTOMS OF VASCULAR HEADACHES

GASTROINTESTINAL	SENSORY	GENERAL
Nausea	Scalp tenderness	Lethargy
Vomiting	Tingling	Washed-out appearance
Cramps or gas	Numbness	Stiff neck
Diarrhea or constipation	Burning	Shoulder pain
Appetite change	Tinnitus	Urination changes
	Odor sensitivity	Light-headed
	Sonophobia	

VASOMOTOR	VISUAL	EMOTIONS
Chills	Blurred	Depressed
Pallor	Diplopia	Irritable
Cold extremities	Spots	Restless
Lacrimation	Zigzag lines	Elated
Nasal drainage or stuffiness	Photophobia	Cry
	Scintillating lights	
	Blind spots	
	Colors	
	Ptosis	

MENTAL	VESTIBULAR	MOTOR
Confusion	Dizziness	Dysphasia
Impaired concentration		Dysarthria
		Imbalance
		Paresis

great number of headache sufferers do not recognize any emotional triggers. Conflict, guilt, and anger, especially repressed anger, can be potent factors in the headache frequency.

Triggers for Vascular Headache

Tyramine	Lights	Conflict
foods	Motion	Anger
Alcohol	Odors	Guilt
Fasting	Medications	Depression
Barometric	Sleep	Dependency
pressure	Hormones	Stress
Physical		
exertion		
Fever		

Combinations of two or more triggers can be additive, and it is the additive effect that is important to precipitation of the migraine.

Cluster Headache Another form of chronic vascular headache is the cluster headache.[8] It is a cyclic disorder that occurs in two patterns. The classic form cycles from headache-free periods to cluster headache periods. The second pattern, chronic cluster, has no headache-free period; but the intensity and frequency of the headaches vary. Neither the etiology nor pathogenesis of this disorder, which occurs more frequently in men than in women, is known. Because many biological rhythms are controlled by central nervous system (CNS) oscillators in the hypothalamus, it is speculated that cluster headache is caused by cyclic biochemical alterations, produced by a transitory malfunction of the oscillatory center. Studies have shown an increase in histamine and serotonin levels in the blood at the onset of the cluster cycle.[22,23]

A *cluster headache* presents as a unilateral, periorbital, overwhelming pain, which develops without warning, lasts for 15 to 60 minutes and suddenly subsides. The eye on the affected side tears, and the nostril on that side drains. The headache tends to occur at specific times during the day, and there may be from one to six or more headaches in 24 hours at the peak of the cluster episode. Episodes tend to occur once a year and last for 4 to 6 weeks. Alcohol, sleep, and weather changes are some of the triggers of this headache.

Muscle Contraction Headache   The most common of the chronic headaches is the muscle contraction headache, which comes from sustained muscle contraction, vasoconstriction, and accumulation of metabolites, all of which cause pain. The vasoconstriction may be a reflex response to the continuously contracted musculature. The vasoconstriction causes a reduced blood flow to the muscles, and the ischemia that occurs as a consequence results in headache. Electromyographic recordings show varying degrees of tension with muscle contraction headache.[5,19] Muscle contraction may be a primary or secondary phenomenon. For some people, chronic, daily muscle contraction headaches may be the result of a central mechanism in the brain that is the source of the pain, rather than irritation and sustained contraction of muscles about the head. This group of headache sufferers has no detectable muscular or arterial abnormality associated with their severe pain.[30] Muscle

contraction headaches very commonly are associated with depression.

Serotonin and norepinephrine levels are depressed in patients with chronic muscle contraction headaches and in endogenous depression. The tricyclic antidepressants that raise the level of these substances are used in the treatment of both these conditions.[22]

The muscle contraction headache is a generalized, steady, nonpulsatile ache. People describe the pain as a feeling of tightness in the forehead, around the head, or the occiput, and as a sensation of tightness and stiffness in the neck and the upper back. The muscle contraction headache that most people experience is a sporadic episode, and is rarely brought to the attention of the health care professional because it is self-limiting and likely to be relieved by over-the-counter analgesics. It is the person who suffers chronic, daily, sometimes continuous, head pain that usually is seen by the health professional.

All types of head pain in their later stages can give rise to muscle contraction. A person can have a headache from a brain tumor, and the muscles about the head can then tighten in response to the pain. Likewise, the person with a migraine also will have muscle contraction pain.

Mixed Headache   Combination headaches are very common. There can be a combination of any of the above mechanisms. A very common mixed syndrome is migraine and muscle contraction headache.[8,33] Some headache experts find that this mixed headache is the most common type encountered in their practices. The mixed headache syndrome occurs when vascular and muscle contraction components occur simultaneously. Independent migraine or muscle contraction headaches are not a mixed headache. The person with a mixed headache has a daily, dull headache, which periodically exacerbates to a more severe migraine. The characteristics of both migraine and muscle contraction are present.

Post-traumatic Headache The post-traumatic, disautonomic headache occurs after marked or mild trauma to the head. There may or may not be obvious evidence of injury to the skull, adjacent soft tissue, or the neck structures. There are three headache patterns:

1. Pain or circumscribed tenderness in a scar or site of impact due to stimulation of pain endings caught in locally damaged tissue
2. A steady sensation of aching pain in a circumscribed area or in a caplike distribution (probably due to sustained neck or head muscle contraction)
3. A throbbing or aching pain occurring in attacks, usually unilateral, and in temporal or frontal regions.[6,37]

These recurrent episodes of pain are due to dilation of the branches of the external carotid artery. Many of these are nonmigraine vascular headaches; however, the migraine process can be triggered or aggravated by head injury. Sometimes the same patient exhibits more than one mechanism of head pain. There can be muscle contraction and vasodilation together, or in combination with scar formation. This headache can become persistent and chronic for months or even years.

Table 8-3 lists the characteristics of the most common acute (secondary) headaches. Table 8-4 lists the characteristics of the most common chronic (primary) headaches.

PSYCHOSOCIAL ASPECTS OF HEADACHES

The nervous system is as sensitive to symbolic threat as to physical threat. The head, which is the center for thoughts and feelings, is the area that frequently hurts when a person is under stress. The stress may come from hostile impulses toward members of the family or some authority figure outside of the family, such as an employer or colleague. It may come from internal conflict, or vacillating feelings of dependency and aggression towards parents, spouse, or work associates. There may be feelings of inadequacy or uncertainty, or emotions (chiefly anger) that are socially unacceptable.

A broad generalization can be made about persons with headaches, particularly those with migraine; they are likely to be perfectionistic and compulsive. Their standards are extremely high and they are unable to either modify them or adjust to changing situations. The families as well as the patients themselves suppress feelings. The inability to express feelings leads to conflict, and this in turn triggers the headache.

Analysis of situations in which a headache occurs often reveals a relationship between the headache and emotional stress. Many clinical observations support the idea that the person with migraine headaches reacts to stressful events in an exaggerated or inappropriate manner. The person who gets migraine headaches usually performs well under stress, perhaps too well, and then experiences a headache when the stress is over.

Severe emotional trauma is found to be the key etiologic factor in some people with headaches. They fail to recognize the relevance of unbearable emotional pain and conflict to their headache problem, and tend to gloss over or avoid elaboration of intense feelings about life events and interpersonal relationships. This becomes an occult emotional trauma.[17] The extreme emotional pain in which the persons perceive themselves as

(*Text continues on page 192*)

TABLE 8-3
CHARACTERISTICS OF ACUTE (SECONDARY) HEADACHES

DISEASE	TEMPORAL PATTERN	LOCATION	QUALITY AND SEVERITY	ASSOCIATED SYMPTOMS	PRECIPITANTS
Intracranial mass lesions Tumor Hematoma Abscess	Intermittent Progressive Early or later symptom	Influenced by site of lesion May be well-localized and may become generalized with progressive increase in ICP	Variable intensity	Pathologic reflexes Papilledema Slowed mentation Dizziness Vomiting Seizures Sensory or motor deficits	None or sometimes changes in head position Valsalva's maneuver Coughing Hematoma may be with or without history of trauma.
Essential hypertension	Almost daily More intense during early morning	Occipital or generalized	Vascular Dull to moderate	BP elevated Episodes of dizziness or blurred vision	Valsalva Jolts to head
Ischemic cerebrovascular disease Embolus Thrombus Infarct Transient ischemic attacks	Usually acute onset Sometimes headaches precede the event	Influenced by site of lesion: contralateral Frontal Occipital Eye	Vascular Usually mild to moderate Infarct commonly painless	Visual disturbances Neurologic deficits	
Meningeal irritation Meningitis Subarachnoid hemorrhage Arachnoiditis Lumbar puncture	Acute onset No previous history except sometimes before subarachnoid hemorrhage if there has been a previous bleeding episode	Generalized and predominently occipital	Intense deep pain Vascular in nature Explosive and intense onset with hemorrhage	Nuchal rigidity Various neurologic deficits Fever Abnormal CSF	Exertion causing Valsalva's maneuver with hemorrhage Upright position lumbar puncture
Toxic vascular	No consistent pattern Usually daily	Diffuse	Pulsating Moderate to severe Increases as fever increases	Malaise Anorexia Fever	Fever-producing disease Alcohol use Hypoxia Hypercapnia Hypoglycemia Altitude Drug withdrawal Toxic substances Vasoactive drugs
Temporal arteritis	Late middle age and elderly Random attacks to persistent daily attacks	Initially localized temporal to generalized frontotemporal Bilateral or unilateral	Deep, burning, throbbing	Tender, nodular temporal arteries Elevated sedimentation rate Later intermittent or permanent visual loss	

TABLE 8-4
CHARACTERISTICS OF CHRONIC (PRIMARY) HEADACHES

DISEASE	TEMPORAL PATTERN	LOCATION	QUALITY AND SEVERITY	ASSOCIATED SYMPTOMS	PRECIPITANTS
Migraine Common	Onset: children to early adulthood Recurrent over a long period with symptom-free intervals between headaches Few hours to few days	Frontal, temporal, parietal, occipital Unilateral or bilateral	Throbbing, pressure Moderate to severe	(see Table 8-2)	(see Table 8-2)
Classic		Classic: unilateral and one side tends to be affected more frequently		Classic: visual scintillations, blind spots or visual field cuts, numbness, and tingling, paresis	
Cluster Episodic (classic) Chronic	Onset ages 20 to 50 Classic: cyclic One to several times a day for 4–8 wk Brief duration, 15 to 60 min Chronic: no free periods	Unilateral behind or one eye or temple	Excruciating Throbbing, sharp	Unilateral lacrimation and rhinorrhea Conjunctival injection Facial flushing Horner's syndrome	Reason for cycles unknown (see Kudrow) Alcohol REM sleep Barometric pressure changes
Muscle contraction	Teens to age 60 Daily dull Many years	Generalized or frontal occipital including neck and upper back	Steady nonpulsatile ache Tightness Bandlike	Fatigue Insomnia Depression Anxiety	Very often no identifiable precipitating factors
Mixed migraine and muscle contraction	Onset ages 20 to 50 Daily, dull intermixed with periodic throbbing	Frontotemporal or occipital, often worse on one side	Dull with periodic severe headache	Irritability Fatigue Associated symptoms of migraine	Same as migraine for the throbbing periods
Post-traumatic	Onset with trauma May last months to years	Site of trauma Caplike Temporal frontal	Varies (see text)	Same as muscle contraction and mixed headache	History of trauma

helpless, hapless victims may not be revealed in the standard headache history. The health professional needs to be sensitive to cues that an occult emotional trauma may exist and may be the precipitating factor in the patient's headache problem.

Chronic headaches are not imaginary or merely psychosomatic, but are real pain, related to a specific psychophysiologic disorder. It is not uncommon to find on the problem list of the health record of the person with headaches several psychophysiologic problems, such as fatigue, colitis, ulcer, dizziness, constipation, and hypertension.

Depression often is associated with chronic migraine and muscle contraction headache. It is academic to discuss whether depression or pain comes first, or whether the pain and depression arise from a common cause. Regardless of the etiology, the patient needs help with both the depression and the pain.

GENERAL HEALTH AND MENTAL HEALTH CONSEQUENCES OF HEADACHES

Chronic headaches sufferers do not have health consequences from the headache *per se*, except for the effect of the pain on the person's spontaneity or sparkle. The effects on health may come from the unresolved psychological conflicts that trigger the headaches. The unrecognized and unresolved issues of dependency, hostility, and rigidity are perpetuated for the person, the spouse, and the offspring if psychological intervention does not occur.

The problem of drug dependence in patients with chronic headaches, particularly migraine or mixed headaches, must be considered. There is the possibility of a rebound reaction of constriction, dilation, and headache from prolonged frequent use of ergotamine and analgesics. Rather than risk getting an extremely painful headache, the person begins taking medications at the first sign of such an event. A daily prophylactic dose of the drugs is used and augmented with additional amounts as the headache seems imminent. To secure continued relief from the onset of headaches, increasing frequency of usage occurs. Recognition of this situation is essential. The symptoms are often increasing frequency of headache, refractoriness of the headache to appropriate preventive medications and fatigue. Headaches occur if the ergot or analgesic is not taken.[33,35] When asked to give up the drugs the person becomes very anxious because of the fear of the pain and of losing the only measure of controlling it.

Other consequences from extensive use of analgesics, particularly acetylsalicylic acid, include gastritis, ulcers, and anemia. Renal function may be affected by continued use of various analgesics as well. The frequent use of ergotamine over a period of time may lead to vasoconstrictive symptoms.

The major consequence of chronic headaches is that they affect the whole family, for they too may have the quality of their lives diminished by the person's headache. Chronic pain causes physical and mental depletion, such as less involvement in the family, job, and leisure pursuits. Family plans, as well as individual plans, frequently may be disrupted by the onset of a headache. Family members become distressed and anxious as they watch a person go through the intense pain of a headache episode. It is also discouraging to live with a person who continuously has pain and has no means of relieving it.

Research on the impact of headache on the life of a person and family is needed. The majority of people with seriously troublesome, chronic headaches do not see themselves as sick and do not exhibit sick role behaviors. Because of their compulsive, perfectionistic nature, people with chronic headaches tend to be very productive and to carry on their responsibilities, particularly in their job and in homemaking. People with chronic headaches realize that they may be incapacitated at any time with an acute headache, and therefore may push themselves to overachieve when feeling well. This overexertion may then itself produce a headache, setting up a vicious cycle. Relaxation and enjoyment are difficult for them to experience.

NURSING ASSESSMENT

SUBJECTIVE DATA

An accurate diagnosis is essential if appropriate and effective therapy is to be provided. The headache history, general health history, neurologic examination, laboratory, and possibly other diagnostic studies, plus follow-up on the patient's response to medications and other treatments, are the factors involved in the diagnosis of headache. The most essential part of the evaluation is the headache history.[24,33,36] The nurse in any setting can be instrumental in obtaining a detailed description of the headache. The essential items of the headache history are listed opposite.

Schedule sufficient time to obtain the particular details of the headache and to begin to establish trust. Measures that can facilitate obtaining explicit details from the patient are: 1) having the person keep a headache record, which can be used both as an assessment tool and a self-monitoring tool (Fig. 8-2), and 2) having the person use a pain-severity scale to describe the headache pain. Examples of both of these tools are given later in the chapter. Characteristics of the pain involve several parameters (see the box on Characteristics). By supplying these descriptive terms, the patient can characterize the headache more accurately. Although

---

Central Components of the Headache Assessment

Number and types of headache patterns
Age and circumstances of onset
Family history of headaches
Characteristics of the pain
    Quality
    Severity
    Location
    Onset and chronology
    Frequency
    Duration
Precipitating factors (triggers)
    Biologic
    Environmental
    Interpersonal
    Intrapersonal
Conditions that predispose, aggravate, and
    relieve
Prodromal symptoms
Associated symptoms
Use and response to medication
Emotional factors

---

patients often assume that a description of the location and intensity of the headache is sufficient, it is not. Neither the location nor the intensity alone are reliable clues to the diagnosis of the pain.

Ask if the headaches have followed the same pattern consistently or if this is a different pattern. Also ask what the patient thinks the cause or the trigger for the headaches is; they often know the cause or trigger. Identify psychosocial issues, such as dependency, marital conflict, and job stresses, because there are both organic and functional aspects of pain. All patients need to be evaluated and treated for both aspects of the pain, or successful control of the headaches will be limited. Determine the current therapy the person is using for headaches and other health problems. Close questioning about medications taken for headaches, particularly anal-

Date/Time	Location	Severity	Associated preceding	Symptoms accompanying	Triggers	Treatment	Relief	Duration	Comments

FIG. 8-2   Headache diary.

gesics, ergotamines, decongestants, and over-the-counter (OTC) drugs, may yield valuable information. The name(s) of specific drug(s), dosage, frequency, and length of time taken should all be obtained, because tapering and discontinuance of these medications are part of the treatment program. The person's headaches may actually be rebound headaches, and it is important to get back to the basic pattern. Headaches also may be a side-effect of prescribed medications, such as vasodilators and bronchodilators, that the person is taking for the other health problems. Untreated conditions such as anemia, diabetes mellitus, or hyperthyroidism may be the etiology of headaches. Knowledge of the etiology of the headache makes for more effective treatment planning.

OBJECTIVE DATA

Every patient with headaches requires a physical and neurologic examination, with particular attention to the head, cervical

Characteristics of the Pain

Quality: Dull, sharp, pressure, throbbing, ache, pounding, tight, band, boring, squeezing, burning, stabbing

Severity: Consider 0 to 5 scale

Location and radiation: Unilateral, bilateral, orbital, temporal, frontal, occipital, neck, shoulder

Onset pattern: Time of day, relationship to events

Chronology (time course): When first began, change in pattern. If the person has daily headaches with episodic acute headaches, distinguish which came first and when each began.

Frequency: Times/day, times/week, times/month, times/year

Duration: Continuous, minutes, hours, waxes and wanes

Conditions that predispose: Fatigue, tension, disrupted routines

Conditions that aggravate: Movement, heat, cold

Conditions that alleviate: Physical activity, sleep

spine, cranial nerves, and mental status, plus cerebellar, motor, and sensory functions.[24,33,36] Note the presence of bruits and muscle tension about the head and neck. In most patients with headache the examination will be normal, and further testing will not be indicated. However, if organic disease is suspected from the history and physical examination, some noninvasive investigations can be done, such as skull x-ray, computerized tomography scan of the brain (CT), and electroencephalogram (EEG).[33] Skull x-rays, which show the anatomy of the skull, are done if one suspects a fracture, sinus disease, pituitary enlargement or any neurologic disorder that affects bone structure. The CT scan of the cranium shows structural disturbances within the brain. It is done in situations in which there are intractable persistent headaches, recent onset of a headache, any neurologic symptom or sign, or changes in the course of the headache symptoms. The EEG shows electrical disturbances of the brain. All the indications for doing a CT scan also apply for doing an EEG, plus any paroxysmal activity, dizziness, loss of consciousness, possibility of substance abuse, memory, impairment or questionable cognitive dysfunction, and any organic brain disturbance.

A blood test panel, which includes hematology, biochemistry, and thyroid function, is done to rule out other diseases that may be aggravating the headache pattern.

The physical and neurologic examination and the diagnostic studies will be normal for the person with chronic vascular and muscle contraction headaches. The person with traction headaches may have an intracranial mass lesion, and this will be demonstrated in the diagnostic studies, particularly the CT scan. There is a high incidence of minor encephalographic abnormalities in the person with migraine headaches.[15] The sedimentation rate will be elevated in a person with temporal arteritis.[1] X-ray films may show osteoarthritis of the cervical spine. Opacities in the sinus areas of the skull x-ray occur with sinus disease.

NURSING DIAGNOSIS

NURSING CONSIDERATIONS RELATED TO THE MEDICAL DIAGNOSIS

What does the nurse need to determine before intervention can begin? The basic question is: Is this headache pattern one that may be indicative of an imminent or progressive life-threatening situation? To assess this, determine if there are signs or symptoms that are indicative of intracranial, life-threatening problems. The questions to ask are: Has this headache been present before? Has it been diagnosed? Is the pattern the same or changed? Patients who have a change in their headache pattern, who have not been diagnosed, or who have neurologic signs, need to be referred to the physician; or the nurse practitioner, through the use of protocols or in consultation with the physician, needs to begin evaluation of the headache.

The National Institutes of Health has drawn up a list of alarm signals for seeking medical attention for the headache sufferer. These signals are reasonable guides for the nurse to use for referral.[27]

- Any headache that comes on suddenly or is marked by excruciating pain
- Any headache associated with fever. This sign is especially ominous if the fever follows the headache rather than, as in the customary pattern of influenza symptoms, merely accompanying it.
- A headache accompanied by convulsions
- Headaches of any strength accompanied by mental or neurologic abnormalities such as blurred or double vision, confusion, loss of alertness or consciousness, loss of bodily function, coordination, or sensation
- A headache following a blow to the head
- Any pattern of headaches localized in the ear or eye
- Any pattern of headaches occurring in an older person who has previously been free of frequent headaches
- Recurring headaches in children
- A pattern of headaches at any age that interferes with routines of living
- Frequent headaches, especially if they exhibit a change in severity or pattern from routine aches of the past

Headaches that progress in frequency and intensity, or that interfere with routines of living, require reevaluation. Additional assistance is needed when the person is using increasing amounts of analgesics, ergotamine, or decongestants.

A sudden, excruciating headache may be from a subarachnoid hemorrhage; headache preceding fever may mean meningitis, and headache and convulsions may be from a mass such as a brain tumor, abscess, subarachnoid hemorrhage, or meningitis. Neurologic impairment may result from a mass such as a tumor, infection, hemorrhage, classic migraine, or cerebral vascular disease. Headache following a blow to the head can be from a subdural hematoma. Headache localized in the ear may mean ear disease; localization in the eye may be referred pain from an intracranial lesion or eye disease. The onset of frequent headaches in the older person may mean temporal arteritis. Recurring headaches that interfere with the routines of living need to be addressed to determine if the etiology of the headaches is the presence of stress or if the headache is a symptom of a physical problem.[7]

The long list of conditions in which headache may be a symptom emphasizes the need for a thorough health history, headache history, and physical examination to diagnose correctly the type of headache, and to establish an effective treatment program. Effective treatment can occur only after a medical diagnosis of the headache has been made. A diagnosis is needed to know what the mechanisms of the headache are so that care can be based on principles related to the particular headache mechanism. This is particularly true for nursing interventions related to patient education about the headache.

NURSING DIAGNOSES

Nursing diagnoses common to the population of people with chronic headaches are: knowledge deficit of mechanisms and management of headaches, pain, self-management deficits, self-esteem disturbance, fear and anticipation of pain, and various other psychological states (e.g., marital conflicts). Alterations in comfort-pain, pain self-management deficit, altered gastrointestinal functioning, increased sensitivities, altered mood, and fear of the pain are common in severe, acute, or recurrent acute headaches.

MANAGEMENT

Effective pain reduction and care require that the nurse know the seriousness of the head pain and the probable mechanism of the pain, that is, vascular, muscle contraction, traction, or inflammation. While the diagnostic workup is in progress, the nurse can use the measures discussed in the following section. Many of the measures will continue to be appropriate after the specific headache mechanism is determined.

There are two basic areas of nursing management: 1) measures to relieve symptoms during the headache episode, and 2) measures to help prevent headache episodes.

MANAGEMENT TO RELIEVE SYMPTOMS DURING THE HEADACHE EPISODE

Nurses working in various settings may be required to assist a patient with a migraine headache that has been triggered by events related to other health problems. For example, a woman with migraine may have a headache precipitated in the postpartum period as the hormonal levels change. This can be an intense migraine. The nurse in a coronary care unit may need to assist a person with a vascular headache due to vasodilating medication given for a coronary problem. The postoperative period can be a time when migraines are triggered because preventive medications are withheld, or the situation is stressful. People with migraine also tend to get a headache whenever they have a fever.

The goals of nursing care during the acute headache episode are:

1. To abort or reduce the pain
2. To promote relaxation of the person, especially the head and neck muscles
3. To reduce the accompanying symptoms
4. To identify possible triggers.

Pain reduction is the same for both the person with acute secondary headaches and the person with a recurrent episode of chronic headaches. A major difference, however, is the identification, monitoring, and treatment of the underlying disease of the secondary headache. Patients with secondary headaches are monitored for changes in neurologic status, fever sources, and possible intracranial hemorrhage. Measures to prevent increased ICP, to reduce fever, and to control infection are instituted. Pain medications that have a sedative effect should be avoided in patients with an altered state of consciousness. Seizure precautions also may be necessary.

Other goals of medical and nursing care are to detect changes, to prevent complications, and provide treatment measures to reduce or reverse the condition that is causing or triggering the headaches.

Therapeutic Relationship

The single most important nursing intervention for the patient in pain is the nurse–patient relationship. The nurse can listen, try to understand, anticipate needs, interpret what is happening, and intervene to improve the situation.

Anticipating the need for light reduction, quiet environment, blankets because of chilling, and information promotes the patient's trust in the nurse, which aids relaxation and enhances the effects of medications administered. The patient needs information about what to expect with treatment. For example, the person who has been given adequate medication for a migraine is likely to experience a decrease in blood pressure and nausea before experiencing a decrease in pain.

Reassurance comes from hearing about what one is experiencing or will be experiencing. Knowledge means control for many patients. Therefore, an explanation of the complex interactions of headache can be an intervention to reassure as well as helping to increase the patient's control over the pain. Patients need reassurance concerning the seriousness of the headache. Many people have the recurring fear that their headaches, particularly when there is an exacerbation of the headache, are symptoms of an underlying brain tumor or impending stroke, yet these fears may remain unspoken. They particularly need to be discussed when there is a history of such an illness in a close friend or relative. Explicit explanation of the results of the neurologic examination and diagnostic studies is needed, along with the assurance that these findings almost definitely rule out a serious problem of the brain. Reassurance of the absence of signs of an organic lesion are given in conjunction with statements that this does not mean the headaches are imaginary.

Pain Reduction Measures

Head Position and Protection Head position and protection both can contribute to comfort. Most people with vascular headaches are more comfortable with the head of the bed elevated because this position reduces the pulsatile nature of the vascular pain. If the ICP is elevated, venous drainage also may be promoted in this position, which reduces the pressure.

When the intraspinal pressure is low, as it is after a lumbar puncture, keeping the person in a supine position can readily relieve the headache.[1] In addition, the caudal displacement of intracranial structures is avoided by the supine position.

Teaching and assisting the person with vascular headaches to avoid the Valsalva maneuver prevents exacerbation of the headache. The Valsalva maneuver enhances the amplitude of pulsations and distends sensitive vessels, and therefore exacerbates the pain.

Identify measures to protect the head from jarring, which prevents headache exacerbation. Many vascular headaches sensitize the head to any jolt; therefore, patients tend to protect their heads by tensing the neck and shoulder muscles.[6,43] This muscle tension, however, is self-defeating. Hence, such measures as letting the person bend, stand, and move at his own pace is helpful.

Sensory Input Heat, ice, pressure, and massage are extremely useful measures for aborting and diminishing head pain. They are so readily available and in such common use that people have a tendency to minimize their value, to the extent that some people have never tried these measures. It may be helpful to place the benefit of these measures in the context of the gate control theory of pain (see Chap. 6). An explanation of this theory can provide the patient with a rationale for the effectiveness of these measures. It can also promote trust and willingness to implement nonmedication interventions. Then the patient will not feel that the pain is being discounted by the recommendation of these measures. In addition, an understanding of the gate control theory can provide the patient with some intellectual control over the pain.

Local heat can provide particular benefit for head pain, particularly muscle contraction pain, alone or as a reflex tightness of neck and shoulders associated with vascular pain. The physiologic effects of local heat result in vasodilation and increased blood flow, a degree of analgesia, sedation, and muscle relaxation. All of these underlying mechanisms are not understood, particularly the analgesia and the sedative effect.[38] Heating pads, hot showers, sitting in the sun, or a warm hand are sources of heat.

Cold has the opposite effect of heat. Cooling the tissues results in vasoconstriction and a relatively mild, cutaneous anesthesia.[38] Ice tends to subdue the pulsating pressure of a vascular headache.

An ice pack about the vascular areas of the head, and a heating pad across the back of the neck and shoulders where the muscles are tight tend to be the most helpful measures. However, whether to use heat or cold and where to place them are determined by one criterion: whatever feels good.

Massage to the neck, shoulders, and forehead is soothing for tight muscles. Massage can increase circulation and relax the muscles, thereby relaxing the person, and reduce the pain. Likewise, local pressure to areas of distended scalp vessels decreases pain by reducing the blood flow and the amplitude of the pulse wave. People will bury their heads in the pillow, apply digital pressure, and even tie belts around their heads. They need to be reassured and given permission to do such "weird," pain-relieving activities.

Relaxation Measures Self-control and pain control relaxation measures are useful during the headache episode. Relaxation techniques, focusing, distraction, guided imagery, or controlled breathing may be very helpful. Examination and discussion of self-talk (i.e., what one tells oneself), and one's emotional responses to headache, are all part of the relaxation regimen.

Coaching in body relaxation measures, such as described in Chapter 6, and audio tapes with relaxation exercises, calm the person and enhance the effects of the headache treatment, as well as relax the head and neck muscles. Personnel in emergency rooms and other settings that frequently treat people with headaches should consider purchasing appropriate relaxation tapes and a tape recorder to enhance the effects of medications and the other comfort measures used.

Medication Medications for a headache given at its onset increase the success rate in aborting the pain. Patients learn this principle. The occasional headache can evolve into a daily headache; along with the increased headache frequency may be increased drug usage. This can perpetuate the increased headache frequency and have health consequences from the use of the drugs. Patients with increasingly frequent headaches should restrain and limit the use of abortive medications. Clinical experience shows that limiting the use of abortive medications to 2 days a week or less avoids the rebound phenomena.

When a person with frequent acute recurrent headaches reports pain, medication should not be the immediate response. The person would benefit from a model for self-care that promotes comfort and relaxation measures to abort and subdue a headache.

The medications prescribed to abort an acute migraine usually include ergotamine (if there are no contraindications for using it) and an antiemetic. At home this is usually used in suppository form. In the emergency room injectable forms are used and an analgesic is often added to the regimen. For persistent, severe headache a steroid, such as dexamethasone, may be added.

Mild analgesics will usually relieve the simple muscle contraction headache. Use of analgesics for cluster headache is problematic because the intensity of the pain requires a large amount of the analgesic. Even then pain relief may not occur, but the person feels drugged for some time.

Comfort Measures The common concern of the headache treatment program is to recondition patients from responding to the onset of headache with a reaction of fear, anxiety, and medication, to one of relaxation and comfort measures first. Learning to verbalize about emotionally charged events that trigger a headache can subdue pain and reduce headache frequency. Calming of the accompanying symptoms is needed for comfort and for reduction of the distress caused by these symptoms, such as lowering the temperature in the febrile state to dampen the forceful pulsations of the headache. The person with migraine may be as restricted by the combination of light, sound, and odor sensitivities, nausea and vomiting, irritability, and chilling as by the head pain. A quiet, darkened room free of odors and sufficient blankets are necessary for the person to relax and get the most benefit and relief. An antiemetic may be necessary to control the nausea, wretching, and vomiting.

Sleep Sleep can help to resolve a headache by itself and also can potentiate the effects of other measures used to reduce the headaches. Therefore, measures to promote sleep and instructions to the person to go to bed and sleep, can enhance the effects of the treatment.

Oxygen Administered by mask at 7 liters for 10 to 15 minutes, oxygen is effective in aborting cluster headaches in a large percentage of people.[22] The mechanism for relief from oxygen inhalation may be the reduction of cerebral blood flow. Because the pain is so intense, these patients usually cannot be quiet: they pace, move around, and do various things. They also are very, very impatient and have difficulty using the oxygen mask unless it gives immediate relief.

First Aid Measures

Many headaches arise from psychological stress and physical exertion. They seldom last long, and if they occur only infrequently and without any significant pattern or intensity, they can reasonably be dismissed as of no consequence beyond the moment. In those situations basic measures like fresh air are useful, because toxic fumes in the air may be the cause of the headache. Other useful measures are rest and quiet, lying down, falling asleep, massage of the neck muscles, a heating pad, hot shower, warm tub, a snack if a meal has been postponed, aspirin, and a cup of coffee. (The coffee is used for its caffeine, but soft drinks may be used instead.) These are used along with the aspirin because caffeine enhances the effect of the analgesic, and caffeine also has a vasoconstrictive effect.[27]

MANAGEMENT TO PREVENT OCCURRENCE OF CHRONIC HEADACHES

The goals in a preventive program for chronic headaches are

1. An understanding of headache physiology and therapy that is sufficient for the patient's satisfaction and effective functioning
2. Patient participation in headache management
3. Identification of headache triggers, responses to therapy and modification of treatment
4. Identification of appropriate methods to manage a headache episode
5. Acknowledgment of personality and psychosocial aspects that affect headache frequency

Frequent Visits

Visits are valuable in establishing trust and a relationship that contributes to mobilizing the person's hope for headache control. Repeated contact with a primary nurse assists the patient to find acceptable interpretations and to understand the headache pattern. The person's increased self-understanding and acceptance is the basis for better self-care practices and headache prevention.

Patient Education

Education about the cause and mechanisms involved in headaches is essential in a preventive program. One study of 100 patients in an outpatient setting asked patients what was most important to them when they came to the doctor.[29] Many of these patients desired an explanation of the cause of the headache. Pain relief was chosen first by only 69% of the patients. Pain relief is an important aspect of treatment, but often it is not the primary concern of the patient.

A planned education program includes three major areas; 1) types of headaches, 2) treatment approaches, and 3) the process of care for the person with headaches. Types of headaches include descriptions of vascular, muscle contraction, rebound, and mixed headaches. These are described from the perspective of the pattern of pain, the associated symptoms, and the triggers. The approaches to treatment include behavioral aspects of preventing the circumstances that result in headaches, behavioral aspects of management of headaches, and the rationale for medications and their appropriate use. Measures to abort pain are used to stop the development of a headache at its onset. Symptomatic treatments include medications and comfort measures. The process of care emphasizes that the patient is an active participant in the care and needs to be informed and educated about headaches. The patient keeps a headache record, implements the plan of care, comes back, and gives a progress report. The program is modified until the most effective and safest program is developed for the person. The patient is told that if rebound headaches are occurring from the current medication regimen, the first phase is to taper and discontinue the medication, and to establish a preventive program for the headache. The rationale for diagnostic studies is part of the patient education. The role of the primary nurse, which includes continued contact, promoting self-understanding and effective self-management of the headaches, is explained. A program for patient education of the person with chronic headaches is detailed in *Neurologic Care: A Guide for Patient Education* by Van Meter.[41]

Headache Diary

A headache diary helps patients to see patterns of their headaches and to recognize triggers. It also helps them give a succinct summary about the pattern to the nurse. The diary includes such items as time of headache onset, characteristics of the pain, and associated symptoms. A model of a diary is given in Figure 8-2. Use of a scale for severity of pain and a scale for the relief experienced from treatment helps to promote mutuality of understanding when talking about the headaches. An example of each is listed (p. 202).

Detailed descriptions of the location of the headache can be noted in the diary by the use of a diagram of the head with numbers for various locations (Fig. 8-3). The patient's consistent use of the pain and relief scale and diagram results in more explicit descriptions of the headaches experienced, with mutual understanding of the terms.

General Health Practices

The general health practices of the person are a major focus in promotion of self-care to prevent headaches. A well-balanced diet, adequate rest, time for relaxation and recreation, physical exercise, along with modification of some behaviors and self-expectations, can reduce the frequency of headaches. A well-balanced diet for the person with vascular headaches requires regular eating times, avoidance of fasting (which can be a trigger),

Pain Severity and Relief Scale

SEVERITY SCALE

0 = No headache
1 = Low level headache that enters aware-
    ness only at times when attention is de-
    voted to it
2 = Headache pain level that can be ignored
    at times
3 = Painful headache but can continue at job
4 = Very severe headache, concentration
    difficult but can perform task of an un-
    demanding nature
5 = Intense, incapacitating headache

RELIEF SCALE

0 = No relief
1 = Minimal improvement of questionable
    significance
2 = Has discomfort but not as severe as be-
    fore taking medication or relaxation
3 = Pain present but not disturbing
4 = Free of pain

moderation in caffeine consumption, and avoidance of the foods that can be "trigger" foods (Table 8-5). Excessive fatigue can be a trigger; therefore adequate rest and an effectively paced schedule are essential. Time for recreation and a reasonable amount of physical activity are also desirable; exercise is a tension reliever. A regular exercise program can dissipate the symptoms of stress, thus preventing headaches. Some people find that exercise done at the onset of headache helps to abort it; others experience an exacerbation of the headache.

Women with migraine may need to avoid using birth control pills or hormone supplements.[21] Many women with migraine either begin to experience headaches or have an exacerbation of their previous headaches after starting to take birth control pills. Stopping the pill or reducing and decycling the estrogen replacement therapy will most likely lower the frequency of migraines.

FIG. 8-3 *Location of pain.*

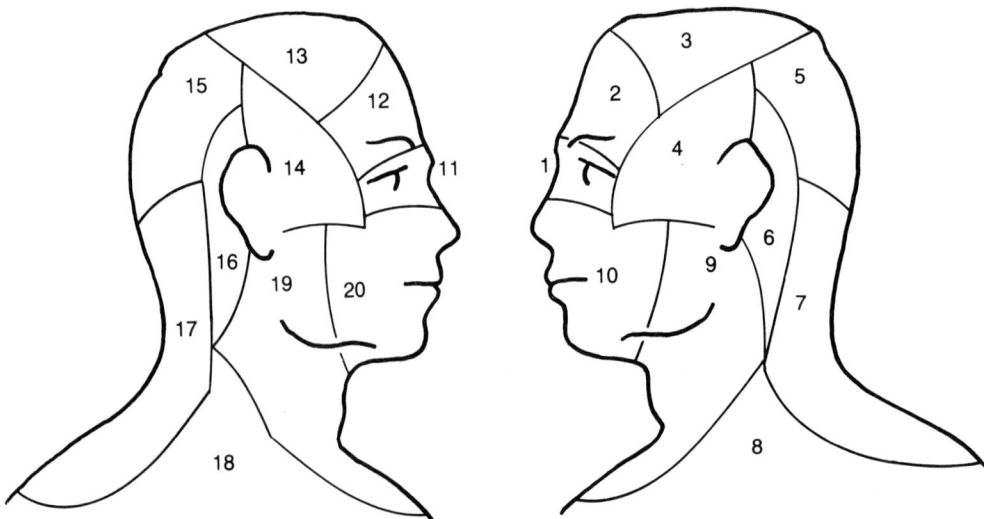

TABLE 8-5
FOODS THAT MAY PROVOKE VASCULAR HEADACHE*

Chocolate	Candy, foods, drinks
Ripened Cheeses	Cheddar, brick, mozzarella, Gruyère, Emmentaler, Stilton, Brie, Camembert, boursin
Alcoholic Beverages	Beer, red wine, sherry, others
Fruits and Their Juices	Bananas, plantain, avocado, figs, passion fruit, raisins, pineapple, oranges and other citrus fruits
Vegetables	Onions, pods of broad beans (lima, navy), pea pods, nuts, peanut butter
Fermented, Pickled, Marinated Foods	Herring, sour cream, yogurt, vinegar
Yeast Products	Yeast extracts, hot fresh breads, raisin coffee cakes and doughnuts
Meats and Nitrites	Bologna, hot dogs, pepperoni, salami, pastrami, bacon, sausages, canned ham, corned beef, smoked fish
Monosodium Glutamate	Chinese food, Accent, Lawry's seasoned salt, instant foods (canned soup, TV dinners), processed meats, roasted nuts, potato chips
Caffeine	Coffee, tea, cola

*These foods contain a vasodilating amine (tyramine, phenylethylamine, or dopamine); monosodium glutamate; caffeine, nitrate or nitrite compounds. Any foods in which aging, bacterial action, molds, or tenderizer is used to enhance flavor, to prepare, or to preserve are likely to contain one of these headache-provoking agents.

The recurrent acute episode for the chronic headache sufferer is most probably a manifestation of a primary headache, but always keep in mind that the person may have an undetected underlying organic reason for the headaches. Effective management of any associated medical disorders is part of the program.

A simpler life-style, with a balanced view of what are reasonable self-expectations, can help to reduce headaches. Recognition of the sources of daily anxieties and how to cope with them, along with reasonable expectations and some behavior modification to deal with compulsiveness and perfectionism, can do much to decrease the stress an individual places on himself.

Supportive Counseling

Counseling is important for many people because of the anxiety, depression, occult emotional trauma, marital conflict, or job stresses that commonly are associated with headaches. A technique to help persons recognize and acknowledge the impact of psychological issues on their headache pattern is to give examples of emotions being translated into physical responses. Such examples are embarrassment, which translates into blushing; anxiety, into sweaty palms; being startled, into palpitations; and fear, into trembling. It is also helpful for them to know that underlying conflicts can affect the headache threshold. When a person is distressed, more headaches are likely to occur, and the headache is more likely to develop into a severe headache. The reverse is also true; when life is calm and things are manageable, the headache is less likely to happen and, if it does, it is less likely to develop into an intense headache. Once these relationships are accepted by the person, counseling will be accepted more readily. It is not uncommon for the process of care of the headaches to be the vehicle whereby much needed, but unacknowledged or resisted, mental health issues are acknowledged and treated.

Control Versus Cure

Chronic headaches result from a physiological predisposition and an overresponsiveness of the body to various internal and external stimuli. As such, they are not curable but they are controllable. This is a basic concept in the management of chronic headaches and one that is essential for the patient to comprehend. The first objective of treatment is to prevent the circumstances that result in headache. Behavioral aspects of care such as identifying and avoiding the triggers, relaxation and stress management techniques, and counseling, are all preventive measures. Preventive medications stabilize the physiological overreactivity to reduce headache frequency. A combination of medications, especially if there is a mixed headache syndrome, may be necessary for a successful program.

Common Medical Therapies for Chronic Headaches

The response to various treatments is highly individual, and each patient's treatment must be tailored to his needs. Adequate dosage and combination of medications are frequently the key to effective pharmacotherapy for the prevention of headaches. Beta-blockers, tricyclic antidepressants, methysergide, nonsteroidal anti-inflammatory agents, calcium channel blockers, phenothiazines, and monoamine oxidase inhibitors are all classifications of drugs used in the prophylaxis of migraine.[7,33]

Medications Used in the Prophylaxis of Chronic Headaches

Propranolol (Inderal) has the greatest efficacy for migraine prevention of all the drugs used.[9] Propranolol is a beta-blocker that prevents the dilation of blood vessels and blocks the aggregation effect of epinephrine on platelets. The dose, as with any other headache preventive drug, needs to be titrated for the patient. The dosage range for propranolol can average between 60 mg to 160 mg per day. A few patients will require smaller amounts and some even larger amounts.

Amitriptyline in combination with propranolol is the most consistently effective drug therapy for mixed migraine and muscle contraction headaches. Amitriptyline alone is most effective for muscle contraction headaches.[33] Reports have indicated that amitriptyline is effective as a pain-preventing agent, exclusive of its antidepressant effect. Other antidepressants in the tricyclic and tetracyclic classifications may be prescribed for the person with muscle contraction headaches.[13]

Dramatic control of classic cluster headaches may be achieved with lithium carbonate, methysergide, indomethacin, chlorpromazine, or a combination of these drugs.[23] A steroid burst is sometimes a means of controlling the cluster exacerbation.

Adherence to medication therapy is not typically a problem because nonadherence has a built-in punishment, pain. Increasing the dosages, however, as a self-care measure sometimes is employed by patients who tend toward substance overuse.

Drugs Prescribed at the Onset of a Headache to Abort Its Development

Ergotamine preparations are the most universally effective for migraine-abortive therapy. However, the side-effects of nausea and vomiting may make it intolerable to some patients. The nausea and vomiting can be treated with an antiemetic. Ergotamine and antiemetics are most effective in suppository form. Isometheptane mucate (Midrin) is a mild, effective abortive medication that may be used for migraine, mixed, or muscle contraction headaches. Very early in the onset of migraine, aspirin or acetaminophen also may abort it but these can lead to overuse. Prolonged migraines (status migrainous) may need steroids like dexamethasone along with the usual abortives to resolve themselves.

A person who seeks help in the emergency room, office, or clinic for severe migraine may need an ergotamine preparation such as dihydroergotamine mesylate, analgesics such as meperidine, or antiemetics such as chlorpromazine, and dexamethasone. Each of these four agents helps to calm a component of the migraine symptomatology. The appropriate combination is critical, as is having the person remain long enough to evaluate effectiveness and to administer additional doses of some parts of the therapeutic program to get complete relief.

Resources for Patients With Chronic Headaches

Many health care professionals have limited knowledge about chronic headaches. Until recently, the study of headaches has not been part of the curriculum of educational programs. Continuing education programs, which frequently focus on chronic pain, now include headache. Research and publications are including this topic as well. There has been little interest and expertise because of the lack of knowledge. The consequence of this lack of expertise on the part of health care professionals has been inadequate headache relief for patients, and patients who are given admonitions that the pain is "all in their heads and they will have to live with it." Some patients stop seeking help; some never have sought help, using only home remedies, and still others desperately try any possible resources as they live anxiously from one headache bout to the next.

Dealing with Headaches (a Time-Life book), is a picture essay of the history, mechanisms, and treatment of headaches.[26] *Freedom from Headaches*, written for the headache sufferer by two physicians, Saper and Magee, devotes a chapter to each of the common chronic headache patterns.[34] Mechanisms, medications, treatment, and self-care are covered. It is an informative book, and is an effective resource for the nurse to gain an overview of chronic headaches before delving into a more complex, physiological treatise on headaches.

The National Migraine Foundation (NMF) is an organization whose purpose is to provide accurate information to people with headaches and the general public.[28] To do this the quarterly *NMF Newsletter* is published. This organization also provides a list of physicians and clinics specializing in the treatment of headaches and supports research on headaches.

Peer-support groups have not yet been developed for headache sufferers, but this might be beneficial. The patients in the country's first inpatient headache treatment program have commented consistently in the patient group discussions on the benefit experienced by them from being in a group with other headache sufferers. For many, it is the first peer sharing-experience about their headache woes and frustrations.

Refractory headaches necessitate the

services of health professionals specializing in headache care. The NMF can provide a list of names of physicians and clinics in a particular locale. The persons named on the list may have an interest in headaches but may not be specializing in the care of this entity. To establish which health professional is likely to be most effective, the persons can ask what percentage of the practice has to do with chronic headaches and what types of services are provided for the patient with chronic headaches. From this the patient can select the most experienced physician and the one that best describes the services provided.

CONCLUSION

THE KNOWN AND THE UNKNOWN

Ongoing care for headaches is essential, as it is for any chronic disease. Modifications in therapy, progress in patient education, and insight are necessary to treat neglected headaches or unsuccessfully treated headaches effectively. Research in headaches is making such strides today that the patient needs to keep in touch with health care professionals to gain the advantage of any improved treatment. The patient can waste time and money going from place to place. Patients go from place to place for two major reasons: the diagnosis and management are not effective, or the focus on refractory headaches as a sign of underlying emotional conflicts is resisted by the patient and family, so they leave to seek help other places.

Elements of a successful treatment program are correct diagnosis of the type of headache, treatment with appropriate medications in adequate dosages and proper route and timing of administration, flexibility of the therapeutic regimen, recognition of multiple mechanisms of headaches, treatment of residual muscle spasm, awareness of physiological and psychological headache trig-

gers, and recognition of the vital role of the clinician–patient relationship. Although much is known about effective methods of treating the person with headaches, there is much to learn.

Questions to be studied range from the minute, biochemical events of the vascular headache, to the incidence of headache in different populations. Research of interest to the nurse might include the following questions: What are the commonly held misconceptions concerning headache in the general population? What are the benefits of a peer-support group for the person with chronic headaches? To what extent do chronic headaches have an impact on a person's life? Which comfort measures are most efficacious for headache relief? What are effective structures and milieux for inpatient headache treatment programs? What does a person suffering acute or chronic headaches most want from the nurse?

Headache care specialists hope that the oversimplification of "a headache is a headache" has been disproven and that an appropriate treatment program will be advocated for each person suffering from frequent headaches.

REFERENCES

1. Adams RD: Headache. In Thorn GW et al: Harrison's Principles of Internal Medicine, 8th ed. New York, McGraw–Hill, 1977
2. Ad hoc committee on classification of headache. Arch Neurol 6:173, 1962
3. Alvarez, WC: Was there sick headache in 3000 BC? Gastroenterology 5:524, 1945
4. Bakal DA, Kaganov JA: Symptom characteristics of chronic and non-chronic headache sufferers. Headache 19:285, 1979
5. Blumer D. Heilbrown M: Chronic muscle contraction headaches and the pain-prone disorder. Headache 22:180, 1982
6. Dalessio DJ: Wolff Headache and Other Pain, 4th ed. New York, Oxford University Press, 1980

7. Dalessio DJ: Classification and mechanism of migraine. Headache 19:114, 1979
8. Diamond S, Medina J: Headaches. Ciba Symposia 3:2, 1981
9. Diamond S, Kudrow L, Steven J et al: Long-term study of propranolol in treatment of migraine. Headache 22:268, 1982
10. Diamond S et al: Panel discussion: The use of analgesics in headache. Headache 19:185, 1979
11. Dorland's Illustrated Medical Dictionary, 26th ed. Philadelphia, WB Saunders, 1981
12. Edmeads J: The headaches of ischemic cerebrovascular disease. Headache 19:345, 1979
13. Fields H, Taub A: Antidepressants for pain. Aches and Pains: Mar 9, 1982
14. Friedman AP: Modern Headache Therapy. St. Louis, CV Mosby, 1959
15. Friedman AP: Headache and related pain syndromes. Med Clin North Am 62:3, 1978
16. Friedman AP: Nature of headache. Headache 19:163, 1979
17. Gill JR, Stein HJ: Occult emotional trauma: A trigger factor to certain headaches (abstr) Headache 22:153, 1982
18. Greden JF: Coffee, tea, and you. The Sciences 6: Jan 1979
19. Haynes SN, Cuevas J, Gannon LR: The psychophysiological etiology of muscle contraction headache. Headache 22:122, 1982
20. Heyck H: Headache and Facial Pain. Chicago, Year Book Medical Publishers, 1981
21. Kudrow L: Hormone therapy and migraine: Cause and effect. Consultant 16:177, 1976
22. Kudrow L: Cluster headache: diagnosis and management. Headache 19:142, 1979
23. Kudrow L. Cluster Headaches. New York, Oxford University Press, 1980
24. Kunkel RS: Evaluating the headache patient: History and work-up. Headache 19:122, 1979
25. Lance JW: Mechanisms and Management of Headache, 3rd ed. London, Butterworths, 1978
26. Murphy W: Dealing with Headaches. Alexandria, VA, Time–Life Books, 1982
27. National Migraine Foundation Newsletter. National Migraine Foundation, 5252 Western Avenue, Chicago, IL, 60625
28. National Institute of Neurological and Communicative Disorders and Stroke: Headache Hope Through Research, Washington, D.C., U.S. GPO, 1971
29. Packard RC: What does the headache patient want? Headache 19:370, 1979
30. Phillips HC, Hunter MS: A psychophysiological investigation of tension headache. Headache 22:173, 1982
31. Pozniak–Patewicz E: "Cephalic" spasm of head and neck muscles. Headache 15:261, 1976
32. Ray BS, Wolff HG: Experimental studies in headache: Pain-sensitive structures of the head and their significance in headache. Arch Surg 42:813, 1940
33. Saper JR: Headache Disorders: Current Concepts and Treatment Strategies. Boston, John Wright PSG, 1983
34. Saper JR, Magee K: Freedom From Headaches. Fireside Press, New York, 1981
35. Saper JR, Van Meter MJ: Ergotamine habituation. Headache 20:159, 1980
36. Sargent JD: Some thoughts regarding diagnosis of functional headaches. Headache 22:186, 1982
37. Speed WG: Post-traumatic headache. National Migraine Foundation Newsletter, 40:1, 1982
38. Stillwell GK: Therapeutic heat and cold. in Krusen F, Kottke F, Ellwood P: Handbook of Physical Medicine and Rehabilitation 2nd ed., Philadelphia, WB Saunders, 1971
39. Traumb YM, Korczyn AD: Headache in patients with hypertension. Headache 18:245, 1978
40. U.S. Department of Health and Human Services: Patients' reasons for visiting physicians: National Ambulatory Medical Care Survey, U.S. 1977–1978. Dept. of Human Services, Vital and Health Statistics, Series 13, No. 56, Dec. 1981
41. Van Meter MJ: Teaching the Person with Chronic Headache. In Van Meter MJ: Neurologic Care: A Guide for Patient Education. New York, Appleton–Century–Croft, 1982
42. Webster's International Dictionary, 3rd ed. Springfield, Mass, G&C Merriam, 1971
43. Wolff HG: Headache. In MacBryde CM, Backlow RS (eds): Signs and Symptoms Applied Pathologic Physiology and Clinical Interpretation, 5th ed. Philadelphia, JB Lippincott, 1970

BIBLIOGRAPHY

Ekbom K: Lithium for cluster headache: Review of the literature and preliminary results of long-term treatment. Headache 21:132, 1981

Glover B et al: Biochemical predisposition to dietary migraine: The role of phenosulphotransferase (abstr.). Headache 22:151, 1982

Graham JR: The migraine connection. Headache 21:243, 1981

Hendler N: Diagnosis and Nonsurgical Management of Chronic Pain. New York, Rave Press, 1981

Napolitano LV et al: Questions and answers about tension headaches. Patient Care: June 30 1980

9

Dizziness
and
Vertigo

Joyce Jenkins

Dizziness is a common problem that has plagued humanity for many years. In spite of its frequency, medical and nursing research is limited regarding its mechanisms and causes. The growth of the space program and its technological advances precipitated scientific interest in the state of weightlessness and its effect on the balance mechanism because astronauts experienced recurring problems with dizziness. Subsequently, the study of dizziness was broadened to include other people who also experienced this troubling problem.[3] In 1965, a study of 864,666 people over 45 years of age, residing in 25 states, was conducted to determine the physical complaints of this age population. The findings indicated that both men and women experience dizziness as a significant medical complaint. Of 24 specific complaints, dizziness was reported fourth in frequency of occurrence among women and seventh in occurrence among men.[13] Some studies indicate that dizziness becomes more common with advancing age; other studies indicate that dizziness is seen more frequently in the young, as well as in older adults.[3,14]

Nurses encounter many patients with the complaint of dizziness in the ambulatory setting, either as a single problem or as an accompanying symptom of other problems. The nurse may be the major health care provider or may be a member of the health team that cares for the patient during various stages of the assessment and treatment process. In either case, it is imperative that the nurse understand the physiological mechanisms, the basis of the multiple pathophysiological etiologies, and the medical and nursing management of dizziness.

DESCRIPTIONS AND DEFINITIONS

The term *dizziness* refers to a disturbance in balance. It is frequently used to describe an array of unpleasant sensations of unreal movement experienced by the patient. These sensations may vary from a mild momentary episode to which the patient will adjust without difficulty, to a more terrifying attack that leaves the patient disabled or frightened.[3] The terms used to describe the milder sensations include giddiness, light-headedness, faintness, wooziness, "swimming sensation in the head," a floating feeling, and blackouts.

Patients also have described dizziness as

a swaying feeling with a slight back-and-forth or a to-and-fro sensation of movement. The more disabling forms of dizziness are less vague in description. Invariably what is experienced is a sensation of either the person or objects in the room moving or revolving in space. Other descriptions are a whirling or spinning in space, a feeling of up-and-down movement of the body, a feeling of the ground and floor coming up, or "everything spinning in circles."

Dizziness and vertigo often are used interchangeably, but actually the symptoms are different and one must distinguish one sensation from another to focus the data base and facilitate the most appropriate management.

Specifically, *dizziness* is the nonrotational feeling of light-headedness, vague wooziness, the nonpainful peculiar feelings in the head, and the sensations of faintness. *Giddiness*, a term used to denote a swaying sensation, also falls in this category.

Vertigo (derived from the Latin verb *vertere*, "to turn") implies a sensation of either the body or its surroundings turning. The term has also been expanded to include a hallucination of movement in any plane.[12] More specifically, the patient experiencing vertigo has a sense of disordered orientation of the body in space. Objects seem to move in a rotary, horizontal, vertical, or oblique manner. In other instances, the sensation is confined to the head, which is felt to be revolving, swaying, or rocking.[5] A similar sensation may be felt by a person who turns around and around several times and then comes to a sudden stop. In addition, there are other sensations that sometimes are discussed with dizziness. A panel of specialists discussing the subject of dizziness categorized the sensations into four basic types:

Dizziness: A vague light-headed feeling

Vertigo: A definite rotational sensation or hallucination of motion
Syncope: A sensation of impending faint or loss of consciousness
Disequilibrium: Loss or impaired sense of balance without the head sensations.[4]

This chapter primarily addresses the first two types.

MECHANISMS OF DIZZINESS AND VERTIGO

ANATOMY AND PHYSIOLOGY OF BALANCE

A state of equilibrium and balance is maintained when opposing forces of motion and gravity are instantaneously and methodically counteracted. The delicate adjustments needed to balance these forces for an awareness of the head and body in space and the rate and direction of head and body movements, including rotation, depend on the interaction of three body systems: vision, proprioception, and the vestibular system. Sensory input from these three systems is closely interconnected in the brain stem to maintain balance and spatial orientation. At least two of these systems must remain intact for a person to function.[4]

In the *visual system*, impulses from the retinas of the eyes are coordinated by oculomotor mechanisms to give information about the position and movement of the body. A person experiencing vertigo and disequilibrium while watching a movie of rotating or rapidly moving objects illustrates the importance of visual input in maintaining sense of balance.

The *proprioceptive pathway* is responsible for the conveyance of those sensations that are peculiarly one's own or within one's

self (*proprio* meaning "own"). Proprioceptors are afferent nerve impulses originated in
receptors in the muscles, tendons, joints, and
the vestibular apparatus of the inner ear. Proprioceptors of joints and muscles are essential to all reflex and postural movements. The
proprioceptors of the neck that relate the
positioning of the head to the rest of the body
are particularly important. The neural structures involved in proprioception are the posterior columns of the spinal cord, the cerebellum, and the vestibular apparatus. The
posterior columns carry stimuli from proprioceptors in muscle tendons and joints to
the cerebral cortex, which determines the
muscles required to contract and in what
strength they are to contract to continue moving in the desired direction. A pattern of impulses is generated by the cerebral cortex,
along pathways to the pons and midbrain,
which relay the impulses over the middle
and superior cerebellar peduncles to the
cerebellum. The cerebellum then generates
subconscious motor impulses along the inferior cerebellar peduncles to the medulla and
spinal cord. The impulses pass downward
along the spinal cord and out the nerves that
stimulate the prime movers and synergists to
contract and inhibit the contraction of the
antagonists. The result is smooth, coordinated movement.

The Vestibular Mechanism

The vestibular apparatus is composed of the
semicircular canals, the saccule, utricle, vestibular nerve, the vestibular nuclei, and the
vestibular portion of the eighth cranial nerve.
Most of these structures are in the inner ear,
so that a review of the anatomical relationships in the inner ear is essential (Figs. 9-1
and 9-2).

The internal or inner ear is also called
the *labyrinth*, because of its intricate series of

canals. It consists of two main divisions: 1) a
bony labyrinth, and 2) a membranous labyrinth that fits into the bony labyrinth. The
bony labyrinth is a series of cavities in the
dense portion of the temporal bone. Its three
areas are the vestibule, cochlea, and semicircular canals (See Fig. 9-2), so named because
of their shape. The bony labyrinth is lined
with periosteum and contains a fluid called
perilymph. This fluid surrounds the *membranous labyrinth*, a series of sacs and tubes
lying inside and having the same general
form as the bony labyrinth. Epithelium lines
the membranous labyrinth and contains a
fluid called *endolymph*.

The vestibule constitutes the oval, central portion of the bony labyrinth. The membranous labyrinth in the vestibule consists of
two sacs called the *utricle* and *saccule*, connected to each other by a small duct (see Fig.
9-2). The walls of the utricle and saccule are
composed of a thin sheet of connective tissue
lined with simple, squamous-type epithelium. Each contains a small flat plaquelike
region called *macula*.

Microscopically, the structure of the
macula consists of differentiated neuroepi-
thelial cells that are innervated by the
vestibular branch of the vestibulocochlear
cranial nerve (eighth cranial nerve). The two
maculae are located anatomically in planes
perpendicular to one another. They possess
two kinds of cell types: receptors and supporting cells. Two shapes of receptor cells
have been identified: one is flask-shaped and
the other is more cylindrical. Both show long
extensions of cell membrane called *stereo-
cilia* (they are actually microvilli), and one
kinocilium anchored firmly to its basal body
and extending beyond the longest microvilli.
Some receptor cells have over 80 such
projections, which are also called *hair cells*.

The supporting cells of the macula, scattered between the receptor cells, are colum-

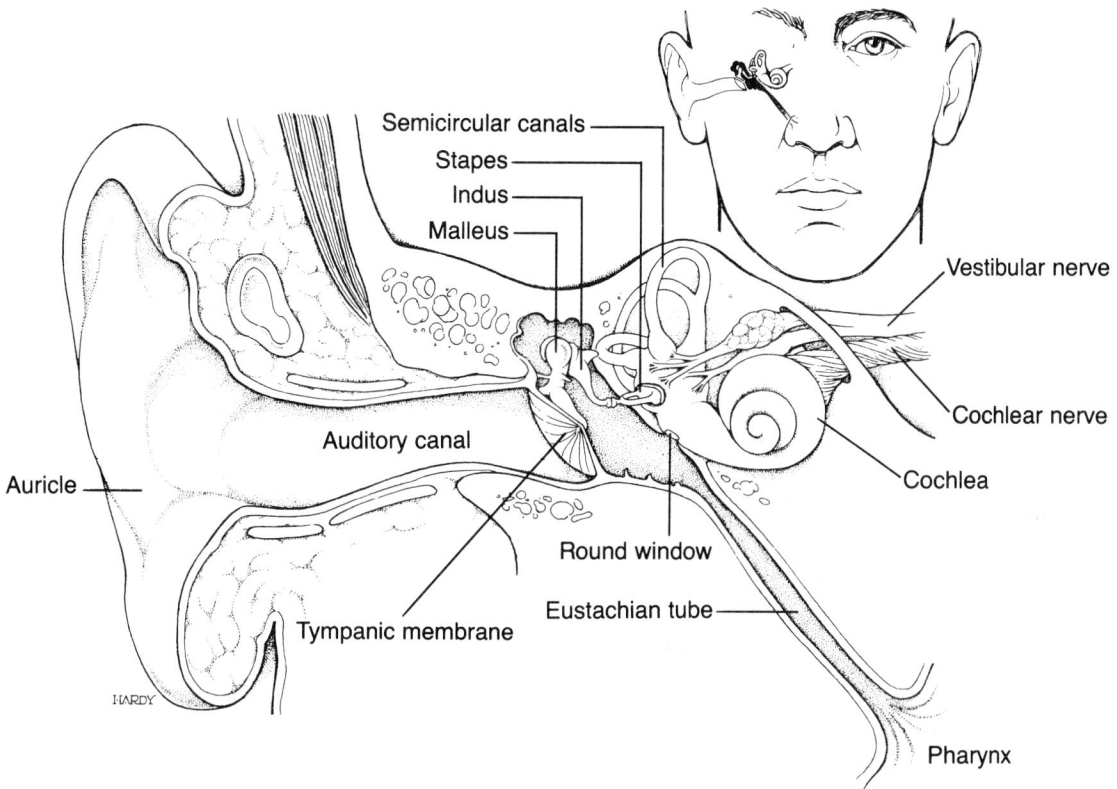

FIG. 9-1 *The anatomical relationship of the external, middle, and internal portions of the ear as seen in a section through the right side of the skull.*

nar and have short microvilli on the exposed surface. Floating directly over the hair cells is a thick, gelatinous glycoprotein layer, probably secreted by the supporting cells, called the *otolithic membrane*. A layer of free particles of calcium carbonate called otoliths extends over the entire surface of the otolithic membrane. When the head tips downward, the otoliths slide with gravity in the direction of the ground. As the particles move, they exert a downward pull on the gelatinous mass, which in turn exerts a downward pull on the hairs and makes them bend. The movement of the hairs stimulates the dendrites at the bases of the hair cells.

The impulse is then transmitted to the temporal lobe of the brain through the vestibular branch of the vestibulocochlear nerve. The utricle and saccule are considered to be sense organs of static equilibrium, which refers to the orientation of the body (mainly the head) to the pull of gravity and the ground.[22]

The walls of the membranous semicircular canals are constructed just like those of the utricle and saccule: connective tissue plus a lining of squamous epithelium. These fluid-filled tubes are situated within the bony canals of the inner ear but occupy only a small portion of the hollow space (See Fig. 9-2). The canals lie in contact with the outer

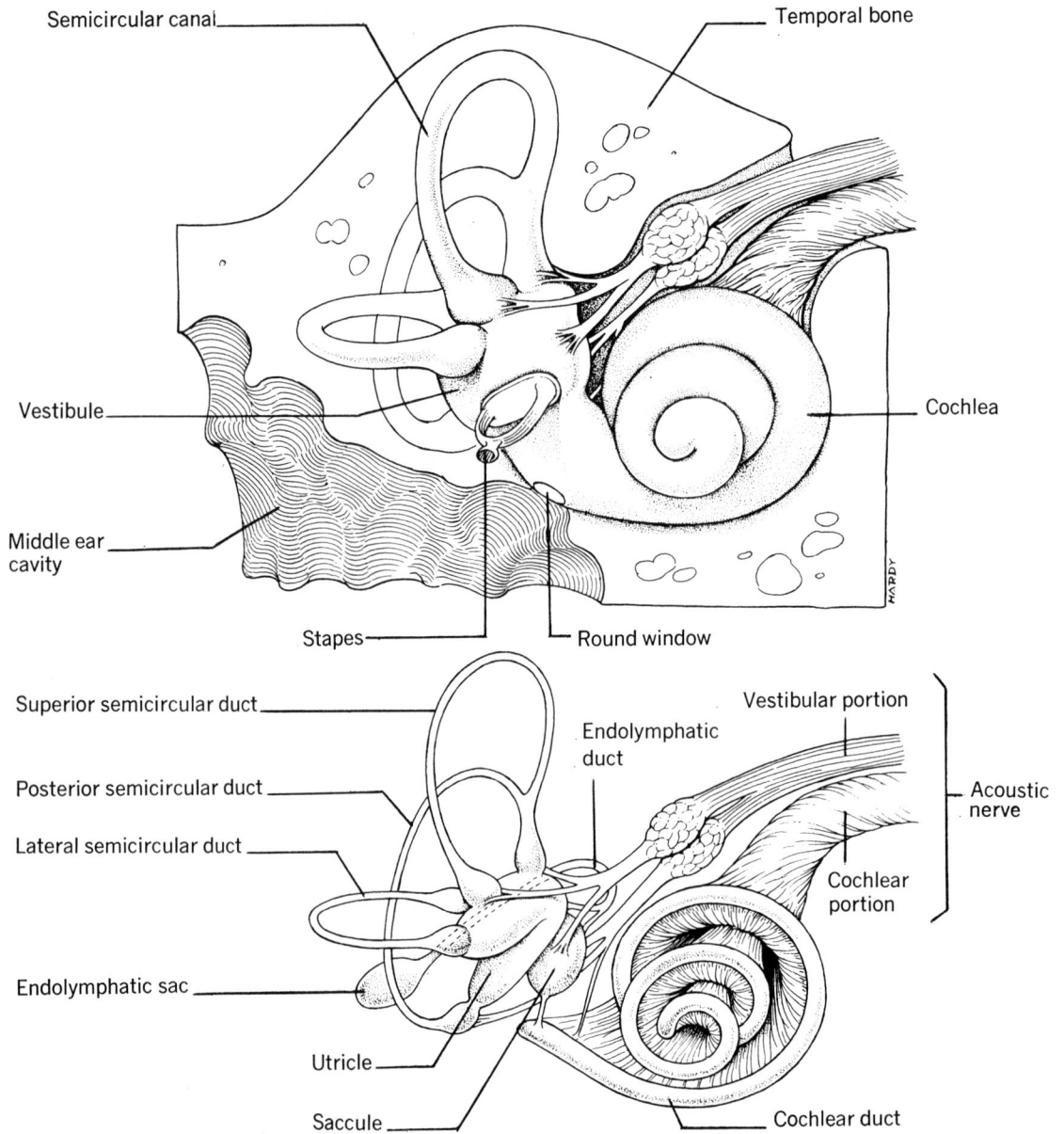

FIG. 9-2 *Above, the bony labyrinth; below, the membranous labyrinth as seen when removed from the bony labyrinth.*

rim of the bony (hair) cells, supporting cells, nerve fibers, and capillaries. They are positioned at right angles to one another in three planes: frontal (the superior duct), sagittal (the posterior duct), and lateral (the lateral duct). This positioning permits detection of an imbalance in three planes. In the ampulla, the dilated portion of each duct, there is a small elevation called the *crista* (Fig. 9-3). Each crista is composed of a group of hair cells covered by a mass of gelatinous material called the *cupula*. When the head moves in the direction or plane of one of the canals, the endolymph in the duct flows over the hairs, bending them in the opposite direction and thus bulging the cupula in the opposite direction. The movement of the hair cells stimulates sensory neurons in the crista, and the afferent impulses pass to the vestibular branch (acoustic) of the eighth cranial nerve (CN VIII). The impulses reach the temporal lobe of the cerebrum and are sent to the muscles that must contract to maintain body balance in the position. Thus the semicircular ducts assist the body in *dynamic equilibrium*, which is the maintenance of the body position in response to a sudden movement.[22,23]

Hypoactivity or hyperactivity of either the right or left vestibular system due to a pathologic condition causes an imbalance of vestibular input to central receptors, resulting in vertigo or disequilibrium.

ETIOLOGY OR POSSIBLE CAUSES OF DIZZINESS AND VERTIGO

Central versus peripheral causes of dizziness and vertigo can be differentiated by those conditions that are due to labyrinth dysfunction (peripheral) and those disorders of the central nervous system (CNS) or other systemic diseases. Once a determination is made about whether the patient is experiencing true vertigo or a nonvertiginous type of dizziness, then further differentiation of symptoms must be done to ascertain whether it is of a peripheral or a central origin (see Table 9-1).

A labyrinthine source of vertigo usually is manifested by sudden paroxysmal attacks of rotary sensations, accompanied by hearing

FIG. 9-3 *Enlargement of the crista.*

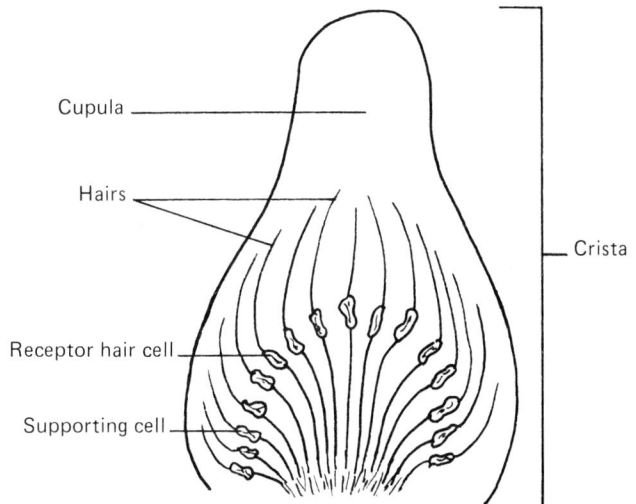

TABLE 9-1
DIFFERENTIAL FEATURES OF PERIPHERAL AND CENTRAL DIZZINESS

CHARACTERISTICS OF SYMPTOMS	PERIPHERAL	CENTRAL
Typical Onset	Sudden, acute, paroxysmal	Gradual, subtle, insidious
Quality (pattern)	Paroxysmal	Seldom, paroxysmal, continuous
Intensity	Usually severe	Mild, seldom severe
Duration	Minutes to weeks	Variable: days, weeks, to months and years
Spontaneous Nystagmus	May be present	May be present
Positional Nystagmus	Usually present in all fields of gaze	Frequently changes in different fields of gaze
Influenced by Head Positions and Movement	Marked, frequently present	Seldom present
Tinnitus	Frequently present	Seldom present
Hearing Loss	Frequently present	Seldom present
Disturbances of Consciousness, Syncope	Seldom present	More frequently present
Abnormal Neurologic Signs	Usually absent	Frequently present

problems, tinnitus, nystagmus, sweating, nausea, and vomiting. A peripheral cause is more likely when the acute symptoms are triggered by head movement, changes in position, a recent history of head trauma, or viral infection.

Vertigo of a CNS origin is more gradual and subtle in onset and, in contrast to a rotatory or whirling sensation, the person experiences a more swaying or seesaw motion and a sense of imbalance. Central origin vertigo is continuous, seldom intense in severity, and varies in duration from days to years. It is often accompanied by other abnormal neurologic signs.

Benign Positional Vertigo

This inner ear problem is caused by calcium oxalate crystals breaking away from the utricle and floating in the endolymph. When the patient changes position, these floaters stimulate the posterior semicircular canal, producing severe, transient vertigo. For example, when the patient looks up or rolls over in bed, they float past the ampulla, causing the vertigo and nystagmus. The usual episode is a severe rotational sensation associated with an abrupt change of position. The duration is brief. This is the shortest and most transient type of vertigo. It usually lasts from 5 to 30 seconds and occurs when the patient looks up, lies down, or rolls over in bed. Diagnosis is made from the history and by reproducing the vertigo and nystagmus.

If the patient is able to avoid the positions that provoke the vertigo, the crystals will remain in a dependent portion of the inner ear and eventually become encased in a thin membrane. The membrane will prevent the crystals from floating and thus prevent the vertigo. Formation of the membrane takes anywhere from 1 to 12 months, during which time the patient usually has intermittent attacks.[18]

Dental Problems

Dental malocclusion and temporomandibular joint (TMJ) abnormalities, due to close proximity of anatomical structure to the vestibular conductive and auditory systems, can cause dizziness. The vestibule may also be involved in the infectious process of an abscessed tooth.

Ear Infections

Dizziness may follow or accompany otitis media, mastoiditis, or an infectious process involving the middle or inner ear. If the ear infection is the cause of the dizziness, it may be accompanied by fullness or pain in the ear and other signs of infection such as erythema, drainage, fluid, and fever.

Vestibular Disorder

Labyrinthitis   The labyrinth is subject to inflammation secondary to bacterial and viral infections, sensitive to the toxic effects of drugs and chemicals, and vulnerable to allergic manifestation of certain foods (e.g., clams and oysters). All types of labyrinthitis result in vertigo with varying degrees of hearing loss, tinnitus, nausea, and vomiting. *Acute labyrinthitis* often follows an upper respiratory infection, with the patient giving a recent history of a head cold, sore throat, "flu," or ear infection. Nystagmus is present, and if the history reveals a recent ear infection the quick component will be toward the unaffected ear. The initial episode of vertigo with nausea and vomiting may last from 12 to 48 hours. The patient may appear pale and diaphoretic and prefer to remain in bed with his head motionless. Even slight movement will cause severe disabling vertigo.[19]

The duration of the episode may be from several days to 2 weeks of prostration and disability, with balance difficulties and brief vertigo with head movement continuing in some patients for weeks to months. The syndrome can be hard to differentiate from a first attack of Meniere's disease. If severe hearing loss has accompanied vertigo, the patient has a 25% chance of ultimately regaining hearing.

Vestibular Neuronitis   Vestibular neuronitis is due to a viral infection of the vestibular nerve. Although the symptoms are similar to those of acute labyrinthitis in its early stages, the major symptom is positional vertigo. The recovery period may last up to 12 months.

Meniere's Disease (Meniere's Syndrome)   Meniere's disease is a common type of labyrinthine disorder in adults, characterized by vertigo, fluctuating progressive unilateral hearing loss, tinnitus, and nystagmus. The vertigo and nystagmus are intermittent with the tinnitus. The hearing loss is more severe during acute episodes and subsides between attacks. Although the exact causes are unknown, some endocrine, vascular, and allergy problems contribute to the disorder. It is thought that the pathology is either an overproduction or underabsorption of endolymph in the cochlear duct, resulting in an increase in pressure in the duct and vestibular system. This increased pressure in turn causes a progressive atrophy of the hair cells of the cochlear or semicircular ducts.[22]

If the cochlear duct is impaired, distortions in the basilar membrane result in roaring and ringing in the ears with hearing loss. From this arises the term *roaring tinnitus*, a symptom experienced by some patients. If the semicircular ducts are involved, a feeling of dizziness and nausea results.

The attacks of vertigo have a sudden onset at regular intervals, are severe to violent in character, and may last from a few minutes to a few hours. The accompanying symptoms are often diaphoresis, nausea, and vomiting, which result in feelings of misery and incapacitation. Remissions may occur, during which time the patient may not experience an attack for several weeks to several months.[21] Meniere's syndrome has its onset most frequently in middle age, around age 50; however, young adults and the elderly can also be affected.

Toxic Labyrinthitis   This condition is caused by the toxic effects of certain drugs on the labyrinths and the eighth cranial nerve. This results in damage to these structures, which is manifested by vertigo, tinnitus, and hearing loss. Streptomycin, the salicylates, quinine, and alcohol are some of the more frequently identified ototoxic agents. If a drug like streptomycin is used over a long period of time it will cause damage to the fine hair cells of the vestibular end-organs, and the result could be a permanent state of disequilibrium. Also, drugs that are used in an abusive way, such as opiates and barbiturates, can cause vertigo from resulting distortions and damage to the vestibular apparatus.

Trauma

Head trauma may cause dizziness related to cerebral concussion, labyrinthine concussion, or a combination of both. This has also been called the postconcussional syndrome or the minor contusion syndrome. Some patients describe a feeling that is not a true vertigo but more of a giddiness in which they feel dazed, unsteady, and faint. Other patients report symptoms that suggest a labyrinthine disorder or vertigo. For example, surrounding objects in the environment seem to move momentarily, and looking upward or to the side may cause a sense of imbalance. Vertigo may be severe, lasting 24 to 48 hours if the temporal bone has been fractured, or transient, if floaters have been dislodged, resulting in benign positional vertigo. Vestibular disorders that result from trauma may last for as long as 12 to 18 months.[9]

Cervical vertigo, in the form of mild dizziness and unsteadiness, results from the pain that follows a whiplash injury or occipital neuralgia. This pain causes neural discharges along the vestibulospinal track. Positional imbalances or unsteadiness may result from trauma to any part of the spinal column.[18]

Cardiovascular Disease

Hypertension   In uncontrolled hypertension, the type of dizziness frequently reported is a swimming or woozy sensation of the head. In some instances, this may be the initial symptom that alerts the patient to the problem of elevated blood pressure. Symptoms are not due to the hypertension directly but to an associated venospasm.

Cardiac Arrhythmias   Symptoms of a cardiac arrhythmia may vary from brief episodes of dizziness, light-headedness, and feelings of faintness to actual syncope. Associated with this are palpitations, fluttering, pounding, or racing of the heart. The cerebral blood flow may also be markedly impaired. Cerebral ischemia is a risk in the older patient whose problems are further complicated by weakness, blurring of vision, paresthesias, and mental confusion. The arrhythmias include transient complete heart block, with Adams–Stokes supraventricular syndrome, Wolff–Parkinson–White syndrome, and paroxysmal supraventricular tachycardia.[21]

Carotid Sinus Hypersensitivity (Carotid Sinus Syncope)   The carotid sinus is normally sensitive to stretch and sensory impulses carried by the nerve of Hering, a branch of the glossopharyngeal nerve to the medulla oblongata. Stimulation of one or both of the carotid sinuses causes three types of responses. The *vagal* type is manifested by a reflex cardiac slowing or sinus bradycardia, sinus arrest, or atrioventricular block. The *depressor* type of response results in a fall of arterial pressure without cardiac slowing. The *central* type of response causes an interference with the circulation of the ipsilateral cerebral hemisphere. Two or all three types of responses may coexist, but it takes only one to result in syncope.[21] Most of the patients with this condition are elderly and have underlying atherosclerotic heart disease, which is detected by ischemic changes on the electrocardiogram (ECG).

An attack can be initiated by relatively minor events such as wearing a tight collar, turning the head, or shaving. The symptoms are a light-headed type of dizziness, sweating, nausea, and pallor, followed by fainting.

Atherosclerotic Obstruction of the Vertebral–Basilar System Vertebral and basilar artery insufficiency from atherosclerosis may cause dizziness and vertigo. This may be suspected in the patient over 50 years old who complains of dizziness or intermittent spontaneous vertigo on turning the neck in a right or left direction backward. The normal person is protected from symptoms because of adequate circulation from the opposite side. In the person with atherosclerosis in one vertebral artery, the turning of the neck may kink the other vertebral artery, producing dizziness, faintness, and in some instances, vertigo. Cervical spondylosis or a vascular anomaly resulting in an extremely small vertebral artery may complicate the condition further.[12]

This problem should be differentiated from benign paroxysmal positional vertigo. The patient with benign positional vertigo experiences symptoms only when the head is moved in a specific position rather than by merely turning the neck.

Subclavian Steal Syndrome This condition occurs when the proximal portion of the subclavian artery branching off the vertebral artery is occluded. This causes a reversal or "steal" of blood flow from the vertebral artery and brain to the subclavian artery and the arm. The resulting ischemia may be aggravated by the use of the arm in movement of exercise. Vertigo and occasionally syncope are among the symptoms of this condition.

Postural Orthostatic Hypotension Postural orthostatic hypotension causes a sensation of light-headedness, general dizziness, or a feeling of impending faintness. Accompanying symptoms may be pallor, dimness or blurring of vision, roaring in the ears, and diaphoresis. The clue to this condition is that the patient experiences these symptoms on rising in the morning or when changing from a lying to an upright position. There may also be a feeling of faintness when standing. Relief is obtained when the recumbent position is resumed or a sitting position is maintained for a few minutes.

The patients most prone to this problem are the elderly who are taking diuretics, other antihypertensive agents, and are on sodium-restricted diets. Physiologically, the decreasing circulating blood volume decreases the venous return to the right heart, lowers the myocardial contractile force, and reduces cardiac output and cerebral perfusion.

The condition may also be idiopathic, accompanying other conditions such as diabetic neuropathy, blood volume loss, prolonged bed rest, varicosities, or symptoms following a sympathectomy.

Anemia The patient with pernicious anemia or an iron deficiency anemia of pregnancy may experience dizziness. Faintness and actual syncope may be symptomatic of a severe anemia from an acute or chronic blood loss. Examples of such problems are duodenal ulcer, cancer of the colon, and metrorrhagia.

Neurologic and Central Nervous System Disorders

Acoustic Neurinoma   This nonmalignant, slow-growing brain tumor originates from the sheath of the vestibular division of the acoustic nerve (eighth cranial) in the internal auditory canal. Its growth continues in the posterior fossa between the pons and the cerebellum and may extend to compress the cerebellum and brain stem. It can also stretch and distort the trigeminal (fifth cranial) and the abducens (sixth cranial) nerves and compress the facial (seventh cranial) and acoustic (eighth cranial) nerves. The initial symptoms develop as a result of pressure on the eighth cranial nerve. The clinical symptoms are a gradual and vague unsteadiness or imbalance, high-pitched ringing in the ears, and unilateral hearing loss. The first symptom may be the patient's increasing difficulty hearing in the involved ear when using the telephone. Initially, the symptoms of cranial nerve involvement may be intermittent, but increase in frequency as the tumor enlarges.

As the tumor growth spreads beyond the internal auditory canal and compresses the brain stem, other neurologic symptoms develop. Facial weakness and loss of the corneal reflex are followed by paresthesias, numbness, paroxysmal facial pain, abnormal taste sensation, and difficulty in swallowing. As pressure on the cerebellum increases, ipsilateral ataxia and problems with coordination may occur. Further growth of the tumor also produces sensory loss and weakness in the extremities as well as the classical symptoms of increased intracranial pressure (ICP) such as headache, diplopia, nausea, and vomiting.

Multiple Sclerosis   Vertigo is the initial complaint in about 7% to 10% of patients with multiple sclerosis, with approximately one third of the patients eventually experiencing brief to severe episodes. The patient is usually between the ages of 20 and 40 and complains of a mild rotatory sensation and vague unsteadiness that may be exacerbated by head movement. Other neurologic signs include blurred vision, transient weakness or numbness in one or both legs, and uncoordination of gait, handwriting, or speech.

Migraine   Headache   (Migrainelike Syndrome)   Vertigo may occur in association with the prodromal stage of a migraine or with the headache itself and is particularly exacerbated by change of posture. Typically the patient will report an aura of diffuse, scintillating scotoma, visual blurring, photophobia, or paresthesia and hemiparesis. This is followed by a throbbing occipital headache, nausea, and vomiting. The symptoms are thought to be due to the constriction and vasodilation of the vertebral basilar system that supplies the peripheral vestibular mechanism of the inner ear, or the central nuclei in the brain stem. The cortex also may be affected.

Seizure   Disorders   In some seizure disorders, particularly those originating in the temporal and parietal lobes of the brain, the aura preceding the seizure may be in the form of an attack of vertigo. The term *epileptic dizziness* has also been used with patients who experience brief episodes of rotatory dizziness with some form of seizure occurring separately. The seizure may vary from periods of altered consciousness without loss of posture, to episodes during which the patient is momentarily unable to move or speak.

In a British study, neurologists found an association between brief episodes of dizziness and epilepsy in young adults in whom dizziness was the primary reason for referral. The results of clinical examination, hearing, and radiologic tests were normal, but electro-encephalograms (EEG) showed abnormalities that pointed to epilepsy. The dizziness occurred in brief episodes lasting only a few seconds, with nausea present in the recovery phase. The attacks were unrelated to external factors or postural changes. Their frequency ranged from about once a week to several episodes a day. The diagnosis was further confirmed by the patients' responses to treatment with anticonvulsant medications.[19] A careful history often leads the examiner to probe more carefully for epilepsy or seizure disorders.

Multiple Sensory Deficits

Multiple sensory impairment can affect several components of the balance system concurrently. The typical patient that experiences the dizzy sensations of multiple sensory deficits is older and may have a combination of chronic diseases affecting the ocular, proprioceptive or vestibular systems, or sensory nerve pathways. There is a loss or confusion of position perspective, particularly when the patient is walking or turning. The patient experiences light-headedness, unsteadiness, or a sense of abnormal motion. It is found most frequently in patients with poor vision, peripheral neuropathy, and cervical spondylosis. The sensory impairment is defined as *multiple* when the person experiences at least two of the conditions concurrently.

Hyperventilation Syndrome

A common cause of dizziness in younger patients is hyperventilation syndrome. During an acute attack, the patient appears apprehensive, diaphoretic, and dyspneic, with complaints of dizziness, chest tightness, and pain. Between acute attacks, a vague light-headedness or woozy type of dizziness, rather than a true vertigo, is the chief complaint. Other symptoms include fatigue, a tingling type of paresthesia of the fingertips, feet, or perioral area. The person with a chronic hyperventilation syndrome may sigh deeply periodically during the encounter. The symptoms are caused by rapid and deep breathing that results in lowered alveolar carbon dioxide concentration and a respiratory alkalosis, thus upsetting the acid–base equilibrium.

The typical profile reveals a person with obsessional and perfectionist characteristics, who is excessively vulnerable to the uncertainties and frustrations of life. These patients are constantly under the stress of meeting deadlines, rushing to be on time, and fearful of falling short of their own exacting standards.[7] The student who strives to be at the top of the class, the ambitious executive, and the creative and gifted wife who has not found fulfillment in the chores of housekeeping or the responsibility of motherhood, are among patients seen with this disorder.

Psychogenic Dizziness

Anxiety and other emotional problems may cause dizziness. The anxious patient is unduly disturbed about symptoms that include a continuous kind of light-headedness and a giddy or "spaced-out" sensation, rather than acute paroxysmal attacks. There is also a history of difficulty with concentration, loss of appetite, and a complaint of being overly tired. The problem is common in adolescent and college-age groups who also admit to poor performance in school. All of these symptoms are signs of depression and anxiety, but these patients often deny the basis of the dizziness as being psychological. Further inquiry reveals problems with either family, school, friends, or undue pressure and stress on the job. The symptoms exacerbate and subside as the problems increase and decrease.

Motion Sickness

Motion sickness is a functional disorder thought to be caused by repetitive, excessive angular, linear, or vertical stimulation of the vestibular apparatus by motion. The symptoms are primarily nausea, vomiting, and varying degrees of dizziness or vertigo. Yawning, salivation, pallor, sweating, and drowsiness may be the warning symptoms of an attack. Specific kinds of motion sickness include seasickness, air, car, space, train, or swing sickness. Anxiety and fright may contribute to the severity of the symptoms.

Prolonged exposure to the offending motion may help some persons to adapt and the symptoms will disappear. In most cases, however, cessation of motion such as getting off a plane, boat, or swing gives immediate relief.

NURSING ASSESSMENT

SUBJECTIVE DATA

Often the patient with dizziness is anxious because of disabling symptoms, fears of a fatal illness, or belief that he has a psychiatric problem. Therefore, it is imperative that the first step in gathering the data base for the nursing care plan is to establish rapport and to give reassurance that the complaint of dizziness is legitimate. This helps the patient to understand that by direct assessment or referral, every resource available will be used to determine the underlying cause of the symptoms.

The most important part of the data base is a detailed and thorough history. It is through careful analysis of subjective information that the most valuable clues are elicited, which will point to the underlying disorder or problem. So important is the specific information that a number of specialists have devised special self-administered questionnaires to be completed by the patient with dizziness facilitating the data-gathering process.[3,4,5,15,18] Some are detailed and some are brief, but all ask the essential questions. The nurse may choose to use one of these tools, but should know that the following information is needed:

Usual Health

Determine what the patient's usual health is; whether he is in relatively good health, feels good most of the time, or has been plagued by acute or chronic problems.

Description of Complaint

Begin by letting the patient know that dizziness means different things to different people. It is important to know what the patient is experiencing. Ask him to try to describe the character of the symptoms without using the word *dizzy*. Do this without excessive prompting to ensure a reporting of accurate subjective information. Sometimes patients have problems articulating the sensations, particularly the light-headed or "spacy" feelings. Assistance can be given by asking if he feels vaguely light-headed, experiences a definite rotational sensation as though *he is whirling and spinning* and the room is stationary, or the sensation that the *room and objects around him are spinning*. Does he have a feeling of a mild, up-and-down seesaw motion or does he experience more of a side-to-side, swaying motion? Ask if he has feelings of faintness or actual spells of "blacking out" or unconsciousness. Has he experienced a feeling of unsteadiness or imbalance without head sensations?

Ask about onset of dizziness. Are the attacks sudden or gradual? Sudden versus insidious episodes give important clues to origin. How frequently do the attacks occur? What is the pattern and duration? Does the dizziness lasts for only a few seconds, minutes, or hours? A CNS tumor causes constant symptoms but positional vertigo lasts only 5 to 10 seconds. Is the patient asymptomatic between attacks?

Obtain specific information about precipitating factors. Does fatigue, exertion, or hunger precede symptoms? Does a particular head or body position precipitate an attack? Find out if there is a relationship between body movement and symptoms. Has the patient been flying or driving recently? If the patient is elderly, does the dizziness occur when changing from a lying to a sitting position? Does turning the neck induce dizziness or other head sensations? Encourage the patient to talk about any recent incidents of motion and movement, however trivial.

Ask about associated symptoms. Find out if there is accompanying nausea and vomiting, hearing difficulty, ear fullness, stuffiness, drainage, or tinnitus. Inquire about headaches and ocular problems, including double or blurred vision, photophobia, or a decrease in visual acuity. Ask about numbness in the face or in the upper or lower extremeties during attacks. Does the patient experience any speech or swallowing difficulties during attacks?

Inquire about attenuating or aggravating factors. Does the patient remember anything that relieves symptoms (e.g., lying down)? Is there anything that makes symptoms worse? Determine the level of incapacitation or disability. Are the sensations mild and fleeting, so the patient can carry on usual activities, or so severe that quiet or recumbency is necessary?

Past Medical History

Review of past medical and surgical conditions may provide valuable clues to the cause of dizziness. Start with recent illnesses. Be especially alert for viral infections involving the upper respiratory system. Ask about ocular problems or changes. Has the patient recently acquired new and stronger lenses? Has there been a recent whiplash or head injury?

In view of the specific systems, inquire about the following:

Neurologic: Seizures, meningitis, migraine headaches, episodes of unsteadiness, sensations of abnormal motion, and strokes, including symptoms suggesting transient ischemic attacks

Cardiovascular: Hypertension, arteriosclerotic disease, other heart problems

Endocrine: Thyroid disorders, including any surgeries, diabetes, episodes of hypoglycemia

Hematopoietic: Anemia or blood dyscrasias, significant blood loss from any cause (e.g., trauma, menstrual disorders)

Musculoskeletal: Problems with ambulation, cervical spine problems, difficulty in walking in the dark

Ask which medications the patient is taking or has taken recently and their relationship with the dizziness.

Inquire about allergies, either ingestion or environmental. Has the patient been exposed to other environmental substances—fumes, paint, toxic chemicals?

Family History

Information about blood relatives with cardiovascular disease should be obtained. Ask about CNS problems such as epilepsy, multiple sclerosis, migraine headaches, and endocrine problems, including diabetes and thyroid disease. Is there a history of psychiatric or emotional problems? All of the conditions have familial tendencies that may uncover the underlying problem.

Habits

Ask about use of caffeine. What is the pattern of coffee drinking? Is excessive coffee drinking replacing regular meals? Caffeine in excessive amounts may contribute to dizziness because of its vasoconstrictive effect. Inquire about smoking habits, both the history and present patterns. Ask about alcohol intake in relation to daily habits and symptoms.

Psychosocial History

In the psychiatric and emotional areas, has the patient experienced any general behavior changes? Is there a history of anxiety or depression? Ask about mood changes and nervousness. In addition to emotional stress, these symptoms could point to organic problems that cause endolymph changes in the inner ear and produce dizziness (e.g., myxedema). Inquire about stress the patient may be experiencing at home or work. It is necessary to know what the nature of the relationships are with family or significant others. To uncover stress-related areas, it may also be necessary to ask about the patient's life-style to develop a profile of a typical day. Ask about travel and the form of travel—boat, airplane, car—and experiences that may have caused a change in inner ear pressure such as mountain climbing, scuba diving, or swimming.

OBJECTIVE DATA

Collection of objective data should begin with initial impressions about the patient. Keen observation, along with the history, will help to determine whether the problem is an organic or a psychiatric, emotionally related problem. Observe the patient's overall appearance, age, behavior, and general affect. Assess the patient's movements and gait for natural balance. Can he walk unassisted without swaying, weakness, or incoordination? Is there evidence of paralysis or spasticity? Is the movement of all extremities normal and free?

Ascertain the quality of the speaking voice and clarity of speech. Note any hoarseness. Is there thickness of speech or difficulty in pronouncing words? Eye contact will detect facial muscle weakness, excessive blinking, or asymmetry of smile.

The Physical Examination

In the physical examination, the nurse should concentrate on those areas that would most likely yields signs that point to the organic causes of dizziness and vertigo: the ocular, labyrinthine, neurologic, and cardiovascular systems.

The following are important components:

Vital Signs Take the temperature, pulse, and respiratory rate. Take the blood pressure in both arms with the patient in supine, standing, and sitting positions. Orthostatic changes are detected by a systolic drop exceeding 10 mm Hg and a diastolic drop exceeding 4 mm Hg. In some elderly persons, the systolic pressure may fall as much as 30 mm Hg when changing from a supine to an upright position.

Check for unequal pulses in the arms and carotid areas.

Eye Examination The patient's ocular system should be tested for acuity, visual fields, fundi, and nystagmus. The nurse should observe for pupil symmetry and note whether pupils are dilated or pinpointed in average room light. Look for prompt consensual constriction of the pupils after direct light stimulus. Determine lid movement, smooth coordinated movements in all six cardinal positions of gaze. Look for ataxia of eye movement on lateral gaze by asking the patient to look rapidly from one side to the other. In multiple sclerosis, as the patient looks from side to side, the eyes will move asynchronously and overshoot the mark before they come to rest again.

Tests for spontaneous or gaze nystagmus are essential in the work-up of every patient with dizziness. Nystagmus consists of a slow and a rapid component. The slow repetitive component toward the midline is the attempt of the vestibular system to compensate for the vertigo. To determine the direction of the nystagmus, look for the direction of the rapid movement. This is the response of the CNS to compensate for vertigo. To test for spontaneous nystagmus, the Nylen–Bárány maneuver is performed (discussed under special tests).

Occasionally, vertical or rotatory nystagmus occurs, indicating a disorder of the brain stem. To check for downward vertical nystagmus, elevate the patient's upper eyelid so that the limbus can be observed.

Bilateral internuclear ophthalmoplegia is another sign that strongly suggests multiple sclerosis. To test for it, ask the patient to follow your finger with his eyes as you move it from side to side. If the adducting eye is weak or shows no movement while the abducting eye moves normally and displays nystagmus, the patient has internuclear ophthalmoplegia. When this sign is bilateral, the cause is probably demyelination in the brain stem. If this sign is unilateral, a neoplasm or vascular disease may be the cause.

Perform a funduscopic examination to determine diabetic and hypertensive retinopathy and abnormalities of the optic disk. Papilledema may be a sign of an acoustic neuroma or of cardiovascular and endocrine disorders.

Ear and Hearing Examination Carefully examine the external canal for discharge and signs of infection. Look for impacted cerumen, foreign bodies, and the presence of blood in the canal. Inspect the tympanic membrane carefully, particularly the upper portion called *Shrapnell's membrane* for perforations or discharge. A patient with chronic otitis media may develop a cholesteatoma, which may erode the surrounding tissue and form a fistula in the semicircular canal.

Hearing tests to determine hearing loss or hearing distortions are necessary for all patients presenting with dizziness and vertigo, regardless of character or severity of symptoms. Many diseases involve both hearing and equilibrium mechanisms, due to the close anatomical relationship between the cochlear and the vestibular portion of the eighth cranial nerve.

Perform Weber's test to determine whether the patient has a conductive or sensorineural hearing loss. Use a tuning fork with a frequency of at least 512 cycles/sec to better distinguish sound and to test the hearing within the frequency range of human speech.

The Rinne test compares the patient's hearing by air conduction and bone conduction. The patient with normal hearing will report that the sounds are louder and clearer in the ear canal through air conduction than by means of the mastoid process through bone conduction. (Chapter 10 contains discussions on the methods to do these tests.)

Hearing discrimination impairment should be tested. With an early acoustic neuroma, a patient may be able to hear pure tones transmitted by the nerve but may not be able to discriminate sounds. He may hear the tuning fork but be unable to understand words. Use a list of phonetically balanced, monosyllabic words (e.g. show, send, smart, rooms). Cover the opposite ear and pronounce the words in a clear reasonably loud voice. Ask the patient to repeat each word after you pronounce it.

With this test, remember that you are not evaluating *whether* the patient hears but *how* he hears. The loss of high frequency sounds often makes speech sound hollow and thick, resulting in the patient's only hearing the last letters like "k" in "nick" or "ow" in "show." If it is evident that the patient's hearing is distorted by the way he is pronouncing the words, then he may have auditory discrimination impairment that may be an early sign of acoustic neuroma.

Nose and Throat Examination   Look for signs of upper respiratory infection or trauma, keeping in mind that colds, flu, sinusitis, and dental problems may cause dizziness. The close proximity of these structures to the vestibular apparatus is also a factor.

Lymph Node Examination   Look for enlarged nodes as well as abnormalities of the thyroid. Do a complete range-of-motion test of the neck to determine if any movements reproduce the dizziness or vertigo.

Cardiovascular Examination   To confirm or rule out a cardiovascular origin of dizziness, assess the cardiac status, using the recommended techniques of physical assessment. Note any arrhythmias, abnormalities in heart sounds, extra heart sounds, murmurs, or bruits in the neck. Listening for bruits is especially important because the patient with occlusive disease may not have other symptoms. It is essential to take time to listen carefully with the diaphragm of the stethoscope over the two areas where bruits are most likely to be heard: 1) the carotid artery bifurcation (at the angle of the jaw and the neck), and 2) the subclavian artery near the origin of the vertebral artery (posterior to the clavicle by at least 3 cm and slightly above the median end of the clavicle).[4]

Neurologic Examination   A thorough neurological examination is essential in the assessment of the patient with dizziness. Besides being an evaluation tool for specific neurologic abnormalities, it assists the provider in determining if the dizziness is of a central or peripheral origin. The necessary components are the assessment of mental status, the 12 cranial nerves, tests of cerebellar functions, and the testing of reflexes, coordination, and gait.

Mental Status   Determine his mental status from the moment there is interaction with the patient. The manner of speech, facial expression, orientation, memory, intellectual performance, and judgment are ascertained best during the interview process. The nurse should be able to distinguish between anxiety-produced behavior resulting from fear of a serious disease, and an affect that would suggest emotional or deep-seated psychiatric problems.

Cranial Nerves   The evaluation of the cranial nerves includes:

- Olfactory (first cranial nerve): Determine the patient's ability to differentiate odors correctly.
- Optic (second cranial nerve): Examination of visual acuity, the optic fundi, and visual fields
- Oculomotor (third cranial nerve): Examination of pupillary constriction, elevation of the upper eyelid, and extraocular movements
- Trochlear (fourth cranial nerve): Evaluation of downward movement of the eye (discussed in examination of the eye and testing of nystagmus)
- Trigeminal (fifth cranial nerve): Ask the patient to clench his teeth to test the contraction of the temporal and masseter muscles. Test the sensory component of the forehead, cheek, and lower jaw on each side for pain. Using a wisp of cotton, test

the corneal reflex for the blink response. Loss of the sense of touch, pain, or temperature on the same side of the face where the corneal reflex is absent may point to a CNS lesion.

- Abducens (sixth cranial nerve): Test for lateral deviation of the eyes when testing for nystagmus.
- Facial (seventh cranial nerve): Have the patient raise his eyebrows, frown, and close his eyes tightly. Have him smile, show his teeth, and puff out his cheeks with his jaw closed. Note whether his smile is symmetric. A late sign of large tumors is unilateral facial weakness.
- Acoustic (eighth cranial nerve): Assessment of hearing loss was discussed in the section on examination of the ear. Additional evaluation of vestibular function will be discussed in the section on special tests.
- Glossopharyngeal and vagus (ninth and tenth cranial nerves): These nerves may be evaluated with the throat examination; however, the significance of abnormalities is noted. Test the patient's gag reflex. Note whether he can phonate without difficulty or hoarseness. Look at the elevation of the uvula at the midline. Note any asymmetry. Unilateral loss of the gag reflex and pharyngeal and palatal weakness provide a clue to an acoustic neuroma and its location. With this tumor, there is displacement of the uvula to the unaffected side with compensatory use of the muscles on that side. The voice is often hoarse due to ipsilateral paralysis of the vocal cords. The patient may also have difficulty swallowing liquids but still may be able to swallow soft and solid foods.
- Spinal accessory (eleventh cranial nerve): Ask the patient to shrug his shoulders against your hand. Note the strength and contraction of the trapezius muscles. Observe the contraction of the sternomastoid

muscles by asking the patient to turn his head to each side against your hand.
- Hypoglossal (twelfth cranial nerve): Look for fasciculations as the patient moves his tongue. Ask the patient to stick out his tongue and look for any deviation, asymmetry or atrophy.

Deep Tendon Reflexes These reflexes must be tested in all extremities on both sides to determine abnormalities. The response of each reflex is evaluated bilaterally for its briskness and ease of elicitation and is compared with the homologous muscle on the other side. The nurse must be aware of normal responses. For instance, a slow relaxation after muscle contraction is observed in hypothyroidism. In testing the knee or quadriceps reflex, if the leg is allowed to swing freely after striking the tendon, it quickly returns to complete rest. In cerebellar disease, hypotonia results in the continued swinging of the leg several times after a single contraction of the muscle *(pendular reflex)*.[17] If a reflex cannot be elicited or if asymmetry is found, the reflex should be tested in several positions to verify its absence, diminished response, or hyperactivity.

A plantar reflex response, or Babinski's toe sign, is indicative of a CNS disorder. Its presence, along with bilateral muscle weakness, hyperactive reflexes, and decreased sensory response may occur with displacement or compression of the brain stem due to an acoustic neuroma. Babinski's sign with hyperactive reflexes and sensory change—particularly the loss of joint position sense—suggests the possibility of multiple sclerosis or a lesion of the spinal cord.

Sensory Perception Decreased sensation is found with diabetic and alcoholic neuropathy. Specific tests to be performed are *position sense*: move the patient's finger or toe and ask him to identify the direction.

Light and deep touch are important as well as vibratory sense.

Motor Function These tests should include strength, range of motion, and gait. The testing of muscle strength and tone in the extremities may be varied and altered to determine adequate motor function.

Cerebellar Function The maneuvers found in the accompanying box, Tests of Coordination and Balance, assist in determining if the dizziness is due to cerebellar pathology. In addition there are special tests with which the nurse should be familiar that reproduce the dizziness or vertigo, thus stimulating or aggravating the pathophysiologic mechanism responsible for the sensation. These tests can often be of great help in deter-

mining or ruling out underlying etiologies. (See Tests That Stimulate Dizziness.)

Laboratory and Diagnostic Studies

A number of laboratory studies should be done if the cause of the patient's dizziness has not been pinpointed. These tests are also necessary to confirm a presumptive diagnosis.

Complete blood count is done to rule out anemia or infection.
Blood glucose is done to rule out or confirm diabetes or hypoglycemia.
T_3 and T_4 determine thyroid deficiency or dysfunction.
Cholesterol and triglycerides tests are done

Tests of Coordination and Balance

POINT-TO-POINT TESTING

With the patient in a sitting or standing position, eyes open and arm extended, ask him to touch the tip of his finger to his nose several times. Have him repeat this with his eyes closed. Then have him touch the tip of his nose and then the tip of your extended finger. Repeat the test, moving the position of your finger. Have the patient do each hand separately. There is awkwardness and dysmetria (overshooting of a mark) in cerebellar disease.

In testing the lower extremities, have the patient in the supine position. Ask him to place his heel on the opposite knee and run the heel down to the shin and foot. Note any tremors or awkwardness. Ask him to point to the opposite foot with each big toe. If an additional test is desired, have him form a figure eight in the air with each foot.

RAPID RHYTHMIC ALTERNATING MOVEMENTS

Ask the patient to pat his thigh with first the palm and then with the back of each hand as rapidly

as possible. Then have him touch each of his fingers with his thumb as rapidly as possible, remembering that the nondominant hand might be slightly awkward.

Assess coordination in the legs by asking him to tap your hand as quickly as possible with the ball of each foot.

ROMBERG TEST

Ask the patient to stand erect with his feet together and his eyes open. If there is unsteadiness or he begins to fall, labyrinthine or severe cerebellar disease should be suspected. Test his balance with his eyes closed. Swaying or falling could indicate impaired or absent labyrinthine function. The patient with decreased position sense can stand relatively well with his eyes open because his vision compensates for the sensory loss, but with his eyes closed he loses his balance.

when a metabolic disorder is suspected or if the patient is symptomatic of or at risk for cardiovascular disease.

Electrolyte levels are taken if there is a suspected cardiovascular problem, if the patient is on diuretics, or is dieting.

Fluorescent treponemal antibody absorption (FTA–ABS) may be indicated if the patient is suspected of having congenital otologic syphilis (syphilitic Meniere's disease).

Electrocardiogram (ECG) is indicated if arrhythmia or cardiac problem is suspected.

Electroencephalogram (EEG) is indicated if the patient's symptoms point to vertiginous epilepsy or any other seizure disorder.

X-rays are needed if symptoms point to mastoiditis, brain lesions, trauma, cervicogenic osteophytes, or spondylosis.

Electronystagmography (ENG) is a method of measuring spontaneous and induced nystagmus. It is usually done by an otolaryngologist when the patient has been referred for persistent unexplained vertigo. One of the advantages of the procedure is that it is objective and provides a permanent record of the patient's vestibular function.

Tests That Stimulate Dizziness

CHANGE IN POSITION

Start with the patient supine. Ask the patient to sit up or stand. Then have him walk a few steps, stop, turn rapidly 180°. Unsteadiness, lightheadedness, or loss of balance may be experienced by patients with multiple sensory deficits. Diabetic or alcoholic neuropathy, postsurgical adjustment following cataract removal, atherosclerotic cerebral disease, or cervical spine disease also may reproduce this type of dizziness. The patient who becomes dizzy when changing from a supine to an upright position, with an accompanying fall in blood pressure, has orthostatic hypotension.

HEAD TURNING

If the head-turning maneuver was not done while examining the neck, you may do it as an additional test to try to evoke reported symptoms. Ask the patient to turn his head to the left and hold it. If vertigo develops, you may suspect a kinking of the vertebral artery, a vestibular disorder, or a problem due to disease or injury of the cervical spine.

NYLEN–BÁRÁNY MANEUVER

The Nylen–Bárány maneuver is a test to determine if the patient is experiencing benign positional vertigo. It is performed by first holding the patient's head between your hands while he is sitting. Turn it 90° to the right, then abruptly but gently carry the head backward to a supine position until it is hanging at about a 30° to 45° angle (Fig. 9-4). Observe the patient's eyes for nystagmus. Rotate the head to the opposite side, then again to the straight position, maintaining each position for about 60 seconds. Watch carefully because nystagmus is delayed for approximately 2 to 20 seconds. The nystagmus is rotatory or horizontal, with the rapid component toward the lower ear in the lateral position. It begins slowly and lasts for only about 60 seconds. Another diagnostic feature of the nystagmus is its *fatigability of response;* that is, repetitive testing or maneuvers results in a reduced-to-absent response, unless the patient is allowed to rest for about an hour. If the etiology is benign paroxysmal positional vertigo, the patient will experience severe vertigo with the nystagmus. This may be accompanied

Tests That Stimulate Dizziness (Continued)

by nausea. This maneuver does not produce nystagmus in normal persons. If positional nystagmus occurs without a delayed onset, and continues as long as the head is held in this special position, then a CNS etiology is suspected. In addition, the nystagmus can be horizontal, vertical, or rotational, changing with the direction of the gaze. This distinguishes it from nystagmus of peripheral vertigo, which is horizontal or rotatory and remains the same in all fields of gaze. Also, the rotation of the head evokes severe vertigo if it is of peripheral origin, whereas the head position does not usually influence the vertigo of central origin.

CALORIC TEST

The caloric test evaluates vestibular function. It is done by a physician experienced in the procedure or by a specialist in otolaryngology or neurology. The purpose is to determine whether the patient's labyrinths are normal, hypoactive, or nonfunctional. It involves syringing each ear with water, just above and just below body temperature *(bithermal method),* or using cold water only, to produce cooling of the labyrinth. When the head is tilted backward about 60°, the horizontal semicircular canal is in a vertical position. Heating and cooling it causes movement of the fluid, due to the convection effect. The brain interprets this movement of fluid as head movement. In response to this, a sideways movement of the eyes occurs to maintain gaze at one spot. The cerebral cortex recognizes immediately that this is abnormal fluid movement, not head movement, and signals the return of the eyes. This results in an *induced nystagmus,* characterized by slow movement to one side and a rapid return. Warming and cooling is done for 40 seconds. In the patient with

normal labyrinthine function, the rapid component of the nystagmus is *away* from the irrigated ear when irrigated with cold water and *toward* the irrigated ear with hot water. The amount of time that the nystagmus is detectable is the test result. Each ear is done separately and gives the examiner an indication of the status of the vestibular apparatus on each side. A slowed response suggests a hypoactive labyrinth, while a repeated injection of water with no resulting nystagmus suggests a nonfunctioning labyrinth.

VALSALVA MANEUVER

Have the patient perform the Valsalva maneuver when it is suspected that dizziness is caused by a sudden rise in the intrathoracic pressure resulting in decreased cardiac output and hypoxia. This occurs in the older patient with compromised cerebral circulation due to atherosclerosis, who may complain of lightheadedness or faintness when coughing, or straining while lifting, defecating, or voiding. It in turn causes a marked fall in venous return to the right heart and decreases the cardiac output. Have the patient do forced expiration with his mouth closed or 15 seconds. This closes the glottis and elevates the intrathoracic pressure.

HYPERVENTILATION

If hyperventilation syndrome is suspected, ask the patient to breathe deeply and rapidly through the mouth for 3 minutes by the stopwatch. Ask him to raise his hand or signal you when sensations or dizziness or other symptoms occur. The patient with hyperventilation syndrome will often complain of dizziness or light-headedness after only a minute of breathing.

NURSING DIAGNOSIS

The nursing diagnosis of the patient with dizziness and vertigo includes accurate and comprehensive data collection, differentiat-

ing between an acute or stabilized process, seeking appropriate physician consultation, and facilitating treatment coordination and follow-up. From the subjective data, the nurse can determine if symptomatology is in-

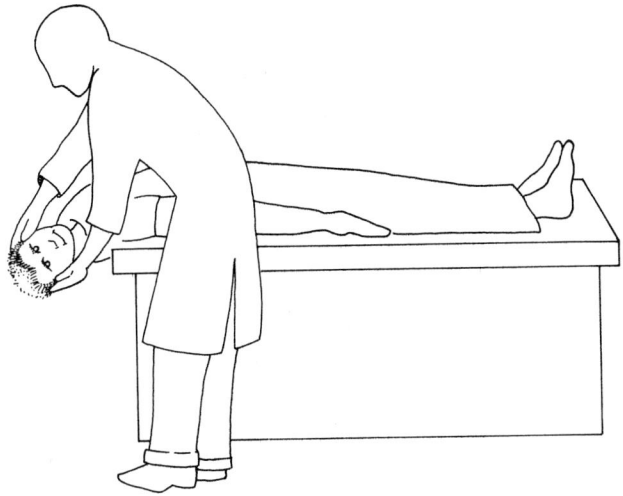

FIG. 9-4 *The Nylen–Bárány maneuver is a screen test for benign positional vertigo.*

dicative of an acute condition or one that suggests a more stable process. The clues of rapid onset of dizziness, along with other symptoms that cause considerable patient discomfort, signal an acute process. The milder, intermittent, and more subtle sensations that require less adjustment and allow the patient to carry on the activities of daily living give more reason to think about a stabilizing, self-limiting condition. The nurse then refines the problem further by distinguishing the revolving spinning sensations of true vertigo from the light-headed sensation of nonvertiginous dizziness.

Physician consultation is appropriate in any phase of the diagnostic and management process. The nurse determines the need by the complexity of the problem and the management skills within her individual scope of practice. The nurse with advanced skills should consult the physician after the preliminary assessment regarding the medical diagnosis, management, and possible referral to a specialist. In the ambulatory setting, referral for the patient with dizziness should be considered when:

- Dizziness occurs following head or neck trauma.
- Dizziness is accompanied by cardiovascular abnormalities.
- The patient has a systolic BP > 200 mm Hg, a discernible cardiac arrhythmia, or a carotid bruit.
- There are findings indicative of a persistent ear infection, hearing problems, or a vestibular disorder.
- Evidence of cervical spondylosis or osteophytes exists.
- Evidence is found of a focal neurologic abnormality or vertical nystagmus, or the patient complains of whirling sensations.
- The patient experiences any sensations with a loss of consciousness.

The nurse is in the unique position of being involved directly in the assessment and management process, or is the liaison person that fosters continuity, provides support, and counsels the patient about the diagnostic and therapeutic plan.[15,27]

Dizziness and vertigo can be frightening and disabling symptoms that cause anxiety irrespective of the complexity of etiology. It is often the fear of the unknown rather than the severity of the symptoms that brings the patient to the health provider for help. If the dizziness is perceived by the patient to be a serious problem, the anxiety may exacerbate the symptoms and add to the physical discomfort.

The coping and tolerance capabilities with these symptoms can be ascertained early in the assessment process. The perceptive nurse will often pick up cues during the history that reflect anxiety and fear that inhibit adjustment. Give the patient the opportunity to verbalize fears and concerns about the effects of the symptoms, diagnostic procedures, and the management of the personal and social environment. Assessment of the coping ability of dizziness must be individualized. The patient with vertigo may be incapacitated by the spinning sensations and accompanying symptoms with peripheral disorders. On the other hand, the nonrotational type of dizziness may not be totally disabling, but just as frightening to the older person or the person whose occupation requires driving, operating machinery, or precision of sight and balance. Interpreting the unknown can create an environment that makes it easier for the patient to participate more effectively in the medical management and self-care regimens. Concise reasonable explanations to questions about dizziness must be given to the patient so that his anxiety is alleviated or kept within reasonable bounds. The nurse can be the key person that helps the patient to explore alternatives to adjustments that must be made in coping with symptomatology or the disease.

MANAGEMENT

The management of dizziness and vertigo is dependent upon identification and management of the underlying problem. The goals are twofold. The immediate goal is to determine the cause and the basis of the pathology. The second, more long-term goal is intervention through the treatment process, which results in the relief and control of the symptomatology. It is reassuring to the patient to be informed of each step so he can see the progression of the therapeutic and management process to resolve the problem.

PATIENT EDUCATION

Since the causes of dizziness are multiple, the counseling and teaching necessary for effective management must be individualized. In some patients, particularly the older person with several chronic problems, education regarding the adjustment to and treatment of those problems may be the major nursing intervention. In other instances, patients with benign disorders often are relieved of a great deal of anxiety by basic explanations and reassurance that the symptoms can be controlled or will resolve in time. Still others are helped by overcoming fears of the unknown by an explanation of the diagnostic procedures involved in the more lengthy work-up.

PHARMACOLOGIC MANAGEMENT

The pharmacologic agents known as *antivertigo drugs* are used to relieve the symptoms of vertigo and the nausea and vomiting that often accompany peripheral causes of labyrinthine malfunction. Some drugs have primarily antihistaminic properties, whereas others have a combination of antiemetic, anticholinergic, and antihistaminic properties.

The effectiveness of the *antihistamines* is related to their anticholinergic activity. It appears that the anticholinergics act on the CNS by a central antagonism of acetylcholine. This blocks the excitatory labyrinthine impulses at the cholinergic synapses in the area of the vestibular nuclei. The *antiemetic* property of the drugs is due to suppression of action on the centrally mediated, nausea-and-vomiting–chemoreceptor trigger zone.[16,26]

Meclizine (Antivert and Bonine) is an antihistamine that helps to prevent nausea. Cyclizine (Marezine) has antiemetic, anticholinergic, and antihistaminic properties. It comes in an injectable form when nausea and vomiting prevent the use of the oral route.

Migral is a drug containing cyclizine, caffeine, and ergotamine tartrate, recommended for its vasoconstrictor action in the treatment of migraine and other vascular headaches. The cyclizine component relieves the dizziness and vertiginouslike symptoms that accompany migraine headaches.

Dimenhydrinate is the chlorotheophylline salt of the antihistaminic agent, diphenhydramine, and comes in several nonprescription forms (Dramamine, Eldodram, and Trav-arex). While the precise mode of action of dimenhydrinate is not known, it appears that the major effect is a depressant action on hyperstimulated labyrinthine function. It is widely used for the prevention of motion sickness.[26]

Diphenidol (Vontrol) is a vestibular suppressant used for severe vertigo. It exerts a specific antivertigo effect on the vestibular apparatus and inhibits the chemoreceptor zone to control nausea and vomiting. Vontrol is used to control symptoms of Meniere's disease and labyrinthitis following middle and inner ear surgery. Because of the possible adverse effects of disorientation, confusion, and hallucinations, its use is limited to patients who are hospitalized or under continuous close professional supervision.

As with any drug, the patient being treated with an antivertigo and antiemetic agent must be aware of the action and side-effects. If an antihistaminic agent is used, the patient should be told about the sedative effects and warned about driving or operating machinery. Anticholinergic effects of these drugs such as blurred vision, dry mouth, and urinary retention should be explained. The patient with closed-angle glaucoma should be told why an antiemetic with anticholinergic effects would be harmful.

The relationship of the time of dosage and its mechanism of action must be explained. The patient with a migraine headache must understand that relief is obtained if the drug is taken before the headache becomes intense. Likewise, the person with motion sickness must know that the drug must be taken *before* sailing or riding to prevent overstimulation of the labyrinth. Most importantly, the patient must know that drugs do not cure dizziness and vertigo but are short-term agents used to relieve the symptoms of the basic disorder.

MEDICAL TREATMENT AND NURSING IMPLICATIONS FOR SPECIFIC ETIOLOGIES

Drug-Induced Dizziness

Dizziness that is induced by a specific drug can only be relieved if the drug is discontinued. In some instances, a smaller dose or weaker strength medication may be sufficient. If the problem is toxic labyrinthitis, immediate withdrawal of the drug may prevent labyrinthine damage. If an agent has been prescribed as treatment-specific therapy, such as streptomycin for an infectious process, substitution of another drug may be necessary to prevent permanent organ damage from the ototoxic effects. Any change in a drug regimen by the physician must be done after weighing the risks of possible damage against use of a less effective agent.

If psychologic dependence on a drug or drug abuse is suspected, then urging the patient to stop use of the drug is not sufficient.

A thorough assessment is essential, with attention given to history of drug use, complications of drugs, and psychosocial data. Physical complaints should be explored with a thorough physical examination. The nurse should recognize that the key to management is the patient's recognition of the problem and the desire to change or seek help. Referral to a program or agency that specializes in drug dependency, coupled with understanding and support, are often the greatest service that can be provided. (For more information on nursing intervention with drug dependency the reader is referred to Chapter 21).

Benign Paroxysmal Positional Vertigo

If benign paroxysmal positional vertigo is caused by a virus, infection, or head trauma, the best advice that can be given to the patient is to try to avoid the position that precipitates the sensations. The condition is self-limited; the patient recovers in 4 to 6 months. If symptoms persist beyond that time, then the patient should be reevaluated to determine other etiologies.

Orthostatic Dizziness

Management of orthostatic dizziness involves alterations in therapy and reassurance that the symptoms can be controlled. In certain susceptible patients, such as the elderly, management is multifaceted.

If the patient is on antihypertensive drugs, careful assessment should determine whether the correct dosage regimen is being followed. A consequence of an incorrect dosage of a sympathetic inhibiting agent like guanethidine is orthostatic and exercise hypotension with dizziness and syncope. The patient must understand that correct dosages, as well as consistent adherence to the therapeutic plan, are essential. If a diuretic has been prescribed, then the patient must

know that taking it prevents fluid overload which, if present, decreases the effectiveness of a medication like guanethidine and increases the severity of orthostatic dizziness.

Often, the most conscientious patient experiences orthostatic dizziness, so the nurse can be supportive and helpful in suggesting ways in which activities can be adjusted to minimize and reduce symptoms. Encourage the patient to slow down body movements, particularly when arising from bed in the morning. Getting out of bed slowly and dangling the legs over the side of the bed before standing are recommended. Also, the patient should be advised to stand slowly. The body adjusts to the change in position better and signals if it is moving too fast by the feeling of weakness or faintness. Lying down and resting until the dizziness passes and then slowly moving again provides relief.

Other suggestions are listed here:

- Encourage the patient to wear support stockings when up, and to move the legs and feet as frequently as possible to prevent pooling of blood in the lower extremities. Movements and exercise should not exceed that which produces symptoms.
- Encourage the patient to perform as many tasks as possible in the sitting position.
- Use blocks to raise the head of the bed about 6 inches to minimize posture changes from the supine to the sitting position.[11]
- Suggest to the elderly male that sitting rather than standing when he urinates or shaves in the morning may be helpful.
- Recommend that the patient avoid heavy strenuous work and driving while symptomatic.

The patient must be monitored frequently to determine whether the physiological adjustments have been made, both in the abatement of symptoms and objective hypotension signs. If the problem persists, consider altering the medication schedule or adjusting the strength so that it is divided, for example 250 mg twice a day instead of 500 mg once a day. Reduction of the dosage or changing to a different drug are other options. Monitoring the patient at each encounter for symptoms, encouraging and supporting the patient during adjustment, and anticipatory guidance for prevention and management during initial treatment stages are important.

Otitis Media and Ear Infections

Vigorous and prompt medical treatment of ear infections often results in resolution of the underlying problem and the abatement of the dizziness. Emphasize the importance of taking prescribed medications, such as antibiotics and decongestants, for the recommended length of time to prevent complications and recurrent infections. Follow-up visits must include evaluation of the middle ear for continued infection, preservation of hearing, and evidence of damage to the inner ear apparatus.

Acute Labyrinthitis

Treatment of acute labyrinthitis is symptomatic. Although the patient may feel quite ill, there is no specific medical therapy because the cause is usually viral. The patient may find relief only in the recumbent position during the acute phase, so bed rest is encouraged as a palliative therapeutic measure. Antiemetic drugs, such as dimenhydrinate and meclizine, along with an advancing liquid diet, are other measures that may be used until the nausea, vomiting, and vertigo have subsided. The patient needs to be reassured that the problem is self-limited, although in some cases the feeling of disequilibrium with certain head movements may last for a few weeks to a few months. In most patients, complete recovery occurs in 3 to 6 months.

Meniere's Disease (Meniere's Syndrome)

Since Meniere's disease has multiple pathophysiological causes, medical treatment is directed at the specific cause for the pathology causing the inner ear disorder. The patient with a medical problem such as an allergy, adrenal pituitary insufficiency, vascular insufficiency, estrogen deficiency, or hypothyroidism responds to the appropriate management of those problems. The patient with Meniere's disease caused by physical or acoustic trauma, stenosis of the internal auditory canal, a viral infection, or idiopathic disease will ultimately require surgery to prevent disabling vertigo and permanent hearing loss.

During an acute attack, symptomatic treatment is essential. The patient feels miserable and appears quite ill. Bed rest may be most effective, since vertigo is minimized in the reclining position. Dimenhydrinate or cyclizine may be helpful in controlling the vertigo as well as the nausea and vomiting. Encourage the patient to take clear liquids and advance to other nonirritating foods as tolerated. Once the acute episode has passed, medications may be continued for a period to reduce recurring vertigo. If, after several months of treatment, the patient continues to have disabling symptoms that interfere with life-style and vocational functioning, surgery may be indicated.

A microsurgical procedure called the *endolymphatic subarachnoid shunt* is the procedure of choice for idiopathic Meniere's disease. It involves decompression and drainage of the canal and is most effective in the patient with recurrent vertigo, pressure, and tinnitus. This procedure requires general anesthesia, takes about an hour to perform, and requires from 2 to 3 days of hospitalization. The postoperative course is mild and relatively painless, with rapid convalescence and few complications, which makes it an option for the older patient. It is especially important that the procedure be performed without delay in patients with bilateral hearing loss, or when the disease involves the only ear with hearing function.

In patients with long-standing disease but some residual hearing function, a vestibular neurectomy may be the surgery of choice. A *vestibular neurectomy* is done through the middle or posterior cranial fossa and eliminates the normal impulses from being transmitted to the inner ear. It provides relief of tinnitus in 50% of people undergoing the procedure, and permanent relief of vertigo in 95% of patients. Further hearing loss occurs in 10% of cases, with complications of cerebrospinal leakage and infection, with infection and transient facial weakness occurring in a small number of patients.[20]

The patient with advanced Meniere's disease, characterized by irreparable and irreversible hearing loss with severe tinnitus, may be a candidate for a *translabyrinthine eighth nerve section*. This procedure markedly relieves tinnitus and vertigo. About half of these patients report improved hearing postoperatively in the opposite ear due to cessation of the tinnitus. This procedure is more complex and is usually performed by a neuro-otologist. Complications, which are infrequent, include bleeding, cerebrospinal leakage, and transient facial weakness. The hospital course for a vestibular neurectomy or eighth nerve section is 4 to 5 days. Postoperatively, patients experience a rapidly subsiding vertigo with a full return of balance in approximately 3 to 6 weeks. Caution should be given concerning rapid body movements, which may cause mild imbalance for up to a year following surgery.[20]

Although most patients with Meniere's disease are treated by an otolaryngologist, the nurse may see the patient during phases of the diagnostic and treatment process. Care of the total patient involves an understanding that Meniere's disease is a chronic disabling condition that causes great physical and emotional discomfort. Because the symptoms can be severe, the patient may become frightened and discouraged easily. The nursing management involves continuous support and counseling of the patient in coping with the symptoms, patient teaching of diagnostic and treatment procedures, and assisting in adjustment of life-style and activities of daily living following surgery.

Cardiovascular Problems

Successful management of cardiovascular problems requires thorough assessment and judicious medical treatment of the basic problem. Patients with aortic valvular stenosis, atherosclerotic destruction of the vertebral–basilar artery system, subclavian steal syndrome, and cardiac arrhythmias usually are managed by a specialist in cardiology or internal medicine. Nursing management involves monitoring of symptoms, and education regarding activities, prescribed medication, and possible surgery. The nurse should monitor patients with arrhythmias for frequency and severity of dizziness, other symptoms, and side-effects from antiarrhythmic agents. Give careful attention to the severity of symptoms before placing the patient on drugs. Some agents, like quinidine, result in tinnitus and vertigo and may intensify a pre-therapy symptom.

The patient with carotid sinus hypersensitivity may require adjustment in medications, particularly digitalis, which seems to aggravate the condition. Treatment of symptoms also may include reminding the patient not to wear clothes tightly around the neck and to avoid sudden turning of the head.

Dizziness as a symptom of congestive

heart failure is relieved when the capacity of the heart to adapt or respond effectively to the pumping demands is restored. This requires increasing the force or strength of contraction and reducing the demands on the myocardium.[6] Specific medical therapy depends on the degree of the failure and the underlying etiology.

Dizziness in the hypertensive patient may be due to symptomatology of the disease or its treatment. If the symptoms accompany uncontrolled or undiagnosed disease, an antihypertensive regimen must be initiated, continued, and carefully evaluated for its effectiveness. The goal of therapy is to develop a plan that reduces the blood pressure, prevents damage to target organs, and is acceptable to the patient. If the dizziness (resulting from orthostatic hypotension) is a result of antihypertensive drugs, adjustments must be made in the drugs or dosages, and suggestions given for preventing symptoms and increasing drug tolerance (see section on orthostatic dizziness).

Neurologic and Central Nervous System Disorders

The patient with dizziness that points to a CNS disease or lesion should be referred to a specialist in neurology. Nursing management of the patient with an acoustic neurinoma may include explanation of normal neurologic functioning, interpretation of dizziness, and other abnormal symptoms, along with the reason for referral.

The most effective management of dizziness associated with migraine headache involves avoidance of factors that precipitate attacks, prophylactic measures to decrease the frequency of headaches, and symptomatic treatment. (An indepth discussion regarding the nursing care of migraine headaches is found in Chapter 8).

Management of a seizure disorder by a neurologist is directed at the etiologic factors, the resulting seizures, the most effective medication, and the impact of the disorder on the patient's social functioning. Patient understanding of the nature of the seizure disorder, the medication program, potential side-effects of drugs, and the danger of not taking the medications as prescribed is essential. Alert the patient to symptoms that precipitate an attack whether they be dizziness, headache, scotoma, or vague feelings of malaise and discomfort. Share education regarding stimulants (specifically alcohol, coffee, and tobacco) that precipitate attacks, and advise the patient to abstain from these agents. In addition, the nurse should emphasize the importance of adequate rest, proper nutrition, avoidance of extreme physical exertion, exposure to infections, and emotionally stressful situations that may precipitate an attack.

The patient with multiple sensory deficits may experience chronic dizziness due to the irreversible pathology of the medical problem. Chronic alcoholism and poorly controlled diabetes of many years standing may result in irreparable sensory loss. Orthopedic and arthritic problems may require surgery to relieve the deficit. In the older person with multiple deficits, correction of one deficit may still leave the patient with the need to adjust to the remaining deficit. Adaptation to sensory loss can be facilitated by increasing the information to other sense organs. The sensation of unsteadiness experienced by the older patient wearing new glasses after cataract surgery may be relieved by encouraging the patient to touch objects when walking until he obtains a feel and sense of surroundings. If dizziness due to vestibular deficits or cervical spondylosis occurs during ambulation, touching a stable object like a chair or table often brings relief and redefines a sense of position perspective. The nurse should explain the chronic nature of the problem and suggest ways in which the patient and family members may initiate safety measures while facilitating adjustment to the condition.

The most important aspect of nursing management in the hyperventilation syndrome is patient education. This requires that the patient understand the association between emotion and stress and hyperventilation, and how overbreathing produces the symptoms. If he is experiencing an acute attack, having him breathe into a paper or plastic bag will provide relief. Increased awareness that hyperventilation is the body's response to excessive anxiety may trigger self-directed behavior changes that result in abatement of symptoms[15] Providing this information helps the patient to gain insight into the cause of the problem, which is the first step in preventing repetitive episodes. In addition, knowing that the physical exam rules out any organic disease reassures the patient.

Paramount to recovery is assessment of personal, social, or work-related difficulties that may be the basis of the anxiety and the psychological distress. Open-ended questions that allow the patient to talk about life in general may be most helpful in establishing an atmosphere of comfort and relaxation, in which deeper-seated issues can be discussed with more ease.

There are also behaviors that will help the patient to prevent acute attacks. Suggesting that the patient be more aware of involuntary mannerisms—sighing, sniffing, coughing, and deep breathing—that signal an impending attack may be helpful. The patient should also try to avoid wearing tight-fitting clothes such as girdles, which encourage habitual thoracic breathing. Prevention also involves learning relaxation techniques—being aware of tense posture and relaxing the head, neck, shoulders, and thorax several times a day is helpful. He should

know that lounging in a chair rather than sitting on the edge is relaxing. Also, he should be more alert to situations that aggravate these habits and postures.[7] The patient should give thought to possible adjustments in his life-style that would allow him to slow down and allow times for activities that are fulfilling physically and psychologically.

In psychogenic dizziness, as in the hyperventilation syndrome, direct treatment toward education of the patient to the relationship between the dizziness and other problems of psychoneurotic origin. Organic causes are first excluded with detailed history and thorough physical examination. The patient may be experiencing symptoms related to depression, due to a chronic medical problem like poorly controlled diabetes, uncontrolled hypertension, or thyroid disease.[22] In addition, the nurse often may uncover in the interview a long-standing history of somatic complaints disproportionate to the medical problem. There may be a history of being treated for anxiety and depression.

Encouraging the patient to talk about problems is therapeutic. Many patients are not aware of the level of stress in their lives. The nurse should realize that the problem may be chronic, so that time should be allotted for continued counseling on a long-term basis. Referral to other professionals may be necessary if it is apparent that the patient is unable to come to a resolution of the problems.

The ideal treatment of motion sickness in susceptible persons is prevention of an attack with antivertigo or antiemetic drugs before exposure to conditions that produce symptoms. The nonprescription agents, meclizine, dimenhydrinate, and cyclizine, are more commonly used. For best results, the medication should be taken approximately 30 minutes before motion-producing activity. Once an attack has begun, resting in a supine position, removing oneself from the offending motion, and taking ice chips for fluid maintenance usually will bring relief.

SUMMARY

Dizziness is a common patient complaint that nurses encounter on a frequent basis in many types of settings. The causes are multiple, and the sensations experienced by patients vary. Knowledge of the possible etiologies, the appropriate assessment, recommended medical and nursing management, and patient education strategies are essential for effective intervention. Understanding of organic and inorganic problems that result in dizziness will help to demystify the management process for the care provider and to alleviate the anxiety and concern of the many patients who experience this symptom.

REFERENCES

1. Beland IL, Passos JY: Clinical Nursing, 3rd ed. New York, MacMillan, 1981
2. Bradbeer TL: Vertigo: In health and disease. Nurs Times 73: 1586–1589, Oct 13, 1977
3. Elin JC: The Dizzy Patient. Springfield, IL, Charles C Thomas, 1968
4. Evaluating complaints of dizziness: Patient Care 15: 23–61, May 30, 1981
5. Facer GW, Maragos NE: The dizzy patient. Postgrad Med, 57 No. 6: 73–77, May 1975
6. Goroll AH, May LA, Mulley AG: Primary Care Medicine. Philadelphia, JB Lippincott, 1981
7. Hill Oscar (ed): Modern Trends in Psychosomatic Medicine 216–217. London, Butterworths, 1976
8. Hudak CM, Redstone PM, Hokanson NL, et al: Clinical Protocols. Philadelphia, JB Lippincott, 1976
9. Isselbacher KJ, Adams RD, Brownwald E et al (eds): Harrison's Principles of Internal Medicine, 9th ed. New York, McGraw-Hill, 1980
10. Barber HO: Diagnostic Techniques in Vertigo. Journal of Vertigo 1, No. 1: 1–16, 1974
11. Kochar MS, Daniels LM: Hypertension Control for Nurses and Other Health Professionals. St. Louis, CV Mosby, 1978
12. MacBryde CM, Blacklow RS: Signs and Symptoms, 5th ed. Philadelphia, JB Lippincott, 1970
13. Mullan DA (ed): Physical complaints of the aging. Geriatrics Marketer 4, No. 4: Apr 1965
14. Orma EJ, Koskenoja M: Postural dizziness in the aged. Geriatrics 12: 49, 1957
15. Pflaum SS: Protocol: Diagnosis and management of dizziness/vertigo. Nurse Prac 3: 27–29 Sept–Oct, 1978
16. Physicians' Desk Reference 36th ed: Oradell, New Jersey, Medical Economics, 1982
17. Prior JA, Silberstein JS: Physical Diagnosis. St. Louis, CV Mosby, 1977
18. Probing physical causes of dizziness: Patient Care 15: 41–102, July 15, 1981
19. A seizure of dizziness: Emergency Medicine 13: 93–94, June 30, 1981
20. Silverstein H: Look for all the causes of dizziness. Consultant 19: 114–115, Apr 1979
21. Spector M: Dizziness and Vertigo: Diagnosis and Treatment. New York, Grune & Stratton, 1967
22. Stephens GJ: Pathophysiology for Health Practitioners. New York, MacMillan, 1980
23. Tortora GJ, Anagnostakos NP: Principles of Anatomy and Physiology, 3rd ed. New York, Harper & Row, 1981
24. Tortora GJ, Evans RL, Anagnostakos NP: Principles of Human Physiology. New York, Harper & Row, 1982
25. Turner JS: The dizzy patient: Diagnosis and treatment. Drugs 13: 382–387, 1977
26. Weiner, MB, Pepper GA, Kuhn–Weisman G et al: Clinical Pharmacology and Therapeutics in Nursing. New York, McGraw–Hill, 1979
27. Whitney FW: Guidelines for neurological consultation. Nurse Prac 7, No. 7: 13–18, July–Aug 1982
28. Wideroe T, Vigander T: Propranolol in the treatment of migraine. Brit Med J 2: 699–701, 1974

BIBLIOGRAPHY

Burnside IM: Nursing and the Aged. New York, McGraw–Hill, 1976

Clairmont AA, Turner JS, Jackson RT: Dizziness: A logical approach to diagnosis and treatment. Postgrad Med 56, No. 2: 139–144, Aug 1974

Drachman DA, Hart CW: An approach to the dizzy patient. Neurol 22, No. 4: 323–334, Apr 1972

10

Communication Deficits

Sue Fink

Communication affects all nursing care. It is through communication that nurses establish relationships, identify problems and strengths, carry out health teaching, and assist people with their responses to actual and potential health problems. Many physical, psychological, and social factors interact to influence one's ability to communicate effectively. While psychological and social factors alone can cause serious disruptions in communication, the major focus of this chapter will be on the nursing assessment and management of people who have communication deficits resulting from sensorineural impairments.

Communication is the complex process by which we interact with our social and physical environment. Through communication we learn about others, our physical world, and ourselves. We also use communication to influence the behavior of others and to alter our environments to meet our needs. Human communication is a dynamic, continuous process without a discrete beginning or ending. While we are generating thoughts and translating them into a code of verbal or nonverbal behavior that transmits our meaning to others, we are simulta-

neously receiving and interpreting messages from others and from our surroundings. Through this continuing process we are able to affect our environment and are in turn affected by it.

The nervous system directs our complex communication patterns. To understand the meaning of another person we must be able to receive sensory stimuli through vision, hearing, and touch. Neural pathways must be capable of transmitting these stimuli to the brain, which in turn must be capable of interpreting their meaning. To convey our meanings to another person we must be able to formulate thoughts and to translate these thoughts into word symbols, gestures, or other actions. The neuromuscular system carries out these translations as speech, writing, gestures, and other behaviors.

Psychological and social factors play an equally important role in determining our ability to understand the meaning of others and have our own meaning understood. To each interaction we bring our own view of our personal world, our self-perceptions, our past experiences, our attitudes, and our values. These unique aspects affect how we express ourselves, how we interpret the stimuli we receive, and often the stimuli to which we attend. The meanings that we attach to verbal and nonverbal behavior are socially and culturally learned. Social factors that affect our ability to understand one another's meaning include not only the language we speak but also the gestures we use, the ways in which we use touch, the distances that we place between ourselves, and the meanings that we attach to the use of time. These symbols that we use for communication have arbitrarily assigned meanings that vary according to our personal, social, and cultural background.

Although speaking and listening are the most common channels used for communication, in many situations several channels are used. While we hear and interpret the words of the speaker, we simultaneously hear and attach meaning to the tone of voice and rate of speech. As we listen, we also see and interpret facial expressions, hand gestures, and body movements. Similarly, we are aware of the distance between us and the use of touch. When one of these channels of communication is unavailable to us we need to rely more heavily on the remaining ones. We must maintain an awareness of the multiple channels used for communication and identify the assets and success of people with communication deficits if we are to promote the optimal use of communication skills.

Hearing Impairments

DEFINITIONS

Terms that are used to describe the hearing-impaired person do not have precise definitions. In general, the term *deaf* is used to describe the person who is unable to make

use of sound stimuli for communication, while the term *hard-of-hearing* is used to describe the person who, with or without amplification, is able to make some use of sound for communication. The deaf can be divided further according to whether the deafness occurred before or after the acquisition of language skills. The term *prelingual deafness* is used to refer to losses that occur before language skills are developed, whereas the term *acquired deafness* is used to describe losses that occur after these skills have been developed. The terms *deaf* and *hard-of-hearing* have been associated with many negative stereotypes and give us little accurate indication of the person's communication ability. Therefore, the term *hearing impaired* is preferred. It is hoped that the use of this term will lead to greater recognition that hearing losses occur on a broad continuum, and the range of behaviors used to cope with these losses is equally broad.

INCIDENCE

Audiometric surveys of the civilian noninstitutionalized population in the United States define *hearing impairment* as the presence of elevated hearing levels for speech in the better ear. According to this definition approximately 7% to 8%, or 11 million adults, have impaired hearing. Although the majority of these people have difficulty only with faint speech, over 2 million adults have difficulty with normal speech, and 1.5 million cannot understand normal or amplified speech. The prevalence of hearing impairment is higher in men than in women, and higher in older people. Approximately one third of people over age 65 have hearing impairments, and in people over age 75 this statistic increases to include almost half the population. These surveys do not include residents of nursing homes. Among nursing home residents the incidence of significant hearing impairments is estimated to be between 30% and 50%. Approximately 216,000 people in the United State have prelingual deafness.[15]

MECHANISMS OF HEARING IMPAIRMENTS

SOUND AND HEARING

The energy generated by the vibration of a tuning fork or the human vocal cords must travel across an elastic medium, usually air, to reach the person and be perceived as sound. Air molecules are in constant random motion, and when the sound generator exerts its motion patterns on the air molecules, they move back and forth in a motion that mimics the vibratory pattern of the generator. Adjacent air molecules are then set in motion, enabling the energy or sound wave to reach the receiver. There are two properties of sound waves that are important to our perception of sound: intensity and frequency. The intensity or pressure of a sound wave is measured in decibels (db) and correlates with our perception of *loudness*. The frequency of the sound wave is measured in hertz (Hz) and correlates with our perception of *pitch.*

When sound waves reach the person, they travel to the inner ear by air conduction and bone conduction. Sound waves reach the cochlea directly by vibration of the skull bones in bone conduction; in air conduction, sound waves travel through the ear. (For a review of the anatomy of the ear, see the introductory material to Chapter 9.) Briefly, the outer ear channels sound waves through the external auditory canal to the tympanic membrane (see Fig. 9-1). The ossicular chain in the middle ear then carries sound energy to the cochlea in the inner ear. The *ossicular chain* is a series of small, interlinked bones including the malleus, the incus, and the

stapes. The malleus is attached to both the tympanic membrane and the incus, which in turn attaches to the stapes. When sound waves set the tympanic membrane in motion, the stapes move back and forth in the oval window, setting fluid in the cochlea in motion. This motion causes hair cell movement in the organ of Corti (the neural end-organ for hearing), and sound energy is converted to a neural response. This neural response travels along fibers of the cochlear branch of the auditory nerve, and to the brain where it is interpreted as sound.

TYPES OF HEARING IMPAIRMENTS

Hearing impairments are classified as either conductive hearing loss, sensorineural hearing loss, or mixed hearing loss. *Mixed hearing losses* have both a conductive and sensorineural component. *Conductive hearing losses* result from interference in the transmission of sound energy through the outer and middle ear. Some of the conditions that may lead to conductive hearing loss in adults include.

Impacted cerumen
External otitis
Tumors or foreign bodies
Otitis media
Blockage of the eustachian tube
Osteosclerosis
Trauma

Many of the conditions leading to conductive hearing loss are amenable to medical or surgical treatment. Typically, the person with a conductive hearing loss complains of sounds being muffled or faint, but has no difficulty understanding if the sound stimulus is loud enough. These people may find it easier to hear in noisy listening situations, such as a sports event or large party, where people tend to speak more loudly.

Sensorineural hearing losses result from damage or disease to any part of the inner ear or neural auditory pathways. Some of the conditions that may lead to sensorineural hearing loss include:

Presbycusis
Noise exposure
Drug toxicity
Infections
Meniere's disease
Tumors of the auditory nerve
Congenital or hereditary factors.

Most sensorineural losses are not amenable to medical or surgical treatment. People with sensorineural hearing loss may have difficulty understanding or discriminating what they hear, even if the stimuli are intense enough to reach their hearing threshold. The situation is similar to a poorly tuned radio station. Turning up the volume makes it louder, but the distortion of sound remains. Although people with sensorineural hearing losses require a more intense stimulus to perceive sound, the level of intensity that is perceived as uncomfortable is often lower than normal. This phenomena is *recruitment* and accounts for the fact that when you speak more loudly in an effort to make yourself understood, the person may complain that you are speaking too loudly.

People with sensorineural hearing losses typically have the most difficulty hearing in noisy listening situations, such as a crowded restaurant or a large auditorium with many reverberating sounds. They are most successful in one-to-one conversations, particularly with family and friends who may have either unconsciously or consciously altered their speaking patterns. This adaptation on the part of family and friends may lead the person to attribute his difficulties to the speech patterns of others, rather than to his own hearing deficits. The person may say that he hears just fine and may feel that the problem is that people talk too fast or do not speak clearly.

Presbycusis, the most common form of sensorineural loss, is more prevalent than any other form of hearing disorder. *Presbycusis* is a progressive, sensorineural loss associated with aging. The loss is usually bilateral and initially affects only high frequencies. As it progresses, the loss may involve both high and low frequencies but will be greater in the higher frequencies. Persons with presbycusis generally retain some residual hearing for low and middle frequencies. They can hear another person speak and understand a portion of what is said. However, misinterpretation of words that are crucial to the meaning of the sentence is common. This is because the consonant sounds that enable us to distinguish between similar words are higher in frequency and lower in intensity than the vowel sounds. The consonant sounds *f*, *t*, *s*, *z*, *th*, *ch*, and *sh* are most severely affected. The person with presbycusis also may have more difficulty understanding people with high-pitched voices. These factors may be part of the explanation for the family's perception that the person hears "when he wants to and who he wants to."

People with mixed hearing losses may present with characteristics of the greater loss, or with a combination of characteristics that are unclear. Audiograms differentiate the varying degrees of conductive and sensorineural loss. It is important to be aware of the possibility of mixed losses to ensure appropriate counseling and rehabilitative efforts.

IMPACT OF HEARING IMPAIRMENTS

There are three dimensions of hearing that play an important part in our awareness of the world around us and our ability to interact with that world. The signal or warning level of hearing alerts us to conditions in our environment. We use our hearing to constantly scan the environment to anticipate and identify changes. This level of hearing tells us when another person is approaching, enables us to identify a mosquito in the dark, and warns us of an oncoming car when our vision is obscured. The absence of unusual sounds, on the other hand, assures us that all is well. When hearing is impaired at the warning level, our ability to make appropriate adjustments and responses in day-to-day living is disrupted.

The background or primitive level of hearing keeps us in touch with our environment, although we are not consciously aware of these sounds and do not need to make a specific response to them. The loss of these sounds isolates the person from the active, living world around him, may lead to feelings of isolation, and is sometimes expressed as a feeling that the "world is dead."

The symbolic level of hearing is used in understanding speech. Impairments at this level of hearing have an impact on relationships with others and may affect self-esteem. When interpersonal communication is difficult, the person may isolate himself from others or may find that others withdraw from contacts with him. Efforts to communicate will be frustrating and ambiguous not only for the hearing-impaired individual, but for the people who want and need to communicate with him as well.

Hearing impairments are a significant loss for the person and for the people significant to him. All parties may go through a period of grieving in adapting to this loss. Denial, anger, and withdrawal characterize stages of this grieving process.

Hearing impairment has been called "the hidden handicap" because there is seldom anything about the person's appearance or behavior that makes the problem obvious to others. The problems of hearing-impaired people have been poorly understood by society, and frequently they have been labeled "retarded," "senile," or "uncooperative." The great efforts of many hearing-impaired persons to deny their disability and keep their hearing aids invisible suggest that there is still more stigma than empathy attached to hearing disabilities.

Most research on adjustment to hearing impairment has focused on people with prelingual deafness. Most adults who are prelingually deaf socialize with other deaf people, marry another deaf person, and are somewhat isolated from people with normal hearing. The majority of prelingually deaf adults, however, live well-adjusted and productive lives. They are not predisposed to major psychotic illness, despite the frequent characterization of the deaf as paranoid.[14]

Little attention has been given to the adjustment problems of the hard-of-hearing, but some studies report a greater incidence of depression among the hard-of-hearing and suggest that the ambiguity of this person's situation leads to a more difficult adjustment.[14,22] The hard of hearing person's ability to engage in successful social interactions may depend largely on the demands of the environment. Factors beyond his control, such as inadequate lighting and noisy backgrounds, will have a negative impact on his understanding. Because listening may require great concentration that cannot be sustained over long periods, successful interactions may have a very limited time span. Although hearing loss frequently is thought to lead inevitably to social isolation, studies of older adults living in high-rise apartments for the elderly do not confirm this. These studies found no correlation between hearing acuity and social involvement.[6,17] The high incidence of hearing impairment among people living in these settings may lead to an improved environment in which both speakers and listeners adapt their behavior to cope with these losses.

NURSING ASSESSMENT

Nurses come into contact with hearing-impaired persons in many different settings and for varying reasons. Both the setting and the reason for the nurse–patient contact will influence the nurse's assessment. When the hearing-impaired person has been hospitalized for another health problem, the nurse's assessment focuses on determining effective means of communication so that a plan of care that meets the person's communication needs can be developed. At other times the patient may talk with a nurse about a hearing problem before seeking any other type of assistance. In this instance, the purpose of the nurse's assessment is to provide a data base for counseling and referral. When the patient already is undergoing rehabilitation, the nurse's assessment may focus on the patient and family's adaptation and identifying specific learning needs. The nurse's clinical judgment will be required in deciding the appropriate focus and comprehensiveness of the assessment of individual patients.

INTERVIEWING TECHNIQUES

During the initial contact with the hearing-impaired adult, the first priority is to assess the person's communication ability. Assumptions must be avoided. The man wearing a hearing aid may use it only to become aware that someone is speaking to him and depend on speech-reading or lipreading for communication. The woman whose daughter speaks to her in sign language may also be able to speech-read or understand written

messages. The altered communication mode that the nurse observes may be due to the daughter's problems rather than the patient's. Many adults with hearing impairments are being seen by the nurse for other health problems and do not readily identify or acknowledge their hearing problem. These people can be identified by the nurse who is alert to the following behaviors that suggest hearing loss:

Frequent requests for repetition
Inappropriate answers
Leaning forward
Turning one ear toward the speaker
Strained facial expression
Need to see the speaker's face
Talking loudly or with a flat voice
Slurring words or dropping endings
Tiring easily and becoming inattentive.

Ask directly whether the person can understand your speech; then offer to speak more slowly, more loudly, or change position. This approach signals the desire to communicate effectively and your willingness to alter your behavior to achieve this. When talking to someone else about the hearing impaired person in his presence, convey this to him and let him know the general topic. Often the person with a severe hearing impairment is accompanied by a spouse or another person who has much of the information that the nurse needs. The nurse can use this person to economize on time and energy of both the patient and herself. However, she must not exclude the patient. Letting the patient know the general topic and providing an opportunity for him to make comments, before directing more specific questions to his companion, is one method of including the patient without tiring him. When a sign language interpreter is needed to communicate with a deaf person, the natural inclination is to focus on the interpreter. The nurse–

patient relationship will be enhanced by avoiding this tendency and maintaining eye contact with the patient. This gesture conveys to the patient your interest in him and his problems.

SUBJECTIVE DATA

General

It is useful to begin the interview by gathering general information regarding age, place of residence, educational and occupational background, and life-style. This information is useful in determining specific listening situations about which you may wish to question the patient.

History

When assessing the history of the hearing impairment, first direct attention to the onset of the hearing problem, the reason the person is seeking attention for the problem (if he is), and any steps that have been taken already to address the problem. In addition, assess the history of factors associated with hearing impairment, including

Other family members with hearing loss
Ear infection, current or past
Upper respiratory infections, current or past
Head and ear trauma
Medications (antibiotics, salicylates)
Noise exposure (work and hobby)
Presence of tinnitus or vertigo.

Patient's Perception of the Hearing Problem

Ask the patient to describe how his hearing has changed. Use open-ended questions to help the patient to describe listening situations that cause the most and the fewest problems. Whether you ask additional questions about specific listening situations will depend somewhat on the amount of informa-

tion the patient has already given you, and somewhat on the purposes of your assessment. The accompanying self-administered questionnaire can be useful in helping the hard-of-hearing person to think about the specifics of his hearing problems. Although these questions can be answered *yes* or *no*, presenting them without a forced choice between these options stimulates people to think about situations that occur in their daily lives. Another useful method of determining the impact of the hearing loss is to ask whether the person has stopped participating in any groups or activities that he formerly enjoyed. Reflective statements that acknowledge the difficulty or losses the patient has experienced provide an opening for the patient to discuss feelings.

Family's Perception of the Hearing Problem

Family members are asked questions similar to the ones suggested for patients. Determine under what circumstances it is most difficult for them to communicate, and under what circumstances it is least difficult. Recall that hearing loss affects not only the person with the loss but also the family. Their own frustrations or anger may prevent the family from viewing the patient's loss objectively. Responses such as, "She never hears anything I say!", or "He hears when he *wants* to!" are best responded to with a reflective statement of how difficult that must be for the speaker. This type of response generally elicits information about family stressors and coping styles that will be more useful in diagnosis and intervention than information gained by further questions about the hearing loss itself.

Hearing Aids

Not all people who have hearing aids wear them. Therefore, ask the person whether he

Hearing Self-Assessment Questionnaire

TALKING WITH ONE PERSON

Can you understand a person seated beside you when you cannot see their face?

Can you understand someone who speaks to you from across the room?

Can you understand someone who speaks to you from the next room?

Can you carry on a conversation with one person in a noisy place, such as a restaurant or a large party?

Is it more difficult for you to understand strangers than it is to understand family or friends?

TALKING IN GROUPS

Do you have more difficulty following the conversation in groups than you do talking with one person?

Are men's voices easier to understand than women's voices?

Do you find yourself becoming tired when conversing in a group?

TALKING ON THE TELEPHONE

Are you able to hear the telephone ring when you are in the same room?

Can you hear the telephone ring when you are in another room?

Do you have difficulty carrying on a telephone conversation?

RADIO OR TELEVISION

Do you have difficulty hearing the radio or television?

When you adjust the volume to suit yourself, do others think it is too loud?

When someone else adjusts the volume, is it loud enough for you?

has ever had a hearing aid. If the person does have a hearing aid, determine when and where it was fitted, when it was most recently evaluated, and the pattern of use. If the aid is currently used determine what, if any, problems are encountered. Also find out if the person knows what to expect of a hearing aid and how to care for it. Can the person manipulate the controls on the aid, change batteries, and insert the ear mold correctly? Does he do these things independently, or does he require assistance?

Rehabilitation Potential

The magnitude of the hearing loss is only one factor in determining a person's potential for rehabilitation. Equally important are his motivation and adaptability, the communication demands in his environment, and the available support from others. When you assess the patient's and family's perception of

the hearing problem, much data about motivation, adaptability, and ability to provide support will be obtained. Similarly, in discussing life-style and the patient's perception of the problem, you will have obtained information about the demands this person's day-to-day environment places on his communication skill. Asking questions about the patient's expectations of treatment and attitudes toward such therapies as hearing aids is also helpful. Attitudes toward aging may be a factor with older adults. Some patients and families may feel that hearing loss is an inevitable part of aging and either believe that nothing can be done or feel it is not worthwhile. Cost may be an important factor for patients of all ages, but particularly for the elderly. While evaluation and surgical treatment usually are covered by health insurance, very few programs cover either evaluation for hearing aids, or the cost of the aid itself. Medicare does not cover these costs. Medicaid offers assistance to qualified persons in some states but not in others. Local charitable organizations may provide some funding, and younger adults may be funded through offices of Vocational Rehabilitation. In addition to assessing the patient's financial status, assess how the person feels about accepting financial assistance when it is needed.

OBJECTIVE DATE

Physical Examination of the Ear

While in some settings nurses will base their referrals and counseling on hearing acuity tests and subjective data, in other settings nurses with skill in physical assessment techniques will conduct the physical examination. The outer ear or auricle is inspected and palpated. A severe external otitis may cause enough edema to impair hearing. The auditory canal and tympanic membrane are inspected with an otoscope. Occlusion of the auditory canal by edema, impacted cerumen, tumors, or foreign bodies may be factors in conductive hearing loss. Inspection of the tympanic membrane may reveal perforations associated with trauma or otitis media, bulging and redness associated with otitis media, or retraction associated with blockage of the eustachian tube. These also may be factors in conductive hearing loss. When the hearing loss is sensorineural, physical findings are usually normal. A complete discussion of examination techniques and normal or abnormal findings is beyond the scope of this chapter. The interested reader can refer to textbooks on physical assessment.

Gross Tests of Hearing Acuity

During the course of the interview the patient's ability to hear and understand has been assessed. Take note of your own tone of voice, distance from the patient, lighting and background noise in the environment, and whether the patient must see the speaker's face. The patient's speech patterns are also assessed. The person who is unable to hear his own voice has difficulty modulating loudness and inflection, and is apt to drop endings or slur words.

Voice tests and the ticking-watch test are further measures that can be used to estimate hearing acuity. Each ear is tested individually, with the opposite ear occluded. Occlusion can be accomplished by either the patient or the nurse placing a finger against the opening of the external auditory canal. The voice tests are conducted with the examiner 1 to 2 ft from the patient's unoccluded ear and positioned so that the patient is unable to see the nurse's lip movements. The examiner says a number in a soft whisper, and the patient is asked to repeat it. If the patient is unable to hear a soft whisper, progressively louder voice tones are used. The ticking of a watch also can be used as a sound stimulus. The farthest distance at which the watch can be heard is measured and recorded. If the patient is able to hear the stimulus of a ticking watch, this is a useful test for determining differences in hearing acuity between the right and left ears. However, since the ticking of a watch is a higher frequency than conversational speech, this test is less useful in estimating functional hearing.

Nurses in some clinic and community settings are taught to use screening audiometers. These machines test only air conduction hearing and they are used to determine whether the person has normal hearing acuity. People who do not have normal acuity are then referred to an audiologist for testing in a sound-proofed room with more sophisticated equipment. Even in a quiet office or room, noise may affect test results, especially in lower frequencies.[2,23]

TABLE 10-1
INTERPRETING TUNING FOR TESTS

	NORMAL HEARING	*CONDUCTIVE LOSS*	*SENSORINEURAL LOSS*
Rinne Test	Positive Rinne Sound is heard twice as long by air conduction.	Negative Rinne Sound is heard longer by bone conduction than air conduction.	Positive Rinne Normal ratio of bone conduction to air conduction with an overall reduction in the time sound is heard.
Weber Test	Sound is heard in both ears equally well.	Sound is heard louder in the defective ear.	Sound is heard louder in the better ear.

Tuning Fork Tests

What the patient has said about his hearing problems will provide clues suggesting whether the hearing loss is a conductive or a sensorineural loss. Tuning fork tests also assist in determining the nature of the hearing loss. A tuning fork with a frequency of 512 Hz is used.

The patient's ability to hear by bone conduction and air conduction is compared in the *Rinne test*. Normally, sound is heard twice as long by air conduction as it is by bone conduction. When the person has a conductive hearing loss, bone conduction will be better than air conduction. This is referred to as a negative Rinne. The Rinne test is conducted by holding a vibrating tuning fork on the mastoid bone until the patient no longer hears the sound; it is then placed 1 inch from the auditory meatus. The patient will continue to hear the sound by air conduction in a positive Rinne.

The *Weber test* makes use of bone conduction and is helpful when the patient hears better in one ear than the other. In this test the vibrating tuning fork is held on the center of the forehead, and the patient is asked whether he hears the sound better or more loudly in either ear. The person with a conductive hearing loss will hear the sound more loudly in the ear with the greatest defect because environmental sounds are blocked from the cochlea on that side. The person with a sensorineural loss will hear the sound more loudly in the ear that has the best hearing because that cochlea or auditory nerve functions best.[3,16] The interpretation of tuning fork tests is summarized in Table 10-1.

Interpreting Audiograms

A basic understanding of audiograms and the methods that audiologists use in testing hearing acuity is helpful to nurses when counseling patients and devising interventions that maximize the use of existing hearing ability. In pure tone audiometry, the person's threshold for sounds presented at various intensities (db) and frequencies (Hz) is determined. Air conduction thresholds are measured by presenting the sounds through earphones; bone conduction is measured by presenting the sound through a vibrating pad over the temporal bone. Pure tone thresholds are plotted using conventional symbols on an audiogram on which normal hearing is

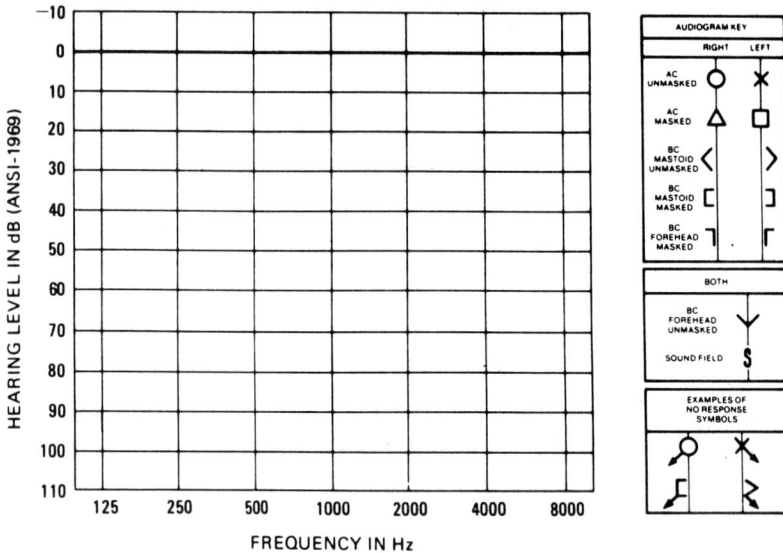

FIG. 10-1 Sample audiogram for recording audiometric results. (Hixon TJ, Shriberg LD, Saxman JH: Introduction to Communication Disorders, p 503. Englewood Cliffs, NJ, Prentice–Hall, 1980)

represented as 0 db (Fig. 10-1). The thresholds from the air conduction tests and bone conduction tests are compared for information about the location of the difficulty. Conductive hearing losses produce an increased threshold by air conduction, but bone conduction remains normal (Fig. 10-2A). When there is a sensorineural hearing loss both bone conduction and air conduction are equally affected (Fig. 2B), while a mixed loss will affect both air and bone conduction with a greater loss by air conduction (Fig. 2C). Since pure tones are not what we use in communication, speech audiometry is used to quantify further how well the person understands speech. The speech reception threshold (SRT) is determined by presenting two-syllable test words at various intensities. The word discrimination score (WDS) is a measure of discrimination rather than acuity. A list of one syllable phonetically balanced words is presented at a level 30 db to 40 db above the person's SRT. This score is expressed as a percentage of words correctly repeated.[3,23]

When interpreting the results of these audiometric evaluations, remember that hearing loss is not equal to hearing handicap. The degree to which the person's ability to communicate is affected is determined by factors such as the demands that his life-style places on hearing and personal adjustment, as well as the degree of loss and the configuration of the loss across frequencies. The average intensity of normal conversational tones at 3 or 4 ft is approximately 45 db, and the audiometric frequencies most critical for understanding speech range from 250 Hz to 4000 Hz. The average threshold for pure tones of 500 Hz to 2000 Hz is termed the *pure tone average* (PTA) and is used in Table 10-2 to estimate the effects of varying degrees of hearing loss on communication. Remember that word discrimination scores are only estimates; in normal listening situations, contextual clues, facial expressions, and gestures may increase understanding. The person with discrimination scores of 80% or better generally experiences no difficulty in conversation, while the person with a discrimi-

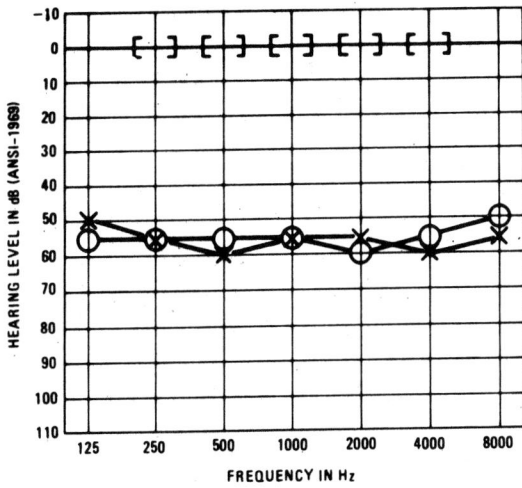

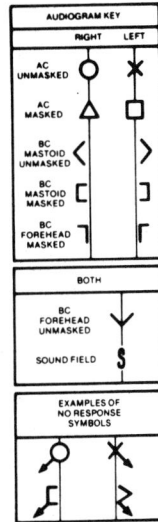

(a)

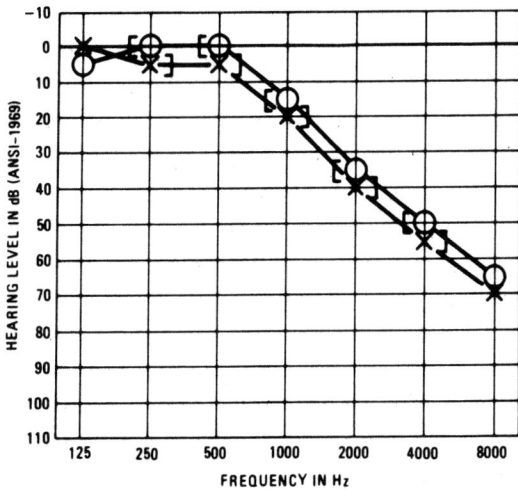

(b)

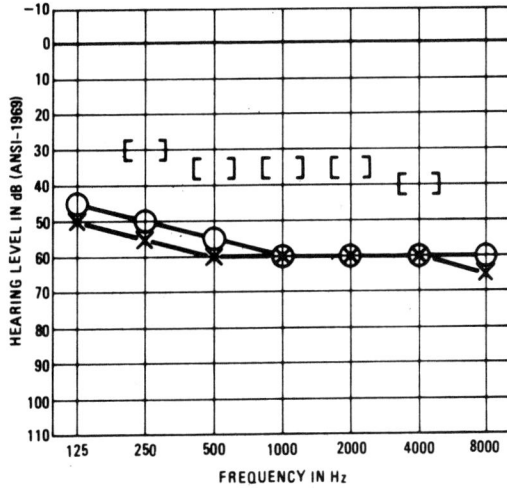

(c)

FIG. 10-2 Audiometric illustrations of three types of hearing loss. (A) Conductive hearing loss, (B) senso-rineural hearing loss, and (C) mixed hearing loss. (Hixon TJ, Shriberg LD, Saxman JH: Introduction to Communication Disorders, p 503. Englewood Cliffs, NJ, Prentice–Hall, 1980)

TABLE 10-2
COMMUNICATION EFFECTS OF VARYING DEGREES OF HEARING LOSS

PURE TONE AVERAGE (BETTER EAR)	ABILITY TO UNDERSTAND SPEECH
< 25 db	No significant difficulty
26–40 db	Difficulty with faint speech
41–55 db	Difficulty with normal speech
56–70 db	Difficulty with loud speech
71–90 db	Understands only amplified speech
> 90 db	Unable to understand even amplified speech

nation score of 50% or less generally has a great deal of difficulty. People with low discrimination scores may not benefit from amplification.[20,23]

NURSING DIAGNOSIS

Assessment data are analyzed to arrive at a nursing diagnosis. In addition to the diagnosis of impaired communication due to sensorineural/conductive hearing loss, several other more specific diagnoses may be made relating to knowledge deficits, alterations in self-concept or social roles, or difficulty that the person or his family experiences in adapting to decreased hearing. Examples of the diagnoses that may be made include:

Knowledge deficit related to resources for hearing rehabilitation
Knowledge deficit related to use and care of hearing aid
Decreased self-esteem related to hearing loss
Altered family and social relationships due to impaired communication.

Nursing diagnosis includes the hearing-impaired person's and family's strengths as well as their problems. Reaffirming these strengths and assisting people to use their strengths in overcoming problems is an important part of nursing management.

MANAGEMENT

GOALS

Assessment data are used to develop individualized goals with the patient. The patient's participation in setting goals is essential for a rehabilitation plan that focuses on maximizing hearing and adapting to remaining problems. Goals may proceed in a stepwise fashion, from acceptance of the hearing loss to a desire for assistance and knowledge of resources, before further evaluation and rehabilitation are undertaken. It is not unusual for the person with a hearing loss to seek evaluation at the insistence of family, friends, or co-workers. The patient's own interest and participation must be stimulated before attainable goals can be established.

FACILITATING COMMUNICATION

Regardless of the reason for the nurse's contact with a hearing-impaired person, the first step is to develop effective communication. Assessment data are used to individualize communication techniques. Notations in the care plan about the person's preferences in routines avoid the frustration of repeated inquiry. The patient's nursing care can be improved if the same staff members are assigned to him as much as possible, and extra time that may be required to meet his communication needs is taken into account when planning assignments or scheduling visits.

Communicating with a deaf person may require written messages or a sign language interpreter. When the deaf person uses only sign language, a smile, a touch, or a gesture can convey concern and interest. Many daily needs can be conveyed by combining facial expressions, gestures, and actual objects or pictures of objects rather than the words that symbolize the object. A sign language interpreter is essential, however, to explain the patient's plan of care, to do health teaching, and to answer his questions. Research studies suggest that the greatest difficulty deaf persons face in meeting their health needs is an inadequate understanding of the health care problems.[11,13] Often a friend or family member is able to serve as interpreter, and the person is most comfortable with this arrangement. When extensive health teaching must be done, it may be preferable to work with a trained interpreter who understands medical terminology and sign language. There are also some patients who do not wish to have family or friends involved in discussion of their illness. Regardless of whether they serve as interpreters, encourage family and friends who are able to communicate in sign language to do so. This provides needed stimulation that enables the deaf person to keep in touch with the world.

The majority of the hearing-impaired persons that a nurse encounters will have some ability to use sound for communication. Assessment data are used to determine how loudly to speak, how close to stand, and whether the person hears better when approached from a particular side. The problems of the hospitalized hearing-impaired person are often compounded by the large number of people with whom he comes in contact. It is not uncommon to see signs on beds or chart covers that read *deaf* or *hard-of-hearing*. Some patients report resenting these signs or being humiliated by them.[11] Determine the person's feelings about this. Remember, signs that merely label do not facilitate communication. A more useful approach is a sign that includes a brief statement on how to communicate effectively with the patient. Other mechanisms that may ease communication for the hospitalized person with a hearing impairment include notes attached to requisitions that go to other departments, telephone calls to the person in another department who will be seeing the patient, and providing an escort who can assist with communication. Institutions that use an intercom system to communicate with patients need to mark the equipment so that anyone answering call lights will know that this person's call must be answered in person.

Establishing effective communications with the hearing-impaired person may require some alteration in the nurse's communication style. Regardless of whether the person has been taught speech-reading or lip-reading, he may depend on visual cues and facial expressions to understand the message. Before speaking be sure that you have the person's attention. This may be done through a gesture or touch. Touch must be used with caution, however, as the person who is unaware of your approach may be startled. Face the light and position yourself so that your face can be seen without strain. For example, when speaking to a person who is seated, sit or crouch so that the listener does not have to continually look up to see your face.

Speaking slowly and distinctly without exaggerating sounds or lip movement will usually be more helpful than speaking loudly. Speaking more slowly provides time for the person with a hearing impairment to assimilate the auditory, visual, and situational cues that he uses to interpret the sounds he is able to hear. While, for some patients, the softspoken nurse will need to increase the intensity of her speech somewhat, shouting should be avoided. Shouting usually will destroy the confidentiality of the

TABLE 10-3
FACILITATING COMMUNICATION WITH THE HEARING IMPAIRED

BEHAVIOR	SPEECH	ENVIRONMENT
Gain attention.	Speak slowly and distinctly without exaggerated lip movement.	Provide adequate lighting.
Face the person.		Decrease background noises.
Position yourself at the listener's visual level.		Decrease visual distractions.
Face the light.	Use short concise sentences.	
Write key words or important instructions.	Rephrase statement if repeating more than once.	
Use appropriate gestures.	Avoid speaking while eating, smoking, or chewing gum.	
Keep hands away from the speaker's face.	Use key words to state the general topic.	
	Clarify whether meaning is understood before going on.	

conversation and may be embarrassing to the patient and others. In addition, the speaker's strain while shouting may be misinterpreted as anger or impatience. Remember that the hearing-impaired listener depends on body language. While writing messages is time-consuming, it is preferable to shouting. Occasionally it is helpful to amplify the sound of your voice by speaking into the diaphragm of a stethoscope while the patient places the earpieces in his ears. Speaking into a rolled newspaper or magazine will also amplify your voice.

The hearing-impaired listener will be able to understand short, concise sentences more easily. Use key words or phrases to introduce the topic to be discussed. Before going on to a new topic, validate whether the patient has understood by questioning or asking him to restate. Write down key words and proper names. Give important instructions in written as well as verbal form. When it is necessary to repeat the same sentence more than once, rephrase it in somewhat different words. Use appropriate gestures while speaking, but avoid hand gestures, which interfere with the visibility of the face. Other behaviors that may interfere with the hear-

ing-impaired person's understanding include gum-chewing, eating, smoking, and nervous mannerisms (e.g., stroking the upper lip or chin).

When communicating with a person whose hearing is impaired, provide an environment which is quiet and calm. Background noises such as radios, television, and other conversations should be eliminated as much as possible. Because the hearing-impaired person needs to attend to visual cues, minimizing visual distractions is helpful. Adequate lighting is also essential for the use of visual cues. Table 10-3 summarizes some of the ways in which behavior, speech, and environment can enhance communication with the person whose hearing is impaired.

HEARING AIDS

The nurse often is involved in teaching patients what to expect from a hearing aid and in counseling them regarding the process of having it fitted properly. A hearing aid is just an aid and cannot restore normal hearing. Even a well-fitted aid has limitations. Distracting background noises are amplified, and distortion of speech sounds may continue. Despite these limitations, amplification of sound through a hearing aid improves the communication ability of many people whose hearing problems cannot be resolved through medical or surgical interventions.

All hearing aids have the same basic components: a microphone to pick up the sound, an amplifier to increase the intensity of the sound, a receiver or earpiece to deliver the sound, and a battery as a power source. Hearing aids differ in three major performance characteristics: gain, maximum power output, and frequency response. The amount of amplification that the hearing aid provides is called the *gain*, and is measured in decibels (db). To prevent discomfort and damage to hearing, aids also have limits on the intensity of the signal they produce. This is the *maximum power output* and is also measured in db. Frequency response is the expression of the range of frequencies over which the hearing aid provides amplification. In addition to these basic characteristics, special features are available that reduce background noise and benefit people with differing amounts of hearing loss in each ear.

Hearing aids also differ in style, and are classified according to where they are worn. The majority of hearing aids in use today are behind-the-ear styles. While early models of the behind-the-ear hearing aid were unable to provide sufficient amplification for people with severe impairments, recent improvements have increased the amount of gain available with this type of aid. This style may not be suitable for people whose manual dexterity is impaired, however, because the smaller controls may be too difficult to manipulate. Eyeglass hearing aids are built into the temple of an eyeglass frame and provide performance characteristics similar to the behind-the-ear aid. This style is preferable for people who wear their eyeglasses contin-

uously. Small hearing aids that fit entirely within the outer ear are available, but are suitable only for mild-to-moderate hearing losses. Hearing aids that are worn on the body consist of a small box, worn in a pocket or attached to a garment, and connected to the earpiece with a thin wire. Body-worn aids are cosmetically unappealing to many users, but may provide a better fit in terms of performance characteristics and ease in manipulation. To achieve maximum performance, all hearing aids should have individually fitted earpieces that are molded to conform to the person's ear canal.

Matching the person's hearing loss with a hearing aid whose characteristics provide improved communication ability is not an exact science. A Department of Health, Education, and Welfare (HEW) task force found that of the 600,000 people who purchase hearing aids each year, a significant number either did not need the aid, were not helped by the aid, or would be better served by medical or surgical treatment. At the time of the study 70% to 80 % of all hearing aids sold were sold without any medical or audiological evaluation.[10] In 1977, the Food and Drug Administration (FDA) established rules designed to protect the hearing-impaired person. These rules require a medical evaluation of the hearing impairment within 6 months before purchasing a hearing aid. However, this examination may be waived by adults, unless one of eight specific conditions exist. These conditions, which require referral to a physician, include:

Visible congenital or traumatic deformity of the ear
Active drainage from the ear in the past 90 days
Sudden or rapidly progressive hearing loss
Acute or chronic dizziness or tinnitus
Unilateral hearing loss of sudden or recent onset

Significant air–bone gap
Visible evidence of cerumen accumulation, or a foreign body in the ear canal
Pain or discomfort in the ear.

Additional rules require that an instruction booklet accompany hearing aids, explaining their use, maintenance, and limitations.[19]

Consumer interest groups have urged hearing-impaired people to seek evaluation, diagnosis, and counsel from physicians and audiologists, and to look to hearing aid dealers for servicing and explanation of the workings of particular aids.[4] When the hearing aid dealer is not providing the evaluation and counseling, this should be reflected in a discounted price. Hearing aids should be rented for a trial period to be certain that they meet the person's needs in day-to-day communication as well as in office tests. A reevaluation of hearing with the aid should be arranged during this trial period, and thereafter evaluation is recommended annually or every other year. Nurses can do a great deal to dispel the myths that persist regarding hearing aids. Whereas few people would dismiss the idea of glasses entirely because "I tried my friend's and it didn't help at all," this is not the case with hearing aids. Similarly, many people do not understand that changes in hearing may require a hearing aid with different performance characteristics. Assistance in locating clinical resources for patients is available through a free pamphlet listing sources of speech and hearing clinical services in your area. It can be obtained by writing to American Speech and Hearing Association, 9030 Old Georgetown Road, Washington, D.C., 20014.

ADAPTING TO A HEARING AID

Once the hearing aid has been fitted, the work of the new hearing aid user has just begun. Sudden introduction of the sounds associated with everyday living may be disconcerting and frustrating to the person who has adapted to the absence of these sounds. The person will need to relearn listening techniques that block out unwanted sound and concentrate on the sounds he wishes to hear. In addition, the person may continue to struggle with the distortions of sound that remain despite amplification. Ideally, the new hearing aid user is involved in an aural rehabilitation program that includes a family member and teaches the person to make maximal use of his amplified hearing as well as providing orientation to the use of the hearing aid. Even in these ideal situations, nurses can be helpful to patients and families by providing support and encouragement. Under less-than-ideal situations, families and patients may have informational needs as well.

There is a great deal of individual variation in the length of time it takes people to adapt to the use of a hearing aid. While a few people are able to adapt within hours or days, the process usually proceeds more slowly. Family members who were not involved in the rehabilitation program may not understand the period of adaptation required, and may express impatience when the patient wears the hearing aid "only a few hours a day" or "only at home." New hearing aid users generally are advised to begin with the aid adjusted to a level that is comfortable, even if that means missing some sounds. Initially, the hearing aid should be used in quieter environments, which provide fewer distractions. While the person concentrates on improving his listening skills he is counseled to avoid becoming overly tired or frustrated. Family members may welcome the nurse's assistance in learning to communicate more effectively. At the same time, encourage all hearing-impaired persons to express their needs openly rather than to expect others to make adaptations without input and feedback from them.

CARE AND MAINTENANCE OF HEARING AIDS

The person who has been fitted with a hearing aid will also need information regarding how to put on the aid, how to adjust its controls, and how to care for the aid. This orientation should be provided by the therapist who fits the aid. Nurses in community settings often will be involved in reinforcing this teaching and making appropriate referrals back to the audiologist or hearing aid dealer. Nurses in hospitals and long-term care settings may provide basic maintenance care in addition to teaching and making referrals, for people who are unable to do this themselves.

Basic care to maintain the hearing aid is not difficult. High temperatures, moisture, and chemicals such as hair spray and insect repellants may cause damage and should be avoided. Since batteries last only 1 to 4 weeks, spare ones must be kept on hand and stored in a cool, dry place to prevent deterioration. It is not necessary to store batteries in the refrigerator, but if they are stored there, bring them to room temperature, and dry them with a clean cloth before inserting them. Batteries are removed from the aid at night and inspected. This prolongs battery life and ensures that a defective, leaking battery will be taken out of service before it damages the aid. Likewise, dead batteries are removed from the aid at once to prevent damage. Battery contacts can be cleaned by rubbing gently with a sharpened pencil eraser.

The ear mold must be kept clean. It can be detached from the tubing and washed in soap and water. Dry thoroughly before reconnecting. If the opening becomes clogged with cerumen, it can be cleaned with a pipe cleaner or small brush. Alcohol and other chemical cleaning solutions are not recommended because they may dry the ear mold and cause it to crack. Avoid twisting the cord on a body-worn hearing aid and bending the tubing on other styles. These are parts of the hearing aid, however, that will require periodic replacement. The cord on a body-worn aid is readily replaced and quite easily damaged. Therefore, people with this type of aid usually keep a spare cord on hand. Replacement of the tubing on an ear level aid is done by the hearing aid dealer.

When the hearing aid produces a weak signal or no signal, there are several checks that can be made by the patient or the nurse before going to the dealer for repairs. Placement of the battery can be checked to make sure the positive contact of the battery is aligned with the positive contact of the aid. Both of these contacts will be labeled with the symbol + . A fresh battery can be tried. Check the ear mold for cerumen accumulation and the tubing or cord for bends, cracks, or twists. If the aid has a telephone setting (T), check to see that the control is in the microphone (M) position. The switch can be moved back and forth to ensure that dust or lint is not interfering with electrical contact. The cord on a body-worn aid can be removed and reinserted, or a new cord tried. If these measures are unsuccessful, arrangement should be made with the dealer for repairs. A fresh battery that deteriorates more rapidly than usual is another sign that the aid should be checked by the dealer.

Hearing aids sometimes produce a high-pitched, whistling sound. This results when sound from the receiver enters the microphone on the aid and is called *feedback*. The sound may be outside the frequency range of the person and therefore inaudible to him. However, when there is feedback, the person generally complains of weaker sound. Feedback that stops when a finger is held over the opening of the ear mold usually is caused by improper insertion or improper fit of the ear mold rather than a problem with the aid itself. Carefully reinserting the ear mold may eliminate the problem. Excessive accumulation of cerumen in the auditory canal may interfere with fit, and will need to be removed by the physician, or according to his instructions. When feedback persists, the mold may need to be refitted.

REHABILITATION PROGRAMS

An awareness of rehabilitation programs and their potential benefits will assist nurses in counseling patients. Rehabilitation of the hearing-impaired adult should be aimed at making optimal use of residual hearing. This is the objective of both auditory training and speech-reading. Auditory training first helps the person to distinguish grossly differing sounds, and then aids in developing the ability to distinguish among more similar sounds. Emphasis is placed on listening skills and using auditory skills to interpret the message when all of the message is not heard. Speech reading concentrates on the use of visual rather than auditory cues. Speech-reading includes lipreading, but teaches the observation of the whole face and body movements as well as the lips. Drill work in speech-reading and auditory training have been used to some extent as isolated therapies. However, rehabilitation programs usually emphasize the general listening and visual attentiveness aspects of these therapies in a total aural rehabilitation program. Speech-training also may be a part of the rehabilitation program. A speech pathologist can assist persons whose hearing loss interferes with their ability to hear their own speech to conserve normal speech or correct problems relating to loudness, pitch, inflection, and rate.

ENVIRONMENTAL AIDS

Hearing plays an important role in warning us about changes in our environment that require us to respond. Devices are available that substitute the visual stimulus of a flashing light for sounds that cannot be heard, such as a doorbell, a telephone, an alarm clock, or a child's cry. In some geographic areas, programs are beginning that train dogs to alert the hearing-impaired person to these sounds. Amplifiers, which can be added to telephone receivers and headphones to improve the ability to hear a radio, record player, or television, are other potentially useful aids. The need for such devices in the home environment is assessed individually.

PSYCHOSOCIAL PROBLEMS

Effective interpersonal communications are an essential foundation for satisfying and productive relationships, and are important to one's self-esteem and self-concept. Successful nursing management must focus on the whole person and his or her adaptation to the hearing impairment. Communication breakdowns caused by the hearing impairment may strain marital or family relationships, and social interactions. Preexisting strains in these relationships may be magnified by the hearing impairment. Many persons and their families will be able to make adaptations with the assistance of a nurse who is able to establish a trusting relationship, listen without judgment, and provide for their informational needs. However, the needs of persons and their families with many preexisting problems or few coping strengths may be better served by appropriate referrals for personal or family counseling.

Communication problems may also have an impact on the person's work role. Some patients may find that improved communication following a rehabilitation program markedly improves their functioning in the work setting. Referrals for vocational rehabilitation will be appropriate for those who find that the communication demands of their current job exceeds their abilities.

Aphasia

DEFINITIONS

Aphasia is a disturbance, resulting from brain damage, in the ability to comprehend and formulate language. It is a disruption in the central coordination of language in the brain, rather than a loss of sensory perception or an interruption in the innervation of the muscles used in speech production. Aphasia is a language problem in which the ability to code and decode the symbols of language are disturbed; it is not a speech problem. The term *dysphasia* is usually used interchangeably with the term *aphasia*. While, traditionally, the prefix *a* is used to indicate complete loss and the prefix *dys* is used to indicate less than total loss, these distinctions seldom are adhered to in the literature or in clinical practice. Even though few people have a total loss of language ability, the term *aphasia* is the one most widely used. Aphasia is a general term used to describe a large variety of problems. Many terms have evolved to describe more specifically the particular difficulties that the aphasic person may experience. Some of the more common terms are

Acalculia: Difficulty with mathematical processes or symbols
Agnosia: Inability to recognize familiar objects or symbols that are perceived by the senses
Agraphia: Inability to write
Alexia: Inability to read
Anomia: Inability to name objects
Apraxia: Inability to carry out planned sequential movements

INCIDENCE AND CAUSES

Disruption or distortion in the cerebral processing of language is associated most often with a cerebral vascular accident (CVA), also known as a stroke. Health statistics reveal that CVA is an important health problem that affects approximately 400,000 people annually and is the third leading cause of death.[15] However, the prevalence of aphasia among stroke survivors is not known. Various clinical studies of stroke patients report an incidence of communication disorders in stroke patients ranging from 20% to 40%, but the type of disorder is not always specified.[15] One clinical study of a series of 850 consecutively admitted stroke patients reports a 21% incidence during the period immediately following the CVA. One to three months later the language disruptions of 2.5% of these patients was still rated as severe.[2] Less common causes of aphasia include traumatic injuries, tumors, and infections. Incidence figures for these causes are also unavailable.

MECHANISMS OF APHASIA

BRAIN FUNCTION IN COMMUNICATION

Although the right and left hemispheres of the brain look alike superficially, it has been recognized since the nineteenth century that in most adults the left hemisphere of the brain is the dominant one for processing language. More than 90% of the population is right-handed, and in 99% of these people the left hemisphere is the dominant one for language. Among those persons who are left-handed, the left hemisphere is dominant in 65%, and the right hemisphere is dominant in 35%.[18]

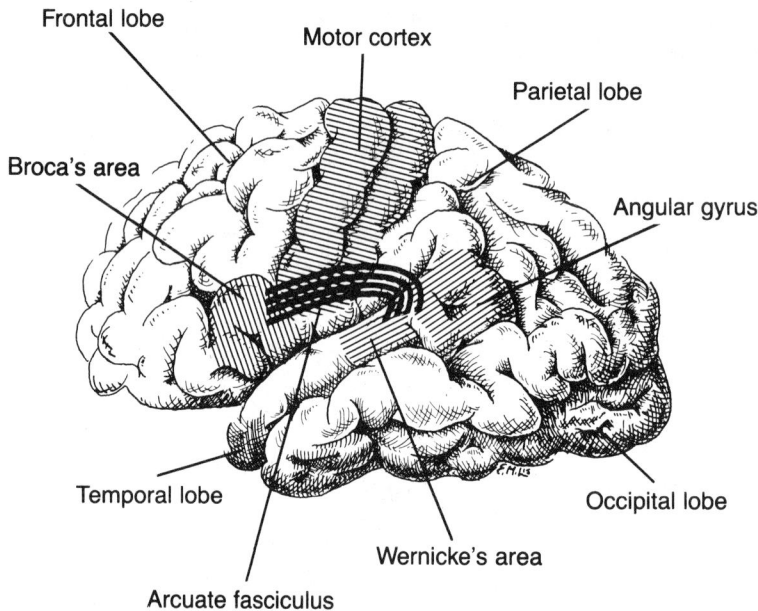

FIG. 10-3 *Language areas in the left hemisphere of the brain. (Louis MC, Povse SM: Aphasia and endurance: Considerations in the assessment and care of the stroke patient. Nurs Clin North Am 15:265, 1980)*

The ability to understand spoken or written messages and the ability to respond to these messages or send a message of our own requires the coordinated functioning of several areas of the cortex. When a message is heard, the neural input from the ear reaches the primary auditory cortex in the brain. Before the meaning of this message can be understood, however, the signal must be processed in the part of the cortex known as Wernicke's area, which lies adjacent to the primary auditory area in the temporal lobe. When the message is a written one, visual patterns from the primary visual cortex are transmitted to the angular gyrus, which arouses the corresponding auditory patterns in Wernicke's area. The angular gyrus lies superior to Wernicke's area[7,8] (Fig. 10-3.)

Sending a verbal message involves the formulation in the mind of the thoughts to be transmitted, the choice of words to be used, and the actual articulation of the message. The formulation of the thought and choice of words is a function of Wernicke's area and the angular gyrus. *Broca's area*, which is located in the lateral posterior portion of the frontal lobe, contains the patterns that control the formation of words. It accomplishes this by exciting adjacent areas of the motor cortex that, in turn, activate the muscles involved in speech. Large nerve fiber bundles, called the *arcuate fasciculus*, carry neural messages from Wernicke's area in the temporal lobe to Broca's area in the frontal lobe.[7,8]

TYPES OF APHASIA

At present there is no universally accepted classification of aphasia. Disagreements in classification stem from divergent views on whether aphasia should be classified on the basis of severity or on the basis of the location of the lesion. The locationist view is most widely accepted and will be used in this chapter to provide a framework for understanding aphasia. However, some reservations regarding this model's usefulness in nursing practice must be noted. The descriptions of brain lesions of individuals may not conform to classical descriptions derived from data about groups. Brain damage often overlaps areas, and therefore the strengths and deficits of the person's communication patterns will not fit clearly into one classification. This is especially so during the time period immediately after the neurologic insult that caused the aphasia, since areas adjacent to the actual lesion often have a temporary loss of function because of edema. One clinical study found that during the acute phase following a CVA, 60% of the aphasic patients had a mixed impairment.

The relationships between the area of the brain that is damaged and the behavioral symptoms that result from the injury have been described most extensively by investigators from the Boston Veterans' Hospital and Boston University and is known as the Boston Classification System. Many diverse forms of aphasia have been classified, but only the most common forms are discussed in this chapter. According to this classification system, aphasias are classified as either fluent aphasia or nonfluent aphasia.

The most frequent nonfluent aphasia is *Broca's aphasia*, which in other classifications is also called motor aphasia, expressive aphasia, anterior aphasia, or apraxia of speech. The spontaneous speech of a person with nonfluent aphasia is slow, labored, and sparse. Normal speech is usually at a rate of 100 to 150 words/minute. The person with nonfluent aphasia may have a rate of only three to twelve words a minute, and even

when it is not this extreme, speech usually is noticeably slower. These few words are often produced with visible signs of struggle such as facial grimaces, gestures, and deep breaths. Phrase length is shortened from a normal six or eight words to one or two words, and the normal rhythm, melody, and inflection of speech is disturbed. The person with nonfluent aphasia speaks in a telegraphic style, leaving out many small, connecting words. Because the words he does produce are usually substantive words, this person is often able to convey a great deal of meaning in very few words. If the brain damage is limited to Broca's area, both auditory comprehension and reading comprehension will be intact. Errors in writing are similar to the ones the person makes in speech. Since the person is able to comprehend, he understands the errors he is making in speech and writing, and thus is often very frustrated.

The most common fluent aphasia is *Wernicke's aphasia*, which has also been called sensory aphasia, receptive aphasia, or posterior aphasia. A lesion in Wernicke's area produces difficulty with both expression and comprehension. Normal rhythm, inflection, rate, and phrase length are preserved in this type of aphasia, so that spontaneous speech is fluent and produced without struggle. While the speech of people with Wernicke's aphasia sounds normal, it is often lacking in content and meaning. For example, the person may say, "I went down to the thing, but it did so I came around." Often lengthy, rambling descriptions are attempted to substitute for a substantive word. For example, the person may say, "I need a...thing for the face... every morning...shave with it." This process is called *circumlocution*. *Paraphrasia*, a substitution of a syllable, a word, or a group of meaningless sounds, is also common. Impaired comprehension is the major deficit found in people with fluent aphasia. This contributes to expression problems because these persons are unable to monitor their own speech. Because they are unaware of their own speech errors, people with fluent aphasia are less apt to be frustrated by their errors, and may become annoyed when other people do not understand them. Reading comprehension deficits are similar to auditory comprehension, and the errors made in writing mirror the speech patterns.

Conductive aphasia is another form of fluent aphasia. When the brain lesion affects the arcuate fasciculus, the connection between the temporal and frontal speech areas is disrupted. Spontaneous speech remains fluent and effortless, and the person comprehends his own speech and the speech of others. The major deficit in conductive aphasia involves finding words. Spontaneous speech and writing both contain many paraphrasias. Because comprehension is normal or near normal, people with conductive aphasia are aware of their speech errors and often become frustrated by them.

Global aphasia is the term used to describe the effects of massive lesions that affect both the anterior and posterior language centers. Since very little brain tissue used for communication is preserved, these people have little, if any, auditory comprehension, and their speech often is limited to repetition of a syllable or a single word. The intentional use of "yes" or "no," and the use of emotion interjections such as "Ah!", "Oh–Oh!" or swearing may remain intact.

RELATED PROBLEMS AFFECTING COMMUNICATION

People who have had brain damage often are left with multidimensional problems that have an impact on their ability to communicate. Hemiparesis or hemiplegia results when the brain damage involves the motor cortex. This most commonly accompanies a nonfluent aphasia, since Broca's area lies adjacent to the motor cortex. When hemiparesis or hemiplegia accompanies a language disorder, the person's dominant hand usually is affected. This may impair the ability to gesture or pantomime as well as the ability to write.

Several types of speech defects may either accompany aphasia or be present without aphasia. Dysarthria is one such disorder that affects the control of peripheral speech muscles. It is characterized by slowness, a weak sound, and uncoordinated speech movements. Speech often sounds garbled. When dysarthria alone is present, the person's speech can be distinguished from that of nonfluent aphasia by the obvious lack of coordination when the person is trying to speak, and the fact that phrase length and rhythm are not disturbed. Dysarthria alone will not interfere with comprehension or word-finding ability, and unless there are motor deficits, the person with dysarthria can write messages. When dysarthria accompanies aphasia it obviously compounds the person's communication problems.

Apraxia, another problem that may be present, is the complete or partial inability to carry out planned, purposeful sequences of movement in the absence of sensory or motor losses. Apraxia can affect speech or other body movements. Apraxia of speech is the same as Broca's aphasia. When apraxia affects body movement, the person may not be able to carry out verbal directions even though his ability to process language remains intact. Apraxia in body movements may interfere with a person's ability to use gestures for communication.

Aphasia often is accompanied by visual field defects. Because lesions that cause aphasia are generally in the left hemisphere, a loss of vision in the right field of both eyes is most common. This loss of vision is called *right homonymous hemianopia.* This vision defect will impair the person's ability to respond to materials that are presented in the right visual field.

IMPACT OF APHASIA

Aphasia is a profound and very abrupt loss that severely taxes the person's ability to cope. Initially, the person is usually fearful, anxious, and bewildered. When he is no longer concerned with mere survival, feelings of frustration, depression, and lowered self-esteem are common. Physical impairments may accompany aphasia and compound the loss. The ambiguity regarding the eventual extent of his residual impairments makes adaptation difficult, and the realization that these impairments may threaten vocational and family security adds to the person's anxieties. Grieving and adaptation are made more difficult by the fact that the recovery period is long, progress is slow and difficult to recognize, and frustrations are frequent.

Impairment in language function affects the whole person. The ability to express needs to others is limited, and the emotional outlet of verbalizing feelings to others is unavailable. Emotional lability frequently is observed in people with aphasia. When speech no longer can be used as an outlet for feelings, the threshold for emotional reactions seems to be lowered so that it takes fewer stimuli for the person to laugh, cry, or become visibly upset. At times, the person himself may not understand what triggered this reaction. Remember too that emotional expressions are a normal part of the grieving process. People with aphasia have also been seen as egocentric because they may be intensely interested in their own concerns and viewpoints and greatly concerned with or-

derliness and schedules. These behavioral changes are thought to be related to the difficulty that the person experiences in expressing his needs and the need to reestablish self-esteem and self-concept. A narrowed focus and ritualistic performance of tasks also is seen as a part of the normal grieving process.

The abrupt changes and stresses of aphasia affect the family as well as the individual. One study that compared the problems of spouses of people with aphasia to the problems of spouses of CVA patients without aphasia found that with aphasia, problems appeared to grow worse over time. The enforced loss of communication due to aphasia affected marital adjustment adversely. Friends of the couple gradually stopped visiting because of their frustration in trying to communicate with the aphasic person, and social isolation of the family unit increased.[12] This study suggests that family members need support in coping with their losses and the changes in family roles. They need opportunities to discuss their feelings and frustrations, as well as concrete suggestions regarding means of reestablishing some level of communication, understanding the reasons for behavioral changes, and increasing their social contacts.

Residual aphasia that persists past the rehabilitation stage has an impact on all aspects of life. The degree to which people with residual aphasia are handicapped depends on their adjustment, and the amount of support from others, as well as the degree of language impairment. Some people with moderate impairments may find that they are able to carry out their usual activities even though everything takes longer or is more frustrating. Others experience changes in work, social, and family roles, all of which threaten their self-concept. Age and family responsibilities also modify the impact of a residual aphasia. The impact on a middle-aged person who is actively involved in earning an income and parenting children is different from the impact on the retired person with grown children. However, motivation and adaptability may differ as well and play an important role in determining the rehabilitation outcomes.

NURSING ASSESSMENT

The extent of the patient's language problem, the reason for seeking health care, and the setting all influence the assessment of persons with aphasia. However, the initial focus is to identify the intact language processes that can be used to establish communication. When the patient is being seen for another health problem, he or a family member may spontaneously report the language problem and the ways in which he is best able to communicate. At other times, the nurse may notice during the interview that the patient is having difficulty understanding or responding. It is best to assess the source of this difficulty as soon as it is noted, rather than struggling on or making trial-and-error modifications during the interview. Assumptions often lead to ineffective behaviors that interfere with the nurse-patient relationship. The person who has difficulty understanding language will not understand a loud voice better, and the raised voice may be interpreted as anger or impatience. Similarly, the person whose comprehension is better than his verbal responses indicate may not be given explanation or instructions he could benefit from, unless the nurse has assessed the problem carefully.

When the patient's ability to use language is severely limited, it is often necessary to get some information from secondary sources, such as a family member. When the patient is hospitalized or is in a long-term care setting, it usually is preferable to talk with the family member away from the bedside. Interviews with recovered aphasic people reveal that they felt that people were always talking *about* them rather than *to* them, a situation that they found very distressing.[21] When the patient is evaluated in his home or in a clinic setting, a separate interview with the family member may not be necessary or desirable. A focus on the patient can be maintained by first communicating with the patient on his level, and then using gestures, eye contact, and seating arrangements to include the patient while the family member responds to questions. Asking questions during the physical examination is sometimes another possibility.

Assessment of the family member's feelings or perceptions should be done privately. The ability of the aphasic person to detect emotional content in speech is generally intact, because this is a function of the right hemisphere of the brain. Patients may become frustrated if they hear that loved ones are upset, but are unable to understand their words.

The nurse should monitor the aphasic person's energy level and frustration level during the assessment. Both frustration and fatigue have an adverse effect on the person's language skills, which can result in inaccurate data. This problem is most likely to occur during the hospitalization period, and can be avoided by completing the assessment in short segments. Endurance is also a factor with some patients seen in the community. It is important to determine priorities in these instances, and to cover areas of top priority first. Morning visits are often best, and return visits should be scheduled to coincide with the time of day when the person is least tired.

SUBJECTIVE DATA

General

Identify the specific type of neurologic injury that the patient has had, the location of the lesion, and the date it occurred. Determine whether the patient is working with a speech pathologist or has in the past. In acute care settings, much of this data will be available on the chart, but in other settings the patient or family should be asked these questions. Collect information regarding the person's social, educational, and vocational background. Knowledge of specific interests and hobbies is useful in planning interventions. Determine the ways in which the patient coped with previous losses and stressors. When the patient is unable to provide this type of data, information can be obtained from the family or close friends, but some of these perceptions may differ from those of the patient.

Patient's Perceptions

Patients with severe impairments may be able to convey anxiety, fear, and frustration through body language and facial expression. A brief, even one word, reflection of the nurse's perception may help the patient to express his feelings. A person with nonfluent aphasia probably understands what is said, and his response may be meaningful despite the fact that it is produced with struggle and limited to a word or two. A calm, unhurried approach that indicates acceptance and concern can facilitate communication.

In addition to providing opportunities for the patient to express feelings, assess the perceptions of the patient whose language skills extend beyond gestures. The exact format of this assessment will be guided by the patient's comprehension and response capability. Soon after the onset of aphasia, assess the patient's understanding of aphasia and provide needed information. As the patient progresses, focus on what he finds most difficult or most frustrating, and then focus on areas of progress. Defining the patient's assets is as important as defining areas of concern. When the nurse is seeing the aphasic person because of a health problem that is unrelated to aphasia, it may be difficult to decide whether to question the patient about his language skills. Acknowledging identified assets provides an opening for the patient to mention concerns, without implying that his language skills are a problem.

Family Perceptions

When the patient's language abilities are so severely impaired that body language and facial expressions are the primary means of communication, family or close friends are often the best interpreters. People who have shared a history of effective communication usually are able to understand each other through nonverbal channels more easily than strangers. However, family members often are so stressed by the patient's serious illness and other related changes in their lives that they are unable to use this capacity without assistance.

Nursing research suggests that the families of seriously ill people share the following needs:[5,9]

- Need for relief of anxiety through explanations of what is happening to the patient
- Need for information about the patient's progress
- Need for support and opportunity to ventilate feelings
- Need to be with the patient
- Need to be helpful to the patient

During the acute state of the patient's illness, assessment is focused first on the family's need for information and explanation. Does the family understand that the patient's problems in understanding and in expressing himself are related to a specific problem in processing language, rather than a generalized mental deficiency? Do they know that some spontaneous recovery from his current impairments can be expected to occur over the next 3 months, and that additional gains can be achieved through therapy? Often informational needs will have to be met or plans made to meet them before proceeding with the assessment. It may not be possible to assess the family's previous communication patterns until their own stress has been reduced. On the other hand, helping family members to see the ways in which they can communicate with the patient and can be helpful to him is often an excellent way to reduce their stress.

When the patient is past the acute stage, the family's perception of problems and strengths provides useful data. Assess whether the family members' own needs are being met and to identify their strengths as well as their concerns.

OBJECTIVE DATA

Neurologic Status

The person with aphasia has suffered a neurologic impairment and needs a complete neurologic assessment, unless he is being seen for another problem and his condition is known to be stable. This assessment includes sensory status, motor status, cranial nerves, and reflexes. The nurse's own background in physical assessment, the setting in which she works, and the availability of current data from the assessment of other health care providers determine how much of this assessment is carried out by the nurse. In all instances, the nurse needs to assess whether hearing, vision, and motor abilities have an

impact on the patient's ability to communicate. Often the available data identify the patient's problems, but the nurse needs to do further assessment to identify assets such as functions that are still intact.

Language Skills

Knowledge of the characteristics of various types of aphasia will assist the nurse in the assessment of language skills. These characteristics are summarized in Table 10-4. Remember that patients will not generally follow these characteristics precisely, and the goal of assessment is to identify both intact functions and problems. Listen carefully to the person's spontaneous speech, and note how long it takes him to respond. Allow enough time for the patient's responses. It takes the person with aphasia a long time to process stimuli and formulate a response. If sufficient time is not provided, responses may not reflect his capabilities. Observe whether the patient seems to understand what is said.

Comprehension can be tested further by giving the patient a simple, one-step direction such as, "Pick up the glass." If he is able to carry out a one-step direction, try two- and then three-step directions. When testing auditory comprehension, avoid giving the patient cues with gestures. Often comprehension is overestimated because the person is able to use situational cues, facial expressions, and gestures to understand what is expected. After auditory comprehension has been assessed, evaluate the patient's ability to understand directions that are accompanied by gestures. For example, give a direction such as, "hand (extend your hand toward the patient) the glass (point to the glass) to me" (point toward yourself). Compare the patient's performance on several different directions given with and without gestures or pantomime. Research has shown that apha-

TABLE 10-4
CHARACTERISTICS OF FLUENT AND NONFLUENT APHASIA

	FLUENT APHASIA	NONFLUENT APHASIA
Spontaneous Speech	Articulated effortlessly Normal rate, rhythm, and inflection Word and sound substitutions are common. Lacks meaning and content Unaware of speech errors	Speech is labored. Rate, rhythm, and inflection are disturbed. Telegraphic speech Able to convey meaning with few words Aware of speech errors
Writing	Word and sound substitutions similar to speech errors	Errors are similar to those made in speech.
Motor Response to Verbal Directions	Impaired except in conductive aphasia May rely heavily on situational cues, gestures, and facial expression	Intact as long as response is within their motor capabilities
Reading	Impaired to the same degree as auditory comprehension	Usually intact (i.e., same as previous level)

sic people respond more accurately and more rapidly to directions that combine verbal messages and gestures than they do either to verbal messages or gestures alone.[1] Reading comprehension can be tested using written one-, two-, and three-step directions, or by using materials at hand (e.g., a newspaper or magazine) and asking questions about content. The choice of methods should be guided by the patient's ability to express himself verbally. It is appropriate for nurses in acute care settings to defer tests of reading comprehension until these tests are pertinent to nursing care. Comprehensive testing frequently is done by the speech pathologist before data on reading comprehension are needed in nursing care. In community settings, reading comprehension is often pertinent to health teaching or interventions to stimulate language development.

The patient's ability to express himself is the other major area of language skills as-

sessment. Note the characteristics of the patient's spontaneous speech, then, assess social gesture speech and repetition. Social gesture speech or automatic speech requires the least linguistic skill and usually remains intact. Examples of this level of speech are social responses ("Thank you," "You're welcome," "How are you?", "Fine"), prayers, familiar rhymes or songs, and swearing. This type of speech is sometimes apparent without prompting, and may seem almost involuntary. It can also be elicited by the nurse's greeting or by beginning a rhyme such as, "Roses are red, violets are..." Repetition is tested by having the patient repeat numbers, words, or phrases. People with aphasia often have more difficulty repeating abstract words and phrases such as "No ifs, ands, or buts," than they may have repeating concrete words and phrases.

The presence or absence of repetition ability is important in planning ways to stimulate language. It is also helpful to assess whether the patient can name objects or pictures of objects. People who are having difficulty with naming sometimes can choose the correct response when offered a choice of responses. They may also be able to describe or demonstrate an object's use despite the inability to say the name. The assessment of writing ability can be deferred during hospitalization unless the patient indicates that he wants to explore this possibility. When working with patients in the community, remember that the ability to sign one's own name is an important skill for managing one's affairs. The importance of assessing the patient's ability to express his needs through gesture and pantomime cannot be overemphasized. Even people who have a lot of verbal ability find this skill useful at times when they are tired or frustrated.

NURSING DIAGNOSIS

Diagnoses are derived from the assessment data. The specific diagnosis, communication deficit due to fluent or nonfluent aphasia, will usually be accompanied by associated diagnoses such as

Difficulty expressing needs due to aphasia
Difficulty understanding verbal statements or questions due to aphasia
Anxiety related to impaired communication
Decreased self-esteem related to communication impairment
Family knowledge deficit regarding successful communication strategies.

In addition to identifying the person's problems, it is important to come to conclusions about his communication assets. The following statements are examples:

Expresses needs with gestures or picture cards.
Conveys meaning in a few words when increased response time is provided.
Family members communicate easily with gestures and single words.

MANAGEMENT

GOALS

When the nurse-patient contact occurs soon after the neurologic injury, the first priorities will be to establish some means of communication and to decrease anxiety. When the patient has passed the initial phase, additional goals may relate to stimulating language development and fostering self-esteem. At any point there may be specific goals that relate to the identified needs of family members.

FACILITATING COMMUNICATION

The communication strengths and deficits of people with aphasia vary widely. Therefore, nursing interventions need to be based on assessment data and should be modified based on an ongoing evaluation. All aphasic people need a calm, unhurried approach and an environment that is as free of distractions as possible when they are trying to communicate. Avoid situations that require the patient to interact with more than one person at a time. Both frustration and fatigue will decrease the person's language skills, and an unsuccessful performance contributes to even greater difficulty in using language. The nurse is often the member of the health care team who is in the best position to provide ongoing assessment of these factors and serve as a patient advocate.

METHODS TO EXPRESS NEEDS

Establishing ways in which the patient can express his needs is a primary concern. For some patients, this may mean simply providing them enough time to respond and listening carefully for the meaning in their few words. Not being given enough time to respond can be frustrating, but allowing the struggle to continue too long can be equally frustrating. Everyone has characteristic ways in which body language and facial expressions are used to convey frustration levels. The nurse needs to become sensitive to each person's pattern. When the patient's frustration is high, attempting to supply a choice for the missing word, making a clarifying statement, or asking if he can use gestures may be helpful. Use assessment data in deciding which approach to try for each person and evaluate the response. If the need is not an urgent one, it may be best to postpone further attempts until the patient has had a chance to rest.

Encourage people who are having difficulty expressing themselves to use gestures along with their speech. Modeling of this behavior by the nurse and positively reinforcing the patient's use of gestures provides this encouragement. When the patient is having difficulty naming objects, a picture board or a simple set of index cards, with pictures of commonly used items, can be helpful. The person with aphasia should be encouraged to express himself at whatever level is within his capability. The nurse should reward his attempts to communicate, as well as his successes. This encourages his continuing efforts. Do not correct expression errors; however, clarifying responses are helpful. Suppose for example that the patient has in his hand a towel, washcloth, shower cap, and bath powder and says to you, "I can find the foap." Your response might be, "You're looking for soap."

METHODS TO STIMULATE LANGUAGE DEVELOPMENT

There are a variety of ways for the nurse to stimulate language development. If the pa-

tient is using picture cards or pointing to objects to express himself, state the name of the object and, if he can, have him repeat the name. Similarly, talking to the person while you provide care stimulates him to use language. The nurse can use words to describe briefly what she is doing or what the patient is doing. Talk to him about concrete things in the environment or topics of interest to him. It is essential, however, that messages be keyed to the patient's ability to comprehend. Otherwise, words become a meaningless barrage rather than a stimulus.

When the patient is having difficulty with comprehension, speak in a normal tone of voice, but slow the rate of speech and speak concisely. Avoid childish language, but choose words carefully so that the message is conveyed in as few words as possible. Provide adequate time for the patient to process what is being said before repeating the sentence. It may be best to wait until he indicates that he wants the message repeated. If the patient misunderstands, let him know in an accepting way that there has been a misunderstanding, and repeat the message. Try different wording if he still does not understand. Monitor both the patient's frustration level and your own, and switch to a nonverbal method when indicated. Switching to a different topic is also sometimes helpful.

Whenever possible, accompany words with gestures and make use of situational cues. For example, the patient who cannot understand a message that it is time for him to get ready for physical therapy (PT) will probably understand easily if a wheelchair is brought to the bedside, along with his robe and shoes, and he is then told, "PT now." The actual object or a picture of the object may help to convey the meaning more easily. If he can follow only a one-step direction, break more complex directions into single steps and let him perform one step before giving him the direction for the next step. When the patient has problems comprehending verbal messages, remember that gestures, facial expressions, voice inflections, and use of touch assume great importance in establishing a trusting relationship and conveying acceptance.

Methods of facilitating communications with the aphasic person extend beyond the modifications that the individual nurse makes in her interactions with the patient. Communicating with this patient and stimulating his language development will require time, and this must be considered in planning assignments or scheduling visits. The needs of the patient are met best by having the same staff members consistently provide his care. Even though specific interventions that are most effective in facilitating communication are written in his care plan, it is not an adequate substitute for care provided by the same nurse. Developing a therapeutic relationship that surmounts the patient's communication deficits takes time. Both the nurse who is providing care and her colleagues need to recognize that communicating with the aphasic person can be frustrating for the nurse. A network of supportive colleagues can provide for the release of these frustrations and enable the nurse to meet her own needs. The view of a more objective colleague sometimes can help the nurse to identify the small steps of progress that have been made. Setting interim goals that lead to the long-term goal is as important for the nurse as it is for the patient.

Many of the mechanisms suggested for the hearing-impaired person that inform others of the patient's communications needs are applicable to the aphasic person as well. Specific information regarding the most effective means of communicating with the person needs to be conveyed, not just the fact that the person has aphasia.

PSYCHOSOCIAL PROBLEMS

Interviews with people who have recovered from aphasia reveal that what they needed most at the onset of their aphasia was information about what had happened and what was going to happen.[21] Written accounts of experiences with aphasia relate that these people felt fearful and bewildered, and had a sense of no longer being a person. The nurse needs to provide explanations which are keyed to the patient's comprehension. The nurse's actions often speak for her, so that she needs to be certain she is sending the message she intends. The gentle way in which the nurse handles the patient when attending to his physical needs, her calm attempts to let him know what is happening, and the respect shown for his privacy all communicate that he is in an environment in which he will receive care and be accepted and respected.

Participating in self-care activities and making decisions about his care are important to the patient's self-concept. Activities that help the patient to assert some control over his environment are to be encouraged rather than resisted. Providing opportunities for the patient to make choices in his personal care and diet are examples of such activities. Grooming is also important to self-concept. Encourage the patient to attend to grooming needs when he is able to and provide positive reinforcement for these behaviors. The nurse attends to these needs when the patient is unable. Most patients will respond to gentle encouragement if they are able physically and emotionally to meet their own grooming and hygiene needs. When this is not the case, providing this care may meet the person's dependency needs. Meeting the person's need for dependency enables him to move forward and begin to function more independently.

Personal possessions are helpful in maintaining a sense of self. A favorite old robe is more meaningful than a new one. Pictures of loved ones and pictures of the patient carrying out favorite activities help to maintain identity. A small bottle of the after-shave lotion he has always used or the cologne she has always preferred are other suggestions that can be made to families of patients in hospitals or nursing homes. The nurse who is visiting the patient in his home can bolster his sense of identity by commenting on personal memorabilia. When the person is not very mobile, family members might be encouraged to move some small, valued possessions to the area in which the patient spends the greatest portion of his time.

FAMILY SUPPORT

A supportive family can be an invaluable asset to the aphasic person. However, to provide this support, their own needs must be met. The nurse is often the member of the health team who has the closest contact with family members and is best able to assess their adaptation. Some families will only need opportunities to verbalize their feelings and concerns and have their informational needs met. Other families will have extensive needs that require referral to a social worker. The nurse can help the family to use effective communication techniques by providing concrete suggestions, and by modeling the behaviors that she suggests in the family's presence.

REHABILITATION PROGRAMS

During the rehabilitation period, the patient and his family will continue to need support. Assessment of the family as a whole and the individuals who compose the family must be ongoing. Some who were coping well may

have difficulty after discharge, and referrals for home assessment and follow-up are nearly always appropriate. The community health nurse will need to decide which of the problems that she identifies are within her range of expertise and whether referrals to other health care providers should be suggested to the family. Speech pathologists, social workers, vocational counselors, and mental health professionals may play an important role in helping the patient and his family to reach their optimal level of functioning.

The speech pathologist is the most intensively involved in assisting the person to regain language skills. Although there is a period of about 3 months in which spontaneous recovery may occur, speech therapy often is begun as soon as the person's medical condition is stable. The speech pathologist's initial evaluation may be an informal one at the bedside when therapy is initiated early. Later evaluations will be a detailed analysis of the patient's language skills. The speech pathologist will also intervene with family members to provide support and counseling. Communication between the nurse and the speech pathologist will help each of them to meet the patient's needs. The nurse can provide data about the patient's day-to-day functioning and identify times of the day during which he communicates most successfully. These will be good times to schedule therapy sessions. The speech pathologist can provide assistance to the nurse to resolve specific communication problems that the patient is having and also suggestions for providing an environment that is conducive to language development. The nurse will need to exercise judgment, however, in deciding whether specific drill work should be reinforced outside of therapy sessions. The patient's need for physical and emotional rest between therapy sessions must be considered.

CONCLUSION

Communication is the process by which we interact with our physical and social environment. The specific examples of hearing loss and aphasia are used to illustrate the impact that communication deficits can have on a person's physical, psychological, and social functioning. The nurse's assessment of a person with a communication deficit focuses on the needs and strengths of both the person and his family. Counseling, teaching, and referrals are important aspects of nursing management. The primary goals of nursing intervention are to improve communication abilities and to assist patients and their families to cope effectively with communication deficits and related problems.

REFERENCES

1. Beukelman DR, Yorkston KM, Waugh PF: Communication in severe aphasia: Effectiveness of three instruction modalities. Arch Phys Med Rehabil 61:248, 1980
2. Brust J, Schafer S, Richter R, et al: Aphasia in acute stroke. Stroke 7:167, 1976
3. Busis S, Paisner H, Wolfson R: Pointers for detecting hearing loss. Primary Care 11:174, 1977
4. Consumers Union: How to buy a hearing aid. Consumer Reports 41:346, June 1976
5. Dracup K, Breu C: Using nursing research to meet the needs of grieving spouses. Nurs Res 27:212, 1978
6. Edsall J, Miller L: Relationship between loss of auditory and visual acuity and social disengagement. Nurs Res 27:296, 1978
7. Geshwind N: Specialization of the human brain. Sci Amer 241:180, 1979
8. Geshwind N: Some special functions of the human brain. In Montcastle VB (ed): Medical Physiology, St. Louis, CV Mosby, 1980
9. Hampe S: Needs of the grieving spouse in a hospital setting. Nurs Res 24:113, 1975
10. Health, Education and Welfare: Final Report to the Secretary on Hearing Aid Health Care. Springfield, VA, U.S. Department of Commerce, 1975
11. Iveson L: To be deaf...views from the people who are. Nurs Care 9, 1976

12. Kinsella G, Duffy F: The spouse of the aphasic patient. In Lebrun Y, Hoops R (eds): The Management of Aphasia. Amsterdam, Swets & Zeitlinger, 1978
13. Lass L, Franklin R, Bertrand W, et al: Health knowledge, attitudes, and practices of the deaf population in greater New Orleans. Am Annal Def 123:960, 1978
14. LeBuffe FE, LeBuffe L: Psychiatric aspects of deafness. Primary Care 6:295, 1979
15. Leske M: Prevalence estimates of communication disorders in the US. ASHA 23:229, 1981
16. Malasanos L, Barkauskas B, Moss M, et al: Health Assessment. St. Louis, CV Mosby, 1981
17. Norris M, Cunningham D: Social impact of hearing loss in the aged. J Gerontol 6:727, 1981
18. Palmer BP: Language dysfunction in cerebrovascular disease. Primary Care 6:827, 1979
19. Rules of the Food and Drug Administration for the Hearing Aid Industry. Washington, DC, General Registry, 9286-9296, Feb 15,1977
20. Schow RL, Christensen JM, Hutchinson JM et al: Communication Disorders of the Aged. Baltimore, University Park Press, 1978
21. Skelly N: Aphasic patients talk back. Am J Nurs 75:1140, 1975
22. Sussman M: Sociological theory and deafness: problems and prospects. In: Health, Education and Welfare: Research on Behavioral Aspects of Deafness, Washington, D.C. Vocational Rehabilitaion Administration, 1965
23. Wiley TL: Hearing disorders and audiometry. In Hixon TJ, Shriberg LD, Saxman JH (eds): Introduction to Communication Disorders. Englewood Cliffs, NJ, Prentice-Hall, 1980

BIBLIOGRAPHY

Berlo DK: The Process of Communication. New York, Holt, Rinehart & Winston, 1960
Blanco K: The aphasic patient. J Neurol Nurs 14:34, 1982
Brookshire RH: An introduction to Aphasia. Minneapolis, BRK Pub, 1973
Clark CC, Mills GC: Communicating with hearing impaired elderly adults. J Geront Nurs 5:41, 1979
Corliss E: Facts About Hearing and Hearing Aids. Washington, D.C. U.S. Government Printing Office, 1971
Corso JF: Presbycusis, hearing aids, and aging. Audiology 16:146, 1977
Corso JF: Auditory perception and communication. In Berin J, Schaie K (eds): Handbook of the Psychology of Aging. New York, Van Nostrand-Rinehold, 1977

Dreher B: Overcoming speech and language disorders. Gerontol Nurs 2:345, 1981

Gardner H: The Shattered Mind. New York, Alfred A Knopf, 1975

Geshwind N: Language and the brain. Sci Am 226:76, 1972

Guyton A: Basic Human Physiology. Philadelphia, WB Saunders, 1977

Heller BR, Gayner EG: Hearing loss and aural rehabilitation of the elderly. Top Clin Nurs 3:21, 1981

Hixon TJ, Schriberg LD, Sarman JH: Introduction to Communication Disorders, Englewood Cliffs, NJ, Prentice-Hall, 1980

Hodgins E: Episode. New York, Simon & Schuster, 1971

Holland A: Treatment of aphasia following stroke. Stroke 10:475, 1979

Holm CS: Deafness: Common misunderstanding. Am J Nurs 78:1910, 1978

Kalb J: Understanding aphasia and the aphasic. J Neurol Nurs 9:15, 1977

LoGrasso GA: Using words without sound. Am J Nurs 80:2186, 1980

Louis M, Povse S: Aphasia and endurance: Consideration in the assessment and care of the stroke patient. Nurs Clin North Am 15:265, 1980

Luey HS: Between Worlds: The problems of deafened adults. Social Work in Health Care 5:253, 1980

Mamaril AP: Sudden deafness, Am J Nurs 76:1992, 1976

Nance A, Ochsner G: Language modality performance patterns in aphasia. J Commun Dis 14:421, 1981

Norman S, Baratz R: Understanding aphasia. Am J Nurs 79:2135, 1979

Pitorowski M: Aphasia: Providing better care. Nurs Clin North Am 13:543, 1978

Pluckhan ML: Human Communication. New York, McGraw-Hill, 1978

Prinz P: A note on requesting strategies in adult aphasia. J Commun Dis 13:65, 1980

Schuell H: Aphasia Theory and Therapy. Baltimore, University Park Press, 1974

Wallhagen M: The split brain: Implications for care and rehabilitation. Am J Nurs 79:2118, 1979

Werner-Beland JA: Grief Responses to Long-Term Illness and Disability. Reston, Va, Reston Publishing, 1980

Weiss CE: Why more of the aged with auditory deficits do not wear hearing aids. J Am Geriatr Soc 21:139, 1973

11

Impaired Mobility

Carol J. Schaupner

Unrestricted and unimpaired mobility is an ability that people usually take for granted. In a healthy state, the person decides when, how, and how much to move any part of the body. Standing, walking, stretching, and other activities are done by choice. However, an alteration in one's physical or mental state of health, always has an effect on the person's mobility. A physical alteration may produce decreased strength and endurance, a state that affects motion. The most severe alteration results in paralysis. A mental alteration may cause a change in desire or motivation to move the body.

Nurses are certain to encounter the problem of impaired mobility while working with people who have alterations in physical and mental function. A diagnosis of impaired mobility produces numerous other problems that result from disuse and affects many body systems.

The purpose of this chapter is to identify patient populations where the diagnosis of impaired mobility is likely to be made, to identify its signs and symptoms, to identify the related effects of impaired mobility, and to discuss nursing management methods to prevent or minimize the effects of impaired mobility.

SCOPE OF THE PROBLEM

Impaired mobility is associated with a wide variety of health problems (Table 11-1). Thus, the nurse frequently encounters the problem in many patient populations.

Impaired mobility may be a direct result of a medical condition such as paralysis, or a result of the prescribed treatment for the condition such as surgery, bed rest, casting, or traction. Postoperative patients who are experiencing severe pain will limit their activity until the nurse intervenes with medication, splinting, breathing, and relaxation techniques, or other nursing interventions. A person with a chronic illness, cancer, or a cardiac problem, for example, often limits activity due to decreased endurance and easy fatigability. The person with a neurologic impairment who has paralysis will have a long-term or permanent degree of impaired mobility that will require readjustment in life-style to compensate for this altered mobility (Fig. 11-1).

Table 11-1
PROBLEMS LEADING TO IMPAIRED MOBILITY

PROBLEM	MEDICAL CONDITION EXAMPLE
Intolerance to activity/decreased strength and endurance	Acute medical conditions: MI's, GI disorders Chronic conditions: Cancer, congestive heart failure, cardiomyopathy, chronic obstructive pulmonary disease
Pain/discomfort	Burns, rheumatoid arthritis, chronic pain syndrome, postoperative pain
Perceptual/cognitive impairment	Brain tumor or trauma, CVA, vision disorders
Neuromuscular impairment	Multiple sclerosis, Parkinson's disease, spinal injury, myelitis
Musculoskeletal impairment	Muscular dystrophy, arthritis, fractures, scoliosis
Depression/severe anxiety	Neurosis, schizophrenia

Sensory deprivation has also been shown to have effects on mobility. Decreased sensory stimuli can lead to a decrease in physical activity. As a person's environment is limited, the variety of sensory input is often limited, causing the person to decrease physical activity.

MECHANISMS OF IMPAIRED MOBILITY

Impaired mobility and its effects have been recognized as a significant problem in medicine and nursing for many years. In 1947, Asher wrote an article entitled, "The Dangers of Going to Bed." In describing the adverse effects of bed rest he concluded, "Get people up and we may save our patients from an early grave."[1] This short sentence has been an enduring reminder to nurses to encourage patients to increase their activity as quickly as possible during an illness or after surgery. A study by Deitrick, Whedon, and Shorr, in

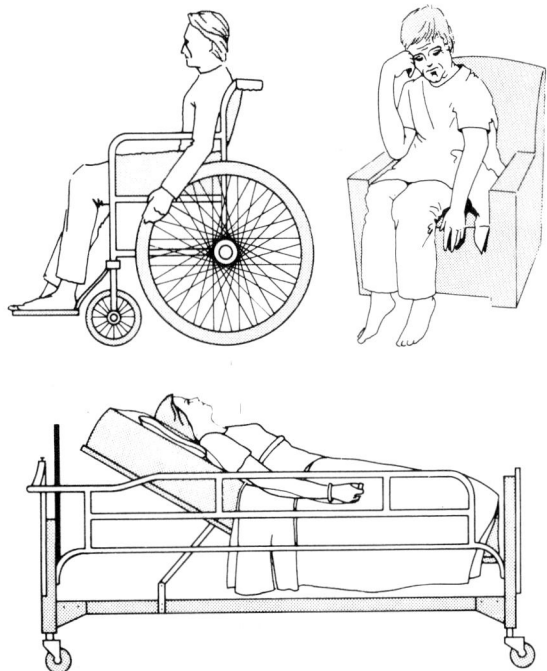

FIG. 11-1 *Impaired mobility may be a result of various conditions.*

1948, used plaster casting for a period of 6 to 7 weeks.[4] This study provided a basis for further immobilization research. Research on the effects of immobilization increased in connection with the space program. Vallbona and colleagues, through a project with the National Aeronautics and Space Administration (NASA), compiled the types of studies that were being conducted to determine the physiological and psychological effects of immobilization.[11] Most studies used bed rest or water immersion for immobilization.

The scope of this chapter does not permit a discussion of all the physiology related to the diverse effects of immobility on body systems. The reader is referred to Browse's,

The Physiology and Pathology of Bedrest, Olson's, "The Hazards of Immobility," and Steinberg's, *The Immobilized Patient,* all of which detail research in the areas of circulatory, respiratory, bone, muscle, joint, skin, and psychological function.[2,8,10] A summary of the major effects of immobility on these body systems is shown in Table 11-2.

MUSCULOSKELETAL EFFECTS

Problems of the muscles and bones may be both the cause and the result of altered mobility. Healthy people confined to bed rest or otherwise immobilized have been shown to develop various effects on muscle and bone.

Table 11-2
EFFECTS OF IMMOBILITY ON BODY SYSTEMS

SYSTEM	POTENTIAL EFFECT
Musculoskeletal	Muscle atrophy, decreased muscle strength and tone, decreased mass, contracture, joint degeneration, osteoporosis
Metabolic	Negative nitrogen balance, hypercalcemia, reduced metabolic rate, anorexia, obesity
Genitourinary	Urinary stasis, infection, retention, renal calculi, altered sexual functioning
Cardiovascular	Increased heart rate, decreased stroke volume, decreased oxygen uptake, orthostatic hypotension, venous thrombosis, dependent edema
Respiratory	Stasis of secretions, altered function of mucous membranes and cilia, ventilation/perfusion imbalance, aspiration
Skin	Pressure sores, excoriation, rashes
Psychological/social	Perceptual alterations (depression, worry, restlessness, dreams), body image change, altered life patterns (job, financial structure, independence/dependence, social isolation, social roles), altered relationships, decreased learning and problem-solving
Gastrointestinal	Constipation

Disuse of a muscle, and lack of contraction and stretch, lead to decreased size of muscle fiber and a resulting muscle atrophy. Muller has reported that an immobilized muscle loses about 3% of its original strength each day. After 7 days, little strength is lost for the remaining period of immobilization.[7]

Contracture is a serious effect of immobilization. *Contracture* is the shortening of muscle fiber because of immobilization in one position and lack of stretch to muscle fibers. For a period of time, contractures are reversible by movement and exercise. Eventually, however, muscle fiber is replaced by fibrous tissue, and normal range of motion cannot be restored (Fig. 11-2).

The most common contractures that occur include hip-flexion and heal-cord contractures. Hip-flexion contractures develop from sitting for long periods in a chair, or in bed with the head and foot of bed elevated. Heal-cord contracture, the classic "foot-drop," is due to the effect of gravity on an unsupported foot in bed. Shoulder, elbow, and finger contractures are also common in persons with paralysis, if intervention by exercise has not occurred.

Contractures result in limitations of a person's ability to function in daily activities. Foot, hip, and knee contractures may impair ambulation. Activities such as feeding, dressing, and grooming may be impaired by contractures of the upper and lower extremities.

METABOLIC EFFECTS

The 1948 study conducted by Deitrick, Whedon, and Shorr was one of the first to measure the effects of immobilization on metabolic functions of healthy subjects. They found significant nitrogen excretion beginning after the 5th to 6th day. There was an average total nitrogen loss of a 53.6 g over the

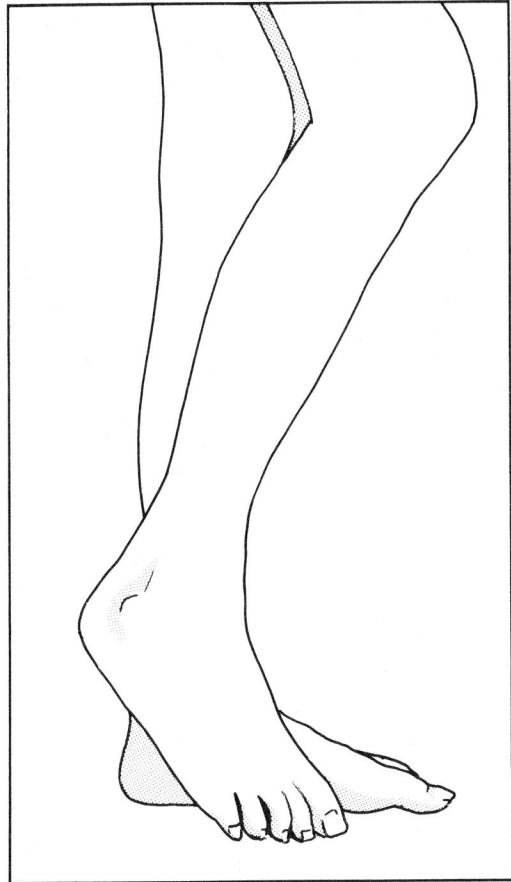

FIG. 11-2 Knee and ankle contractures.

6 to 7 weeks of the study.[4] Browse relates several studies that substantiate the disuse atrophy that occurs with bedrest.[2] The decreasing muscle bulk provides the source of protein catabolism, resulting in the excretion of nitrogen. Thus, the need for protein-replacing diets is evident.

Metabolic changes due to immobility that predispose to renal stone formation were found by Deitrick and co-workers.[4] These include increased calcium excretion combined with constant urine volume, a slight rise in urinary pH, and a constant citric acid level.

Anorexia is a potential problem with immobility. Deitrick's subjects showed a tendency toward loss of appetite. Anorexia may be because of decreased energy expenditure, change of diet, or contributing physical and psychological factors related to the cause of immobility.

Obesity may become a problem when immobility is prolonged. Decreased metabolic rate, decreased energy expenditure, and a consistent or increased food intake will result in weight gain. Obesity can be an added severe impairment to a person with altered mobility.

CARDIOVASCULAR EFFECTS

The most significant effects of immobility on the cardiovascular system are a decrease in resting heart rate and stroke volume (i.e., a general decrease in myocardial performance), a decline in maximal oxygen uptake, orthostatic tolerance changes, and venous thrombosis. A general deconditioning occurs after a period of immobilization. Oxygen intake is an indicator of physical fitness. Studies reported by Steinberg show oxygen uptake declined by 27% after 20 days of bed rest. Tilt-table tests have demonstrated the orthostatic response to immobilization. The heart rate rises, blood pressure falls, and fainting may occur. Steinberg has an excellent description of the pathophysiology involved in orthostatic hypotension.[10]

Another vascular effect of immobility is venous thrombosis, which can lead to a life-threatening or fatal pulmonary embolus. However, immobilization is only one of many factors that contribute to venous thrombosis; pressure on the vein and damage to the vessel wall, change in blood coagulability, and change in blood flow are also contributing factors.[10]

Dependent edema is a potential complication of immobility. Increased fluid collection in the tissues and decreased fluid return through the vascular system can result when extremities are in a dependent position. The normal pumping mechanism for the fluid is decreased, due to change in the muscle pressure on the veins.

RESPIRATORY EFFECTS

Immobilization has not been shown to produce basic changes in pulmonary function, or in the mechanics of air exchange in healthy people.[10] However, there are circumstances of illness that have direct effects on respiratory function when the patient is immobilized. In general, the effects of immobility are due to position changes of the respiratory system. Browse describes the function of the cilia and the movement of mucus in the bronchioles as protective mechanisms against respiratory infection. In the supine position, the bronchiole is on its side. Gravity draws the mucus downward causing pooling and a reservoir for infection while the upper side of the bronchiole becomes dry, which also predisposes to infection (Fig. 11-3).[2]

Aspiration is a potential problem that often is associated with immobility. Neuromuscular conditions that produce impaired mobility may affect the mechanisms of swallowing. In this instance, aspiration of food or secretions occurs more easily if the person is not sitting up.

GASTROINTESTINAL EFFECTS

Constipation, a frequent complication of decreased mobility, is the result of several factors. Although peristalsis in the intestine is unaltered, work of the accessory abdominal muscles to aid in the passage of stool is decreased. Other factors that contribute to constipation are change in habits including change of diet, and decreased fluid intake,

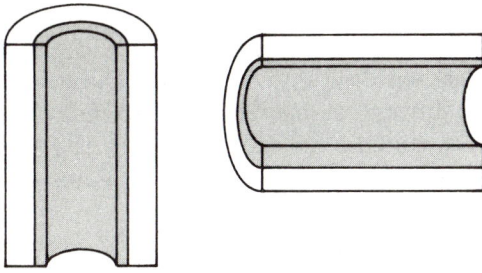

Vertical   Horizontal

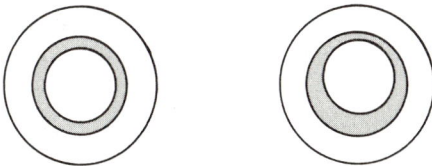

FIG. 11-3   The effect of gravity on the distribution of mucus within a bronchus. (Browse NT: The Physiology and Pathology of Bedrest, p 60. Springfield, Illinois, Charles C. Thomas)

leading to harder stool with a loss of bulk. Use of a bedpan instead of commode chair or toilet alters the physiologic position for defecation. The helpful effect of gravity is decreased or eliminated. Lack of privacy for defecation in a hospital setting also contributes to constipation.

FIG. 11-4   The effect of posture on the drainage of the kidney. (Browse NT: The Physiology and Pathology of Bedrest, p 83. Springfield, Illinois, Charles C. Thomas)

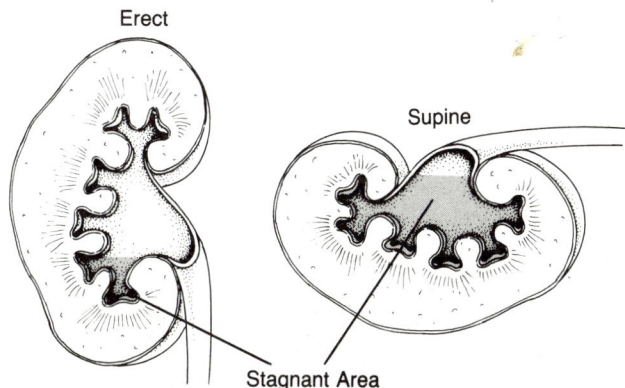

Constipation, if allowed to continue, leads to fecal impaction. Loose or watery stool passed around an impaction may confuse caregivers unfamiliar with this problem. When this continues, it leads to greater impaction or bowel obstruction, especially in the elderly.

GENITOURINARY EFFECTS

Impaired mobility produces effects on the renal system and voiding mechanisms. Urinary stasis occurs in the kidney in the recumbent position (Fig. 11-4). Stasis increases the possibility of urinary tract infection. Increased calcium excretion through the urinary system, combined with other factors (discussed under Metabolic Effects), contributes to the formation of renal stones.

Urinary retention may be a problem if impaired mobility causes an inability to assume a position that is physiologically best for voiding. Diseases of the central nervous system (CNS) may alter a person's voluntary control of voiding, which may lead either to incontinence or retention. A person may postpone voiding to avoid pain if movement is painful or if privacy is not adequate, leading to a type of urinary retention.

Neurologic conditions, for example, motor sensory changes from a spinal cord in-

Erect

Supine

Stagnant Area

jury, may produce physiologic changes in sexual function. In other conditions, decreased energy and endurance and a general change in level of physical fitness will influence sexual function. The basis for the effect on sexual function may be the psychological effects of immobility. Factors such as change of priorities, inner-directed concerns, and feelings of dependency and isolation from others produce a change in a person's usual pattern of sexuality and sexual functioning.

SKIN INTEGRITY

The effect of immobilization on skin, the body's protective covering, is an important area for nursing assessment and intervention. Altered skin integrity is a nursing diagnosis that may have several causes, a primary cause being pressure associated with immobility. The older terms *bedsore* and *decubitus ulcer* have been the labels used for this nursing problem for years.

Pressure sore is a more descriptive term because it incorporates the cause of the skin breakdown—pressure. Pressure on subcutaneous tissue occurs when the body weight and the force of gravity make contact for a prolonged period against surfaces such as a bed or chair. Tissue changes begin to occur within 1 hour of continuous pressure. Tissue damage and varying degrees of pressure sores occur when the pressure is allowed to continue.

Pressure sores vary in severity. First de-

gree pressure sores are evident by a reddened area or reactive hyperemia that does not disappear within 1 hour of relief of the pressure. If no preventive measures are taken, the skin breaks down and leads finally to late-stage pressure sores, which are open ulcers with bone involvement.

The most vulnerable areas of pressure sore development are places where tissue is compressed against bony prominences, such as the trochanters, ischial tuberosities, ankles, heels, and so forth (Fig. 11-5), (see also Fig. 13-2).

The combination of degree of pressure and duration of time contribute to the rapidity of breakdown. Normal intracapillary pressure is 25 mm Hg. Sitting pressures on bony prominences may go to 300 mm Hg or higher.[10] The factors of shearing force, friction, moist skin, poor nutritional state, edema of tissue, and decreased or lost sensation all contribute to the development of pressure sores.

PSYCHOSOCIAL EFFECTS

Zubek and McNeil found psychosocial effects such as vivid and complex dreams, worry, fright, and restlessness directly related to a prolonged recumbent position.[13] Zubek reported that adding the restriction of visual and auditory stimulation to the immobilized condition produces even greater behavioral impairment. There was increased norepinephrine excretion in their subjects

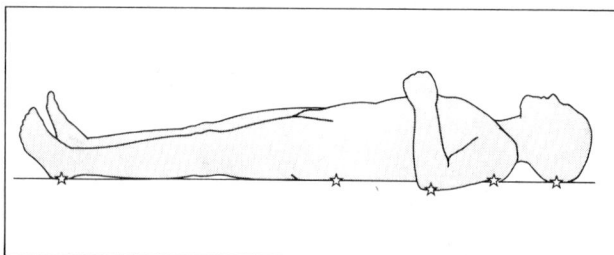

FIG. 11-5 Starred areas show where patient is most vulnerable to pressure sores in supine position.

and increased generalized emotional tension.[12]

The severe effects that neurologic disabilities have on mobility are discussed by Carlson. These effects include alteration of life pattern, disruption of coping, and impact on significant others. There are also changes in self-perception, including self-concept and body image.[3]

Hammer and Kenan describe intellectual, emotional, and social effects of immobilization. Intellectual effects include decreased motivation to learn, retain, transfer, and generalize information, as well as uninterest and loss of attention to activity. Emotional effects include loss of personal worth, fear, guilt, anger, and frustration. Body image changes result from dealing with weight loss, atrophy, and new postures (e.g., sitting in a wheelchair). Social effects include isolation, change in social interaction, and change in social roles.[5]

Psychological and social effects of immobility have important implications for nursing intervention. A patient may become more isolated if immobility continues, and socially isolated if friends and family are not able to make frequent contact. Social roles, such as spouse, lover, or parent are altered by the person's confinement and immobility, and thus will have an effect on their interpersonal relationships. A person's financial structure or that of his family may be altered significantly if immobility causes a change in that person's ability to work. If this leads to a decreased income, it will likely lead to additional stress for the person with impaired mobility.

NURSING ASSESSMENT

Acquiring subjective and objective data by assessment is the basis for forming a nursing diagnosis. The nurse must ask herself: Does this person have a problem with mobility? If so, knowing that many other problems are related to an alteration in mobility, does this person have evidence of related problems?

Table 11-3 indicates areas for assessment to document a diagnosis of impaired mobility. Objective data is obtained by physical examination and directly observable events. Subjective data includes health history, statements by the person relating to the level of activity, medical diagnosis, and environmental, mental, and emotional factors.

SUBJECTIVE DATA

The person's description of activities of daily living (ADL) provides data about his ability physically to perform the tasks of getting out of bed, bathing, dressing, grooming, eating, and other daily activities. Areas to assess are alteration in performance of ADL, assistance or equipment needed, and length of time that activity can be performed before fatigue sets in.

Pain

Pain is a factor that contributes to altered mobility. Ask: Does the person have pain? In what location? Is it constant or intermittent,

Table 11-3
ASSESSMENT DATA: MOBILITY

SUBJECTIVE DATA	OBJECTIVE DATA
Health history	Height and weight
Level of ADL	Range of joint motion
Endurance	Muscle strength
Duration of problem	Muscle bulk, tone
Age	Bed mobility
Pain	Balance (sitting and
Mental function	standing)
Sensory input	Involuntary movements
Body image	Reflexes
Environment	Gait
(effect on movement)	

sharp or dull? Does anything relieve it? Is it limiting activity?

Mental Function

An examination of mental function should be done when evaluating immobility. A person with decreased responsiveness may be unable to move voluntarily. A person with brain damage, whether due to trauma, tumor, or infarct, may have motor function deficits. A person with a memory loss may need prompting and direction in motion and activities.

Emotions

Depression may cause an alteration in mobility. The depressed person is likely to be less active, and may even be immobile, whereas the anxious person is often more active or even agitated.

Body Image

Body image change often accompanies altered mobility. A person who must now use a wheelchair restructures his body image. A person with brain trauma may have perceptual deficits and altered body image owing to the brain damage. A person whose joints are visibly changed because of arthritis also will have a change in body image.

Body image change also may be a factor that leads to a change in mobility. Obese people may limit activity because of feelings about their body, leading to a decreased activity spiral. Persons with skin disorders or suffering from the aftermath of severe burns may limit their environment and activity based on their body image.

Environmental Factors

A person's mobility may be limited by the physical environment. An elderly person may find it difficult to carry out activities because the bed is too high or the toilet too low. A person in a wheelchair is confronted with architectural barriers. The wheelchair cannot go up stairs, or the buttons on an elevator are too high. Assessment of the person's perception of the environment provides essential data.

Is the environment fostering sensory deprivation? Is the person confined to bed in traction or in an early postoperative state? Does the person's environment contain stimulators—sound, color, or points of orientation like calendars and personal belongings?

OBJECTIVE DATA

Height and Weight

Height and weight are important to determine the possibility of problems for a person in a state of altered mobility. Excess weight makes moving more difficult. Obesity or underweight contribute to skin problems. Very tall patients may have more difficulties if a shorter person needs to assist with transfers.

Range of Motion

Test range of joint motion by asking the person to move the joints and observe the extent and ease with which this is done. Is there stiffness, pain, or limitation in motion? If the person is unable to move the joints, the examiner moves them through range of motion, assessing the factors of mobility and limitation. The joint should be supported by placing hands above and below the joint being tested. Limitations in movement are measured with a goniometer, which gives the degree of immobility.

Muscle Strength, Bulk, and Tone

Muscle bulk may be assessed by observation, by comparing muscle size bilaterally, and by measuring muscle circumference. Assess muscle tone by acquiring a feel for resistance of the muscles when extremities are moved through range of motion. Test muscle strength by testing individual muscles or muscle groups that perform various functions. A muscle's ability to overcome resistance by the examiner is tested. For example, to test the muscles that perform the function of elbow flexion, the patient flexes the elbow; the examiner provides resistance by trying to straighten the elbow while the patient continues to try to flex further. If the elbow is able to flex further, the muscle has overcome resistance. A commonly used muscle grading scale is:[9]

5 (Normal) Complete range of motion against gravity with full resistance
4 (Good) Complete range of motion against gravity with some resistance
3 (Fair) Complete range of motion against gravity
2 (Poor) Complete range of motion with gravity eliminated
1 (Trace) Evidence of a slight contractility, no joint motion
0 (Zero) No evidence of contractility

Bed Mobility and Balance

Muscle and joint function can be observed in a person's ability to carry out movement. Is the person able to roll from side to side in bed, or move from the foot to the head of the bed? Can the person sit at the side of the bed unsupported and maintain that position against resistance? Ability to stand and to maintain a standing position when the examiner provides some resistance must also be assessed. These observations are essential to determine a person's level of functional ability.

Involuntary Movements or Reflexes

Observations should be made of any tremors or spasticity in the extremities. These may be spontaneous or elicited by stimulation of touch. Testing for the presence of normal

muscle reflexes or the presence of abnormal reflexes (e.g., Babinski's reflex) gives data of a possible neurologic basis for a state of altered mobility.

Gait

General ability to ambulate is observed. What is the posture? Is there balance and symmetry of movement? Are there contractures of hip, knee, or ankle? Is there any pain on ambulation? The nurse can refer the patient to a physician or physical therapist to do a detailed assessment of gait if a problem is detected.

Environmental Restrictions

Environmental restrictions on movement can be observed. Is the person confused or combative? Is he wearing a jacket or hand restraints? Is there a cast or traction?

Potential Problems Related to Mobility

Guidelines for assessment data for potential problem areas related to impaired mobility are seen in Table 11-4. Subjective data include *any* perceptions or statements that the person has about these areas. Assessment may reveal a current problem, such as shortness of breath, that may be related to chronic obstructive pulmonary disease, which affects mobility. The data also will reveal current or potential problem areas related to altered mobility. For example, a finding of no bowel movement for 5 days in a person whose previous pattern has been every other day and who has been on bed rest for 2 weeks, indicates constipation related to immobility.

NURSING DIAGNOSIS

Nursing diagnoses are determined from the data. The Task Force for Classification of Nursing Diagnosis has defined some possible

Table 11-4
ASSESSMENT DATA: PROBLEMS RELATED TO IMPAIRED MOBILITY

SYSTEM	SUBJECTIVE	OBJECTIVE
Respiratory	Dyspnea Ventilation assistance Medications	Respiratory rate Depth Lung sounds Secretions Oxygen
Cardiovascular	Chest pain Dyspnea Medication Pain in extremity	Heart rate, rhythm, sounds BP Edema Warmth Swelling Erythema in an extremity Homans' sign
Skin integrity	Pruritis Cosmetics Medications	Sensation Color Turgor Lubrication Lesions Tone
Gastrointestinal	Intake Eating patterns Food preferences Bowel movement history Medications	Bowel sounds Abdominal tone, mass Anal sphincter tone Bulbocavernosis Anal wink reflex
Genitourinary	Voiding patterns Output Urgency Pain Sexual function history Medications	Bladder distention Genital appearance Anal reflexes
Psychosocial	Life-style Relationships Sexual attitude and patterns Behavior patterns Dependency/independence coping style Emotions expressed, communication pattern, learning potential, interests/activities, finances	Verbalizations Facial expressions Body position Observed interactions

causes for the diagnosis of impaired mobility:[6]

Intolerance to activity/decreased strength
    and endurance
Pain/discomfort
Perceptual/cognitive impairment
Neuromuscular impairment
Musculoskeletal impairment
Depression/severe anxiety

Persons with head trauma and decreased level of consciousness, for example, are unable to move their extremities voluntarily or move their bodies in bed. The diagnosis: impaired mobility related to decreased level of consciousness. An obese person who spends most of the day watching television, never exercises, feels embarrassed by his body size and shape, and has been limiting social contacts because of this embarrassment, would be diagnosed as having impaired mobility related to obesity and body image.

A person with a spinal cord injury who is unable to move the lower extremities voluntarily has impaired mobility related to loss of muscle innervation.

The effects of impaired mobility give rise to many related nursing diagnoses, for example:

Pressure sore related to immobility
Constipation related to altered mobility
Altered sexual patterns related to immobility
Altered social roles and financial status re-
    lated to immobility

DURATION

Before intervention is planned, factors such as the duration of the problem and its impact on the person's life-style need to be considered. A problem such as a spinal cord injury causes chronic immobility problems, and intervention should be planned that takes this into consideration. Problems like depression or pain may cause intermittent difficulties over a short or long period of time. Some problems, such as immobility related to postoperative pain, are temporary.

ACUITY

Acute situations limit the type of intervention that may occur. For example, in an acute flare-up of rheumatoid arthritis, joints are not exercised as they are when the disease is quiescent. A person immediately after a myocardial infarction increases the level of activity and exercise gradually. Range-of-motion exercises are limited when a person has an unstable spinal cord fracture until stabilization is complete.

RESOURCES

Factors such as the setting in which intervention occurs and the resources available have an impact on what degree and type of intervention are possible. Intervention may occur in a rehabilitation center, hospital clinic, or home. A person's medical insurance (i.e., state or federal coverage) influences the type of support services that the person will be able to receive.

In addition to nurses and physicians, health professionals such as physical therapists, occupational therapists, respiratory therapists, and social and vocational counselors are available to work with people with impaired mobility. Family and friends are essential support systems for a person with impaired mobility. Their assistance is needed both to help restore mobility and to cope with related problems.

Intervention relies heavily on the person's perception of his needs and assistance available from support systems. People with impaired mobility have varying needs for assistance with activities. A functional level classification has been suggested:[6]

CLASSIFICATION OF FUNCTIONAL LEVEL

0   Completely independent
1   Requires use of equipment or device
2   Requires help from another person for assistance, supervision, or teaching
3   Requires help from another person and equipment or device
4   Is dependent, does not participate in activity

This classification provides a quick way of identifying what level of assistance a person requires, which in turn allows intervention to be planned accordingly, allowing for independence, yet providing necessary support.

MANAGEMENT

A nursing management plan contains three concepts: collaboration with the patient, education, and action. These three concepts continue throughout management implementation. The patient must collaborate on the plan, have knowledge of his needs, the program itself, and any equipment necessary to meet these needs. He must take action himself or with the assistance of others. Two key areas in the management of a person with impaired mobility are providing mobility and support measures.

PROVIDING MOBILITY

If a person is able to perform any movements in bed, encourage him to do so. When those abilities are absent, the nurse or other support person must do these activities.

Positioning

A person must be turned and positioned in bed frequently enough to prevent the occurrence of pressure areas and to facilitate lung expansion. Turning is generally done every 2 to 4 hours but should be individualized, based on how the person responds to this time schedule.

Proper bed position is one in which the joints are supported in functional positions, avoiding abnormal weight on joints. Extremities need to be positioned in a way that prevents pressure on areas prone to skin breakdown. Extremities also are positioned to facilitate stretch of certain muscles, such as at the shoulder and hip. (References for illustrations of proper positioning are included in the bibliography.)

Range of Motion

Joints need to be moved through their range-of-motion twice a day. If done passively, take care to support the joint being moved. It should be moved only to the person's tolerance, which may be limited by pain or excessive stiffness (Fig. 11-6). Three repetitions of a movement are usually sufficient for maintaining range of motion. Patients should be given time and encouragement to complete programs taught by physical therapists.

Transfers and Sitting

An activity that is essential to regaining mobility is sitting (Fig. 11-7). It is a step on the way to further mobility, increases endurance, furthers the effects of gravity on body functions, distributes pressure more equally, and provides a psychological change of perspective.

For people requiring assistance in moving from the bed to a chair, nurses and other helpers need to use proper transfer techniques. A transfer can be either a safe and efficient operation, or one that is frightening and puts the patient and nurse at risk. The most essential elements of a good transfer are planning how it will occur (so that both parties know how to proceed), balance, maintaining a good base of support, using leg and

FIG. 11-7   Patient is shown in the progressive stages of mobility.

thigh muscles, and keeping the back straight (Fig. 11-8). Nurses and those caring for people who are unable to transfer independently need to know good transfer techniques so that they are not injured, and also to ensure that the transfer is safe and efficient for the person requiring assistance. (References for illustrating proper transfer techniques are included in the bibliography.)

Ambulation

Ambulation is the next activity of progressive mobility. This may begin with a few steps, increasing to the person's tolerance. Support devices are often necessary initially, or may be necessary for long-term use. De-

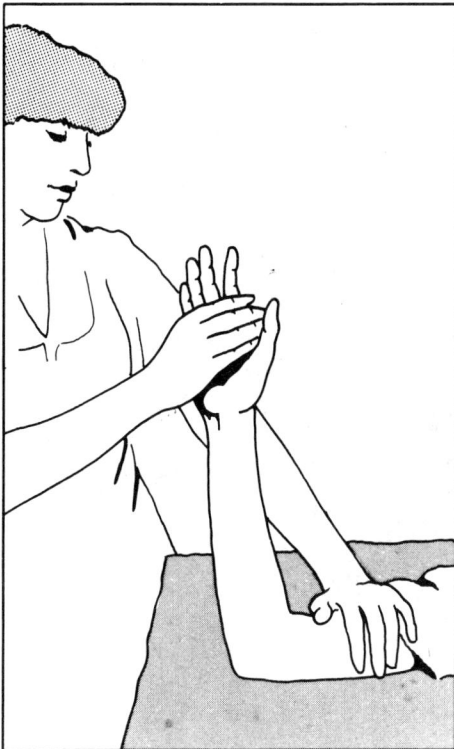

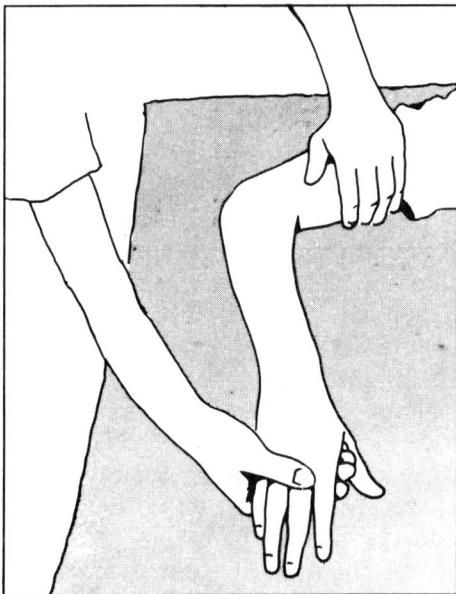

FIG. 11-6   Moving shoulder and elbow joints through range of motion.

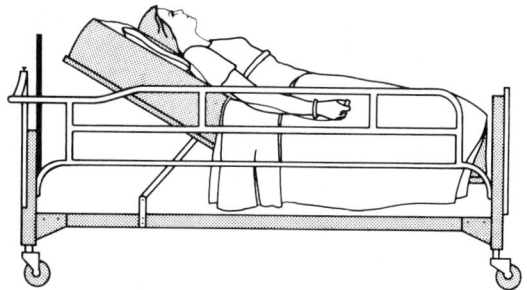

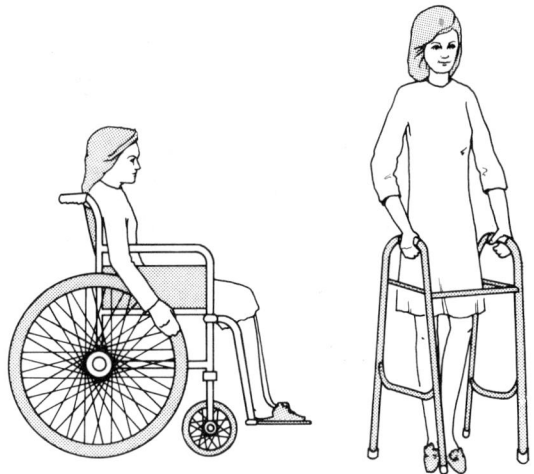

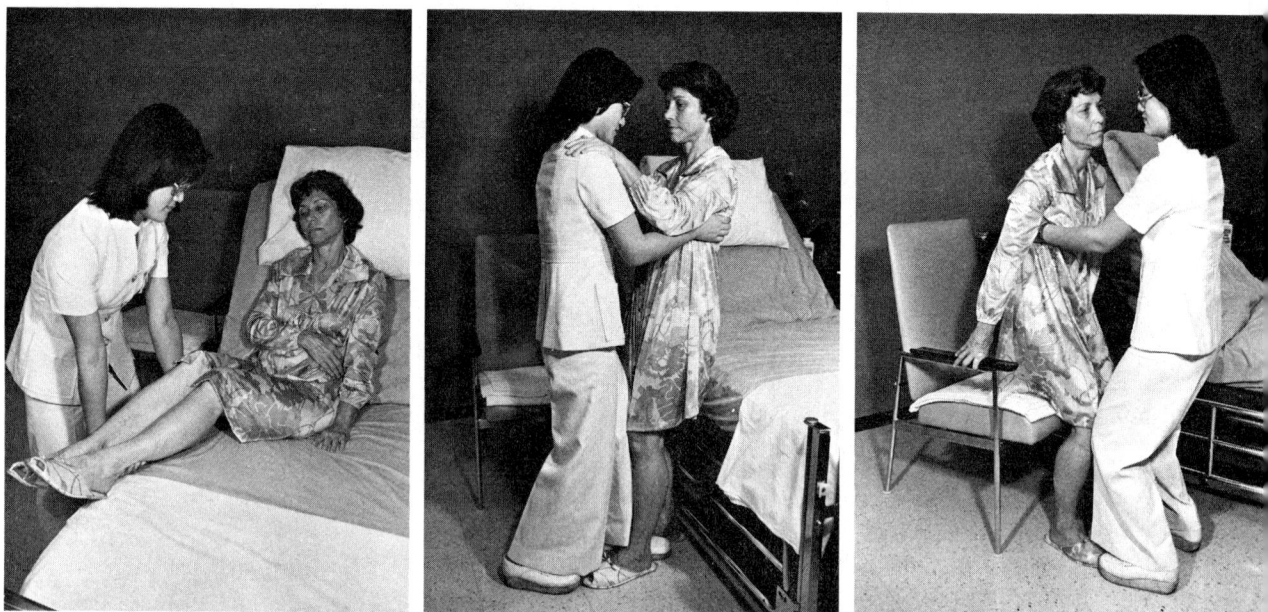

FIG. 11-8   *Proper body mechanics in a transfer technique. The nurse must keep a straight back and use her leg muscles.*

vices are used to increase a person's range of mobility and to provide necessary support.

Wheelchairs provide mobility on a temporary or permanent basis. Wheelchairs may be standard for those who have the ability to propel them with their upper extremities or with electric power. Wheelchairs also may be custom-made for sports that require different speeds and centers of gravity. Varying disabilities require different features, such as one-side drive for hemiplegics or altered balance for amputees.

Walkers have four-point bases of support for stability in ambulation. Some have wheels for people who are unable to lift and place the walker in front as they ambulate. Crutches are designed to give support to persons who have upper extremity strength, but have an alteration in the ability to bear weight on the lower extremities. Canes provide support on one side of the body, safety,

and stability when minimal assistance is necessary.

Exercise

When assisting a person from a state of immobility to maximum mobility, the person needs to use motion abilities in a gradually increasing manner. Daily living activities provide range of motion, endurance, and strengthening. Physical therapy appointments provide structured time for a person to work on gradually increasing mobility through range of motion, strengthening exercises, transfers, and ambulation training.

Bed exercise programs prescribed by therapists are important activities for the patient to complete in nontherapy time periods. Nurses can assist patients to carry out activities learned in therapy sessions and put them into practice 24 hours a day (Fig. 11-9).

Recreational activities are also a way to

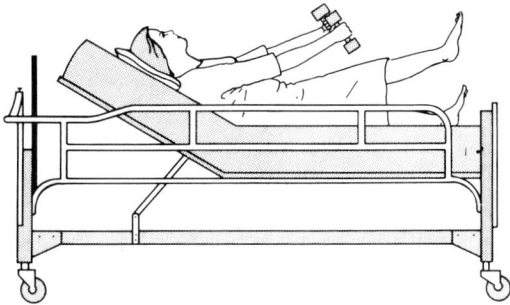

FIG. 11-9 In-bed exercise program.

increase a person's mobility. Getting out of bed and participating in an activity provides opportunity for physical motion. A quadriplegic who is swimming gains a different perspective on his abilities than when he is lying in bed.

SUPPORT MEASURES

Many support measures and assistive devices are available for a person with impaired mobility. They are designed to help prevent the complications that can occur in potential problem areas and to provide greater functional ability.

Positioning Aids

Devices are available to support body parts in good alignment. Foam rubber wedges, head supports, and other items help provide proper body positioning. Pillows are usually the most readily available and widely used positioning aids. Devices made of hard or soft plastic, lined with foam rubber to form a boot held on the foot with Velcro straps, are designed to help prevent foot-drop contracture and to relieve pressure on the foot and ankle area. These are generally more effective in relieving pressure and are not a substitute for good range of motion to the ankle joint.

Slings often are used for people with loss of function of an upper extremity. These should be used to support the shoulder joint against gravity when the person is sitting or standing. They should not be left in place for long periods, or contracture of the elbow and shoulder may occur.

Pressure Relief Devices

Devices for minimizing the occurrence of pressure sores are helpful and numerous. The air-fluidized bed, with air causing constant motion of silicone beads, can provide some advantages to persons with impaired mobility. Water and air mattresses also can be used if the person finds them satisfactory. The most easily obtainable and economical cushion or bed mattress is one made of foam rubber. Many in the "egg crate" style are available. Plain foam rubber is often adequate if the person adheres to a regular schedule of pressure relief by turning or lifting.

Other wheelchair cushions include silicone-filled pads, and water- or air-filled cushions. All have advantages and disadvantages. A person should consider convenience, ease of handling, and expense, in addition to effectiveness in relieving pressure.

Elastic Stockings

Elastic stockings help to prevent dependent edema and thrombus formation when a person is strictly immobilized. Although elevation of the lower extremities and exercise are more effective in managing these problems, some people must wear elastic stockings on a long-term basis.

Respiratory Therapy

Persons with greatly impaired mobility may need assistance, either by the nurse or respiratory therapist, in keeping their lungs clear and expanded. Regular coughing and deep breathing are basic practices. Use of devices such as inspiratory spirometers aid in expanding the lungs. Specialized treatment, for example, intermittent positive pressure or an ultrasonic nebulizer, may be needed if a person has problems with copious secretions or atelectasis. People with dyspnea may benefit from oxygen therapy. Many patients learn to administer their own treatments or use of oxygen.

Assistive Devices for Activities of Daily Living

Many devices now exist to help a person with impaired mobility perform activities of daily living (ADL). Occupational therapists specialize in evaluating, recommending, and instructing people in the use of these devices. Nurses should be familiar with these devices to make recommendations to patients and assist them in learning how to use them. Numerous catalogs are available through occupational therapy departments, libraries, and publications for persons with disabilities. These catalogs contain pictures of equipment and ordering information. Examples of this equipment include a universal cuff to strap on to the hand to hold objects when finger grasp is impaired, adapted eating utensils, grooming aids, dressing sticks, adapted kitchen utensils, and raised toilet seats.

INTAKE OF FOOD, FLUIDS, AND MEDICATION

Food, fluids, and medications all have an important role in managing the potential problems associated with impaired mobility. A well-balanced diet is essential for good health, especially when a person has a problem with mobility. Capacity for exercise is altered, so that a person must consume calories adequate to maintain a desired weight. Overweight can be an added burden in moving one's body, and underweight can limit strength.

A diet sufficient in fruits, vegetables, and other sources of bulk is essential to prevent constipation. When mobility is severely impaired, additional measures are needed. These include the addition of natural laxatives such as prune juice or medications like stool softeners, mild laxatives (senna, psyllium hydrophilic mucilloid), and suppositories. A natural, nonmedicated bowel program is the most desirable if it can be obtained. A fluid intake of 2000 ml a day or greater is desirable to prevent constipation. The primary principles of bowel management are to plan regular intervals of evacuation, usually every other day; to provide a stimulus to gastrointestinal motility, (i.e., in a position conducive to evacuation on a toilet or commode chair); and to keep the stool consistency soft and easily passable. If regular attention is given to bowel evacuation, constipation need not be a problem.

Fluid intake is also a consideration in managing renal and urinary problems. A fluid intake of 2000 ml or greater per day is helpful in preventing accumulation of calcium deposits in the kidneys. The acidic properties of cranberry juice are thought to have an effect on the renal system to lessen the possibilities of stone formation and infection.

Fluid intake is a consideration for people with altered urinary elimination. People doing intermittent catheterization must balance their intake with their catheterization schedule, so as not to distend the bladder. People with indwelling catheters need a high daily fluid intake to maintain a flow of urine through the urinary system to prevent stagnation and further infection. People who have difficulty getting to a toilet or commode sometimes tend to decrease their fluid intake for the sake of convenience. The nurse needs to observe if this is occurring and help to find ways to make voiding convenient.

Medications are sometimes necessary to

manage voiding problems associated with immobility. A patient with neurologic damage to the voiding mechanism may need either cholinergic medication (bethanechol chloride) to promote bladder emptying or anticholinergic medication (propantheline bromide), to eliminate spasticity of the bladder. Urinary tract infections, which are frequent complications of immobility, are treated with antibiotics; urinary antiseptics may be used to help prevent these infections.

Other medications used in altered mobility are those used to control pain and muscle spasticity. These medications frequently cause depression as a side-effect. A person's reactions to medication need to be observed closely to determine if the detrimental side-effect outweighs the desired effect.

PSYCHOLOGICAL AND SOCIAL INTERVENTION

Impaired mobility has profound effects on a person's psychological and social structure. Hammer and Kenan describe an immobilization cycle. This cycle begins with immobilization leading to confinement, sensory deprivation, and dulling of the sensory processes, leading to further internal immobilization.[5] Looking at the process of immobilization as a cycle lends itself to identifying points of intervention in that cycle to prevent adverse effects.

The establishment of a therapeutic relationship between the health care provider and the patient can produce a positive effect on the patient's psychological outlook. Use of all health professionals, nurses, physicians, social workers, therapists, and psychologists can provide a wide range of services to patients.

Nurses can lessen the effects of a person's confinement. Opportunities can be made for the person to maintain social interaction and relationships. Privacy can be facilitated. Getting a person up out of bed is a powerful act toward encouraging activity. Encouraging independence and promoting physical activity can counteract some of the restlessness and tension seen in patients with immobility. Intervention to promote activity covers a wide range, such as medicating and providing encouragement for a postoperative patient to ambulate, or sensitively eliciting the feelings of someone regarding his sexual needs and functional abilities and directing him to qualified counseling if necessary.

Sensory deprivation and dulling of the sensory processes can be lessened through structuring of the environment. As many sights and sounds of the person's life as possible should be in his altered environment. Technology has brought advances for sensory stimulation. In addition to radio, television, and tape recorders, small computers and electronic games are available as stimulators. Encourage personal belongings in the environment and contact with family and friends. Body image issues often surface when a person is given access to mirrors and is encouraged in grooming and dressing.

To achieve control over the problem of impaired mobility and its related problems, the person must have knowledge of those problems and their management. In providing education, consider the effect of immobility on learning and problem-solving.

Interventions that meet people's immediate needs have to occur before successful learning can take place. If a person is focusing on his weakness and inability to walk, he will not be receptive to extensive teaching. If concerns about sexual functioning are not addressed, the person probably will retain little information on other subjects. When the "immobilization cycle" is broken by interventions that foster sights, sounds, interactions, and activity, the potential for successful learning is greater.

CONCLUSION

The diagnosis of impaired mobility is multifaceted. Impaired mobility to varying degrees is seen in a wide variety of patient situations. Problems related to impaired mobility touch every aspect of a person's life. Nurses need to approach the problem of impaired mobility with an awareness of the extensive effects it can have on their patients. Intervention must begin early to keep a person mobile and to prevent a spiral of adverse effects.

REFERENCES

1. Asher AJ: The dangers of going to bed. Br Med J 2:967, 1947
2. Browse NL: The Physiology and Pathology of Bedrest. Springfield, IL, Charles C Thomas, 1965
3. Carlson CE: Psychosocial aspects of neurologic disability. Nurs Clin North Am 6:309, 1980
4. Deitrick JE, Whedon GD, Shorr E: Effects of immobilization upon various metabolic and physiologic functions of normal men. Am J Med 4:3, 1948
5. Hammer R, Kenan E: The psychological aspects of immobilization. In Steinberg FU (ed): The Immobilized Patient: Functional Pathology and Management. New York, Plenum Press, 1980
6. Kim MJ, Moritz A: Classification of Nursing Diagnoses: Proceedings of the Third and Fourth National Conferences. New York, McGraw–Hill, 1982
7. Muller EA: Influence of training and inactivity of muscle strength. Arch Phys Med Rehabil 51:449, 1970
8. Olson EV: The hazards of immobility. Am J Nurs 4:780, 1967
9. Riley L: Musculoskeletal system. In Judge RD, Zuidema G (eds): Clinical Examination: A Physiologic Approach, 3rd ed, p. 287. Boston, Little, Brown & Co, 1974
10. Steinberg FU: The Immobilized Patient: Functional Pathology and Management, p. 11–32. New York, Plenum Press, 1980
11. Vallbona C, Vogt FB, Carders D et al: The effect of bedrest on various parameters of physiological function. In: Part I: Review of the Literature on the Physiological Effects of Immobilization. Washington, DC, National Aeronautics and Space Administration, 1965
12. Zubek JP et al: Behavioral and physiological changes during prolonged immobilization plus perceptual deprivation. J Abnorm Psychol 74:230–236, 1969
13. Zubek JP, McNeil M: Perceptual deprivation phenomena: role of the recumbent position. J Abnorm Psychol 72:147, 1967

BIBLIOGRAPHY

Ford J, Duckworth B: Moving a patient safely, comfortably. Part 1: Patient positioning. Nurs 76 1:27, 1976

Ford J, Duckworth B: Moving a patient safely, comfortably. Part 2: Transferring. Nurs 76 2:58, 1976

Kennedy M, Pfeifer G: Current Practice in Nursing Care of the Adult. St. Louis, CV Mosby, 1979

Krusen F, Kottke F, Ellwood P: Handbook of Physical Medicine and Rehabilitation, 2nd ed. Philadelphia, WB Saunders, 1971

Martin N, Holt N, Hicks D: Comprehensive Rehabilitation Nursing. New York, McGraw–Hill, 1981

Millen H: Body Mechanics and Safe Transfer Techniques. Detroit, Aronsson Printing, 1978

Norris WC, Noble CE, Strickland SB: Spinal Injury Learning Series. Jackson, University of Mississippi, 1981

Rantz MJ, Courtial D: Lifting, Moving and Transferring Patients, 2nd ed. St. Louis, CV Mosby, 1981

Rusk H: Rehabilitation Medicine, 4th ed. St. Louis, CV Mosby, 1977

Sana J, Judge R: Physical Appraisal Methods in Nursing Practice, 2nd ed. p. 339. Boston, Little, Brown & Co., 1982

Spencer W et al: Physiologic concepts of immobilization. Arch Phys Med Rehabil 46:89, 1965

Stryker R: Rehabilitative Aspects of Acute and Chronic Nursing Care, 2nd ed. Philadelphia, WB Saunders, 1977

Urosevich PR (ed): Coping with Neurologic Disorders: Nursing 81 Books. Springhouse, PA, Intermed Communications, 1981

Urosevich PR (ed): Providing Early Mobility. Nursing 81 Books. Horsham, PA, Intermed Communications, 1981

12

Fever

Wilma Geels

HISTORICAL PERSPECTIVE

Fever is one of the oldest and most widely recognized manifestations of disease. Hippocratic writings contain precise descriptions of the fevers associated with malaria, bacterial pneumonia, and enteric disorders. The humoral theory of disease, which said that fever was due to the excess of bile, was the predominant medical belief through the eighteenth century.[3]

The systematic investigation of fever and temperature regulation began much more recently. In the late nineteenth century the French physiologist, Claude Bernard, discovered through scientific studies that the sources of animal heat came from the metabolic processes of the body. He also identified the role of the autonomic nervous system in regulating body temperature through changes in the flow of blood to the body surface. Thermoregulation was thus one of the key concepts in Bernard's theory of homeostasis, the belief that there is a constancy of the *milieu interieur* through the operation of dynamic mechanisms. It was also during this period that the role of the central nervous system (CNS) in regulating temperature in both health and fever was identified.

Instruments to measure temperature accurately were not developed until the seventeenth century, when the mercury thermometer first came into use. Its use as a diagnostic tool in medical practice became popular in 1871 on the basis of Wunderlich's writings, in which he advocated the taking and recording of patients' temperatures on a regular basis.[10]

Human beings are not unique in their ability to develop fever. It occurs in all mammals, reptiles, birds, amphibians, and fish. Because the ability to develop fever arose so early in evolution and is a common feature of animal life, many scientists believe it must have value as an adaptive or defense mechanism. Whether this is true has not yet been proven.

Regulation of body temperature and the changes that result in fever, its pathogenesis, assessment, and management are the focus of this chapter. Although other hyperthermic disorders are also discussed, the emphasis is on fever as a nonspecific manifestation of disease. The great variety of diseases that give rise to fever are not discussed, except when used as examples.

DEFINITIONS

To understand the phenomenon of fever, it is necessary to define some terms:

Fever: An elevation of body temperature above the normal range (99.4°F or greater) usually due to disease. Thermoregulatory mechanisms are functional but act to maintain an elevated temperature.

Pyrexia: Fever

Malignant hyperthermia: A severe rise in body temperature in which thermoregulatory mechanisms are not functioning

Defervescence: The period of subsidence of fever back to the normal temperature range

Homeothermy: Ability to maintain a constant temperature despite fluctuations in the environmental temperature. Mammals and birds are homeothermic (warm-blooded).

Poikilothermy: Variation in temperature according to that of the environment. Reptiles and fish are poikilothermic (cold-blooded).

Pyrogen: Any substance that can produce a fever

Endotoxin: Toxin from gram-negative bacteria, which acts on phagocytic cells to produce and release endogenous pyrogen.

Endogenous pyrogen: A protein released from phagocytic leukocytes that acts as a common mediator from immunologic, toxic, or infectious agents, and through interaction with heat-sensitive neurons in the anterior hypothalamus acts to raise the set-point of the hypothalamic thermostat.

MECHANISMS OF FEVER

NORMAL TEMPERATURE REGULATION

Human beings and other mammals and birds are *homeotherms.* Their body temperature is held constant despite great fluctuations in the environmental temperature, because their basal metabolic rate is high enough to regulate their internal temperature through changes in the amount of heat produced and lost by the body.

Reptiles and fish, on the other hand, are *poikilotherms.* Their temperatures vary with that of the environment, and therefore they need to rely on external sources of heat to maintain a relatively constant internal temperature.

Body temperature is a measurement of the balance between heat loss and heat production (see later in chapter). The ability of a person to maintain an internal body temperature within narrow limits (97°F–99°F), even though the environmental temperature may vary widely, is necessary for the person's safety and survival. It is accomplished through a negative feedback system, in which circulatory and neuroendocrine mechanisms are activated. The central mechanism for sensing temperature changes is located in the hypothalamus, which acts as a thermostat. Neurons in this area respond to changes in the temperature of the blood flowing through the hypothalamus by sending impulses to the heat-losing center in the preoptic area of the anterior hypothalamus, or to the heat-producing center in the posterior hypothalamus. When one center is activated, the other is depressed.

SOURCES OF HEAT PRODUCTION

Heat is being produced continuously in the body through the metabolism of all cells.

Metabolic activity, which is the total of all chemical reactions within the cells, is increased with the ingestion of food and through contraction of skeletal muscle. At rest, the greatest amount of heat is generated in the liver, but during exercise by far the greatest amount of heat production comes from the skeletal muscle. Heat produced by muscular activity is of particular significance because it can be adjusted according to need, whereas heat generated as a by-product of cellular metabolism is obligatory. The amount of heat generated by the skeletal muscle with exercise can increase the metabolic rate up to 20 times what it is at a resting state. The heat-dissipating mechanisms cannot keep pace with this acute increase in heat production, and the body temperature may rise to as high as 104°F. Because this elevation is not associated with disease and is usually of short duration, it is not considered to be fever.

A cold environment activates temperature-regulating mechanisms in the body, resulting in heat production and heat conservation. *Shivering* is a rhythmic contraction of muscles throughout the body. It can be a very effective means of heat production, generating up to four times the normal amount of heat.[8]

Hormones also have an effect on heat production and may be stimulated by cold. Thyroxine can increase the metabolic rate to as much as 100% above normal. The increase develops gradually, but its effects are long-lasting. Norepinephrine and epinephrine, on the other hand, produce a rapid increase in the metabolic rate, but their effects are short-lived. Strong emotions, such as anger, stimulate the sympathetic nervous system, which causes the release of epinephrine from nerve endings and the adrenal glands.

Heat conservation mechanisms in response to cold include cutaneous vasoconstriction and piloerection. The amount of blood flow through the skin can vary greatly, from almost nothing to as much as 30% of the cardiac output. With peripheral vasoconstriction, blood flow to the skin is greatly restricted, thus conserving heat in the core of the body. *Vasoconstriction* is a more precise mechanism used to conserve heat because of the fine-tuned elasticity of the blood vessels; whereas shivering, which is an all-or-nothing reaction, provides only a crude adjustment. *Piloerection*, or goose bumps, also occurs with cold. Although this is not an effective method of raising body temperature in human beings, in lower animals it acts as an insulator by entrapping a layer of air next to the skin, so that the amount of heat lost to the environment is lessened. Conservation of body heat can also be increased by the person's behavior. The amount or kind of clothes worn can act as insulation, and the indoor environmental temperature can be adjusted so that a stable body temperature is maintained.

SOURCES OF HEAT LOSS

Just as large amounts of heat are generated in the body, large amounts also are lost, usually in equivalent amounts. Thus, under normal conditions, the person is in *heat balance*. Four methods by which heat is lost from the body are radiation, conduction, convection, and vaporization, all of which function interdependently.

Radiation is the transfer of heat from one object to another with which it is not in contact. It accounts for approximately 60% of total heat lost from the body when the person is at complete rest under normal temperature conditions. The human body radiates heat in all directions, as do all objects and walls in a room. Consequently, radiation as a means of heat loss is only effective if the body temperature is greater than that of the surroundings. In a cold environment, heat loss through radiation may be detrimental to physiologic functioning. Because heat loss is proportional to surface area, a person in cold surroundings can reduce the amount of heat lost from the body by curling up, thus reducing the surface area exposed to the cold.

Conduction, the transfer of heat from one object to another with which it is in contact, occurs only as long as there is a temperature gradient. Because this gradient quickly disappears, the amount of heat lost in this way is very small. If, for example, a nude person sits in a metal chair, heat will be lost by conduction only when the temperature of the chair surface is lower than that of the body.

Convection is the removal of heat by air or water currents. As heat is conducted to air or water, convection currents carry it away. An increase in current velocity causes convection to occur more rapidly; thus, convection enhances heat loss by conduction. Convection also is effective only when there is a temperature gradient, with the surrounding temperature cooler than that of the body.

Vaporization, or evaporation of water, is the fourth physical process by which heat loss occurs and is the most important one when the ambient temperature is greater than the body temperature. Vaporization occurs almost constantly through insensible perspiration and through the respiratory passages. When both the ambient temperature and the humidity are high, vaporization does not occur as rapidly as in dry air, because the air is already saturated with moisture. As a result, people feel more uncomfortable on a hot, humid day because their ability to dissipate heat is less effective.

A high environmental temperature activates temperature-regulating mechanisms, which results in increased heat loss and decreased heat production. The body has a rich supply of cutaneous blood vessels, which when dilated carry heat away from the interior to the body surface, where it can be dissipated. The amount of blood flow to the body surface is under the control of vasomotor reflexes and can be adjusted with a great degree of precision, depending on the body's needs. Under ordinary cool conditions, the blood flow to the skin is about 400 ml/min in the average adult, but with maximum vasodilatation this flow can increase to 2800 ml/min.[8]

Sweating, including insensible water loss, is another mechanism activated by heat. It provides water to be vaporized, which results in loss of heat from the body. Persons who are born without sweat glands will have great difficulty maintaining a stable body temperature in hot weather and are prone to heat stroke, which is often fatal.

Insensible water loss from the skin and lungs is approximately 600 ml/day. In hot weather, however, the unacclimatized person can lose up to 700 ml/hr, and with acclimatization this can be increased to 1500 ml/hr. This occurs because of increased output from the sweat glands, not through the development of new ones. Also, as a person becomes acclimatized, the amount of sodium chloride in the sweat decreases, because of an increased production of aldosterone. As a result, after 4 to 6 weeks of exposure to high temperatures, the sodium chloride loss is 3 to 5 g/day, instead of the 15 g/day prior to acclimatization.

A small increase in the amount of heat lost from the body can occur with an increase in the respiratory rate, but this is not significant in human beings. Table 12-1 summarizes these temperature-regulating mechanisms.

REGULATION OF BODY TEMPERATURE: THE HYPOTHALAMIC THERMOSTAT

Maintenance of body temperature within a relatively narrow range is under the control

Table 12-1
TEMPERATURE-REGULATING MECHANISMS

TEMPERATURE-INCREASING MECHANISMS	TEMPERATURE-DECREASING MECHANISMS
SOURCES OF HEAT PRODUCTION	SOURCES OF HEAT LOSS
Exercise	Radiation
Increased basal metabolic rate	Conduction
Specific dynamic action of food	Convection
Hormones (estrogen and testosterone)	Vaporization
MECHANISMS ACTIVATED BY COLD	MECHANISMS ACTIVATED BY HEAT
Shivering	Cutaneous vasodilatation
Cutaneous vasoconstriction	Sweating (sudomotor)
Piloerection	Increased respiratory rate
Increased output of thyroxine, norepinephrine, and epinephrine	

of the hypothalamus and is the result of a negative feedback system, which has three elements. First, there are *sensors* or *receptors*, located in the hypothalamus, that sense the existing central temperature. Heat-sensitive neurons, located in the preoptic area of the anterior hypothalamus, increase their firing rate when there is a rise of temperature of the blood circulating through the area. Likewise, cold receptors, located in the posterior hypothalamus, skin, and spinal cord, increase their output with a drop in body temperature. The second element of the negative feedback system is the *effector mechanism*, consisting of the vasomotor, sudomotor, and metabolic elements, all of which have been discussed previously. The third element in the system is the *integrator* or *controller mechanism*, also located in the hypothalamus, that determines whether the temperature is too high or too low and activates the appropriate mechanism to maintain a constant set-point of central temperature.[15] The *hypothalamic thermostat* is the term used for this thermoregulatory mechanism. Precisely how this thermoregulatory integrator works is not known.

NORMAL BODY TEMPERATURE

Normal temperature refers to the core body temperature and not the temperature of the skin, which varies according to that of the environment. The most practical way to measure the core temperature accurately is either orally or rectally, areas that have a rich blood supply and therefore reflect the temperature of the hypothalamus.

Most people think of the normal body temperature as 98.6°F, but this belief is only partially accurate. More precisely, 98.6°F is the normal body temperature for most adults when taken orally in the middle of the day. Normal temperature, which ranges between 97°F and 99°F, varies according to the time of day. The temperature is generally lowest in the early morning and gradually rises until it peaks in the late afternoon. This is true even for most people who work at night and sleep during the day.

Other factors that have an influence on normal body temperature are sex, age, and disease. Sexual differences in body temperature are mainly due to hormonal influences. Both estrogen and testosterone increase the rate of metabolism and thus body temperature. Estrogen also increases fat deposition in the subcutaneous tissue, which acts as insulation for women. Thus women maintain their internal temperature more evenly than do men, who tend to be more lean and muscular. Another difference is that premenopausal women will have a rise in body temperature of 0.5°F to 1.0°F at the time of ovulation, due to the effect of progesterone. The mechanism by which progesterone affects the body temperature is not known.

Age also influences normal body temperature. Both the very young and the very old have difficulty maintaining a normal temperature with extremes in environmental temperature; the young because their thermoregulatory mechanisms are not yet fully developed, the elderly because their peripheral circulation is decreased because of the effects of aging.

Fever, an elevation of body temperature due to disease, causes an increase in the rate of cellular metabolism. For each 1°F rise in temperature, the metabolic rate increases 7%.[7] This increase in heat production through increased metabolic rate has the tendency, therefore, to heighten a fever. A lower body temperature, on the other hand, slows down the rate of metabolism and heat production, which in turn lowers the body temperature still further.

PATHOPHYSIOLOGY OF FEVER

Fever has had a long history as a hallmark of disease. In fact, for many centuries fever and disease were considered synonymous. But only in more recent times have the mechanisms and functions of fever become more evident through scientific investigation.

Fever is not an unregulated elevation of body temperature. It is a resetting of the hypothalamic thermostat to a higher set-point in response to a variety of stimuli. Stimuli capable of inducing a fever by raising the set-point are known as *pyrogens.*

When the set-point is at a higher level, the person will feel cold until the internal temperature reaches that of the set-point. The mechanisms usually activated by a cold environmental temperature are now used to bring the body temperature up to its new set-point. Peripheral vasoconstriction and shivering occur as a means of conserving heat in the core of the body. The person whose temperature is rising may also curl up in bed under heavy blankets until he feels warm, that is, when the body temperature coincides with the new higher set-point. If the set-point has changed rapidly, the person may even experience shaking chills until the high temperature has been reached, at which time he will feel neither hot nor cold even though his temperature may be as high as 103°F. As long as the pyrogen that caused the elevation in the set-point continues to act, the body temperature will be regulated at this higher level, usually with the same diurnal variation as occurs normally.

Once the precipitating factor is no longer in effect, the set-point is lowered back to normal with the result that the person suddenly feels hot, perspires profusely, and experiences peripheral vasodilatation, which dissipates the heat from the body.

ENDOGENOUS PYROGEN

Numerous substances have been found to cause fever experimentally in animals, both vertebrates and invertebrates. Collectively, these fever-producing substances are known as *pyrogens* and include gram-positive bacteria and some of their exotoxins, gram-negative bacterial endotoxins, pathogenic fungi, certain steroids, antigen–antibody complexes, and a number of nonorganic substances.[5] Almost all fall under one of three categories of fever-producing substances: infectious agents, immunologic substances, and toxic substances.

Although the fever induced by these different agents has varying characteristics, such as time and duration of onset, degree of elevation, and duration, the mechanism by which fever is induced is similar in all. These substances trigger the production of *endogenous pyrogen* (EP), a protein mediator produced by phagocytic leukocytes, which acts on the hypothalamic thermostat to raise the set-point. The precise method by which EP interacts with the thermoregulatory mechanism is not known (Fig. 12-1).[4] EP may directly alter the activity of the heat-sensitive neurons in the hypothalamus, or it may act through an intermediate substance, like prostaglandins. Injection of prostaglandins into the hypothalamus causes a rapid rise in temperature; the antipyretic effect of aspirin is

FIG. 12-1 *Pathogenesis of fever.*

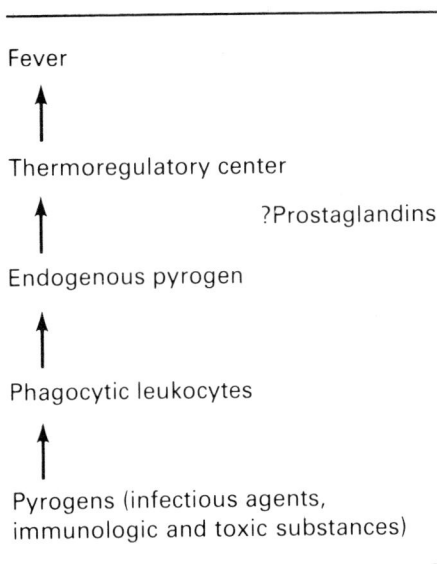

Fever

↑

Thermoregulatory center

↑   ?Prostaglandins

Endogenous pyrogen

↑

Phagocytic leukocytes

↑

Pyrogens (infectious agents, immunologic and toxic substances)

thought to be due to its inhibitory effect on prostaglandin synthesis. The exact role of prostaglandins in fever however has not yet been elucidated and is currently a matter of debate.[7]

DEHYDRATION

In addition to endogenous pyrogen as a direct cause of fever, dehydration can also cause a rise in body temperature, partly because there is a decrease in the amount of fluid available for sweating, but also through a direct effect on the hypothalamic thermostat.[8] Dehydration as a cause of fever is more important in infants than it is in adults, in whom it has rarely been shown to be the cause of fever.[14]

FUNCTION OF FEVER

Does fever serve any purpose? Is it either harmful or beneficial to its host or is it neither? Because the ability of the organism to develop fever began early in evolution and has continued up to the present time, this trait would seem to have survival value. For many years fever was thought to be beneficial. Hippocrates thought that fever helped the body to fight infection. Fever therapy was used to treat many diseases, including gonorrhea and syphilis. Even though fever therapy has had some value, the question of whether naturally occurring fever associated with disease is beneficial is not proven by that fact.

Only in recent years have experiments provided information concerning the adaptive value of fever. Laboratory experiments with lizards (which are poikilotherms) injected with live bacteria demonstrated that those lizards placed in a high environmental temperature, and who therefore developed a fever, survived longer than those in cooler surroundings, who did not develop a fever.

Thus, in that class of animals, fever clearly has been shown to have survival value.[10]

Whether this is true for human beings, who are homeothermic, and whether it is true when the fever is not experimental but an accompaniment of disease, has not yet been proven. Such studies would be difficult, if not unethical, to do; therefore, at present one can only speculate on the adaptive value of fever. Fever may help the infected host by increasing the activity of the body's defense mechanisms, such as increased activity of phagocytes. Fever does require a considerable expenditure of energy, which would be maladaptive for survival if fever were harmful to the host. Therefore, authorities believe fever *does* have survival value, even though this has not been demonstrated in human beings.

The belief that fever *per se* is harmful and should be treated coincided with widespread availability of antipyretic drugs at the end of the nineteenth century.

High temperatures can have detrimental effects, especially in the elderly, whose energy reserves are more limited. Fever increases the metabolic rate, and causes loss of weight and nitrogen excretion. The work and rate of the heart are increased. For every 1°F temperature elevation, the heart rate is increased by ten beats per minute. Headache, myalgias, and arthralgia often accompany fever, along with a general feeling of malaise and unpleasant warmth. Fever blisters, which usually occur in the mouth during febrile periods, are caused by a virus that seems to be activated by heat.[2]

MALIGNANT HYPERTHERMIA

Body temperature is elevated in both fever and hyperthermia, but these terms are not synonymous. In fever, the thermoregulatory mechanisms are still operating but at a higher set-point. *Hyperthermia,* on the other hand, is an elevation of temperature that occurs when the core body temperature is higher than that of the hypothalamic thermostat, and therefore is not under its control. It results from the inability of the body to dissipate its heat load. Heat production exceeds heat loss, either because of increase in heat production or because of a reduction in the activity of the heat loss mechanisms (e.g., radiation or evaporation).

There are three categories of hyperthermia:

1. Exercise hyperthermia
2. Hyperthermia due to inadequate heat dissipation
3. Hyperthermia resulting from pathologic or pharmacologic impairments of the thermoregulatory mechanisms.

Exercise hyperthermia occurs after vigorous exercise and is the result of the internal heat load produced by the exercise itself. It can occur even though the person is in good physical condition. Symptoms include muscle cramps and muscle spasms and a rise in temperature. It is usually a benign condition, since it is self-limiting, ending when the exercise is terminated; therefore, no treatment is needed other than fluid and electrolyte replacement.

Hyperthermia due to inadequate heat dissipation occurs with heat stroke. Heat stroke is a serious disorder that is not self-limiting. If it is not treated, the body will continue to store heat, causing lethal elevations of temperature. Heat stroke occurs only in hot, humid environments and is accompanied by a lack of sweating. It occurs most often when a person has not been acclimated to working in such an environment and thus has a limited adaptive capacity. The heat-dissipating mechanisms, such as peripheral vasodilatation and sweating, fail, because the body is unable to maintain an adequate, circulating blood volume in the peripheral vessels. Because the working muscle and the cutaneous circulation require large portions of the cardiac output, the heart is unable to meet the demands.[16] The person with heat stroke may become dizzy, then delirious, and eventually may lose consciousness. The body temperature rises to 106°F or higher. Such an extreme elevation is very damaging to body tissues, especially the brain, liver, and kidneys, causing local hemorrhages and degeneration of the parenchymal cells.[8] Treatment must be immediate and drastic, but even with treatment, the mortality rate is high. Because the hypothalamic thermostat has not been reset to a higher level, aspirin, which acts directly on the hypothalamus, is not an effective treatment for heat stroke. Whole-body cooling by immersion in ice water or by sponging the skin is recommended. Additional treatment consists of supportive therapy to treat circulatory collapse and fluid and electrolyte loss.

Hyperthermic disorders resulting from pathologic or pharmacologic impairments include hypothalamic lesions, such as those resulting from a cerebral vascular accident (CVA) or tumor invasion, malignant hyperthermia due to anesthesia and other pharmacologic agents, and hypermetabolic disorders such as "thyroid storm." These conditions are relatively rare and like heat stroke require immediate intervention by whole-body cooling if death is to be prevented.

NURSING ASSESSMENT

SUBJECTIVE DATA

Fever is a common manifestation of many diseases and disorders, ranging from acute infection, in which the temperature rise may be abrupt and severe, to some others, in which there is a low-grade fever that persists for weeks. Before a diagnosis can be made, a thorough history and physical examination are necessary. When taking the patient's history, obtain information about the fever itself: its duration, highest elevation, and daily pattern. Some people are aware immediately when their temperature rises, whereas others may be unaware of the presence of a fever for some time. Ask the patient when the fever started and what the first symptoms were.

Note associated signs and symptoms, such as weight loss, lack of appetite, nausea and vomiting, cough, headaches or other pain, diarrhea or constipation, a feeling of weakness and lethargy, or general malaise. The patient may have a feeling of generalized discomfort. The nurse also should ask the patient questions pertaining to his occupation, current medications taken, recent foreign travel, and recent surgical operations or other illnesses. Any one of these things may be a contributing factor to the person's fever.

OBJECTIVE DATA

Begin the physical examination by noting the person's overall appearance. Does the person look sick, flushed, dehydrated, in pain? Examination of the abdomen for masses, the lungs for decreased breath sounds or adventitious sounds, and the skin for lesions or petechiae, are part of the standard work-up in looking for the cause of the fever. A mass in the abdomen may be indicative of a neoplasm. An enlarged spleen may be because of infection, lymphoma, or leukemia. An enlarged liver may indicate a liver abscess or metastatic cancer. If both the liver and spleen are enlarged, the cause may be chronic infection, leukemia, lymphoma, or cirrhosis. Palpation of the lymph nodes should also be carefully done. Tender, enlarged lymph nodes usually indicate the presence of an infection, while non-tender nodes would lead one to suspect a malignancy.

Obtain an oral or rectal temperature. A temperature record kept by the patient for several days can provide information regarding the pattern of the fever. A number of fever patterns, such as intermittent, remittent, sustained, and hectic or septic patterns, have frequently been described in both nursing and medical texts. Definitions of fever patterns follow:

Intermittent: The temperature is elevated for periods of time but falls to normal at some time each day.
Remittent: The temperature rises and falls each day but does not return to normal.
Sustained: The temperature is elevated with less than a 0.5°F variation during a 24-hr period.
Relapsing: Short, febrile periods are interspersed with longer periods of normal temperature.
Hectic or septic: Fever in which there are wide variations of at least 2.5°F each day.

Even though these fever patterns frequently are described in books, there is little consistency between specific diseases and certain fever patterns. Musher and his colleagues studied large numbers of patients with fever, both prospectively and retrospectively, and found that, with few exceptions, fever patterns were not helpful in diagnosis. Patients who had either intermittent or remittent fevers because of infection usually followed a diurnal pattern of higher temperature in the late afternoon, and patients with CNS damage were more likely to have a sustained fever pattern, but overall there were many variations in the patterns.[12]

Increased blood pressure, pulse, and respiratory rates usually accompany a fever, because of the increased metabolic rate that speeds up all body processes. Measure these vital signs at the same time the temperature is taken. If the fever is due to a drug reaction, however, these accompanying signs and symptoms are less prominent.

PARACLINICAL DATA

Diagnostic studies that may be helpful are complete blood count (c.b.c.), chest x-ray, urinalysis, blood cultures, cultures of other body secretions and fluids such as urine and sputum, and surgical or other traumatic wounds. There are a multitude of other tests that may be needed to make a diagnosis, depending on the information obtained in the history and physical examination.

NURSING DIAGNOSIS

Diagnosis of the medical disorder causing the fever is primarily the responsibility of the physician. The nurse should be aware of those patients who are at risk for developing fever and should observe them for associated signs and symptoms. The nurse is also responsible for determining the route and frequency of temperature checks, for their accurate and prompt recording, and for reporting abnormalities.

FEVER ASSOCIATED WITH DISEASE

Disease categories that often give rise to fever are:

All infectious diseases
Mechanical trauma
Neoplastic diseases (e.g., Hodgkin's disease and leukemia)
Hematopoietic disorders

Vascular disorders (e.g., CVAs, pulmonary embolus, and myocardial infarction)

Immunologic disorders, including collagen diseases and drug fevers

The common features of these diverse conditions is their ability to cause tissue damage, which in some way stimulates the release of pyrogens, which act on the thermoregulatory mechanism to increase the setpoint. Febrile illnesses almost never cause temperature elevations above 106°F, which is the critical safety level. Above that level, irreversible tissue damage occurs. Temperatures below that level in an otherwise healthy adult are well tolerated if supportive therapy is given. Furthermore, failure to develop a fever in the presence of severe infection is usually a poor prognostic sign.[2]

FEVER RELATED TO POSTOPERATIVE SOURCES

After a surgical operation, the patient often has a low-grade fever of 99.4° to 100°F for 2 or 3 days, which may be because of tissue damage. A marked temperature elevation during that time, however, is usually due to atelectasis. There are a number of reasons why the postoperative patient is at risk for atelectasis. Coughing and deep-breathing exercises are painful; so the patient is apt to breath shallowly. The narcotics used for pain control are also respiratory depressants and thus lead to shallow breathing. Furthermore, the anesthetic agents used in surgery can be irritating to the respiratory passages, causing an increase in mucus secretion. If this is not cleared by coughing and deep-breathing, atelectasis and fever result.

Later in the postoperative period, other causes of fever are urinary tract infection, wound infection, or thrombophlebitis. Diag-

nosis of these conditions usually is not difficult because of their prominent associated signs and symptoms.

FEVER OF UNDETERMINED ORIGIN

Fever of undetermined origin (FUO) is defined as a temperature of 101°F or greater, on numerous occasions that lasts 3 or more weeks and for which a cause has not been found after 1 week of in-hospital evaluation.[6]

Esposito and Gluckman, in a comprehensive review of patients with FUO, concluded that only a small number of those patients are never diagnosed. Of those patients who were undiagnosed at the time of discharge from the hospital, most defervesced spontaneously and were not later found to have serious disease. Most of the patients whose initial diagnosis was FUO eventually were found to have a common disorder, with fever being an atypical manifestation. One of the distinguishing features of patients with FUO caused by an underlying disease is prominent weight loss. FUO unaccompanied by weight loss is usually due to a benign, self-limiting disease.[6]

FACTITIOUS OR SPURIOUS FEVER

Factitious or spurious fever is not a common problem, but when it occurs, it can be difficult to diagnose and treat. Patients who have factitious fevers fall into one of two categories: those with an elevated temperature because of thermometer manipulation, or those who have a real but self-induced fever because of ingestion or injection of some pyrogenic substance into their bodies. Diagnosis of factitious fever is often difficult and arrived at only after a prolonged and costly evaluation.

Methods used to fake a fever are use of

external heat on the thermometer, heating the oral cavity by holding hot liquids in the mouth just before the temperature is taken, shaking the thermometer, and using friction on the thermometer by rubbing it between one's hands. Except for heating the oral cavity, the methods of faking a fever rely on the use of a mercury thermometer. The electronic thermometer in use in many hospitals is not subject to manipulation by the patient.

The nurse should be alert to the possibility of factitious fever in the patient with FUO under the following conditions:[11]

Lack of normal diurnal variation in the temperature variation
Normal pulse rate in the presence of an abrupt rise in temperature
Rapid defervescence without diaphoresis
A temperature recording of 106°F or higher (rarely occurs in adults)

Patients who have a fever because of self-induced infections may be detected through blood cultures that grow numerous kinds of bacteria, and especially those that rarely cause bacteremia in an otherwise healthy adult. Patients with self-induced infection often have an underlying psychiatric disorder, and treatment of their illness is difficult and complex.[1]

MANAGEMENT

Because of its long association with disease, the presence of a fever is alarming to both patients and health care personnel, and the immediate response may be to treat the fever. This is not always necessary or even desirable because of its possible adaptive value. Treatment of the fever before determining its cause may mask clues that would lead to a diagnosis. In addition, the measures used to

treat fever can themselves have harmful effects. Thus, unless the temperature elevation is life-threatening, it is preferable to determine the cause of the fever before treating it.

Patients tolerate moderately high temperatures (104°F or less) remarkably well, unless they are elderly or debilitated, in which case the increased energy demands on the heart may lead to cardiac failure. For the otherwise healthy adult, interventions to treat the fever itself are not necessary as long as fluids and electrolytes are replaced and the patient's nutritional status is monitored.

MANAGEMENT OF POSTOPERATIVE FEVER

The patient with postoperative atelectasis often develops a fever. In this case it is the atelectasis that needs to be treated, not the fever. Surgical patients need to cough and deep breathe at regular intervals, and to become progressively more active.

If the fever source is an indwelling catheter, it needs to be removed promptly and, if possible, not reinserted. Thrombophlebitis, another cause of postoperative fever, is treated with bed rest, elevation of the extremity, and local heat. Surgical wound infections as a cause of fever usually occur 5 to 7 days postoperatively. The wound usually is opened to allow for drainage, is packed, and it then heals by secondary intention. Although the nurse can do little to prevent wound infections, she should be alert to early signs and symptoms, such as redness, tenderness, or purulent discharge from the wound.

ANTIPYRETICS AND HYPOTHERMIA MEASURES

Antipyretics lower the temperature by resetting the hypothalamic thermostat back to its normal level. They are not usually given unless the temperature is 102°F or higher. When used, they are more effective if given frequently and in small doses to avoid large temperature swings. The goal should not be to return the temperature to normal, but only to a point at which energy demands on the body are lessened.

Whole-body cooling by sponging, immersion, or hypothermia machines is the treatment of choice in heat stroke, along with vigorous massage of the skin, which brings more blood to the body surface and so helps to dissipate the heat load.[9] Whole-body cooling also is used in cases in which the patient's fever is high (103°F or greater) and is dangerous to the patient's health. When used to treat fever, use whole-body cooling in conjunction with antipyretics. If antipyretics are not also used, the body's heat-conserving mechanisms, such as shivering and vasoconstriction, will be activated. Only when the body's thermostat has been reset will the other temperature-lowering methods be effective.

SUPPORTIVE THERAPY AND COMFORT MEASURES

Patients with temperature elevations need periods of quiet and rest to reduce the energy demands on the body. Comfort measures such as good hygiene and removal of damp bedding and wet gowns should be routine.

Supportive therapy includes fluids and electrolyte replacement and nutritional support. Increased sweating that occurs with fever can cause a fluid loss of up to 3 liters a day. Sodium chloride also will be lost through perspiration and must be replaced. Broth and Gatorade are good sources of fluids and electrolytes, but if the patient cannot take fluids orally, replacement will need to be given intravenously. Fluid replacement should be sufficient to produce at least 1000 ml urine per day.

The increased metabolism that occurs with fever will lead to loss of weight unless the patient takes in additional calories. Unfortunately, the febrile patient is often anorexic or may even have nausea and vomiting. If he is able to eat, encourage high-calorie, high-protein foods. If a dietitian is available, he or she should be consulted for advice and suggestions about the palatability and nutritional value of various foods. If the fever does not continue for more than a week and if the patient is otherwise healthy, a decreased food intake can be tolerated by most patients for this period of time. If lack of caloric intake persists, more drastic measures, such as total parenteral nutrition, will need to be started. Generally however, fluid and electrolyte replacement is more urgent than is caloric replacement. Severe dehydration will occur long before there is a critical weight loss.

TEMPERATURE-TAKING ROUTINES

Monitoring the febrile patients' temperature is the principal way to determine whether the therapeutic measures are effective. In general, the higher the temperature, the more frequently it should be taken, especially if it is rising rapidly. In such cases, a battery-powered rectal probe should be inserted so that the temperature can be monitored continuously without disturbing the patient.

At other times, unless contraindicated, oral temperature readings are as accurate as the rectal temperature, provided the thermometer is placed correctly, in the sublingual pocket, and is left in place for a sufficient length of time (7 minutes if one is using a mercury thermometer).[13]

If the temperature is measured rectally by a mercury thermometer, an accurate reading can be obtained in 3 minutes. In most people the rectal temperature is approximately 1°F higher than the oral temperature and the axillary temperature is about 1°F lower than that of the oral cavity. If one is to get an accurate axillary temperature, the thermometer must be left in place at least 10 minutes. Because it does not reflect as accurately the core temperature as do the other two areas, axillary temperatures should be used only when the oral and rectal routes are not available.

PATIENT EDUCATION

Many people do not know when to seek medical help for a fever or how to treat it properly themselves. Whether the person with a fever should obtain medical help depends both on the degree and duration of the fever, and the presence of other signs and symptoms. Temperatures of less than 104°F for 2 or 3 days in an otherwise healthy adult are not harmful, but if other signs and symptoms such as jaundice, prolonged vomiting, or enlarged lymph nodes are present, advise the person to get medical care. Such signs could be indicative of a potentially serious illness requiring medical intervention. Or if the person who has a cold for a week and continues to have a cough also suddenly develops a fever of 102°F, medical care should be obtained to rule out pneumonia.

SELF-CARE MEASURES

If the person is at home, he should be advised to drink large amounts (3 liters a day or more) of fluid and to eat high-calorie, high-protein foods, such as milk shakes and eggnog. Keep physical exertion to a minimum, although most people with a fever will not want to be very active. Fevers associated with self-limiting diseases such as viral infections usually do not need medical attention. Antipyretics are not necessary, but if the person wishes to take them for symptomatic relief, he should be advised to take them at regular intervals until the temperature drops to 101°F, rather than to 98.6°F.

Tell the person to take and record his temperature at regular intervals and to report acute elevations above 103°F. If the fever persists or if more worrisome signs and symptoms arise, such as persistent vomiting, the person may need to be hospitalized for evaluation and care.

SUMMARY

Body temperature is a measurement of the balance between heat production and heat loss, and is maintained within a narrow range through a complex, negative feedback system. Fever, a nonspecific sign of disease, represents a rise in the set-point of the hypothalamic thermostat in response to the action of pyrogens on the thermostat.

Fever by itself is not diagnostic of any one disease; however, its presence is usually indicative of some disorder in the body. Assessment and diagnosis of the cause of fever are necessary before treatment is begun. Whether treatment of the fever itself is warranted is controversial. Antipyretics should not automatically be used unless the temperature is dangerously high. Supportive measures such as fluid and electrolyte replacement and nutritional support are necessary for the patient's comfort and welfare.

REFERENCES

1. Aduan RP et al: Factitious fever and self-induced infection. Ann Intern Med 90:230–242, 1979
2. Atkins E: Fever, In: MacBryde CM, Blacklow RS

(eds): Signs and Symptoms, 5th ed. pp 451–475. Philadelphia, JB Lippincott, 1970

3. Atkins E, Bodel P: Clinical Fever: Its history, manifestations, and pathogenesis. Fed Proc 38:57–63, 1979

4. Atkins E, Bodel P: Fever. N Engl J Med 286:27–34, 1972

5. Bernheim HA, Block LH, Atkins E: Fever: Pathogenesis, pathophysiology, and purpose. Ann Intern Med 91:261–270, 1979

6. Esposito AL, Gleckman RA: A diagnostic approach to the adult with fever of unknown origin. Arch Intern Med 139:575–579, 1979

7. Ganong WF: Review of Medical Physiology, 10th ed. Los Gatos, CA, Lange Medical Press, 1981

8. Guyton AC: Textbook of Medical Physiology, 6th ed. Philadelphia, WB Saunders, 1981

9. Keush GT: Fever: To be or not to be. NY State J Med 76:1998–2001, 1976

10. Kluger MJ: Temperature regulation, fever, and disease. In Robertson D (ed): International Review of Physiology, Environmental Physiology III, Vol 20. Baltimore, University Park Press, 1979

11. Lee R, Atkins E: Spurious fever. Am J Nurs 72:1094–1095, 1972

12. Musher D et al: Fever patterns: Their lack of clinical significance. Arch Intern Med 139:25–1228, 1979

13. Nichols GH, Kucha D: Taking adult temperatures. Am J Nurs 72:1091–1093, 1972

14. Petersdorf RG: Alteration in body temperature. In Wintrobe MM et al (eds): Harrison's Principles of Internal Medicine. New York, McGraw–Hill, 1974

15. Snell ES, Atkins E: The mechanisms of fever. In Bittar EE, Bittar N (eds): The Biological Basis of Medicine, Vol 2. New York, Academic Press, 1968

16. Stitt J: Fever versus hyperthermia. Fed Proc 38:39–43, 1979

BIBLIOGRAPHY

Benzinger TD: The human thermostat. Sci Am 204:134–144, 1961

Davis–Sharts J: Mechanisms and manifestations of fever. Am J Nurs 78:1874–1877, 1978

Dinarello C: Production of endogenous pyrogen. Fed Proc 38:52–56, 1979

Dinarello C, Wolff SH: Pathogenesis of fever in man. New Engl J Med 298:607–612, 1978

DuBois EF: Fever and the Regulation of Body Temperature. Springfield, IL, Charles C Thomas, 1948

Erickson R: Oral temperature differences in relation to thermometer technique. Nurs Res 29:157–164, 1980

Kluger M: Fever and survival. Science 188:166–168, 1975

Simon HB: Extreme pyrexia in man. In Lipton J (ed): Fever. New York, Raven Press, 1980

13

Skin Changes

Penelope Paul
Judith Holcombe

Skin changes are among the most common symptoms that people experience. In 1979, 30,650,000 visits to physicians' offices resulted from symptoms involving the skin, hair, and nails.[69] Overall, skin rashes were the ninth most common reason for seeing a physician. The estimate of the amount of money Americans spend each year on emollients is $300 million.[75]

Actual or potential impairment in skin integrity has important implications for peoples' physical and psychosocial well-being. Loss of integrity compromises the functions of the skin. Of particular significance is the threat of infection. Skin changes can be associated with much discomfort, in the form of pain or itching. The fact that many skin changes are highly visible and difficult to conceal may affect peoples' perceptions of self and their ability or willingness to participate in social activities.

Through the application of the nursing process, nurses have significant roles in the assessment and management of actual or potential skin changes and their effects on persons. It is not within the scope of this chapter to discuss the assessment and management of all skin changes; however, we will focus on four skin changes that frequently concern nurses: dry skin, rashes, decubitus ulcers, and wounds. In the discussion of each of these problems, emphasis is placed on the causative and contributing factors and the nursing management. The psychosocial impact of skin changes in general are addressed in the chapter on body image changes.

MECHANISMS OF SKIN CHANGES

NORMAL STRUCTURE AND PHYSIOLOGY

The skin is the largest organ in the body. It provides the interface between the body and the environment. As such, intact skin serves a number of important functions. Sensations such as touch, which are mediated by cutaneous nerves, provide necessary information about the environment. The skin provides a barrier to the introduction of foreign materials, including microorganisms. However, based upon investigations with rats, it is possible that chemical contaminants in the environment, such as chlorophenothane (DDT) and polychlorinated biphenyl (PCBs), readily penetrate intact skin.[10] Particularly in dark-skinned persons, the skin provides an effective screen against ultraviolet radiation from the sun. Within the skin and in the presence of sunlight, the precursor 7-dehydrocholesterol is changed to vitamin D, which enhances absorption of calcium from the gastrointestinal tract and is necessary for normal bone physiology. The skin prevents excessive loss of body fluids. Through dilatation and constriction of cutaneous blood vessels and changes in the quantity of perspiration secreted, the skin is important in the regulation of body temperature. A less well-known function of the skin is its role in glucose metabolism. The skin may contain enough glu-

cose to equal half of the amount in blood; thus, the skin may play a role in glucose metabolism by serving as a reservoir.[4]

The structure of the skin is uniquely adapted to fulfill these functions. As indicated in Figure 13-1, the skin consists of two primary layers, the epidermis and dermis, with the subcutaneous tissue lying beneath the dermis. The epidermis, the outermost layer, varies in thickness from the palms and soles, where it is thickest, to the eyelids, where it is very thin. The thickness of the epidermis is significant because skin areas with thicker epidermis are more resistant to allergens and irritants than are areas with thin epidermis.[69]

FIG. 13-1 Normal skin.

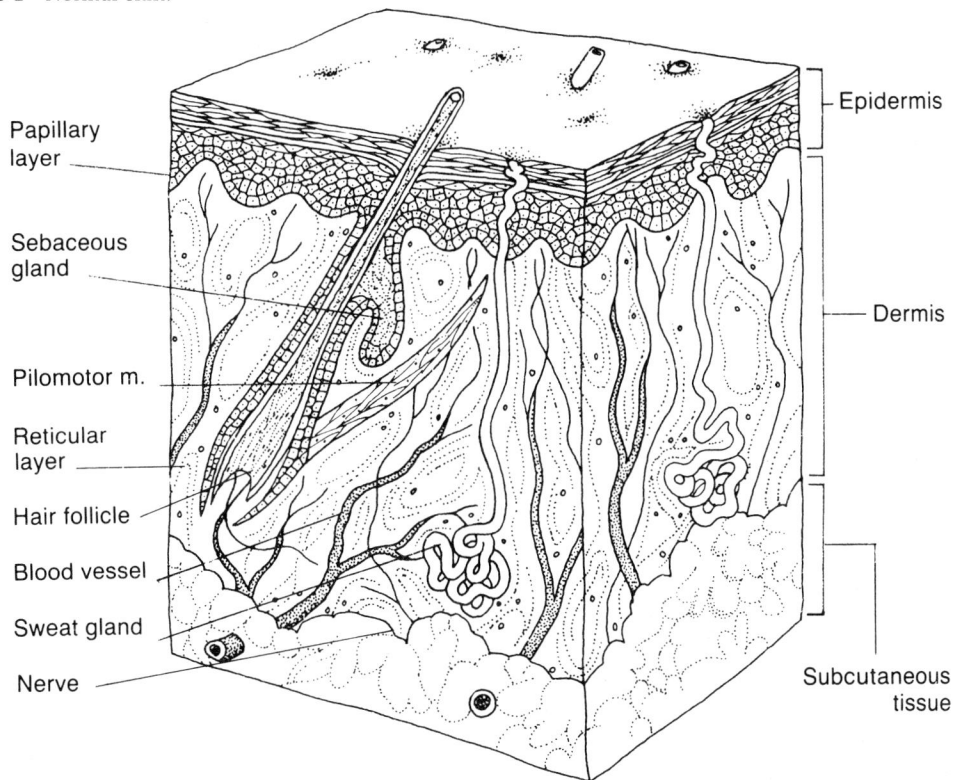

The three major cell types of the epidermis are the keratinocytes, melanocytes, and Langerhans cells. The keratinocytes, or squamous cells, are the most important cell type. They form *keratin*, which is the protein that makes up the stratum corneum, or outermost layer of the epidermis, and provides the structural protein of the hair and nails.

The keratinocytes are located in the basal cell layer, the innermost part of the epidermis. As the cells divide, one of the daughter cells migrates through the epidermis to the surface. During its transit through the epidermis, which takes approximately 26 days, the cell undergoes change, losing its nucleus and becoming one of the dead horn cells that make up the stratum corneum.[73] The rapid turnover as horn cells are shed and replaced is important to the accomplishment of the primary purpose of the stratum corneum: to provide a barrier to the entry of environmental substances into the body.

The melanocytes are also found in the basal layer. These cells synthesize *melanosomes*, which produce melanin. *Melanin*, the pigment that gives color to eyes, hair, and skin, is a very effective sunscreen that absorbs radiation from the sun.[10]

The number of melanocytes is the same in albinos and in persons with dark skin.[11,83] Variations in skin color are determined by the size and distribution of melanosomes. In blacks melanosomes are larger than in whites, they more actively produce melanin, and they may be found throughout the epidermis rather than just in the basal layer. Tanning results from the production of melanosomes that are larger than usual. *Vitiligo*, which is manifested as depigmented patches that may occur particularly in dark skin, results from localized destruction of melanocytes and their pigment-producing ability.

The Langerhans cells, the final cell type, are found in the middle layer of the epidermis, which is called the *stratum malpighii*. Their function remains a subject for investigation, but they may be important in immune reactions.[83]

The dermis, which lies directly beneath the epidermis, provides support and nutrition to the epidermis. The most important cells making up this mass are the *fibroblasts*, which produce *collagen*, the protein substance that gives the skin most of its strength and ability to resist stress. The fibroblasts also synthesize elastic fibers that give the skin the ability to return to its original shape when stretched. An additional function of the fibroblasts is the production of *ground substance*, which is found between the collagen and elastic fibers and serves as a cushion and lubricant.

The dermis, which is richly supplied with blood vessels and nerves, is the source of nourishment for the epidermis, which contains no blood vessels or nerves. The dermis contains two vascular plexuses, one of which is located near the epidermis and the other near the subcutaneous tissue below the dermis. There are many interconnections between the two plexuses. Stimulation of postganglionic fibers of the sympathetic nervous system results in constriction of dermal blood vessels to conserve body heat and excitation of the pilomotor muscles to produce "goose flesh." Blood can be shunted from arterioles to venules in the plexuses, bypassing the capillaries where heat exchange with the environment occurs.

Nerves in the dermis transmit sensations of touch, pressure, temperature, itch, and pain. The sensation experienced is determined by the frequency with which impulses are transmitted, the number of nerve fibers that are stimulated, and factors in the central nervous system (CNS) that may serve as inhibitors or reinforcers.[100] Itch and pain derive from similar nerve fibers. Stimuli of low intensity tend to produce the sensation of itching, whereas stimuli of higher intensity may be experienced as pain.[73]

To reach the dermis, blood vessels and nerves pass through the subcutaneous tissue. The subcutaneous tissue consists primarily of *adipose tissue*, which provides a cushion to protect deep structures from trauma and a layer of insulation to help retain body heat.

The skin appendages, or *adnexa*, include the hair, nails, eccrine glands, apocrine glands, and sebaceous glands. The color of hair results from the distribution of melanosomes. The hair becomes gray as a result of a smaller number of melanocytes producing few melanosomes. The growth of hair is cyclic. At any one time approximately 90% of scalp hairs are growing; this percentage decreases with age, especially in male pattern baldness.[83]

Toenails grow more slowly than fingernails. Both grow more rapidly during the day time and in hot weather.[73] It takes approximately 6 months to replace a fingernail; a toenail takes about a year.[11] The calcium content of nails increases with age or trauma.

Eccrine glands are present in the skin all over the body except for the nail beds, lip margins, clitoris, labia minora, and glans penis. They are particularly numerous on the palms of the hands and the soles of the feet. The major function of these glands is to help maintain body temperature by producing perspiration, which evaporates from skin surfaces. This function is controlled by the sympathetic nervous system. In extreme circumstances, 6 liters of fluid containing sodium chloride, potassium, glucose, urea, and lactose can be lost through evaporation of perspiration.[11] Whereas heat stimulates all eccrine glands, emotions are important in the stimulation of the glands of the palms, axillae, and forehead.

The apocrine glands serve no clear function in human beings. They are present primarily in the axillae, where the ducts empty into hair follicles. Apocrine glands are present to a lesser extent in the mons pubis, perineum, genitalia, face, scalp, and abdomen. Modified glands are also present in the ear, where they produce cerumen. The secretion from apocrine glands in the axillae is milky and free of odor until acted upon by bacteria. The odor is strongest in adolescence and young adulthood and becomes less noticeable with age.

Sebaceous glands are present in the skin all over the body except for the palms and soles. They are most numerous on the face, scalp, upper chest, and upper back. Sebum, which consists of lipids that coat the skin and hair, has limited antibacterial and antifungal properties. In contrast with the eccrine glands, the secretion of sebum is not controlled by the nervous system. While the pituitary gland may be necessary for the functioning of these glands, the androgens primarily control the size and activity of the sebaceous glands.[100]

THE SKIN AND AGING

That the skin and its appendages change with age is well known. Americans spend millions of dollars each year in an effort to deal with their concerns about wrinkles, graying hair, and male pattern baldness. Although much has been written about skin changes and aging, there is a great need for more research in this area. Kligman wrote: "Neither plastic surgeons nor dermatologists know anything about the anatomy of the wrinkle."[58]

Changes that are known to occur with aging involve the epidermis, dermis, and skin appendages. The epidermis of exposed skin changes more than that of unexposed skin. The thickness of the epidermis becomes more variable with age, but overall it does not change. The number of functional melanocytes decreases. As a result, the skin may be less effective as a barrier to ultraviolet light.[43] Another potentially significant finding reported by Gilchrest is that the number of Langerhans cells decreases, beginning in young adulthood. The loss of these cells may contribute to the decrease in immunological responsiveness of the skin of the elderly.

The thickness of the dermis and the amount of collagen it contains decrease with age. The remaining collagen becomes stiffer. Where the skin has been damaged by ultraviolet light, the amount of ground substance increases. The overall result, primarily from the decrease in collagen, is skin that has less strength.

In the young adult the dermis interdigitates with the epidermis. In older people the junction between the epidermis and dermis becomes flatter. As a result, the area of contact between the epidermis and dermis is decreased, which may result in less effective transport of nutrients and increased susceptibility to shearing forces.[43]

The number of small blood vessels in the dermis decreases with age. This change is enhanced by exposure to sunlight. Kligman found that in skin areas that are exposed repeatedly, including the face and the back of the hands: "the vessels of septa- and octagenarians are so sparse and tortuous that one wonders how the overlying epidermis survives."[58] The nerves of the skin show little change with age.[71]

The graying of hair results from fewer melanocytes. Both the hair and nails of older adults grow more slowly than the young. With age, the number of hair follicles decreases. According to Gilchrest, the primary factor in balding is a change from thick, well-pigmented hairs to short, fine hairs with little pigment.

The aging process affects the functioning of the glands within the skin. The elderly have fewer eccrine glands, and the degree of perspiration produced in response to heat is variable.[17] Among women, sebum production decreases following menopause. Men have less change in the amount of sebum secreted because the functioning of the sebaceous glands is dependent upon androgens.[17,47] Some authors attribute dry skin, or xerosis, which is common in old age, to decreased sebum production.[18,47,98] However, this relationship is controversial. According to Gilchrest there is no direct relationship between decreased sebum production and xerosis. There are no known clinical effects of decreased sebum production.[43]

Although some skin changes with aging are inevitable, the rate at which skin ages varies with hereditary factors and exposure to the elements, especially ultraviolet radiation. The sun is responsible for most of the visible changes associated with degeneration of the skin,[59] especially among individuals who have fair skin, blue eyes, and blond or red hair.[17] In contrast, black skin is more resistant to damage by sunlight and tends to deteriorate later in life.[96] Thus, young white men and women, who spend much time in the sun with little protection from ultraviolet radiation, may pay for this pastime later with prematurely aging skin. The relationship between excessive exposure to sunlight and skin cancers is also well established.[17,31,43,47]

DRY SKIN

Dry skin is very common, especially as one grows older. It may be a localized problem, which is more likely in areas with little hair such as the waist or lower legs.[89] On the other hand, the skin may be generally dry and tight all over the body. In the affected areas the skin is not only rough, dry, and scaly, but it may also itch. Moreover, scratching only tends to intensify the itching.[58] Dry skin, especially when scratched, may develop breaks in the surface, resulting in loss of the skin's integrity as a barrier to environmental agents and opening the way for the entry of microorganisms.

An understanding of the causative and contributing factors in the development of dry skin is necessary before the problem can be managed appropriately. Skin becomes dry due to loss of water. If water is lost from the skin surface more rapidly than it is replaced, the skin surface will dry out. Water is lost through evaporation. Perspiration and diffusion of water from underlying tissues are potential sources of water to the skin surface. At one time it was thought that a natural barrier to water loss existed at or near the base of the stratum corneum in the epidermis.[12,13] More recent evidence suggests that the tightly packed horn cells serve as the barrier that resists the diffusion of water.[75]

Environmental factors are important to the maintenance of moisture in the skin surface. Blank concluded that high temperatures and flowing air are important factors in the loss of moisture from the skin. However, the environmental circumstance that is most important in producing dry skin is a low relative humidity.[12] Gaul and Underwood agreed that the moisture content of air is an important consideration in relation to dry skin. They indicated that the important considerations are dew point and barometric pressure. *Dew point* was defined as the air temperature at which water vapor in the air begins to condense. Based upon their investigations, they concluded that the condition in which chapping is likely is a change from a high dew point and low barometric pressure to low dew point and high barometric pressure. Chapping was enhanced by exposure to wind, water, and soap.[41]

Other factors contribute to dryness of the stratum corneum. Exposure to lipid solvents, such as alcohol, in combination with water, alters the stratum corneum so that it is less able to absorb water from the environment. As a result, it becomes dehydrated and brittle.[12] Van Scott and Lyon investigated the effects of soaps and detergents on skin. They studied samples of dry, powdered keratin that was exposed to 1% solutions of various soaps and detergents. To varying extents, the soaps and detergents altered the physical properties of the keratin. The investigators indicated that sebum may provide a small amount of protection, but its benefits are overwhelmed by the action of soaps and detergents.[93]

Two other effects of soap are "defatting" and change in the pH.[90] The pH on the surface of normal skin is between five and six, and maintenance of the pH in this range may be important in the control of skin bacteria.[9] This normal acid condition is altered by exposure to the alkalinity of soaps. The length of time it takes for the normal acidity to be restored depends upon the amount of soap used, the duration of exposure, and the extent to which the soap is removed by rinsing. The effects of soaps on skin lipids and on pH are factors in skin irritation caused by soaps. Soaps may also affect the barrier function of the skin by increasing the permeability and allowing alkali and other irritants to reach more deeply into the epidermis.[90]

RASHES

The cause of a rash is often difficult to determine.[14] Generalized rashes that develop quickly are commonly due to medications. Certainly, when a person on a new medication develops a rash, drug reaction should be suspected. This type of prompt reaction usually occurs when the person has had previous exposure to the offending medication. When a patient takes a medication for the first time, it takes about 10 days for hypersensitivity to develop.[35] Sometimes a person has a prompt reaction to a medication without having taken the drug previously. For example, penicillin is normally found in small amounts in milk and may cause sensitization, resulting in an allergic reaction when penicillin is prescribed for the first time.[35] Among the medications and substances that may cause a rash are barbiturates, codeine, morphine, digitalis preparations, insulin, salicylates, toothpaste, medicated chewing gums, and vitamins.[29] Two of the leading causes of skin rashes are semisynthetic penicillins and whole human blood.[3]

Numerous systemic diseases may cause generalized skin rashes. Infectious diseases such as rubella, rubeola, and chicken pox are associated with generalized rashes. In syphilis, the chancre at the site of infection is followed by the generalized skin eruptions of secondary syphilis. Persons with Hodgkin's disease may have generalized redness of the skin and pruritus. Pruritus may also be a prominent symptom in uremia and in diseases associated with obstruction of bile flow.

The etiological factors associated with localized rashes are also numerous. Medications may produce fixed drug reactions in which erythema or plaques develop in specific areas of the body. The reasons for the specific locations in which the reactions occur are unclear.[63] The etiology of localized rashes is usually something other than systemic disease or allergic reactions to medications or food.[29]

Rashes resulting from skin contact with allergens and irritants often follow recognizable patterns. Many nurses are familiar with the lesions resulting from contact with poison ivy, sumac, or oak. The linear pattern of the vesicles is uncommon among skin lesions.[79] Many other substances may cause skin reactions. The perfume in many cosmetics may produce dermatitis. Ingredients of deodorants, antiperspirants, hair dyes, hair bleaches, nail polish, and lipsticks, to name just a few, may serve as skin irritants and produce rashes in the areas where they were applied. Nickel, which may be a constituent of jewelry, eyeglass frames, or brassiere clasps, can produce dermatitis in a characteristic pattern where the metal contacts the skin.

Occupation exposure to substances that can cause skin irritation is frequent. Nurses and physicians may develop problems following exposure to substances such as medications, rubber gloves, antiseptics, iodine, and soaps. Dentists may develop dermatitis from contact with soaps, local antiseptics, and disinfectants. Gardeners may have skin reactions after working with fertilizers, insecticides, and plants such as chrysanthemums and tulips. Paints, turpentine, paint thinners, and epoxy resins may cause problems for painters.[31] The homemaker may be prone to hand dermatitis resulting from contact with irritants such as water, detergents, bleach, and other household cleaning materials. Women with dual roles of nurse and homemaker may be particularly likely to have chronic problems resulting from exposure to irritants both at work and in the home.

Materials used in making clothing and shoes may produce dermatitis. For example, the dyes and finishes used for synthetic fabrics can cause irritation, whereas cotton does not tend to produce skin irritation. Dermatitis resulting from clothing is more common in people who are obese, have dry skin, perspire heavily, or wear tightly fitting clothes.[31] Synthetic rubber, which is used in making products such as gloves, boots, and underwear, may cause skin irritation. According to Jordon and Bourlas, underwear with elastic that was washed with laundry bleach can cause skin irritation which occurs because the bleach reacts with a component of the elastic to produce a strong allergen.[54]

Some rashes are associated with hot weather. The inflammation seen in *intertrigo* results from the retention of heat and moisture where two skin surfaces rub together. It is particularly likely to affect obese people. Another skin problem associated with hot weather is *miliaria,* or "prickly heat," a condition in which the eccrine glands are obstructed.

Many rashes, including miliaria, are associated with pruritus. Americans spend about $11 million annually on topical agents for pruritus, other than corticosteroid preparations.[16] The cause of the itching may be local, as in miliaria, dry skin, or contact dermatitis, or it may be a systemic disease. In degree of discomfort the sensations may vary from annoying to unbearable. Scratching, in an effort to relieve the sensations, is associated with bacterial infection, which further complicates the problem.

DECUBITUS ULCERS

Decubitus ulcers represent a challenging problem for nurses and a source of increased morbidity and mortality to patients. Development of a decubitus ulcer adds to the cost of hospitalization. The estimated cost of treating a severe decubitus ulcer is $7,500 per month.[20] The ultimate cost in terms of physical and emotional effect on the patient is immeasurable.

Decubitus ulcers or pressure sores are localized areas of cellular necrosis. These ulcers occur most frequently in persons who are confined in bed, are debilitated, or have decreased motor or sensory function. Any

---

Common Pressure Points by Position

Supine: Sacrum, coccyx, spine, heel, elbow, scapula, and occipital bone
Prone: Kneecap, sternum, crest of pelvis, ribs, and male genitalia
Lateral: Greater trochanter, ribs, medial and lateral malleolus
Sitting: Tuberosities of pelvis

---

condition that interferes with circulation to the cells will affect the function of the cell. For the cell to remain healthy, it must receive receive nutrients and eliminate waste continually. Prolonged or excessive pressure reduces or obstructs blood flow depriving the cell of nutrients and, if not relieved, results in cellular damage and ultimately in cellular death.[60]

Most authorities agree that it is pressure that causes tissue necrosis. Pressure on the skin is transmitted to underlying structures and interferes with blood flow. Any pressure above the capillary pressure, which normally is approximately 20 mm Hg to 30 mm Hg, will begin the breakdown process.[48,60] Tissues over the bony prominences in the weight-bearing areas are particularly subject to injury. People experience pressure exceeding 30 mm Hg on weight-bearing areas in both sitting and lying positions.[66] Landis found that a person sitting on an unpadded wooden chair has a capillary pressure of 300 mm Hg over the ischial tuberosities.[61] The pressure to the human buttocks lying on an innerspring mattress is approximately 70 mm Hg.[48]

Lindan and colleagues found that when persons with ideal body weight were in the supine position, the sacrum, buttocks, and heels were the points of highest pressure. In the prone position the knees and chest were the highest pressure areas. The sitting position produced the greatest pressure points over the ischial tuberosities.[66]

Some common sites for decubitus ulcer formation are shown in Figure 13-2. High-risk areas vary according to the patient's position.

The greatest percentage of decubitus ulcers occurs in the lower portion of the body. Lindan and co-workers reported that 75% of pressure sores were found to occur over the sacrum, greater trochanters, and tuberosities of the pelvis.[66]

The duration of pressure must also be considered. Decubitus ulcers most often occur after long periods of continuous moderate pressure.[6] Verhonick, Lewis, and Goller used thermography to measure the temperature in body areas subjected to pressure. A *thermogram* provides a picture of peripheral circulation and temperature. The investigators found that the longer pressure had been applied, the greater the time required for the skin temperature to return to normal.[94] Kosiak and Husain found that constant pressure of 60 to 70 mm Hg produced pathologic changes within 1 to 2 hours; however,

FIG. 13-2 *Skin care is particularly important over bony prominences.* (King EM, Wieck L et al: Illustrated Manual of Nursing Techniques, p 401. Philadelphia, JB Lippincott, 1981)

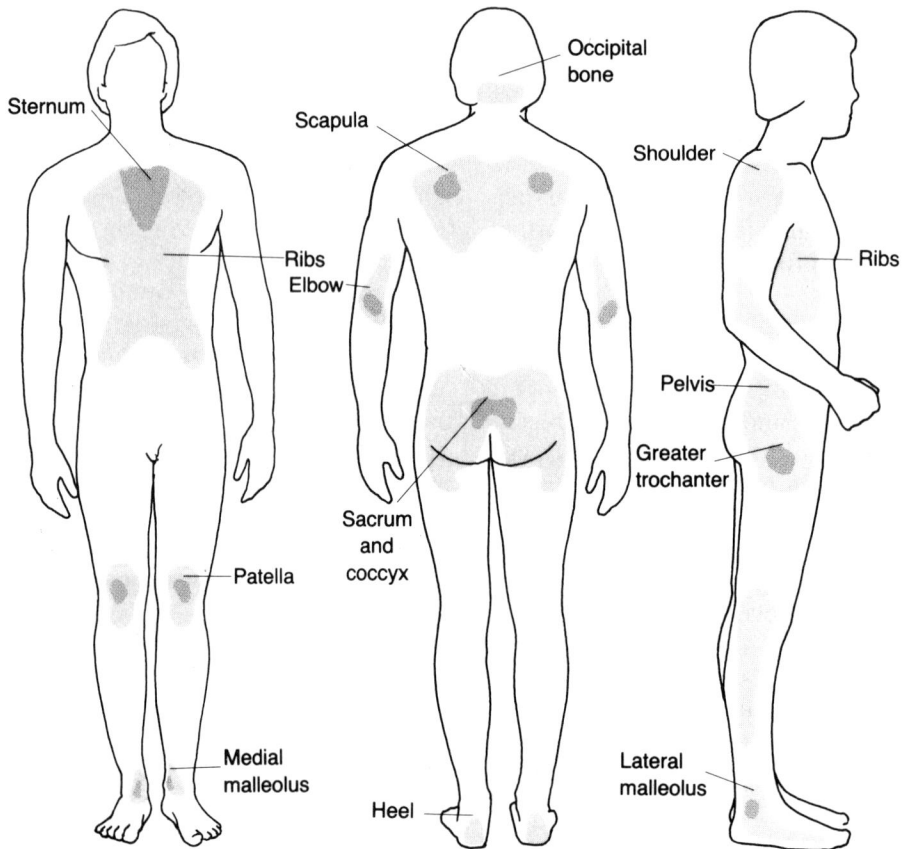

Kosiak demonstrated that tissue could tolerate much higher pressures (up to 240 mm Hg) with little cellular damage if pressure was periodically removed for 5 minutes.[53,60]

Shearing force is the second important factor contributing to decubitus ulcer formation. *Shearing* occurs when two or more layers of tissue slide in opposite directions, causing small capillaries to kink, stretch, or tear. For example, when the head of a patient's bed is raised more than 30 degrees, the patient slides toward the foot of the bed. Because of friction between the skin and the bed linens, the skin stays in a fixed position while the underlying tissue shifts. The resulting damage to capillaries reduces the circulation of oxygen to the area and predisposes the person to pressure necrosis. Pulling a patient across the sheets rather than lifting also creates a shearing force.[76] Elderly patients are especially prone to the effects of shearing forces as a result of the decreased interdigitation between the epidermis and the dermis.

Specific nutritional alterations also contribute to decubitus ulcer formation. Anemia decreases the delivery of oxygen to the cell. As a result, tissue ischemia and cellular necrosis become more imminent. Decreased ascorbic acid level increases capillary fragility and delays tissue healing.[6] In the absence of adequate protein, tissue healing does not occur. Hypoproteinemia contributes to the development of edema, which interferes with the cell–capillary exchange by increasing the distance between the cell and the capillary.[46] Edematous tissues have less elasticity and resiliency and are more susceptible to injury.[6]

Both overweight and underweight persons may develop pressure areas. The underweight person has reduced natural fat padding over bony prominences to protect the skin. The larger skin folds of the overweight person provide a warm, dark environment that is conducive to skin breakdown. The extra weight over the bony prominences of the heavy person can further obstruct blood flow to the cells.[46] Dehydration, with the subsequent loss of skin turgor, increases the risk of skin breakdown.[2]

Decreased mobility is a significant contributing factor in pressure sore development. Healthy people change their positions frequently in response to discomfort that occurs from compression of the skin and subcutaneous tissues. Exton–Smith and Sherwin studied the relationship between spontaneous bodily movements in elderly patients during sleep and subsequent decubitus ulcer formation. They found that persons with high mobility scores during the night did not develop decubitus ulcers. Conversely, persons with low mobility scores or those whose scores decreased on successive nights developed decubitus ulcers.[34]

Illness, injury, or medications can alter a person's level of consciousness. Decreased awareness of discomfort from pressure may eliminate the person's ability to change positions. Thus, persons with decreased motor or sensory function are especially prone to pressure sores. Siegel, Vistnes, and Laub reported that the incidence of decubitus ulcers in paraplegics and quadraplegics ranged from 24% to 85%, and 7% to 8% of deaths in those patients could be directly related to pressure sores.[82] Other factors, such as arteriosclerosis and nicotine from heavy smoking, both of which reduce blood flow to the tissues, may predispose a person to decubitus ulcers.[46] In a study by Williams, more men than women developed pressure sores. This may be due to the difference in fat distribution in men and women.[99]

Any object that compresses the underlying tissue can also contribute to ulcer formation. Objects that can produce this effect include buckles, braces, splints, tight restraints, casts, intravenous fluid tubing, and catheter tubing. Wrinkled sheets and foreign objects in the bed or chair can also increase pressure and obstruct blood flow.[46]

Perspiration, urine, and feces add moisture to the skin, promoting maceration. A poorly ventilated mattress covered with impermeable rubber or plastic increases localized sweating and maceration. In a study by Exton–Smith and Sherwin, incontinence was found to be the single most useful indicator of the risk for patients' developing pressure sores. Improper hygiene encourages growth of bacteria normally found on the skin. Ischemic tissues provide a good growth medium for bacteria. If bacteria invade ischemic tissues, destruction and ulcer formation occur more quickly.[34]

Friction injury, with the resultant loss of the epidermis, causes a break in the integrity of the skin.[6] Dry skin can cause cracks in the skin, providing a portal of entry for bacteria. Scratching can result in a denuded area of the epidermis resulting in loss of the barrier function of the epidermis.

Illnesses that produce fever can also increase a person's risk for decubitus ulcers. For each degree centigrade above normal that the body temperature increases, the metabolic rate goes up by 10%.[64] Thus, a higher metabolic rate increases the demand for oxygen in areas already compromised by pressure.

WOUNDS

Wound healing is a complex process that usually works efficiently to restore skin integrity. However, a number of factors affect wound healing and must be considered in the management of wounds. First, an understanding of the process of healing is necessary.

When a person develops a wound, whether from an injury or surgery, a series of events begins that ultimately leads to the restoration of skin integrity. The disruption of blood vessels due to the injury causes blood to leak from the damaged vessel. The result is decreased intravascular pressure and increased pressure in the tissues surrounding the vessel, which inhibits further blood loss. The elastic fibers in the vessel retract, which also decreases blood loss. Platelets adhere to the damaged endothelial cells of the vessel. The platelets rupture, releasing adenosine diphosphate, which results in the aggregation of more platelets to produce a platelet plug. At the same time, thromboplastin from the damaged tissues activates prothrombin, to form thrombin. Thrombin, in turn, acts on fibrinogen, resulting in the formation of fibrin which, in combination with the aggregated platelets, forms a fibrin clot. These processes are accomplished within 1½ to 4½ minutes.[27,40,72]

Inflammation of the damaged tissues is a necessary prelude to repair. Small vessels in the injured area dilate and become more permeable. Leukocytes accumulate at the site of injury. The leukocytes, especially polymorphonuclear leukocytes, migrate into the tissue and move to the site of injury, where phagocytosis and digestion of bacteria and foreign matter occur.[95]

Within 3 to 4 days of the injury, macrophages begin to appear in large numbers. These are primarily responsible for cleaning up the area by ingesting necrotic tissue, red blood cells, and fibrin. Macrophages may also ingest platelets.[38,51] An additional and important function of the macrophages is stimulation of fibroblast replication and neovascularization.[38,51,52] Fibroblasts, along with ascorbic acid and lactate ion, are necessary for collagen formation, which begins on the 2nd day and reaches a peak around the 5th to 7th day. In part stimulated by hypoxia, the blood vessels, which are closest to the wound, sprout capillary buds, which grow to revascularize the injured area. This growth of blood vessels provides more oxygen, which facilitates further production of collagen.[52]

In the injured area, collagen lysis, as well as collagen formation, occurs. Collagen in injured tissue and new, weak collagen formed in the early stages of healing are lysed. For normal healing to occur, there must be a balance between collagen formation and lysis.

Wounds heal by first, second, or third intention. Most surgical wounds heal by first intention. The epidermis heals by epithelialization, which occurs in the first 24 to 48 hours after the wound is closed.[69] Through mitosis, epidermal cells are produced at the wound edges. These cells migrate into the wound, using fibrin strands as bridges. Migration occurs, until cells from the sides of the wound meet. At that point the cells proliferate vertically, adding to the thickness of the layer and restoring the barrier function of epidermis. The dermis heals through revascularization and collagen formation.

During the first days after surgery the tensile strength of the incision is limited, but the thickness of the incision is greater than it will be later. This thickness is called the healing ridge. When the ridge is present throughout the length of the wound by the 7th or 9th postoperative day, dehiscence is unlikely.[52] For a period of 6 months to 1 year the structure of the collagen in the scar is remodeled, resulting in increased tensile strength with less collagen.[52,69]

The processes that occur when wounds heal by second intention are the same, but healing takes longer. Depending upon the size of the wound, epithelialization takes about 6 weeks.[36] It is significant that epidermal cells will migrate only over living tissue. Therefore, necrotic tissue inhibits healing. As granulation occurs, the surface collagen has little tensile strength, whereas the collagen deeper in the wound is more mature and stronger.[52] *Contraction* of the wound is a helpful process by which the wound is made smaller by stretching the surrounding skin to partially cover the wound. Healing by second intention or third intention, in which a wound that was initially left open is later closed, results in larger scars.

Numerous factors influence the healing of wounds. For a wound to heal there must be an adequate blood supply. Healing increases the need for oxygen, which is necessary for collagen formation and epithelialization.[32] Inadequate blood supply and hypoxia inhibit healing significantly and increase the likelihood of infection.

Many nutrients are necessary for wound healing, including the following:

All amino acids
Adequate calories
Essential fatty acids
Ascorbic acid
Vitamin B complex
Vitamin A
Vitamin K
Calcium
Zinc
Iron
Copper
Manganese
Molybdenum
Chromium

Age may affect healing. Older adults are more likely to have compromised circulation, and may have some degree of malnutrition. Aging may slow the process of fibroblast replication and collagen formation. Levenson, Seifter, and Van Winkle indicate that persons over age 45 have higher rates of dehiscence than younger patients.[65] In a study by Cruse and Foord, patients age 66 and over had the highest rates of postoperative infection, while those from ages 1 to 14 had the lowest rates.[25]

Other health problems that the patient has may affect healing. Diabetes mellitus is a prime example. Hyperglycemia and lack of insulin interfere with cellular functions in healing. The functioning of leukocytes is affected in diabetics, especially when the disease is out of control.[50] In general, diabetics are more likely to develop wound infections.

Medications that the patient is receiving may hinder healing. Corticosteroids delay wound healing by increasing the lysis of collagen and by decreasing the patient's ability to resist infection. Medications used in cancer chemotherapy may inhibit protein synthesis and increase the risk of infection. Birth control pills that contain progesterone and estrogen may slow collagen synthesis and decrease the tensile strength of wounds.[52]

Obese persons may have problems with healing because of the relative inadequacy of the blood supply to adipose tissue.[78] Obesity also is associated with higher rates of infection and with dehiscence.[25,37]

Besides obesity, other factors associated with increased risk of wound disruption include malnutrition, inadequate suturing, distention, infection, vomiting, strenuous coughing, malignancies, and dehydration.[37] One noteworthy indicator of wound disruption is increased serosanguineous drainage from the wound.[23]

Changes in wound drainage also are seen in infections. According to O'Bryne, the following are changes that suggest an infection: redness; swelling; thick, creamy discharge, regardless of color or smell; increased tenderness; and deep pain in the surgical area. Aerobic infections tend to occur around the 5th postoperative day and produce a characteristic fever pattern with elevations in the afternoon or evening and a return to normal by morning. Drainage from a wound infected with aerobes will have a

musty odor. Symptoms from infections caused by anaerobes usually occur 6 to 8 days after surgery. A putrid or acrid odor is usually present with anaerobic infection.[74]

NURSING ASSESSMENT

Careful assessment provides the basis for establishing nursing diagnoses and identifying appropriate interventions when working with people with actual or potential skin changes. Assessment depends upon expertise in history-taking and skills of inspection and palpation.

SUBJECTIVE DATA

The description that the patient provides about skin changes usually contains a wealth of information. Family members also may give useful data. A person with a skin change may have had the problem for a period of time. Consequently, the person may have identified effective measures for dealing with the problem. This information can provide helpful clues for establishing a nursing diagnosis and determining the appropriate management.

Ask the person to describe as fully as possible the nature of the problem, its onset, and its progression. The information sought should include answers to the following questions:

How does the person describe the nature of the skin change?
When did it begin?
Where was the person at that time?
What did it look like, smell like, feel like?
What part or parts if the skin were involved?
Has the person or a family member ever had a problem like this one?
What symptoms are associated with the problem?

Does it itch?

Is it painful?

Does it weep?

What has the individual found that makes it better? Worse?

Take a general health history, including any skin problems that the person has had previously, as well as the health of family members. The person's work and hobbies should be explored to identify exposure to irritants. The usual manner of caring for the skin is important. This information should include the frequency and type of bathing, soaps used, and agents that the person uses on the skin.

Explore the person's feelings about skin problems. The high visibility of skin lesions can result in significant emotional reactions. Skin changes, especially if they involve the face, may cause the person to be very self-conscious and uncomfortable in contact with other people. The person may have noted negative reactions by other people, who are frequently concerned that skin changes are contagious. For example, the person with hand dermatitis may have found that others are hesitant to shake hands. When giving change in a store, the clerk may be very careful not to touch the hand of the customer with dermatitis. Thus, the person's concern about appearance and the reactions of others frequently produces major disruptions in psychosocial well-being.

OBJECTIVE DATA

Careful description of skin changes is necessary to provide baseline data to be used in assessment of the progress or lack of progress in managing the problem and to facilitate communication among nurses and other health professionals.

In inspecting the skin, good lighting is essential. Describe the size and shape of le-

sions. A clear ruler is helpful in determining the size of lesions. Indicate any pattern of the lesions. For example, lesions may be linear, as in poison ivy. Lesions associated with ringworn are annular, whereas other skin changes appear in clusters. Describe the distribution of lesions and their locations as exactly as possible in relation to body structures. Palpate skin changes to determine if lesions are flat or raised, moist or dry, warm or cool, rough or smooth, mobile or fixed.

The use of correct terminology is important when describing skin changes. Terms are defined in Table 13-1. As indicated in the table, macules and patches are not palpable, while papules and nodules can be felt. An *erosion* is a superficial skin lesion, but an *ulcer* is a lesion that penetrates more deeply than the epidermis. The information in Table 13-1 also facilitates differentiation among vascular and purpuric lesions.

Special skill is needed in examining the skin of dark-skinned persons. The natural skin tones may mask changes in skin color. Asking the individual and family members to describe any changes in the usual skin tones is one useful approach. Some skin changes are more easily identified by inspecting the mucous membranes. Petechiae, for example, may be observed more easily on the buccal mucosa. However, with practice, skin changes in dark skin can be noted. Color changes are often seen in the loss of the usual red tones of the skin. For example, in cyanosis the underlying skin tones may change from red to gray. Assess jaundice by observing the color of the sclera. However, these observations can be misleading because dark-skinned people may have carotene in the subconjunctival fat, giving the appearance of jaundice. Differentiation between jaundice and carotene deposits may be made by observing the color of the anterior palate using bright daylight. If the palate is not yel-

(*Text continues on page 324*)

TABLE 13-1
DESCRIPTION OF SKIN CHANGES

PRIMARY LESIONS *(May arise from previously normal skin)*

CIRCUMSCRIBED, FLAT, NON-PALPABLE CHANGES IN SKIN COLOR	PALPABLE ELEVATED SOLID MASSES	CIRCUMSCRIBED SUPERFICIAL ELEVATIONS OF THE SKIN FORMED BY FREE FLUID IN A CAVITY WITHIN THE SKIN LAYERS
Macule—Small, up to 1 cm.* Example: freckle, petechia	*Papule*—Up to 0.5 cm. Example: an elevated nevus	*Vesicle*—Up to 0.5 cm; filled with serous fluid. Example: Herpes simplex
Patch—Larger than 1 cm. Example: vitiligo	*Plaque*—A flat, elevated surface larger than 0.5 cm, often formed by the coalescence of papules	*Bulla*—Greater than 0.5 cm; filled with serous fluid. Example: 2nd degree burn
	Nodule—0.5 to 1–2 cm; often deeper and firmer than a papule	*Pustule*—Filled with pus. Example: acne, impetigo
	Tumor—Larger than 1–2 cm.	
	Wheal—A slightly irregular, relatively transient, superficial area of localized skin edema. Example: mosquito bite, hive	

320

SECONDARY LESIONS (Result from changes in primary lesions)

LOSS OF SKIN SURFACE

Erosion—Loss of the superficial epidermis; surface is moist but does not bleed. Example: moist area after the rupture of a vesicle, as in chickenpox

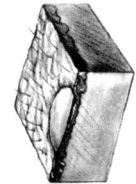

Ulcer—A deeper loss of skin surface; may bleed and scar. Examples: stasis ulcer of venous insufficiency; syphilitic chancre

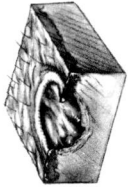

Fissure—A linear crack in the skin. Example: athlete's foot

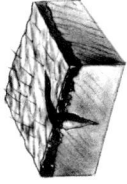

MATERIAL ON THE SKIN SURFACE

Crust—The dried residue of serum, pus or blood. Example: impetigo

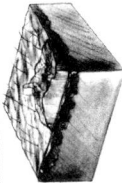

Scale—A thin flake of exfoliated epidermis. Examples: dandruff, dry skin, psoriasis

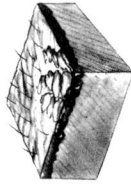

MISCELLANEOUS

Lichenification—Thickening and roughening of the skin with increased visibility of the normal skin furrows. Example: atopic dermatitis

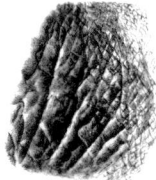

Atrophy—Thinning of the skin with loss of the normal skin furrows; the skin looks shinier and more translucent than normal. Example: arterial insufficiency

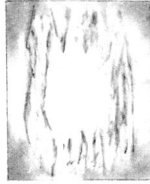

Scar—Replacement of destroyed tissue by fibrous tissue

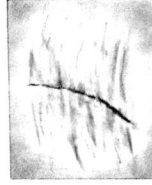

Excoriation—A scratch mark

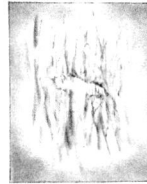

Keloid—A hypertrophied scar

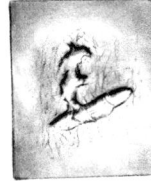

(continued)

321

TABLE 13-1 (continued)
DESCRIPTION OF SKIN CHANGES

	VASCULAR			PURPURIC	
	CHERRY ANGIOMA	SPIDER ANGIOMA	VENOUS STAR	PETECHIA	ECCHYMOSIS
	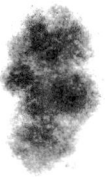	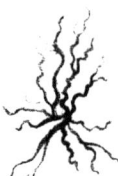			
Color	Bright or ruby red; may become brownish with age	Fiery red	Bluish	Deep red or reddish purple	Purple or purplish-blue, fading to green, yellow and brown with time
Size	1–3 mm	Very small, up to 2 cm	Variable, from very small to several inches	Usually 1–3 mm	Variable, larger than petechiae
Shape	Round, sometimes raised, may be surrounded by a pale halo	Central body, sometimes raised, surrounded by erythema and radiating legs	Variable. May resemble a spider or be linear, irregular, cascading	Round, flat	Round, oval or irregular; may have a central subcutaneous flat nodule

Pulsatility	Absent	Often demonstrable in the body of the spider, when pressure with a glass slide is applied	Absent	Absent	Absent
Effect of pressure	May show partial blanching, especially if pressure is applied with a pinpoint's edge.	Pressure over the body causes blanching of the spider	Pressure over center does not cause blanching	None	None
Distribution	Trunk, also extremities	Face, neck, arms and upper trunk, almost never below the waist	Most often on the legs, near veins; also anterior chest	Variable	Variable
Significance	None; increase in size and numbers with aging	Liver disease, pregnancy, vitamin B deficiency, occurs in some normal people	Often accompanies increased pressure in the superficial veins, as in varicose veins	Blood extravasated outside the vessels; may suggest increased bleeding tendency or emboli to skin	Blood extravasated outside the vessels; often secondary to trauma; also seen in bleeding disorders

(From Bates B: A Guide to Physical Examination, 2nd ed., p 48–50. Philadelphia, JB Lippincott, 1979)
* Authorities vary somewhat in their definitions of skin lesions by size. Dimensions given in this table should be considered approximate, not rigid.

lowish, the color of the sclera is probably due to carotene.[77]

ASSESSMENT OF DECUBITUS ULCERS

In view of the many causative and contributing factors for decubitus ulcer formation, it is important to assess the skin at the time a person is admitted to any health care facility. This assessment will identify persons with potential skin problems so that preventive measures can be initiated. Additionally, persons with actual skin problems can receive early treatment. Based on their previous experience, Andersen and co-workers maintained that most decubitus ulcers occur soon after admission.[82]

Given the causative and contributing factors for decubitus ulcers, Gosnell recommended that assessment include the following categories of information: mental status, continence, mobility, activity, nutrition, skin appearance, skin tone, and skin sensation. Assessment in these categories will facilitate identification of patients at risk for skin breakdown.[44]

Hebert and Alterescu recommend using a pressure ulcer record to document the location of skin irritation.[49] (One such record uses a drawing of the body on which ulcer areas can be shaded.) Any form used to document potential areas of skin change should include the date of assessment and the size of the involved area. With this information it is easy to note increases or decreases in the size of the ulcer. Note the patient's favored position, and carefully assess the high pressure areas.

Reddened areas of the skin should suggest the potential for skin breakdown. The patient should be kept off the reddened area and must be turned every 2 hours. Gently massage the reddened area to increase circulation to the area and assess to note if the redness disappears after massage. If tissue damage has occurred, the redness will not fade after massage.

Ischemia from pressure causes the skin to appear pale. When the pressure is removed, blood rushes into the area and causes a reactive hyperemia. (Note how long the redness lasts.) Redness that does not fade in 15 to 20 minutes is usually one of the earliest signs of tissue damage. These visual changes may not be apparent in the dark-skinned person.

Areas at risk for the development of decubitus ulcers should be gently palpated to determine increased warmth. An area of circumscribed warmth that lasts for more than 15 minutes after pressure is removed should be suspect for decubitus ulcer formation. Redness and increased warmth are the first signs of a potential pressure sore. If untreated, the skin may take on a bluish discoloration, followed by bulla formation. Subsequently, craters may develop in the skin.

NURSING DIAGNOSIS

Actual and potential impairment of skin integrity are among the nursing diagnoses specified by the National Conference on Classification of Nursing Diagnosis. Three defining characteristics of actual impairment of skin integrity were identified: disruption of the skin surface, destruction of skin layers, and invasion of body structures.[57] Many conditions can result in this diagnosis. Four health problems in which one or more of these defining characteristics are demonstrated: dry skin, skin rashes, decubitus ulcers, and wounds.

MANAGEMENT

The management of impairment of skin integrity depends on the type of impairment identified. This section focuses on the management for dry skin, skin rashes, decubitus ulcers, and wounds.

DRY SKIN

Nursing management to prevent or treat dry skin is based upon recognition of the causative and contributing factors which are applicable to an individual patient. Since loss of water is the major factor causing dry skin, nursing management is directed toward conserving or replacing moisture. The patient's environment is an important consideration. Because lack of humidity in the air, most commonly due to heating and air conditioning, causes increased evaporation of water from the stratum corneum, the nurse should discuss ways to increase humidification with the patient. Humidifiers are also helpful, as are pans of water on radiators or at registers of forced air heating. The humidity should be increased, particularly in rooms where the person spends the most time, such as the living room, den, or bedroom. Bathrooms and kitchens tend to have naturally higher humidity because of the frequency of activities in these rooms, which puts moisture into the air.

It is helpful for the patient to use a humidity gauge. If one is not available, a rough estimate of humidification can be obtained by the speed with which plants dry out or handwashed clothes dry. Also, static electricity tends to be more of a problem when the humidity is low.

The ways in which the person cares for the skin affect dryness. Because bathing, especially with soap, promotes dry skin, bathing less frequently and with less soap is desirable. Daily sponge baths can be taken, with complete tub baths or showers less often. If this alternative is unacceptable to the person, other approaches still may help to decrease the dryness of skin. Bubble baths and rubbing alcohol should be avoided. Warm water is better than hot water. The use of just water with no soap is helpful. Superfatted soaps may be of some benefit, but they are expensive to use. Any soap the patient uses will contribute to dryness and should be removed by thorough rinsing.

When giving bed baths to patients, limiting the use of soap and changing the water as often as necessary helps to prevent the drying and irritating effects of soap left on the skin. Spoor found that bathing with water and a bath oil that mixes with water, using no soap, was an effective approach even with very dry skin.[85] Oatmeal baths are soothing for dry, irritated skin.

The care of the skin after the bath is important in preventing loss of additional moisture through evaporation. Pat the skin dry, rather than rubbing it with a towel. While the skin is still moist, apply a film to prevent or limit evaporation of water. Several alternatives for providing this film barrier are suggested in the literature. Petroleum jelly is one of the most effective agents in providing a film that is impermeable to water.[87] Cripps and Friberg recommend the use of Aquaphor or Eucerin cream to retain moisture and decrease dryness.[24,39] Collar and Brown suggest mineral oil, vegetable oil, and vegetable shortening. Their suggestions are likely to be the least expensive.[22] Wells reported that oils, such as Alpha-Keri and Lubath, are effective.[98] Brown and colleagues conducted a demonstration project and found that warm water soaks and massage with mineral oil were effective in treating dry skin on the feet of a sample of nursing home residents.[15]

Although convenient to use, lotions are not generally considered to be as effective in managing dry skin as other agents.[24,98] To be effective the agent used must be rather viscous.[81] Lotions that are liquids have limited ability to provide the film to prevent the loss of moisture.

An additional nursing measure, adequate fluid intake, may be helpful. Diffusion of water from underlying structures may provide some moisture to the stratum corneum. This source of water suggests the usefulness of maintaining an adequate fluid intake.

Clearly, there is a need for additional research to evaluate the relative benefits of various approaches to the nursing management of dry skin. Such research would help to clarify which measures are effective, economical, and acceptable to people.

Because the elderly are especially likely to have problems with dry skin, it is important for nurses to impress upon persons in this age group the need to change skin care habits to prevent or decrease dryness. One needs to recognize, however, the resistance people may feel toward changing habits of personal hygiene that have been practiced for many years. Careful explanations may be necessary before the person demonstrates a willingness to attempt a new approach. Motivation to try something new may be increased by the suggestion of more comfortable skin that is more attractive both in appearance and feel.

RASHES

Rashes are usually easy to observe, sometimes difficult to describe, and often puzzling regarding their etiology. As discussed in the assessment section, descriptions of lesions need to be explicit, clear, and definite to be meaningful. Determination of the etiology of a rash requires careful observation and questioning of the person and family and may require consultation with a physician.

Rashes and the accompanying pruritus may significantly impair the integrity of the skin. Nursing management is directed toward preventing or minimizing the extent of the problem.

Where the etiology of a rash is clearly identified, important aspects of management may be evident. For example, when a rash is caused by an irritant or allergen, avoidance of the substance is clearly an important aspect in treating the problem. Referral to a physician is indicated when the etiology is unclear or complex, or when prescription medications may be needed to promote early resolution of the rash. Patch testing of the skin may be useful in confirming the etiology of the rash.

Nurses play an important role in health teaching for sensitive persons. Health teaching often is directed toward preventing skin problems. To avoid the dermatitis resulting from exposure to poison ivy, care should be taken to avoid plants with leaves growing in groups of three. When exposure can be anticipated, clothing that covers the arms, legs, ankles, and feet should be worn. Prompt bathing of skin that has been in contact with the plants may decrease the severity of the reaction. The clothing worn should be removed by turning it inside out and then laundered. People clearing the plants from infested areas should never dispose of them by burning.

Some people find it helpful to use "hypoallergenic" cosmetics. The absence of perfumes may prevent some cases of contact dermatitis. The use of gloves and other protective clothing may prevent or decrease exposure to irritants at work, while one is doing household chores, or when one is gardening. While not 100% effective, protective creams containing silicone provide barriers to irritants.[5]

Hand dermatitis resulting from contact with soaps, detergents, and cleansers can be prevented or managed by sensitive persons, but the changes in their routine require adjustment. Most important in the management of the problem is avoidance of contact with irritants. The approaches discussed in the section on dry skin are helpful. For many activities, rubber gloves must be worn. The gloves should be inspected regularly for holes. Because the rubber gloves allow perspiration to accumulate, cotton gloves should be worn inside the rubber gloves and changed frequently as they become moist with perspiration or water. Activities for which the gloves are needed should be alternated with activities that do not require this protection. Gloves should be worn when using household cleaning products. They may also be needed when bathing or shampooing the hair. Preparing some fruits and vegetables, such as potatoes, tomatoes, squash, and citrus fruits, can cause irritation. For many people with dermatitis, wool is an irritant.

Obese persons should try to avoid intertrigo during hot weather. Cotton underwear is useful because it absorbs perspiration. Dressing sponges or cotton squares placed between skin folds will increase the absorption of moisture. Talcum powder may be helpful, but caking can result if it is left in place for prolonged periods or if perspiration is heavy. Cornstarch should not be used because it can be metabolized by microorganisms, and it may result in the growth of organisms such as *Candida*.[3] The maintenance of a cool environment through the use of air conditioners and fans is certainly desirable. Areas where skin folds rub together should be observed regularly for signs of inflammation and infection. In these warm, moist areas bacterial infections can begin readily.

Miliaria is also helped by a cool environment. Avoiding excessive or tight-fitting clothes is useful. The person should keep the skin as clean and dry as possible. Unfortunately, there is no immediately effective method of restoring the flow of perspiration.[75]

Pruritis is an annoying problem for the person and can be difficult to manage. When pruritus is attributed to localized problems, removal of the causative factor or factors should relieve the sensations (e.g., treating dry skin will alleviate the associated itching).

Admonishing the person not to scratch is necessary, but the discomfort associated with pruritus makes it difficult to avoid scratching or rubbing areas that itch intensely and continuously. Keeping fingernails short will help to decrease the damage. Because people often scratch without realizing they are doing so, family members can help by watching for scratching and remind the person to avoid doing so.

Nursing measures should be tried to increase the person's comfort. Awareness of itching is increased with inactivity and at night. Therefore, working with a person to identify enjoyable activities may serve to provide distraction during the day and a sufficient degree of fatigue to permit sleep at night.

When appropriate, the pruritus associated with intertrigo and itching around the anus or vulva may be helped by gentle bathing. Among patients confined to bed, using limited amounts of soap and rinsing thoroughly may help to prevent pruritus associated with soap left on the skin.

People who itch should avoid wearing rough clothing, particularly wool, over the pruritic area. Avoidance of overheating may help to keep the sensation from worsening. In some situations it is possible to substitute the sensation of cold for itching by applying cold compresses to pruritic areas.[16,29] The application of lotion may be an easy method of accomplishing a similar result because of the cooling effect that occurs as the water in the lotion evaporates. Oatmeal baths are soothing and provide gentle cleansing of the skin. Either old-fashioned oatmeal or a product such as Aveeno may be used. Cornstarch baths may also be useful for their soothing, antipruritic effects.

When nursing management is not effective in relieving the pruritus, referral to a physician is indicated. Referral should also be made when a systemic cause for the pruritic condition is suspected.

DECUBITUS ULCERS

Most nursing textbooks recommend measures to prevent development and promote healing of decubitus ulcers. However, many of the suggested measures were developed as a result of skin improvement in a small number of cases. Few controlled studies have been conducted that support or refute the efficacy of many measures described in the literature. Coker reported that there are 143 devices and 2,200 topical preparations used with varying degrees of success to prevent and treat decubitus ulcers.[20] The number and diversity of approaches for decubitus ulcer care reflect the magnitude of the problem and suggest that the search for the optimal method of management has not been found.

The most important aspect in the management of decubitus ulcers is the relief of pressure over bony prominences. A procedure for turning the patient at 2-hour intervals should be established. If the patient always is turned in the same direction and the same sequence of positions, nursing personnel will automatically know which direction to turn the patient and which position is next. For example, if the person is always turned to the right (or the left), then all four recumbent positions will be used before returning to the original position. Otherwise, it is possible that the patient will be placed in the same position twice before all positions are used. The goal of such a procedure is to increase the length of time the patient is off

each area. However, if any signs of skin breakdown are present, the patient should not be positioned in a way that will cause pressure to the involved area.

Several activities of the nurse can contribute to skin injury and subsequent pressure sore development. Jewelry and fingernails can cause skin abrasions. Nurses must use utmost care when placing their hands under the patient to move or lift the individual. Injury is less likely when the nurses' nails are short. When providing direct care, avoid or remove jewelry, especially rings with stones or designs that produce sharp edges.

The patient's bed should be clean, dry, and free from wrinkles or foreign objects. Always lift rather than slide or pull the patient in bed. A lifting sheet may alleviate the tendency to pull or slide the patient. Avoid elevating the head of the bed more than 30° for patients at risk for developing decubitus ulcers. Raise the patient's feet against a padded footboard to prevent shearing, which can result from sliding down in the bed. Rubbing the skin with lotion that lubricates the skin and prevents friction will also decrease shearing force.

Topical Agents and Debridement

Alcohol has been recommended to dry and toughen the skin. Because alcohol causes local vasoconstriction and a resultant decrease in circulation, it should be used sparingly. Although tincture of benzoin has been recommended to toughen the skin, disadvantages probably outweigh its usefulness. The substance remains sticky even when dry and can cause the patient's skin to adhere to the sheets. When the patient moves, the superficial layers of skin can peel away. Benzoin can also act as an irritant to some patients.[49]

Numerous agents and devices are used to prevent reddened skin from progressing to pressure sores. Berecek, Hebert and Alterescu, Kavchak–Keyes, and Mikulic have provided useful methods of categorizing these agents and devices.[7,49,56,68] Tables 13-2 and 13-3 incorporate this information. The topical agents are presented in Table 13-2.

If the skin is intact, a topical ointment, washing with soap and water, gentle massage, frequent turning, and relief of pressure will usually result in healing. The same approach can be used if the skin is broken but not draining. Occlusive dressings such as Stomahesive or other gelatin products are recommended for the incontinent patient to prevent further damage from urine or feces. Also, Stomahesive will adhere to denuded skin areas and may stimulate granulation tissue formation.[49]

If the wound is draining, an absorptive agent may be used, in combination with cleansing and relief of pressure. DiMascio reported that healing of decubitus ulcers occurred when a dextranomer (Debrisan) was used.[30] Debrisan seems to promote healing by simultaneously absorbing exudate and cleansing the area, a combination that decreases wound drainage, inflammation, and edema, with a resultant increase in circulation to the ulcer.

The product is supplied as a sterile insoluble powder that can absorb approximately four times its weight in water. Dextranomer also absorbs the products of collagen, tissue breakdown, and bacteria, which allows wound healing without crusting. Wash the involved area with mild soap and water and rinse thoroughly. Apply Debrisan directly to the lesion if the contour permits. A paste of Debrisan and glycerin can be placed on gauze and then applied to the lesion twice daily.

DiMascio found that granulation tissue formed in the presence of gram-negative or gram-positive organisms without prior clearing of the infection with antibiotics. However, before effective healing, surgical or enzymatic debridement was needed if necrotic tissue was present.

Gelfoam powder and compressed pads placed inside decubitus ulcers produced successful healing, according to Lang and McGrath.[62] Karaya is another absorptive agent that can be applied in powder form directly on the wound with a Karaya-gum ring encircling the area. Wallace and Hayter reported healing of decubitus ulcers in 66 of 69 patients. Complete healing occurred in all but three patients.[97]

To promote healing, cleanse infected wounds with an antiseptic such as acetic acid, povidone–iodine, or hydrogen peroxide. Obtain wound cultures so that appropriate antibiotic therapy can be instituted.[45]

Before granulation can occur, debridement of the ulcer area may be necessary if necrotic tissue is present. Several types of debridement have been successfully used. Although surgical debridement is the most rapid and effective, patients experience blood loss. Biochemical debridement can be accomplished using proteolytic, fibrinolytic, or collagenolytic enzymes. These agents should not come in contact with surrounding tissues and are discontinued when debridement is complete.[21]

Wet-to-dry dressings will also accomplish wound debridement. As the moistened dressing dries, necrotic debris adheres and will be removed with the dressing.[19] Lasers have been used to debride decubitus ulcers. Bleeding is less with this technique than with surgical debridement. With this approach, necrotic material is vaporized and bleeding vessels can be cauterized.[88]

Two other topical agents have been used: insulin and Op-Site. Effectiveness of the topical application of insulin to speed the healing of decubitus ulcers was investigated by

TABLE 13-2
TOPICAL AGENTS USED TO PREVENT OR TREAT DECUBITUS ULCERS

AGENTS	ACTIONS	SPECIAL CONSIDERATIONS
Topical Treatments		
Creams and lotions	Softens skin; may relieve skin itching	Gently pat area of application to remove excess.
Vitamin A and D preparation (Sween Cream, Desitin, Diaparene)	Soothing effect; may promote healing	Not effective for severe decubitus ulcers
Aluminum-containing antacids	Soothing and drying effect	Produces alkaline environment, which supports bacterial growth. Magnesium-containing antacids have less soothing and drying effects.
Gelatin products (Stomahesive, Orabase)	Provides soothing protective coating; absorbs drainage	Stomahesive will adhere to weeping tissue. Orabase is more easily removed.
Absorptive Agents		
Dextranomer (Debrisan)	Absorbs drainage	Effective with profusely draining wounds
Karaya	Absorbs drainage	Acidic, which discourages bacterial growth. Should be in contact with draining wound
Absorbable gelatin sponge (Gelfoam)	Absorbable, hemostatic sponge. Supports growth of new tissue	Dressing changed every 3–7 days. Gelfoam remains in place when dressing is changed.
Aluminum-containing antacids	Will dry small amounts of drainage	See topical treatments.
Debriding Agents		
Wet-to-dry dressings	Mechanical debridement as dried dressing is removed	Dressing placed against wound surface should not contain cotton.

Van Ort and Gerber in 1976.[92] In a pilot study with a small sample, patients who received topical insulin to their pressure sores experienced an increased rate of healing. However, in a later publication, the two investigators warned that topical insulin was a questionable therapeutic intervention that can cause hypoglycemia and coma.[42] The reader is reminded that any drug is considered to be a new medication when it is used for a new

TABLE 13-2 (continued)
TOPICAL AGENTS USED TO PREVENT OR TREAT DECUBITUS ULCERS

AGENTS	ACTIONS	SPECIAL CONSIDERATIONS
Hydrogen peroxide	Loosens necrotic materials through effervescent action	Will remove healthy tissue as well as necrotic. Use only in open areas where oxygen bubbles can escape.
Enzymes	Chemical debridement	
Collagenase	Digests collagen	Do not apply to normal skin.
Fibrinolysin and desoxy- ribonuclease (Elase)	Digests fibrin of blood and wound exudates	Before applying Elase, clean wound with hydrogen per- oxide or saline.
Sutilains ointment (Travase)	Proteolytic enzyme	Before using Travase, irrigate wound with saline or water to remove antiseptic or heavy metal antibacterials that will deactivate this en- zyme.
Antimicrobials Acetic acid (.25% strength)	Effective against gram-negative and gram-positive organisms	Inexpensive. Can be made from vinegar. May irritate sur- rounding tissue
Hydrogen peroxide	Effective against anaerobes	See debriding agents.
Povidine–iodine	Effective against spores, vi- ruses, fungi, gram-positive, gram-negative organisms, and anerobes	Check for iodine sensitivity. May increase iodine level in the body
Miscellaneous Insulin	Thought to promote healing	Not FDA-approved for de- cubitus ulcer care. May cause alteration in blood glu- cose level
Polyurethane	Provides a moist environment, which encourages granulation	Dressing can remain in place 3–4 days

purpose, and it must be tested and approved by the Federal Food and Drug Administration (FDA). Topical application of insulin has not been approved by the FDA.

A self-adhesive, transparent, polyurethane dressing such as Op-Site has been recommended for decubitus ulcer care. This nonporous dressing prevents the escape of fluid but is permeable to air and water vapor, which prevents anaerobic bacteria buildup.

A moist environment is created which is thought to accelerate granulation and epithelialization. Ahmed reported improvement in 65 patients with superficial and deep ulcers using Op-Site.[1] To use Op-Site the pressure sore should be cleansed, rinsed with saline, and dried thoroughly. Select a piece of Op-Site 2 to 3 inches larger than the wound since the dressing will not adhere to the wound. The transparent dressing allows continuous assessment of the ulcer. In Ahmed's study the Op-Site remained in place for 3 to 4 days unless it began to leak or became dislodged. A subjective decrease in the time required for dressing changes was also reported.

Physical Devices

There are numerous physical devices that can be used to treat pressure sores either alone or in combination with topical agents. One type of physical device that should not be used is the foam rubber doughnut or air-inflated rubber ring. This device increases pressure in the surrounding tissue and decreases oxygen supply to the ulcer. Some physical devices that are in use are presented in Table 13-3.

Heat often is applied by a 60 watt or 75 watt lamp, which is placed from 45 cm to 60 cm (18–24 in) from the ulcer and left in place for 10 minutes.[56] The resultant vasodilation of arterioles in the area causes an increased blood supply, which brings additional nutrients for tissue healing.[7] A hair dryer will provide warm air, which has a drying effect and also increases circulation.[28]

Hyperbaric oxygen (HBO) also has a drying effect, which is thought to control infection. Epithelialization and possibly capillary growth are enhanced.[56] HBO also helps to differentiate necrotic from viable tissue.[91]

In addition to heat and HBO, other physical devices are available that support all or part of the body. Sheepskins are one of the most frequently used devices. The construction of the sheepskin, whether real or synthetic, allows air circulation to keep the skin dry. Best results occur when the sheepskin is placed in direct contact with the skin. Sheepskins also are thought to distribute pressure over a larger area of the body and to reduce friction.

Davis reported an improvement in decubitus ulcers when patients were placed on sheepskins.[26] First the ulcers were surgically debrided and then placed in direct contact with the sheepskin. However, in their study Bliss and McLaren cited disadvantages of sheepskin when one third of the subjects experienced a worsening of their ulcers.[14] Natural and synthetic sheepskin caused the patients to be hot and uncomfortable. Additionally, sheepskins are destroyed by repeated washings.[49]

Eggcrate foam pads are used in an attempt to disperse pressure over a large portion of the body. Gel pads, which are similar in consistency to human fat, add protection over bony prominences. Thus, pressure is reduced in high-pressure areas and dispersed over a broader area. Souther, Carr, and Vistnes found variations in effectiveness among commercially available pads.[84]

Steffel, Schenk and Walker studied a number of pressure relieving devices, including alternating pressure mattresses, water-filled mattresses, and air-filled mattresses. Thirteen patients, who were at risk for decubitus ulcer formation, each tested five devices that were evaluated by the subjects and their caregivers. Factors evaluated included: cost, stability, dimensions, ability of subjects to assume various positions, extent to which the device made subjects warm or cool, tendency to cause bouncing, noise,

TABLE 13-3
PHYSICAL DEVICES USED TO PREVENT OR TREAT DECUBITUS ULCERS

DEVICES	ACTIONS	SPECIAL CONSIDERATIONS
Physical (Heat)		
Lamp (60-watt bulb)	Increases circulation to involved area and has a drying effect	Place light bulb 18–24 in from patient. Apply 1–2 times a day for 10 min. The skin and lamp should be checked every 5 min.
Hair dryer	Increases circulation to involved area and has a drying effect	For heat, set dryer on warm. Check skin and appliance setting every 5 minutes. For drying effect only, remove heating element.
Hyperbaric oxygen	Increases oxygenation of involved area. Encourages epithelialization	Small chambers that fit over the extremities are available.
Physical (Supportive)		
Sheepskin	Provides aeration and absorbs moisture. Disperses pressure over wider area	Real sheepskins are expensive and may be difficult to clean; effectiveness of synthetic sheepskins is reduced with multiple washings.
Eggcrate foam pads	Disperses pressure over a larger area	A protective sleeve is recommended for incontinent patients.
Gel pads	Pad has a consistency similar to human fat. Disperses pressure over a larger area	Available in a variety of sizes
Alternating Pressure Device	Alternates pressure points	All parts of the patient's body must be in contact with the device. Pillows, supports, or sheepskins will negate its effect.
Water mattress	Disperses pressure	Different types are available. May decrease the patient's mobility
Air-fluidized bed (Clinitron)	Provides uniform support of entire body	The unit is expensive and heavy.
Others		
Timing devices	Auditory reminder for patients to change positions	

ease of cleaning, leakage of fluid or air, weight, mechanical reliability, and linen displacement. Findings indicated a positive correlation between the subjects' and the caregivers' ratings and rankings of the devices.[86]

Steffel and colleagues found that soft or unstable devices such as air or water-filled mattresses, on which the head of the bed could not be adjusted, altered the subjects' abilities to engage in self-care activities. Devices that were higher than the bed interfered with the patients' abilities to perform independent transfers, especially if the device was also unstable. The subjects reported feeling cold on fluid-filled mattresses and warm on air-filled beds. (Many newer models of the devices are now equipped to permit appropriate heating and cooling.) Another problem with some of the devices was noise. An additional finding was that some devices caused problems with linen displacement.[86]

A few of the numerous approaches to decubitus ulcer care have been described. Most of these approaches are based on intuition, subjective assessment, or testing with small samples. Research is needed that clearly demonstrates which of the agents and devices are effective in what circumstances and at what cost. Acceptability to patients and caregivers also must be addressed.

WOUNDS

Actions that will promote wound healing begin in the preoperative period. Aside from the problem requiring surgery, patients should be as close as possible to their optimal state of health. In relation to wound healing, it is very important to consider the patient's nutritional status. Another potentially changeable situation with implications for wound healing is smoking. Platelet function is affected among people who smoke; the result is an increased tendency for coagulation and obstruction of small blood vessels. Additionally, smokers may have less ability to transport oxygen to the tissues.[78] Clearly, these two problems could affect the blood and oxygen supply to the wound.

The preoperative preparation of the surgical site is important in relation to wound healing. Seropian and Reynolds conducted a study on the incidence of postoperative wound infections when the operative site was prepared by using a depilatory versus shaving with a razor. In analyzing the results with 406 patients, they found that 5.6% of the patients who were shaved developed infections, in comparison to 0.6% of the patients prepared using the depilatory and 0.6% of the patients who received no preparation. They concluded that microscopic injury to the skin by shaving was the reason for these statistically and clinically significant differences.[80]

Practices in preoperative disinfection of the skin vary. In their review of disinfecting agents, Kaul and Jewett concluded that the ideal agent and technique do not exist.[55]

The efforts during the preoperative period are directed toward optimizing wound healing postoperatively. Although many surgical wounds heal without difficulty by first intention, management of the wound and dressings are helpful in promoting healing. The major purpose for dressings is to protect the wound. Edlich and co-workers conducted laboratory experiments in which they swabbed the surface of sutured wounds with *Staphylococcus aureus* or *Escherichia coli*. They found that swabbing with the organisms during the first 48 hours after the wounds were created resulted in infection. By the third day, however, resistance was sufficient so that infections did not occur. This research suggests that standard surgical dressings on nondraining wounds may serve no purpose by the third postoperative day.

Additionally, it is important to use particular care, including strict aseptic technique, when wounds are treated or dressed during the early postoperative period.[33]

Op-Site can be used as a dressing. One advantage it provides is that it keeps the wound moist, which is helpful because moisture promotes more rapid epithelialization.[8,52]

In some circumstances, wound healing is delayed. This result is most likely when the patient has complicating problems (e.g., malnutrition). Nursing management of wounds in which healing is delayed is complex and time-consuming. Most often these wounds have become infected. Infection is more likely in wounds with dead space, necrotic tissue, or hematomas.[32] Infected wounds usually are opened and kept open until the infection subsides.

Management of these open wounds focuses on controlling the drainage, cleaning the area, and dressing the wounds appropriately. Management of the drainage is affected by the presence or absence of drains, which are frequently inserted at the time of surgery. The purpose of a drain is to relieve a potentially harmful collection of fluids, such as pus, bile, gastric and pancreatic secretions. However, when fluids are not localized, the presence of a drain may be more hazardous than prophylactic. A drain acts as a retrograde conduit for the entry of skin contaminants.[33]

The chance of infection is reduced with the use of a closed drainage system. The area around the drain site should be carefully cleaned, using aseptic technique. Dunavant suggested that skin protection should be used if the drainage is excessive or contains irritating substances.[32] Protection can be achieved with skin barriers and pouches. Some of the effective skin barriers are not sterile and would be altered structurally or chemically by sterilization. Thus, the benefits produced by the skin barriers must be weighed against the risk of possible infection. Dunavant has not found that infections from nonsterile skin barriers are a problem. Some of the commonly used skin barriers include: Stomahesive, Premium Barrier, and Karaya paste.

Several manufacturers produce pouches that can be sterilized without damage. A pouch provides additional skin protection and allows the drainage to be collected for measurement. The skin surrounding a drain site should be gently cleansed, thoroughly rinsed, and patted dry. A skin barrier of choice should be applied according to manufacturer's directions. The pouch is applied over the skin barrier. A drainage tube and collecting device can be attached to the lower end of the pouch and reinforced with tape to prevent leakage.

Many of the methods used to treat decubitus ulcers also are appropriate for treating open wounds. If a wound contains exudate or necrotic tissue, cleansing and debridement are indicated. Wound irrigations with antimicrobial solutions may be ordered (see Table 13-2). Debrisan produces a chemical cleansing of wounds. (The technique for using Debrisan was described in management of decubitus ulcers.) However, if the wound contains necrotic tissue and crusts, the area must be debrided.

Chemical debridement can be accomplished with proteolytic enzymes. After the wound is cleansed, rinsed, and dried, the wound is slightly moistened, a thin coating of the enzyme is applied, followed by a loose moist dressing. Follow this technique three to four times each day until debridement is accomplished. Wet-to-dry dressings, previously discussed, produce a mechanical debridement. When debridement is complete or is no longer desired, a nonadherent dressing may be placed over the wound. Op-Site may be useful in this situation.

One advantage of Op-Site is its transparency, which permits observation of the wound without disturbing the dressing. All wounds, whether infected or noninfected, closed or open, must be closely monitored for signs of progress or lack of progress toward wound healing. Only in this way can appropriate management be determined, which will help the patient to regain the integrity of the skin.

SUMMARY

Few people during life escape skin changes and their effects. To a greater or lesser extent these changes affect the physical and psychological well-being of the individual. They also carry a financial cost in over-the-counter prescriptions, visits to physicians, and prescription drugs and devices.

Much more needs to be learned concerning the management of skin changes. Many different approaches are used, but frequently protocols have been established on the basis of little empirical evidence to support the efficacy of measures. Clearly, it is important for nurses to conduct research and to work with researchers in other disciplines to gain further knowledge about these skin changes. In this way the care received by patients will be improved, and skin integrity maintained or restored as quickly as possible.

REFERENCES

1. Ahmed MC: Op-Site for decubitus care. Am J Nurs 82:61, 1982
2. Andersen KE, Jensen O, Knorning SA et al: Prevention of pressure sores by identifying patients at risk. Br Med J 284:1370, 1982
3. Arndt KA: Manual of Dermatologic Therapeutics, 2nd ed. Boston, Little, Brown & Co., 1978
4. Arndt KA, Jick H: Rates of cutaneous reactions to drugs. JAMA 235:918, 1976
5. Beach WJ: Skin protective preparations. Cutis 13:638, 1974
6. Berecek KH: Etiology of decubitus ulcers Part a. Nurs Clin North Am 10, No. 1:157, 1975
7. Berecek KH: Treatment of decubitus ulcers Part b. Nurs Clin North Am 10, No. 1:171, 1975
8. Besst JA, Wallace HL: Wound healing: Intraoperative factors. Nurs Clin North Am 14, No. 4:701, 1979
9. Bettley FT: Some effects of soap on the skin. Br Med J 1:1675, 1960
10. Bickers DR, Kappas A: Metabolic and pharmacologic properties of the skin. Hosp Pract, 9 No. 5:97, 1974
11. Binnick SA: Skin diseases: Diagnosis and management in clinical practice. Reading, MA, Addison–Wesley, 1982
12. Blank IH: Factors which influence the water content of the stratum corneum. J Invest Dermatol 18:433, 1952
13. Blank IH: Further observations on factors which influence the water content of the stratum corneum. J Invest Dermatol 21:259, 1953
14. Bliss M, McLaren R: Preventing pressure sores in geriatric patients. Part I. Nurs Mirror 123:379, 1967
15. Brown MM, Boosinger J, Black J et al: Nursing innovation for dry skin care of the feet in the elderly: A demonstration project. J Gerontol Nurs 8, No. 7:393, 1982
16. Burgess PR, Dobson RL: Pruritus, pain, and sweating disorders. J Invest Dermatol 73:495, 1979
17. Carsen RA: Aging skin: Understanding the inevitable. Geriatrics, 30, No. 2:51, 1975
18. Carney RG: The aging skin. Am J Nurs 63:110, 1963
19. Chang LF: How to succeed with wet-to-dry dressing. RN 42:63, 1979
20. Coker KE: The intermittent air-fluidized bed and the neurologically impaired patient. J Neurosurg Nurs 11:31, 1979
21. Cooagenase. Drug update. Nurs 3, No. 10:35, 1973
22. Collar M, Brown MS: Over-the-counter drugs for skin disorders. Part 2: Dry skin, eczema, psoriasis and antiseborrheic preparations. Nurs Pract 2, No. 5:14, 1977
23. Cooper DM, Schumann D: Postsurgical nursing intervention as an adjunct to wound healing. Nurs Clin North Am 14, No. 4:713, 1979
24. Cripps DJ: Skin care and problems in the aged. Hosp Pract 12, No. 4:119, 1977

25. Cruse PJ, Foord R: A five-year prospective study of 23,649 surgical wounds. Arch Surg 107:206, 1973
26. Davis L: Sheepskins and decubitus ulcers. J Med Assoc State Ala 29:164, 1959
27. Dempsey H: Hemostasis. In Menaker L (ed): Biologic Basis of Wound Healing. Hagerstown, Harper & Row, 1975
28. Denholm DH: The hair dryer treatment for decubiti. Can Nurse 70:33, 1974
29. Derbes VJ: Rashes: Recognition and management. Nurse 8, No. 3:54, 1978
30. DiMascio S: Debrisan for decubitus ulcers. Am J Nurs 79:684, 1979
31. Domonkos AN, Arnold HL, Odom RB: Andrew's Diseases of the Skin, 7th ed. Philadelphia, WB Saunders, 1982
32. Dunavant MK: Wound and fistula management. In Broadwell DC, Jackson BS (eds): Principles of Ostomy Care. St. Louis, CV Mosby, 1982
33. Edlich RF, Rodeheaver GT, Thacker JG et al: Technical factors in wound management. In Hunt TK, Dunphy, JE (eds): Fundamentals of Wound Management. New York, Appleton–Century–Crofts, 1979
34. Exton–Smith AN, Sherwin RW: The prevention of pressure sores: Significance of spontaneous bodily movement. Lancet 2:1124, 1961
35. Feingold DS, Bachta M: Common skin diseases seen by the internist. DM 25, No. 7:1, 1979
36. Finley JM: Practical Wound Management. Chicago, Year Book Medical Publishers, 1981
37. Flynn ME: Influencing repair and recovery. Am J Nurs 82:1550, 1982
38. Flynn ME, Rovee DT: Promoting wound healing. Am J Nurs 82:1543, 1982
39. Friberg H: Minding moisture stores of the skin. Patient Care 11:153, 1977
40. Frommeyer WB: Blood coagulation. In Menaker L (ed): Biologic Basis of Wound Healing. Hagerstown, Harper & Row, 1975
41. Gaul LE, Underwood GB: Relation of dew point and barometric pressure to chapping of normal skin. J Invest Dermatol 19:9, 1952
42. Gerber RM, Van Ort SR: Topical application of insulin to pressure sores: A questionable therapy. Am J Nurs 81:1159, 1981
43. Gilchrest BA: Age-associated changes in the skin. J Am Geriatr Soc 30:139, 1982
44. Gosnell DJ: An assessment tool to identify pressure sores. Nurs Res 22:55, 1973
45. Gruber P, Vistnes L, Pardoe R: The effect of commonly used antiseptics on wound healing. Plast Reconstr Surg 55:472, 1975
46. Gruis ML, Innes B: Assessment: Essential to prevent pressure sores. Am J Nurs 76:1762, 1976
47. Hanna MJD, MacMillan AL: Aging and the skin. In Brocklehurst JC (ed): Textbook of Geriatric Medicine and Gerontology, 2nd ed. Edinburgh, Churchill–Livingstone, 1978
48. Hargast TS: Understanding pressure sores. Reprinted from Paraplegia News, April 1979. Rehab Nurs 6, No. 3:23, 1981
49. Herbert P, Alterescu V: Pressure necrosis. In Broadwell CL, Jackson BS (eds): Principles of Ostomy Care. St. Louis, CV Mosby, 1982
50. Hunt TK: Disorders of repair and their management. In Hunt TK, Dunphy JE (eds): Fundamentals of Wound Management. New York, Appleton–Century–Crofts, 1979
51. Hunt TK, Andrews WS, Halliday B et al: Coagulation and macrophage stimulation of angiogenesis and wound healing. In Dineen P (ed): The Surgical Wound. Philadelphia, Lea & Febiger, 1981
52. Hunt TK, Van Winkle W: Normal repair. In Hunt TK, Dunphy JE (eds): Fundamentals of Wound Management. New York, Appleton–Century–Crofts, 1979
53. Husain T: An experimental study of some pressure effects on tissues with references to the bed sore problem. J Pathology and Bacteriology 66:347, 1953
54. Jordan WP, Bourlas MC: Allergic contact dermatitis due to underwear elastic. Arch Dermatol 111:593, 1975
55. Kaul A, Jewett J: Agents and techniques for disinfection of the skin. J Enterostomal Therapy 8(5):19, 1981
56. Kavchak–Keyes MA: Treating decubitus ulcers using four proven steps. Nurs 7, No. 10:44, 1977
57. Kim MJ, Moritz DA (eds): Classification of Nursing Diagnoses. New York, McGraw–Hill, 1982
58. Kligman AM: Perspectives and problems in cutaneous gerontology. J Invest Dermatol 73:39, 1979
59. Knox JM, Cocherell EG, Freeman RG: Etiological factors and premature aging. JAMA 179:630, 1962
60. Kosiak M: Etiology of decubitus ulcers. Arch Phys Med 42:19–29, 1961
61. Landis EM: Microinfection of capillary blood pressure in human skin. Heart 75:209, 1930
62. Lang C, McGrath A: Gelfoam for decubitus ulcers. Am J Nurs 74:460, 1974
63. Langer R: Drug eruptions. In Binnick SA: Skin Diseases: Diagnosis and Management in Clinical Practice. Reading, MA, Addison–Wesley, 1982
64. Levenson S: Nutrition. In Hunt TK, Dunphy DE

(eds): Fundamentals of Wound Management. New York, Appleton–Century–Crofts, 1979

65. Levenson S, Seifter E, Van Winkle W: Nutrition. In Hunt TK, Dunphy JE (eds): Fundamentals of Wound Management. New York, Appleton–Century–Crofts, 1979

66. Lindan A, Greenway RM, Piazza JM: Pressure distribution on the surface of the human body. Arch Phys Med Rehabil 46:378, 1965

67. McLemore T:1979 summary national ambulatory medical care survey. Advance Data 66:1, 1981

68. Mikulic MA: Treatment of pressure ulcers. Am J Nurs 80:1125, 1980

69. Millikan LE: Skin anatomy in wound healing. Ear Nose Throat J 60:10, 1981

70. Mitchell AC: Black skin: An historical, psychological and health care perspective. J Cont Educ Nurs 10:28, 1979

71. Montagna W, Carlisle K: Structural changes in aging human skin. J Invest Dermatol 73:47, 1979

72. Moreno H: Platelet function. In Menaker L (ed): Biologic Basis of Wound Healing. Hagerstown, Harper & Row, 1975

73. Noojin RO: Dermatology. Flushing, NY, Medical Examination Publ., 1977

74. O'Byrne C: Clinical detection and management of postoperative wound sepsis. Nurs Clin North Am 14, No. 4:727, 1979

75. Parrish JA, Suskin RR: Skin reactions to environmental agents. J Invest Dermatol 73:501, 1979

76. Reichel S: Shearing force as a factor in decubitus ulcer in paraplegics. JAMA 166:762, 1958

77. Roach LB: Color changes in dark skin. Nursing 7, No. 1:48, 1977

78. Schumann D: Preoperative measures to promote wound healing. Nurs Clin North Am 14, No. 4:683, 1979

79. Schwartz L: Common skin problems. In Bullough B (ed): The Management of Common Human Miseries. New York, Springer–Verlag, 1979

80. Seropian R, Reynolds BM: Wound infections after preoperative depilatory versus razor preparation. Am J Surg 121:251, 1971

81. Shelmire JB: The influence of oil-in-water emulsions on the hydration of keratin. J Invest Dermatol 26:105, 1956

82. Siegel RJ, Vistnes LM, Laub DR: Use of water bed for prevention of pressure sores. Plast Reconstr Surg 51:31, 1973

83. Silvers DN: The skin: Basic pathophysiology. In Domonkos AN, Arnold HL, Odom RD (eds): Andrew's Diseases of the Skin, 7th ed. Philadelphia, WB Saunders, 1982

84. Souther SG, carr SD, Vistnes LM: Wheelchair cushions to reduce pressure under bony prominences. Arch Phys Med Rehabil 55:460, 1974

85. Spoor HG: Measurement and maintenance of natural skin oil. NY State J Med 58:3292, 1958

86. Staffel PE, Schenk EA, Walker SL: Reducing devices for pressure sores, Nurs Res 29:228, 1980

87. Steigleder GK, Raab WP: Skin protection afforded by ointments. J Invest Dermatol 38:129, 1962

88. Stellar S, Meijer R, Walia S et al: Carbon dioxide laser debridement of decubitus ulcers. Ann Surg 179:230, 1974

89. Sullivan ND, Basler RSW: Geriatric dermatology. In O'Hara–Devereaux M, Andrus LH et al (eds): Eldercare. New York, Grune & Stratton, 1981

90. Thorne N: Cosmetics and the dermatologist. Br J Clin Pract 19:111, 1965

91. Torelli M: Topical hyperbaric oxygen for decubitus ulcers. Am J Nurs 73:494, 1973

92. Van Ort SR, Gerber RM: Topical application of insulin in the treatment of decubitus ulcers: A pilot study. Nurs Res 25:9, 1976

93. Van Scott EJ, Lyon JB: A chemical measure of the effect of soaps and detergents on the skin. J Invest Dermatol 21:199, 1953

94. Verhonick PJ, Lewis DW, Goller HO: Thermography in the study of decubitus ulcers. Nurs Res 21:233, 1972

95. Volanakis JE, Freeman DG, Stroud RM: Acute inflammation and its chemical mediators: Hypersensitivity reactions. In Meanker L (ed): Biologic Basis of Wound Healing. Hagerstown, Harper & Row, 1975

96. Waisman M: A clinical look at the aging skin. Postgrad Med 66:87, 1979

97. Wallace G, Hayter J: Karaya for chronic skin ulcers. Am J Nurs 74:1094, 1974

98. Wells TJ: In geriatric patients: That "minor" skin problem could be trouble. RN 41, No. 7:41, 1978

99. Williams A: A study of factors contributing to skin breakdown. Nurs Res 21:238, 1972

100. Worobec SM, Solomon LM: Structure and function of the skin. In Solomon LM, Esterly NB, Loeffel ED (eds): Adolescent Dermatology. Philadelphia, WB Saunders, 1978

14

Diarrhea and Constipation

Patricia Natale
Howard Beckman

Alterations from usual patterns of bowel function occur at one time or another for everyone. These changes can include a wide spectrum of variation and may reflect disease process or normal physiologic response to variables such as diet, activity restriction, environmental change, and psychosocial stressors. Regardless of etiology, the nurse practicing in any setting must be able to evaluate and manage the response of the person to altered bowel function.

The intent of this discussion is to view the whole person response to intestinal function rather than focusing on the symptom itself. The central point will be the person's perceived experience of diarrhea or constipation and the effect of these changes on daily life activities. Although knowledge of anatomy, physiology, and pathophysiology is important, we feel that effective nursing management is derived from involvement of the person in health care and the subsequent understanding of the alteration of bowel function from the patient's perception.

The goal of this chapter is to present data that will facilitate the nurse's understanding of those variables that affect bowel habit alterations and function. Constipation and di-

arrhea are viewed as symptomatic of physiologic responses to normal or pathologic variables. Information relevant to diarrhea and constipation will be presented separately. (Laboratory and radiographic diagnostic procedures will not be discussed in detail since this material is presented thoroughly in other sources.) Resources for in-depth discussion of specific diseases are provided in the bibliography. The nursing process is used as a model for organization of information.

FACTORS AFFECTING BOWEL FUNCTION

Before discussing specific mechanisms involved in constipation and diarrhea, consider the multiple factors that affect bowel function.

Physiology

The small intestine is responsible for nutrient absorption. Digestive enzymes initiate the process of degrading complex carbohydrates, protein, and fats in the stomach. The duodenum, jejunum, and ileum absorb more fully digested nutrients. For example, the terminal ileum absorbs fat-soluble vitamins D, E, A, and K. Absorption of carbohydrates occurs in the form of mono- and disaccharides. Proteins are absorbed as amino acids, and fats as mono- and diglycerides.

Small intestinal dysfunction can cause significant nutritional deficiency. Because the majority of intestinal material is absorbed in the small bowel, it is the major mechanism in fluid and electrolyte balance. Disease of the small bowel results in large volumes of fecal content being delivered to the colon.

Functions of the colon include absorption of fluid and electrolytes (proximal colon) and storage of feces (distal colon). Material in the colon is gradually exposed to intestinal surfaces by a series of weakly propulsive, mixing muscular contractions. Stool is propelled toward the anus by alternating contraction and relaxation of colonic segments. These events, called *mass movement*, occur two to three times a day, usually 10 to 20 minutes after eating. When stool is forced into the rectum the resulting distention produces the desire to defecate. Mass movements are caused by the duodenocolic and gastrocolic responses, which are initiated by filling of the duodenum and stomach with food. This response explains the common need to defecate at or shortly after eating. Other stimulants include irritation of the intestinal mucosa, stimulation of the parasympathetic nervous system, and overdistention of a colonic segment.

Defecation occurs when the internal anal sphincter is inhibited and the external anal sphincter (under voluntary striated muscle control) is relaxed. Parasympathetic signals intensify peristaltic activity and are enhanced by other stimuli (e.g., the Valsalva maneuver). If a person does not wish to defecate, the external sphincter is tightened, the defecation reflex diminishes and usually does not return for several hours. When tim-

ing is more convenient, defecation reflexes can be initiated by deep inspiration (beginning the Valsalva maneuver) to force fecal content into the rectum and elicit new reflexes by means of increased distention. However, these reflexes are not as effective as those that arise naturally.[16] As stool remains in the colon, more fluid is absorbed; the stool becomes harder and more difficult to pass. Consequently, simply ignoring the urge to defecate can cause constipation.

Age

As one grows older, atrophy of muscle and mucosa occur. Muscle function becomes less efficient, probably due to morphological changes in autonomic ganglia. Loss of cerebral cortical inhibition may contribute to fecal incontinence. As the nervous system ages, peripheral nerve conduction is impaired, producing inadequate motility, delayed feedback control of hormonal and enzymatic release, and reduced sensitivity to pain and intestinal sensation; thus, the ability of the elderly to tolerate space-occupying lesions in the colon with little discomfort. Reduced vasomotor response to exercise, ingestion, and emotion are additional factors that place the older person at risk for altered bowel function.[1]

Activity Level

Exercise is thought to enhance propulsive colonic motion. It is not unusual for runners to notice unplanned urges for defecation while exercising. Reduction in usual exercise levels reduces muscle tone, and thus interferes with elimination patterns. This response often is noted when people are on bed rest for acute illness or restricted activity levels following musculoskeletal injury. Wakefulness increases bowel motility; sleep decreases it.[16]

Nutrition

Eating is probably the major stimulus affecting secretion and motility of the intestines. Currently, much has been written about the poor nutritional quality of western diets. For example, sugar consumption in Great Britain has increased 20-fold since 1750.[18] Also, use of white flour and grain products that have been denuded of fibrous coats is widespread. Burkitt has studied the diet of various cultures extensively.[8] He has shown that decreased fiber causes less bulky stools, a condition that leads to increased intraluminal pressures and prolonged transit time. He also suggests that low-fiber diets contribute to the development of appendicitis, diverticular disease, colon cancer, and polyps. By way of explanation, Burkitt states that chronic low-fiber diets cause small stools, making the descending colon contract too firmly. This action leads to muscular hypertrophy and diverticula formation. Difficult evacuation with associated straining increases venous pressure and favors hemorrhoid development. Authorities also believe that absence of fiber slows transit time, which then prolongs the contact between carcinogens and colonic mucosa. One beneficial action of fiber is believed to be its binding of water in the intestine to form a gel. The result is a bulky, soft stool that is easily passed.

Fiber is classified into two major groups. Structural forms, cellulose and lignin, are termed *crude fiber* and are not believed to be very effective. Noncellulose polysaccharides (dextrins, algal polysaccharides, pectins, and hemicellulose) are called *reserve* or *storage fibers* and provide the most effective dietary sources.[25]

In unprocessed carbohydrate foods, each cell is surrounded by an envelope of fibers. Refining breaks down the cellular wall and exposes its starchy interior. For example, white bread has had its fibrous portions of wheat kernel removed. Baked or canned fruits lose most of their fiber as a result of cooking. Specific food sources and suggestions for dietary manipulation will be discussed later.

Adequate hydration is also necessary for bowel function. Adults probably require at least 2 to 3 liters of fluid daily and, when that amount is reduced because of impaired intake or body loss, stool is more difficult to pass. Finally, a less frequently recognized cause of constipation is fever.

Psychosocial Factors

Both review of the literature and clinical experience reveal a myriad of psychosocial factors relating to change in bowel habits. This discussion begins with elements relating to toileting, habit, and cultural conscripts, and will conclude with considerations of the more general tenets of symptom meaning and somatization.

Culture   Toileting practices and rituals are learned behaviors for all of us. Most of us have set ideas about how often, how much, and in what way stool "should" be passed. Bowel function often is used as a barometer of general health, and alterations in bowel function cause concern. Research reveals a lack of consensus about how many stools per day is normal. The continuum ranges from several daily defecations to two to three bowel movements weekly. Authorities agree that overconcern about defecation is not desirable.

Use of the bowel as a health barometer contrasts with prominent western cultural ideas about toileting. Members of this culture regard feces as unclean. Defecation is completed in private and is not an acceptable topic for social conversation. Discussion with patients having diarrhea from irritable bowel syndrome (IBS) reveals that the most difficult part of the syndrome to deal with is embarrassment from bowel odor and noise occurring with flatulence or explosive stools. Many of these people avoid use of public restroom facilities for just those reasons. One of our patients scheduled all of her shopping and personal business so that she would not have to use a public bathroom.

Anthropologists assert that these attitudes arise from the predominance of the European bourgeoisie and its refinement of social habits. Prosperity, democracy, frequency of bathing, and cleanliness appear to be linked concepts in the value structure in the United States.[28]

Other cultures show evidence of similar attitudes. Indian people suffer ritual impurity as a result of contact with excreta and reproductive fluids. Any habit or action that leads to a state of impurity evokes disapproval from others.[20]

An example from anthropological research serves to underline the importance of understanding the influence of culture on toileting habits. In rural India, an attempt was made to improve sanitation by constructing latrines for villagers' use. It was reasoned that this would reduce fecal contamination of drinking water and reduce disease. The latrines were specially adapted to the local squatting posture used to defecate. However, the villagers did not use their new latrines even though they understood the rationale for their use. Researchers later realized that the prevalent custom of defecating in open fields was linked to social activity. Every morning and evening the village women went in groups to the open fields to relieve themselves, to exchange advice and news of the day and bathe with water from tanks located in the fields. Thus, the habits of toileting and bathing were linked to community sharing and routine. Use of latrines would clearly disrupt these linkages.[28]

Another cultural influence is diet. Constipation is almost unknown in African cultures where foods include nuts, fruits, and other high fiber sources.[8]

Toileting Toileting posture can directly influence the process of defecation. In many Eastern cultures the posture utilized is squatting. This position increases intra-abdominal pressure and enhances propulsion of the fecal bolus. The modern commode with a high seat reduces the impact of the squatting position. The bedpan requires an anatomical position that is almost opposite to squatting. If one adds the psychological impact of dependence and embarrassment occurring when defecating in a pan, it is clearly not an efficacious device. Halpern estimates that straining at stool increases up to sixfold when using a bedpan.[17] Implications for bedpan use with bedridden patients are obvious; it is doubly important to increase dietary and other modifications in such instances.

Self-concept Self-concept as defined here includes body image, role performance, self-esteem, and personal identity.[21] Attitudes about body image affect bowel function, particularly if bowel products are viewed as unclean or symbolic of health in some way. These views then become part of perceived symptom meaning and are important assessment data for the nurse provider. If alterations in bowel activity are perceived to impinge on gender identity, activities as spouse, wage-earner, or adult, those changes are likely to be perceived as significant by the patient. Consider the implications of the use of a "diaper" on a bedridden adult incontinent of stool. One of our patients with IBS suffered insult to his sense of adulthood and maleness because he feared to use the standing position to void for 8 years. He stated he could never tell when he would have involuntary diarrhea and thus chose to void while seated.

Stress Almy's work has clearly linked stressful events to bowel function.[2,3,4] He demonstrated sigmoidoscopic bowel changes when healthy subjects were given distressing news or when highly emotionally charged events were discussed. Other investigators have noted the association between stress and bowel function.[13,24,36,37]

Clinically, in our work with IBS patients, we have found symptom exacerbation during times of stress. Sometimes the stress is quite obvious—death of a loved one, school performance, or job deadlines. At other times, as with multiple life changes, anniversary reactions, or travel, the event may be less overt. Kirsner asserts that when emotional tension is sustained and when the person has difficulty adapting to the stressor, bowel symptoms are likely to increase.[22]

Connection to stressful events may or may not be apparent to the patient or nurse. Remember the concept of *somatization*, which is the unconscious expression of emotional pain through altered bodily function. One example is the tension headache. Persons who somatize persistently are thought to be expressing conflict through their bodies because the perception of the feeling on a psychic level is too threatening to themselves. It is extremely important for the nurse to remember that these physical sensations are as intense as any other. Such sensations are not "all in the patient's head" or imagined. Many people assume that stress-related illnesses and discomfort are not real. Many patients have described a sense of not being believed by a health provider when the patient is told that symptoms are stress-related.

Thus, it becomes vital to know about a patient's developmental level, life changes, role function, life events, losses, gains, and the characteristic manner with which the person deals with these stressors. The former data will expand the nurse's understanding of bowel alteration from the patient's viewpoint, whereas the latter will influence nursing management. Almost all of our IBS patients developed their initial symptoms concurrent to significant developmental change, such as adolescence and midlife, or during events perceived as personal loss. Usual coping strategies during these times were insufficient.

Symptom Meaning When a person's bowel alteration is perceived to interfere with life activities, it acquires additional significance. For the executive who cannot conduct meetings without leaving the room because of diarrhea, this symptom jeopardizes productivity and job security. For people who change the way they dress, adopt loose fitting clothes to disguise the bloating that accompanies constipation or carry changes of clean clothes or wear disposable diapers, this symptom is perceived as a threat to their self-image. For those who avoid travel or select shopping areas specifically for availability of bathroom facilities, the symptom impinges upon recreational or other role function. For this discussion, the term *symptom meaning* is used to encompass all of the connotations of an alteration in body function for a person.

Symptom meaning is also derived from a person's past experience. Persons who have had experience with constipation and bowel carcinoma are likely to be more concerned about constipation. Successful strategies previously used to control bowel alterations are likely to be employed again and, if not successful, the person tends to experience anxiety that the symptom reflects serious pathology. A provider should ask patients routinely if they think they know what the symptom cause is or if they are concerned about a specific etiology. These concerns are often ameliorated just by verbalizing them or when the provider can address them specifically. Even if the provider cannot assuage the patient's anxiety, addressing it conveys a caring attitude that is vital to the helping relationship.

Secondary Gain   Secondary gain may become an element in any physiologic alteration. Changes in body function can become the reason for avoiding work or social responsibilities. Our IBS patients report that their family and friends increase sympathy and attention during symptomatic periods. If a person is able to avoid stressful events or gain increased attention from significant others, a reward is built into each symptom experience: thus the term *secondary gain*. One investigator believes this phenomenon is a learned, conditioned response.[36] In the American culture sympathy from others and freedom from normal responsibilities are socially appropriate responses to illness. However, in some people this normative behavior can increase the reward of illness and thus reinforce the likelihood that the symptom will continue. Many people have early learning experiences in which illness was given special attention. When this becomes a pattern, they may begin to use body function to gain gratification from others. These patterns of getting positive outcomes from symptoms are usually unconscious and not part of the person's awareness.[36]

Assessment of secondary gain is difficult and must be accomplished over time. As the helping relationship is established, the provider usually develops a sense of how the patient gains attention from others and what activities are avoided because of symptoms. Ask the patient to view the symptom as an "advantage" and to list positive aspects of each symptom experience. The "advantage" can then be more fully discussed. Again, this discussion is only appropriate to a fully developed helping relationship.

Diarrhea

INTRODUCTION

Diarrhea is a disorder striking in both its present-day as well as historical impact. Many of the fears and anxieties caused by diarrheal diseases today have their roots in the descriptions of epidemics of cholera in novels, films, and stories. Other images in literature provide quite a different picture. An example is Molierè's lead character in the comedy, *The Imaginary Invalid*, a man preoccupied with frequent bowel movements to the exclusion of all other focuses on life. Although the character's pathology is exaggerated, preoccupation with bowel movements has received much attention in psychoanalytic theory. Additionally, a nurse may find discussing a patient's bowel habits in detail may call up either the nurse's or patient's negative feelings, opinions, and judgments about the concern. The result may be an unconscious desire to avoid an in-depth exploration of the patient's problem.

Although cholera is no longer seen in the United States, significant time and expense is spent each year on the diagnosis and treatment of diarrheal disorders. The impact of this concern is exemplified in the following statistics. From 1977 to 1978, the most recent year for which data is available, the National Center for Health Statistics reported that 4,846,000 physician office visits were initiated by a primary complaint of diarrhea.[27] In addition, 1,281,000 visits for abdominal pain, cramps, and spasms were evaluated to be a result of diarrheal disease. In all, 4,341,000 office visits received a final primary diagnoses of diarrheal disease. Of these patients, 55% to 65% gave a history of an acute problem; the remainder of the presentations were chronic.[27] In addition, many authors cite diarrhea as the most common adverse effect of prescribed medication. The remainder of this section focuses on defining the condition, offering guidelines for evaluation and suggesting a variety of treatment plans that use a biobehavioral perspective of practice.

Diarrhea may be defined as the frequent or increased passage of unformed stools. The stools may be watery or simply semiformed. Volume is not a major aspect in defining diarrhea, although it is important in its evaluation. Change from "normal" for each individual is a major determinant in defining diarrhea because variability in bowel habits is so great. By using the rather vague terms *increased* and *semiformed*, the definition challenges the nurse to engage the patient in clearly defining bowel habits, discussing changes that have occurred, and allowing nurse and patient to work jointly in defining the patient's perception of the problem. Expanding this simple definition provides clues to the impact of this concern on the patient. Part of the history-taking process about this concern includes an exploration of the effect of the diarrhea on the patient's ability to carry out expected day-to-day activities, how the disorder affects the patient's body image, and the disorder's impact on the person's perception of wellness. In defining the condition, sufficient time must be spent to satisfy the patient of the nurse's concern and quality of assessment. Possible starting points for discussion may center around the patient's perception of the problem, the impact of the problem, or the diagnosis the patient feels has caused the diarrhea. Many times, if the initial fears of diagnostic possibilities can be identified, they can be addressed and considered before they disrupt the provider–patient relationship.

MECHANISMS OF DIARRHEA

Diarrhea may be conceptualized most effectively in two ways: 1) the mechanism of the production of the diarrhea and 2) the rapidity of the onset. There are four major mechanisms to the formation of diarrhea stools:

1. Excess osmotic load
2. Active or passive secretion of water and electrolytes
3. Impaired intestinal absorption
4. Altered bowel motility

OSMOTIC LOAD

Excess osmotic loads result from the ingestion of material that is poorly absorbed from the gut lumen. The increased osmotic load in the small intestine results in increased intestinal retention of fluids. These materials may be laxatives, for example, lactulose, ingested foods such as lactose in those with lactase deficiency, or electrolytes that are usually readily absorbed. Sorbitol, used in sugarless gums and candies, is another osmotic culprit. The increased fluid load surpasses the absorptive capacity of the colon, with resultant diarrhea. In general, the intestinal mucosa loses water in excess of sodium. The small bowel contents are hyperosmolar when compared to the serum osmolality, and the diarrhea is large volume. These diarrheal states characteristically stop with the avoidance of the offending medication or food product.

ACTIVE OR PASSIVE SECRETION

Secretory diarrhea may be either passive or active. Passive secretion is less common and less severe. Traditionally, there is local lymphatic or venous obstruction resulting in increased intravascular hydrostatic and intracellular pressure. These differential pressures result in the transudation of water into the intestinal lumen. Examples of etiologic mechanisms are portal hypertension, intestinal ischemia, and some types of mucosal inflammation. The more common and severe active secretory diarrheas have been the subject of intense research during the 1960s and 1970s. [12] The stimulation of mucosal intracellular enzyme systems, notably cyclic AMP, seems to be responsible for the active transport of electrolytes into the intestinal lumen. A remarkable number of stimulators seem to affect this final common pathway. Examples are bacterial toxins produced by *Vibrio cholerae*, Salmonella, and *Escherichia coli*; intestinal hormones such as vasoactive intestinal polypeptide, glucagon, calcitonin, and cholecystokinin; tumors such as villous adenoma; and diseases associated with mucosal damage, such as ulcerative colitis and Crohn's disease. The result is a voluminous, isosmotic diarrhea that is not diminished by fasting.

IMPAIRED INTESTINAL ABSORPTION

An average American consumes 300 g of carbohydrates, 70 g of fat, 90 g of protein, and 2 liters of water daily. Additionally, salivary, gastric, biliary, pancreatic, and mucosal secretions add 7 liters of water per day to intestinal contents, resulting in a water load of 9 liters per day. The small intestine is able to reabsorb up to 15 liters to 20 liters of water per day resulting in a dramatic reserve capability. Disorders that alter small intestinal mucosal integrity sufficiently to cause a markedly decreased functional absorptive surface can overcome the bowel's large reserve capacity and result in large-volume diarrhea. Examples of such disorders are

amyloidosis, celiac disease, and giardiasis. Since the output in this type of diarrhea depends on the intake, fasting may partially reduce the degree of diarrhea. The integrity of water secretion assures isotonic stool compared to plasma. As stated earlier, with sufficient intake, the volume of stool may be large.

ALTERED BOWEL MOTILITY

Because of the limitations of technology, altered motility is probably the least understood of the mechanisms involved in the pathogenesis of diarrhea. There is data to show that in IBS, the baseline electrical activity of the gut is distinguishable from control subjects. [35] This electrical activity influences the frequency of intestinal contraction and the propagation of intestinal contents. Both the frequency and effectiveness of contractility in patients with IBS has been shown to be abnormal. These aspects of motility have been shown to be sensitive both to gastrointestinal hormones as well as psychosocial stress. Additionally, motility disorders have been identified in patients with connective tissue diseases like progressive systemic sclerosis and in metabolic diseases like diabetes. The major point is that in a significant group of people, those with IBS and, probably in many normal people, stimulation of the intestinal tract by an extensive network of central nervous system (CNS) innervation may result in gastrointestinal responses to stresses, for example the college student who develops diarrhea at examination time. These disorders are more often associated with smaller volume diarrheas.

Researchers feel that these four mechanisms either alone, but more often in combination, are responsible for the clinical diarrheal syndromes.

CHRONICITY

In addition to pathophysiologic mechanisms for the formation of diarrheal stools, chronicity is the second major method for evaluating a complaint of diarrhea. Generally, symptoms may be classified acute, chronic, and intermittent. *Acute* is defined by the presence of symptoms for less than 2 weeks. Characteristically, infectious diarrheas are acute, systemic illnesses are chronic, and psychosocially exacerbated diarrheas are intermittent. Common disorders causing these presentations are listed in Table 14-1. Aspects of these disorders will be discussed further under evaluation.

NURSING ASSESSMENT

HISTORY

The history is by far the most critical aspect in the evaluation of diarrheal disease and all too often is inadequately sought. The first step is to clarify the patient's description of the diarrhea to develop a common perception of the concern. For example, a person worried about colon cancer may feel one semiformed stool per day qualifies as diarrhea. While such a concern may not be considered a "valid" complaint, historical information such as a change in diet or preoccupation with cancer may explain the patient's symptom sufficiently to allow the nurse and patient to consider the problem resolved and to alleviate the patient's anxiety and symptoms. Once the problem has been appropriately defined, information needs to be collected on the onset of the disorder, the circumstances surrounding the onset of symptoms, and the chronicity of symptoms. Questioning should be open-ended to allow the patient an opportunity to present any possible contributing factors. Changes in diet, life experiences, new medications,

TABLE 14-1
CLINICALLY IMPORTANT CAUSES OF DIARRHEA

ACUTE	CHRONIC	INTERMITTENT
Viral gastroenteritis	Ulcerative colitis	IBS
Bacterial toxin-induced	Crohn's disease	Lactose intolerance
Staphylococcus	Postoperative dumping	Intussusception
E. coli	Laxative abuse	
Clostridium	Pancreatic insufficiency	
Bacterial invasion	Lactose intolerance	
E. coli	Drug-induced	
Shigella	Giardia lamblia	
Salmonella	Diabetes mellitus	
Campylobacter	Amyloidosis	
Yersinia	Postoperative fistula	
Drug-induced (see Table 14-2)	Villous adenoma	
Hyperthyroidism	Carcinoid syndrome	
Ulcerative colitis	Gastrinoma	
Parasitic	Radiation enteritis	
Ameba	Chronic fecal impaction	
Giardia lamblia		

travel, and exposure to others with similar symptoms are important examples. Follow-up closed-ended questions later on in the interview still allow the identification of precipitating factors to be uncovered, if these are not volunteered in the opening aspects of history-taking. Specific questioning too soon in a visit often prevents a patient from offering important information that is *not* recovered with more specific questioning.

The number and timing of stools must be sought. Nocturnal diarrhea awakening the patient or resulting in night soiling is considered most consistent with pathological diarrhea. Diarrhea that causes a sense of urgency and rectal fullness is commonly of large bowel origin. The character of the stool is critical in the assessment process. Watery, voluminous stools suggest secretory or osmotic diarrheas of small bowel origin. The presence of red blood suggests colonic inflammation as seen with ulcerative colitis or amebic dysentery, while melanotic diarrhea (black, tarlike stool) is associated with proximal colonic disease such as carcinoma or inflammation of the small bowel. Voluminous, pale, foul-smelling stools suggest small intestinal malabsorption. Diarrhea alternating with constipation suggests impaction, obstruction, and IBS.

In acute onset diarrheas, duration of symptoms is usually not a problem, but rapidity of onset provides useful information. Acute, rapid-onset diarrhea usually can be traced to an offending agent or event. Examples include bacterial toxins from a dinner of chili, or potato salad eaten at a picnic. In such situations, others would also have developed symptoms. Other examples are traumatic events such as examinations, divorce, job change, or relocating. Acute, but less rapid-onset diarrhea suggests the accumulation of an offending agent. Examples are bacterial overgrowth with E. coli on a foreign

trip or infestation of *Giardia lamblia*, a parasite that inhabits the small bowel. These symptoms may develop gradually, 7 to 10 days after the trip or exposure. In chronic diarrheas, one approach to chronicity is to ask when the client remembers *not* having diarrhea. This is important since chronic diarrheas associated with malignancy usually will manifest other symptoms within a year, and systemic disease such as amyloidosis may evidence signs of malnutrition. Psychophysiologic diarrheas, on the other hand, are characteristically intermittent, with variable time periods between symptomatic episodes. Often, however, patients define the condition as chronic since the problem has, in fact, gone on for years. Careful history-taking will therefore allow differentiation of chronic continuous diarrhea from chronic intermittent diarrhea. The intermittent diarrhea, as opposed to continuous diarrhea, rarely leads to weight loss, anorexia, fever, or other evidences of malnutrition or systemic disease.

After the amount, chronicity, and character of the stool have been defined, the setting in which symptoms occur needs to be addressed. Major issues to investigate include changes in diet, environment, life experiences, and psychosocial structure. Examples of dietary change may include the following:

Increased fiber from unexpected sources (e.g., fruit coming into season)
Increased lactose in patients with borderline or decreasing lactose tolerance
Increase in amount of coffee, tea, or caffeinated beverages consumed
Spicier foods while the patient was on a trip to a foreign country.

Environmental changes may be subtle, and careful questioning regarding habits and activities must be sought specifically while one is taking a history. Travel has become a major factor in etiologic considerations of diarrheal disease. A notable example is *tourista*, an acute diarrheal syndrome caused by strains of *E. coli*. Characteristically, the diarrhea is associated with abdominal cramping and lasts fewer than 10 days. Infectious diarrheas during trips outside the United States often are caused by drinking nonbottled water, or water in the form of ice added to beverages, or salads and fruits that are prepared by being washed in tap water. These habits need to be sought specifically, since patients may state that they resided in a first-class hotel in a major city and refuse to accept the possibility of their having consumed contaminated foods. As travel involves more rural settings or local dining, the risks of contracting diarrheal diseases increase. Other forms of infectious diarrhea can be contracted closer to home.[33] Water has been contaminated by *Giardia lamblia* in both the United States and Canada. This parasite resides in the small intestine and causes diarrhea. The diarrhea may begin weeks or months after exposure, therefore the travel history should include trips for 6 months before onset of symptoms. Another important environmental factor in acute diarrhea is the location at which foods were eaten. Outbreaks of food poisoning occur after picnics, restaurant meals, and catered affairs. Seek information regarding others with similar symptoms who attended such a gathering, because a significant percentage of the people usually become symptomatic. Other environmental issues include increase in alcohol consumption, increase in cigarette consumption, change in medication use, and exposure to heavy metals in the workplace.

Psychosocial issues and changes in life experiences need to be sought. Major life events such as divorce, retirement, deadlines for work, home, or school may precipitate attacks in patients with IBS. It must be remembered that events are interpreted differently by people, so that any life change should be considered. One must avoid judging the event by one's own value system. Perception of stress at work, home, or school, loss of expected support systems, loss of sense of control over life events all may be involved in exacerbations of psychophysiologic diarrheal states and will be discussed in the management section. These issues are best identified with open-ended questions, but do not take negative responses at face value. Questions like, "Sometimes stress has been associated with diarrhea, have you noticed factors like that recently?" may allow protected issues to be discussed.

Aggravating and alleviating factors can help to identify causes of diarrhea as well as suggest potential treatment possibilities. Symptoms that stop with fasting suggest osmotic diarrheas, and offending dietary agents may then be sought. Symptoms that improve at home suggest psychophysiologic responses to school or work. Symptoms relieved by lactose-free diets or abstinence from caffeine or nicotine implicate those agents.

Specific symptoms associated with the onset of diarrhea can help to implicate specific disorders etiologically in diarrheal disease. Fever suggests infectious or inflammatory diseases; weight loss with chronic diarrhea suggests malabsorptive syndromes and cancer. Epigastric pain radiating to the back suggests pancreatic diseases such as cancer or gastrinoma. Periumbilical pain suggests small bowel disease. Episodes of wheezing and flushing are associated with carcinoid tumors. Arthritis is seen with ulcerative colitis, Crohn's disease, and Whipple's disease. Vomiting is seen with partial bowel obstruction, peptic ulcer, and infectious gastroenteritis. Diarrhea alternating with constipation suggests cancer, impaction, intussusception, volvulus, or IBS. Heat intolerance, smooth skin, and anxiety are seen in hyperthyroidism. These are, of course, just a few examples and are intended as a usable framework. For a complete description of differential diagnosis the reader is referred to Spiro's *Textbook of Gastroenterology*.

Medication history, both prescription and over-the-counter (OTC), should be sought. Overall, diarrhea is felt to be the most common adverse effect of medication. Consider drug effect when any patient taking a new medication (for less than a month) develops diarrhea. Table 14-2 is a list of medications that list diarrhea as a common adverse effect. Remember that almost any drug has been reported to cause diarrhea in certain people. Two issues are of major note here. First, the use of laxatives in the United States is staggering. Many laxative preparations are available as OTC preparations and may not be identified by patients as medications. Additionally, use of home remedies such as mineral oil, prunes, or enemas may not be information that is volunteered and so must be sought. Second, a serious complication of those patients taking antibiotics is

the development of pseudomembranous colitis. This disorder is caused by bacterial overgrowth of *Clostridium difficile* in the gut, resulting in an inflammatory diarrhea that becomes bloody and, if untreated, can, result in death. Patients on antibiotics who develop diarrhea should be monitored closely for the development of fever, bloody diarrhea, abdominal pain, and white blood cells in the stool, because early treatment with oral vancomycin is impressive in curing the disorder.

Family history and past medical history can provide clues to the etiology of diarrhea. Previous history of systemic and metabolic diseases such as diabetes mellitus, hyperthyroidism, amyloidosis, chronic pancreatitis, and gastrinoma provide clues as to recurrence of disease. Surgery such as partial gastrectomy or vagotomy suggest the dumping syndrome, which results in osmotic diarrhea. Many of these disorders may be familial, so that disease in a family member will increase the likelihood of less common diseases in an individual patient. Examples of this include diabetes, lactose intolerance, and gastrinoma.

From this summary, the importance of a

TABLE 14-2
COMMON DRUGS THAT CAN CAUSE DIARRHEA

ANTIBIOTICS	LAXATIVES	ANTACIDS	MISCELLANEOUS	OVER-THE-COUNTER DRUGS	OTHERS
Amoxicillin, ampicillin	Bisacodyl	Magnesium trisalicate	Calcitonin	Alcohol	Enemas
Clindamycin, lincomycin	Cascara	Magnesium hydroxide (found in most antacids)	Cholestyramine	Caffeine	
Cephalosporins	Castor oil		Cholinergic agents—Urocholine	Nicotine	
Chloramphenicol	Magnesium citrate, milk of magnesia		Colchicine	High osmolar nutritional products, (e.g., Sustacal, Isocal)	
Tetracycline	Phenolphthalein		Digitalis (toxic doses)	Sorbitol	
Neomycin (orally)	Psyllium hydrophilic mucilloid		Lactulose		
	Senna		Guanethidine		
	Sodium sulfate		Quinidine		
			Theophylline		

complete, well-constructed, and open-ended history should be apparent. Failure to gain critical information may result in expensive, complicated, and unnecessary procedures being performed on patients. The history allows a categorization of the disorder into the categories *acute, chronic,* or *intermittent* and allows the mechanism to be explored; that is, osmotic, secretory, exudative, or motility disorder. Specific disorders and likelihood of specific disorders frequently can be determined. Rapport and empathy can be established so that a potentially embarrassing concern may be discussed freely and openly. The result is the beginning of a therapeutic relationship that is mutually satisfying to the needs of both the nurse and patient.

PHYSICAL EXAMINATION

The physical examination adds to the information obtained through the history. First, observe for signs of toxicity: fever, chills, vomiting, tachycardia, hypotension, lethargy, confusion, and weight loss, all suggesting the need for rapid intervention. Observe behavioral characteristics. Are there signs of anxiety or depression? Does the patient maintain eye contact, cry easily, appear preoccupied with the illness, or seem to enjoy being ill? Inspect the skin for the smooth, shiny texture of hyperthyroidism, the laxity of dehydration, or the excess tissue seen when people have chronically lost weight. Does the patient appear malnourished (seen with malabsorption syndromes or cancer)? Examine the abdomen for distention, either localized from obstruction or generalized with an adynamic ileus. Are bowel sounds increased or decreased, is a mass present, or is there tenderness? In acute diarrhea these findings may suggest intestinal infarction, partial obstruction, or infectious gastroenteritis, whereas in chronic diarrheas such posi-

tive findings suggest malignancy. The rectal examination is of considerable importance. Inspection of the anus may show stricture from previous surgery or inflammation, fistulous tracts associated with Crohn's disease, or prolapsing tumor. Digital examination may show rectal cancer, villous adenoma, impaction, blood, or segments of tapeworms. Observe a stool specimen for the presence of blood, white blood cells, or mucus. Lastly, a thorough general examination may uncover findings of any of the many disorders associated with diarrhea mentioned earlier. This issue is critical because, although the patient may visit the provider or be admitted with a primary diagnosis of diarrhea, major additional findings of potentially much greater importance may be overlooked.

THE INITIAL LABORATORY INVESTIGATION

Although a major discussion of laboratory testing in diarrheal disease is beyond our scope, a number of commonly used tests are shown on Table 14-3. Choice of tests is directed by information obtained during the history and physical examination, as well as the chronicity of the disorder.

NURSING DIAGNOSIS

Nursing diagnoses relating to diarrhea should focus on the whole-person response to the disorder. Understanding of the diarrhea from the person's perspective is necessary before management is attempted. Assessment statements should reflect the status of the person and the etiology involved. Those diagnoses included here are intended to be categories of diagnosis but not specific statements and are not presented in order of priority. Using them as a guide, the reader

TABLE 14-3
COMMONLY USED TESTS IN EVALUATION OF DIARRHEAL DISORDERS

TEST	RESULT	SUGGESTED GROUP OF DISORDERS	EXAMPLES
White blood count with differential	Elevated segmented granulocytes	Infection, inflammation	Ulcerative colitis Salmonellosis
	Elevated eosinophil count	Parasitic disease	Amebiasis
Hematocrit	Decreased	Anemia, colitis	Colitis, cancer, malabsorption
Sedimentation rate	Elevated	Infection, inflammation	Crohn's Disease Campylobacter enteritis
Blood glucose	Elevated	Impaired insulin utilization	Diabetes mellitus
Electrolytes (Na, K, Cl, CO_2)	K^+ decreased	Secretory diarrhea	Villous adenoma, Shigellosis
Serum amylase	Elevated	Pancreatic disease	Acute, recurrent pancreatitis
Serum alkaline phosphatase	Elevated	Biliary obstruction Hepatic dysfunction	Common duct stone pancreatitis, cancer
Stool Culture	Pathogenic bacteria isolated	Bacterial diarrhea	Salmonella, Shigella, Yersinia, Campylobacter
Stool for Ova and Parasites	Pathogenic parasite identified	Parasitic infestation	Amebiasis Giardiasis
Stool Hemoccults	Blood in stool results in positive test	Infection Inflammation Infiltration	Shigellosis Ulcerative colitis Colon cancer

will probably be able to construct additional statements relative to individual situations. Diagnostic categories are in boldface type for easy reference.

Alteration in Bowel Function: Diarrhea is probably the initial conclusion. The patient's definition of diarrhea, that is, liquid, explosive stools 5 or 6 times in 12 hours is helpful. This definition can then be used in outcome evaluation. It may also be helpful to use some indicator of duration or progress of the symptom.

Because of associated abdominal cramping or skin irritation that often accompanies diarrhea, diagnoses should reflect **alteration in comfort level.** These statements should include specific location of discomfort, that is, the abdomen or perirectal area.

The patient's attempts at management of symptoms is reflected in **self-care activity** diagnoses. Orem defines *self-care activity* as those practices that people use on their own behalf to enhance health and well-being.[29] Self-care is based on thoughtful judgment

TABLE 14-3   (continued)
COMMONLY USED TESTS IN EVALUATION OF DIARRHEAL DISORDERS

TEST	RESULT	SUGGESTED GROUP OF DISORDERS	EXAMPLES
Stool for leukocytes	Present	Infection Inflammation Infiltration	Yersinia enteritis Crohn's disease
Barium enema	Mucosal irregularities Stricture formation	Inflammatory bowel disease	Crohn's disease Ulcerative colitis
	Mass lesion	Tumor	Villous adenoma, colon cancer, polyp
	Obstruction	Structural defect	Volvulus, intussesception
Barium swallow with small bowel follow–through	Intestinal abnormality	Chronic small bowel disorders, often causing malabsorption	Whipple's disease, sprue, amyloidosis, scleroderma
	Peptic ulcer	Hyperacidity syndromes	Gastrinoma
	Mass lesion	Tumor	Adenocarcinoma, cardinoid tumor
	Blind loop	Previous surgical intervention	Vagotomy and partial gastrectomy, ileal resection, intestinal bypass
Sigmoidoscopy with biopsy	Mucosal inflammation	Infection, inflammatory diseases	Amebiasis, Ulcerative colitis, Antibiotic colitis
	Mass	Tumor	Adenocarcinoma Villous adenoma
Lactose tolerance test	Plasma glucose	Lactose intolerance	Lactase deficiency

leading to deliberate action appropriate to the individual. This behavior evolves from one's interpersonal relationships, communication, and culture.[20] Those activities used can be stated specifically or summarized as to category (e.g., diet, analgesia). Often self-care is initiated from knowledge about the body. The nurse should document the **information level** about normal bowel function; that is factors including "normal" patterns, effects of diet, exercise, ritual, drugs, and hydration. The amount of information may be indicated as inadequate, incorrect, or adequate. It is extremely helpful to document self-care activities that are assets, for example, an adequate information level. These assets can then be supported or expanded with further nursing management. Additionally, focusing on the strengths of the patient presents the nurse with the picture of a person capable of dealing with health rather than diagnoses that consist only of deficit-related statements.

The life-threatening complications of diarrhea usually are related to fluid and electrolyte alterations and are managed by the physician. **Alteration in fluid/electrolyte balance;** hypokalemia, dehydration is one example of a statement in this category. Additionally, the nurse is responsible for assessing potential risk factors for dehydration or electrolyte imbalance. These risks are present in the aged or the chronically ill person when oral intake is inadequate or when other fluid loss occurs, as with fever or vomiting. If more than 5% of body weight is lost by these processes, risks are significant and management with a physician is mandatory.

Effects of bowel dysfunction on **activities of daily living** reflect a person's response to diarrhea. Attempts should be made to document effects on major life activities. Alterations in mobility can reflect the need to plan activity according to availability of toileting facilities. Hygiene, grooming, and dress changes can be quite dramatic. One of the authors' patients wears disposable diapers and carriers a large handbag containing extra diapers, clean clothing, and disposable washcloths. Interference with social or recreational activities reveals other life-style changes patients make. Changes in scheduling or omission of social activities outside the home or immediate family can be significant. Impact on work or family responsibilities and self-concept are important indicators of **perceived role function** during symptomatic periods.

Note the status of **factors affecting normal bowel function**. These factors include

Exercise
Hydration
Toilet habit/ritual/position
Diet
Medication use.

For example, alteration in bowel function related to frequent laxative intake, bed rest,

and bedpan use is indicative of some of these specific elements.

Earlier in this discussion, the concept of stress as an influence on bowel function was explained. Consequently, diagnostic statements must describe the patient's current **level of concern** or **anxiety** about the diarrhea, which includes the concept of **symptom meaning.** For example, anxiety related to perception of diarrhea as a cancer symptom reflects on symptom meaning. Note current **situational or maturational stressors.** The individual's coping repertoire, usual coping response, or stress-reducing activities can be documented in several ways. One might wish to describe the strategies specifically as in the diagnoses: coping strategies, withdrawal, worrying, or the nurse can simply evaluate stress-reducing activities as "adequate." When examining coping responses, consider those resources or support systems that support a person during change. Statements should describe the resource and its accessibility, as well as the person's willingness to use the support. For example, support system; willing to use adequate family and financial resources summarizes these elements.

Make any diagnosis of **secondary gain** cautiously, because this label can be stereotypic and bias-laden. These biases occur because health providers forget that intrapsychic mechanisms leading to rewards of illness behavior usually are not deliberate or manipulative. It is helpful to recall that people cope in the best manner that they are able given their circumstances and perceived options. Consequently, any avoidance or reward associated with diarrhea can be included in diagnoses relating to coping behavior. For example, "coping response: avoidance of stressful work situations," states the behavior clearly. Nursing management in this example may be directed at assisting the patient to examine additional options of changing the work situation or relaxation exercises to reduce the stress.

Completing the nursing diagnoses are statements that relate to success of mutually determined nursing management. Note initially the **patient's level of readiness** to take remedial action. For example, if a person is unwilling to change his diet or to begin exercising, it is extremely helpful to know that *before* planning begins. This category of diagnoses contains those strategies that are current options for management as perceived by the patient.

Potential barriers to adherence to nursing management can include cultural, financial, communication, or comfort factors. These statements flow from queries that simply ask the patient which factors may interfere with the proposed plan. Conversely, **facilitators of adherence** are those assets or resources that enhance patient participation in the regimen. When identified, these facilitators can be reinforced or supported. The person's perception of the significant others' response to diarrhea is important. Consider the impact on a person if family or spouse become angry when diarrhea interferes with activity levels.

MANAGEMENT

In this discussion, goals of nursing management are proposed and strategies to meet these goals are outlined. Goals are derived from the proposed categories of nursing diagnosis set forth in the preceding section. Goals and criterion measures are stated and then discussed in detail.

Goal Restore normal elimination pattern, evidenced by reduced number of stools, and passage of formed brown feces.

Goal Restore hydration and electrolyte balance, evidenced by moist mucous membrane, stable body weight, urine output equal to or greater than 500 to 800 ml/24 hr, normal serum sodium, potassium, chloride, and carbon dioxide levels.

Strategies If the patient with diarrhea has had no significant vomiting, no chronic illness, is less than 65 years old, has stable body weight or demonstrated less than 5% body weight loss, is afebrile and shows no fecal leukocytes or occult bleeding, management by the nurse is appropriate. The initial steps of intervention are dietary. During diarrhea without undue emesis, fluid intake should approach 3,000 to 4,000 ml/24 hr. Low-fat liquids are preferred since fatty foods can cause adherence of bacteria to mucous membrane and prolong inflammatory processes.[15] Milk products should be avoided because a transient lactose intolerance develops when colonic mucosa are inflamed and there is a temporary decrease in lactose synthesis.[6] Weak tea with honey, the water in which rice has been cooked, jello, cola beverages, bouillon, and ices are all appropriate foods. When considering amount of intake, small, frequent feedings are judicious. It is helpful to recall that a standard popsicle contains 30 ml to 69 ml of fluids and an ice cream scoop of fruit ice about 120 ml. Replacement fluids should be adequate sources of calories, potassium, and sodium. Commercially available products that contain potassium also may be helpful; Gatorade is one such product. A chart of potassium-containing foods is presented in Table 14-4. Any standard nutrition text will provide a more comprehensive listing.

The diet should progress to solids as tolerated, beginning with cooked rice, cooked cereals, bananas, saltines, and plain baked or boiled potatoes. Again, small frequent meals are wise. New foods should be added slowly over a 24 to 48-hour period. To this regimen,

TABLE 14-4
POTASSIUM FOOD LIST

FOOD	PORTION	POTASSIUM (mg)
Meat		
Hamburger	3 oz	310
Chicken	1 breast	710
Fruit		
Orange	1 medium	360
Banana	1 medium	630
Cantaloupe	1/2 melon	880
Raisins	1 cup	1150
Juices		
Orange	8 oz	440
Prune	8 oz	620
Vegetables		
Corn	1 cup	230
Tomato	1 medium	340
Spinach	1 cup	600

white meat of chicken or turkey and noodles can be added until there is no diarrhea for 24 hours. A bland, low-fat diet should be followed for the next 24 to 48 hours. The normal diet should be resumed gradually.

If the cause of the diarrhea is determined to be stress-related or if IBS is diagnosed, a high-fiber diet should be instituted after the initial episode is resolved. A high-fiber diet is discussed in detail in the section concerning nursing management of constipation.

During the recovery period, assess body weight, temperature, fluid intake and urine output daily. If the patient is managed in the home, teach the family or significant others these measures, as well as specific parameters or symptoms that may merit further physician attention. To facilitate adherence to the diet, consider food preferences, financial status, and the patient's need for assistance with meal preparation. It may be reassuring to both patient and provider to monitor progress by telephone during the acute period.

When there has been more than 5%

weight loss, significant vomiting, fever over 102°F, chronic illness, alterations in electrolyte levels, positive fecal leukocytes, frank or occult blood, physician management is indicated. Additionally, if vomiting occurs with an intake of clear liquids, medical consultation should be sought. The patient should take nothing by mouth, and should be evaluated for hospitalization or intravenous hydration. Assessment of measures of hydration and electrolyte balance should be made as previously discussed.

If the patient is found to be lactose intolerant, symptoms often are precipitated by the quality of lactose. For example, patients may have symptoms from cold foods rather than warm, or lactose-containing foods taken on an empty stomach. Because aged cheddar cheese contains little lactose, effects may vary according to the type of cheese consumed. For the tube-fed person, substitute lactose-free Ensure or Isocal for standard mixtures. Transient, secondary lactose intolerance develops in some cases of enteritis, hyperthyroidism, following gastrointestinal surgery, and during concurrent neomycin or quinidine therapy. The dietary management of diarrhea caused by lactose intolerance consists simply of avoidance of lactose-containing foods. Individuals have varying capacities for digesting lactose, so some experimentation on the patient's part is necessary. Reading labels to discern their lactose content is necessary. A partial listing of these foods follows:

Beverages: All milk (including buttermilk and acidophilus); instant coffee; drinks with chocolate or malted milk; cordials and liqueurs

Cheeses: Lowest content includes aged natural cheeses, Brie, Stilton, and others

Meats: Organ meats, cold cuts with dry milk added (all kosher meats are milk-free)

Canned Fruits and Vegetables: Read labels.
Bread: Read labels.
Desserts: Ice cream, sherbet, cakes and cook-
ies made with milk, chocolate, caramels,
butterscotch, packaged cake mixes
Miscellaneous: Salad dressing

Yogurt contains about 60% of the lactose found in milk. If home-made, allowing for longer fermentation will reduce lactose content.[6]

Two OTC medications that may prove helpful are Lactaid and Lactozyme. If added to milk, these lactose products will hydrolyze 70% of the lactose; if the amount is doubled, 90% of the lactose can be broken down. These products are clinically useful, do not affect milk shelf-life, and add about 20 cents to the cost of one quart of milk.[6]

Goal   Reduce discomfort, evidenced by verbal statement of the patient, reduced interference with sleep, and reduced skin inflammation.

Strategies   Nurses have long battled the effects of diarrhea to surrounding skin. The reader probably has a favorite effective regimen. Whatever the treatment, the area must remain free of stool and wetness. Skin protection can be achieved with petrolatum, zinc oxide, or vitamin A and D ointment applied locally. Sitz baths after every stool or for 20 minutes four times a day promote healing and reduce discomfort. Gently wash and dry the area after every stool. Exposure to a heat lamp or air hastens drying. Daily inspection should include presence of signs of infection or extension of the maceration process.

Abdominal discomfort accompanying diarrhea can be ameliorated by a mild analgesia and local heat application.

Medications can be of some assistance in adding bulk to the diarrheal stool. Local agents like adsorptive clays (kaolin) adhere to bacteria and carry it out through the stool. Pectin, a plant product used with kaolin, soothes irritation and absorbs water. Other absorbent drugs are polycarbophil, carboxymethylcellulose, and psyllium. These bulking products do not decrease stool frequency but do allow a more formed bowel movement. Absorbing agents taken for diarrhea should be taken with one third glass of water instead of the 8-oz dose prescribed for constipation. Tetracycline should not be taken concurrently since its particles are also bound and will be excreted before it will be absorbed. Bulking products are of most benefit with mild-to-moderate diarrhea or traveler's diarrhea, conditions caused by noninvasive bacteria attached to mucous membrane surfaces with intact intestinal mucosa.[32] Additionally, bulking agents are valuable medicines for psychophysiologic responses, in which diarrhea alternates with constipation.

Systemic agents like opiates reduce intestinal motility and prolong the transit time. Belladonna relaxes intestinal smooth muscle and relieves spasm. Diphenoxylate (Lomotil) and loperamide (Imodium) are commonly used derivatives of synthetic meperidine that do not cause dependence and are relatively free of central nervous sytem (CNS) side-effects. These agents are contraindicated in bacterial enteritis because they reduce bowel activity and delay intestinal capacity to excrete the pathogen. Consequently, the bacteria have more time to increase local damage and enter the bloodstream.[31]

Traveler's diarrhea may be prevented by single daily doses of doxycycline (Vibramycin), which appears to be excreted into the small bowel where the bacteria congregate. If taken while one is traveling this agent prevents diarrhea and its effects last 1 week after it is discontinued.[32] Subsalicylate bismuth (Peptobismol) given in 2-oz doses every 6 hours has been found to be as effective as prophylactic doxycycline. It appears to have an anti-inflammatory, antisecretory action that prevents pathogenic attachment to the gut wall.[11]

Peppermint oil was used in one double-blind study to reduce the severity of abdominal cramping but had no effect on stool frequency. Its action is thought to relax smooth muscle.[30]

Bloating, eructation, flatulence, and abdominal discomfort that may accompany diarrhea can be sources of embarrassment as well as discomfort. In diarrheal disorders, abdominal pain and bloating are most often because of increased intestinal gas formation by colonic bacteria. The symptoms also may be due to a motility disorder that impedes the propulsive movement of gas through the bowel, plus an exaggerated pain response to gut distention by volumes of gas.[31] Management consists of information about the condition, avoidance of voluntary belching, low-fat diet, and avoidance of nonabsorbable carbohydrates.[7] Sorbital, found in sugar-free chewing gum, apples, grape juice, raisins, prunes, bananas, and carbonated beverages is felt by one author to cause bloating.[15]

Postantibiotic diarrhea occurs during or up to 4 weeks after a course of antibiotic treatment. A list of antibiotics causing diarrhea is found in Table 14-2. An increased incidence is associated with advancing age. When the drug is discontinued symptoms resolve within 3 to 14 days. Lomotil is contraindicated because it appears to aggravate severity.[5] Monitor each patient closely since increased severity, fever, abdominal pain, or bloody stools suggest the development of pseudomembraneous colitis, a potentially fatal condition. Patients with particularly severe diarrhea or those with signs of toxicity must be evaluated by a physician. Oral vancomycin has been found curative in this condition if begun early in the course of the disease.[5]

Goal Adequate information about normal bowel function, evidenced by verbal statements of the patient or significant other.

Goal Improved status of factors influencing normal bowel function, evidenced by 1½ hours vigorous exercise weekly, fluid intake of 2000-3000 ml/24 hr, maintenance of toilet rituals, and adherence to negotiated diet.

Strategies Principles that nurses use when educating others apply in this instance as well. All information is adapted to the person's level of readiness and ability to comprehend. Small amounts of information, given frequently with reinforcement in writing, are best recalled. Use of significant others for reinforcement of teaching is also helpful. Remember that anxiety reduces perception and comprehension, so that only brief essential facts should be presented at these times. This information should be reinforced at a time when anxiety is reduced. Instruct patients and family about normal bowel physiology, structure, and function. Explain the specific cause of the diarrhea. Pictures are helpful and enhance learning by involving more than one sensory modality. If possible, ask the patient to draw a picture of the bowel during symptomatic periods. These drawings can be used later when teaching relaxation exercises and imagery. Present skin care and hygiene measures to prevent urethral/vaginal contamination in women. Patient and family can use various methods of odor control. Chlorophyll tablets are quite effective. If privacy and other toileting habits are of concern, problem-solving and negotiation can help. The patient should be given a set of written instructions outlining the dietary modifications presented earlier in this discussion. If reading is a problem, there is usually a support person who can help with this function. If not, pictures are helpful. Complications of the diarrhea should be carefully outlined and explained.

Discuss specific criteria for provider attention and write this down. For example, if loss of weight of more than 5 lb or fever over 102°F occurs, the health provider should be contacted.

Diet, hydration, exercise, and ritual changes necessary to control diarrhea may mean life-style alteration on the part of the patient. For this reason, these changes are best negotiated on an individual basis. For example, using the usual activity level as a baseline and asking whether the patient is willing to exercise briskly for 20 minutes 5 times a week is a starting point. From there, the patient clarifies what changes are acceptable and adherence to the regimen is facilitated. Additionally, the person is actively involved in decision-making and control of one's health care.

Goal Reduce anxiety about diarrhea, evidenced by verbal statements, calm facial expression, smooth, coordinated, nonagitated movements, and vital signs within normal limits.

Goal Support or enlarge coping repertoire, evidenced by verbal statements of reduced perceived stress, regular practice of negotiated stress relieving activity, and reduction in bowel symptoms.

Goal Return to usual activities of daily living, evidenced by verbal statements of patient or significant other.

Strategies People vary in their level of readiness to take remedial action, even when it is clear what remedies are indicated. Some people wish a great deal of control and input into their health care, others prefer very little and are content to rely on specific direction. Regardless, once the nurse is aware of the readiness of the individual, this level should be supported and acknowledged. If the readiness state involves a life-threatening situation to self or others, referral for psychiatric evaluation is necessary. Otherwise, negotiation can proceed by the nurse using simple

queries of the patient such as, "Are you willing to ...?" Patients who wish more direction usually will tell the provider clearly, "I don't know; you're the nurse, you tell me."

Those persons who make statements about the relationship between their bowel symptoms and stressful events benefit from further discussion and counseling. Useful strategies include active listening, support, and ventilation, all of which facilitate the development of rapport and emotional release for the patient. If a person is able to identify a specific situational problem, for example, if a decision is to be made, then value clarification and problem-solving techniques can be used. Specific strategies depend on the individual nurse's expertise. Referral for counseling also may be appropriate. These discussions should begin with the concept of psyche–soma inseparability. Use an example, "Remember a time when you have been badly scared. Your mouth got dry, your heart beat rapidly, etc. That's because your mind realized the threat to yourself, sent signals that released chemicals into your blood that caused those bodily sensations." This technique enhances the understanding that stress-related sensations are not imaginary.

If a person is not willing to see the connection between stress and body function, begin efforts at implementing stress-relieving activities and increasing socialization. Exercise, relaxation exercises, meditation, or visualization can be negotiated, taught, and practiced.[34] Negotiations center on patient willingness to practice formerly effective techniques or to learn new skills. Visualization is used extensively in the author's nursing practice. Working from a description or picture of the patient's perception of his bowel, patients are taught to form mental images to counteract symptomatic perceptions. One patient described her bowel as twisted and knotted during a period of diarrhea. After practice, she was able to reduce discomfort by picturing the knots opened and un-twisted by a warm, healing energy. People with strong religious belief systems who relate periods of prayer or meditation are usually able to use those images very richly. Those patients unable to use visualization can benefit from simple relaxation tech-niques. (If the reader wishes more informa-tion about imagery, refer to Chapter 6.) In addition, McCaffrey, Bry, and Samuels have written thorough discussions and their work can be found listed in the bibliography.

Strategies useful for management of acute anxiety are described elsewhere. As-sessing verbal/nonverbal signs is vital. Active listening, ventilation, support, diversion, and exercise are useful. If the patient is in a panic state or elicits tendencies to harm self or others, psychotherapeutic referral should be made.

Return of the person to usual activities of daily living is an effort dependent on the pa-tient and support system. Once it is deter-mined that resumption of activity is desired, the nurse and patient need to determine what resources are available if help is needed; what specific assistance is required and which resources the patient is willing to use. Strategies for these considerations are rooted in problem-solving. The provider as-sists the development of a specific statement of the problem and explores possible options and their consequences, risks, and benefits to the person. Finally, reinforce the patient's ef-forts using either a patient-chosen reward or statements by the provider acknowledging the patient's efforts toward the goal.

Goal   Reduce potential barriers to ad-herence, evidenced by patient verbal state-ments that the regimen is being followed.

Strategies   Adherence to treatment reg-imen is a complicated and highly researched area; however, research does not reveal spe-cific areas consistently effecting positive ad-herence outcomes. If the patient is able to predict prescriptions that are not possible to follow, renegotiating the plan is appropriate. Financial restrictions may necessitate adap-tation of some strategies. Cultural factors, like home remedies, values about toileting, and emotional expression are deeply rooted influences of health behavior. If a patient does not possess adequate information or ra-tionale to follow the management plan, ad-herence may be difficult. Regimens tend to be used when they are simple, contain fewer treatments or medications, and do not inter-fere with life-style patterns.[9]

Constipation

INTRODUCTION

Constipation is a nearly endemic affliction of western civilization. The major factor ap-pears to be the decreasing amounts of crude fiber in western diets, as described earlier. Constipation is felt to be the most common reason for self-medication in the United States. Laxatives represent a multimillion dollar business in the United States. For those caring for geriatric patients, constipa-tion is clearly one of the concerns most frequently voiced. As with diarrhea, the metaphors surrounding the symptom of constipation are direct and enlightening. Common descriptions used by patients to elaborate on their state are ''plugged up,'' ''uptight,'' ''can't let go,'' or ''stuffed.'' Freud's description of anal compulsive be-havior has certainly received much atten-tion. The concern about constipation, then, reflects many social, environmental, anatom-ical, and psychological factors. The knowl-edge and interrelationship between these various factors provides an understanding of the condition and a guide for evaluation and therapy.

The definition of constipation should be considered in a fashion similar to diarrhea. A common definition of *constipation* is bowel movements fewer than 3 times per week, or individual bowel movements of less than 35 g. Again, normal variation is remarkable. This definition was the result of large-scale sampling that defined significant variation from the mean.[10] The most critical factor in the definition of constipation is a sense of variance with the particular individual's "normal" bowel habits. When elicited, this information suggests a variation that requires explanation. In defining the concern and discussing its relevance, the nurse has begun the alliance needed with the patient to evaluate and treat the factors responsible.

MECHANISMS OF CONSTIPATION

The pathophysiology of constipation is multifactorial, but centers on these issues:

Volume of fecal material being transported
Transit time
Anatomical integrity of the intestinal lumen
Neuromuscular integrity of the anorectal defecation response
Heeding the urge to defecate

As described earlier, the *quantity* of fecal material affects the quality of the colonic contractile response. Large, bulky stools have a decreased transit time and stimulate neuromuscular responses to defecate. Diets that are inadequate in volume, fiber, or liquid thus predispose to constipation. Of these, fiber has received the most attention. Nonwestern societies often consume a significant percentage of their diet as unrefined food,

resulting in a large crude-fiber content.[8] Normal bowel habits in such cultures are in the order of 2 to 3 large, bulky stools per day.

Transit time is a factor that depends upon the motility characteristics of the colon. An increase in transit time results in more time available for the reabsorption of water in the colon, resulting in the generation of smaller volumes of fecal material, which further increases transit time. Disorders affecting transit time are motility disorders such as IBS, in which contractions are dissynchronous; electrolyte imbalance and medications that inhibit the muscular activity of the colon; and physical activity, which has been found to decrease transit time.[10]

Anatomical integrity is the most critical aspect in the evaluation of constipation because the disorders involved are both life-threatening and potentially curable. Intraluminal masses may partially or totally obstruct passage of stool. Complete obstruction results in the absence of stool passage and other physical signs that will be discussed later. Partial blockage delays transit and, depending on location, can alter the character of the stools. Typical intraluminal obstructions are listed in Table 14-5. A major form of obstruction is luminal narrowing secondary to stricture. In this instance, mucosal infiltration or postinflammatory scarring results in a nondistensible segment of colon, which impairs transit. Symptoms in these conditions tend to be constant or progressive.

The act of defecation is dependent on a number of factors. First, the rectum must fill with fecal contents. Second, sensory innervation must be intact, to sense the rectal distention. Third, efferent stimulation of the internal and external anal sphincter must be intact to allow defecation. Fourth, the person should be positioned so that with release of

TABLE 14-5
CAUSES OF CONSTIPATION

PSYCHOSOCIAL FACTORS	MEDICATIONS	METABOLIC ABNORMALITIES	NEUROLOGIC DISORDERS	STRUCTURAL ABNORMALITY	PSYCHOPHYSIOLOGIC DISORDERS
Ignoring call to defecate, lack of time Travel (unfamiliar environment), inadequate toilet facilities Lack of exercise Dehydration Inadequate, low-fiber diet	(see Table 14-6)	Hypokalemia Hypercalcemia Hypopituitarism Hypothyroidism Porphyria	Autonomic neuropathy—diabetes mellitus, paraneoplastic Chagas' disease Meningocele Tabes dorsalis Multiple sclerosis Parkinson's disease Myotonic dystrophy Paraplegia (trauma, tumor, polio) Progressive systemic sclerosis	Rectal prolapse Hemorrhoids Rectal carcinoma, adenoma Fecal impaction Foreign body Colonic carcinoma Volvulus Pregnancy Stricture (diverticulitis, ischemic colitis, chronic ulcerative colitis, Crohn's disease, tuberculous enteritis, fistulous abscess, gonorrheal proctitis, corrosive enemas, endometriosis, anal fissure, radiation, postoperative adhesions)	IBS

the sphincters, defecation can occur. Pathophysiologic disruption can occur at any point in this process. Neuropathic disease may disrupt the sensation of a distended rectum; examples are multiple sclerosis or spinal cord injury. Neuromuscular disease may inhibit the release of the anal sphincter. Positioning, as with the use of bedpans, may make defecation much more difficult. Lastly, the urge to defecate may be ignored. These responses may be conscious, as with persons exposed to unsanitary bathrooms while traveling, or unconscious, as a way of expressing anger or hostility.

NURSING ASSESSMENT

HISTORY

As with diarrhea, the history of concern about constipation is the critical aspect of assessment. Two major issues need to be pursued; first is chronicity. Has constipation always been a problem, or is there a significant change in bowel habits? Second, what other symptoms are present? Chronicity is important because of the difference between disorders responsible for constipation since childhood versus a recent change in bowel habits. Constipation since childhood or adolescence usually has its roots in toileting behavior, diet, or psychosocial stressors. When sought, the history usually provides ample evidence of these problems. Because of the ability to cure colon cancer if found at early states, a recent change in bowel habits must be recognized as an extremely important signal. In adults over the age of 45, constipation of recent onset should result in consideration and exclusion of the diagnosis of colon cancer. Other structural disorders also may cause recent alteration of bowel habits and must be considered. Similarly, other disorders and psychosocial factors also may be implicated. These factors are listed in Table 14-5.

Once chronicity has been established, symptoms associated with constipation must be sought. Structural lesions may be associated with abdominal pain, increased bowel sounds (called *borborygmi*), and abdominal distention. If lesions are located distally in the descending colon, stool may be pencil-shaped or of narrowed caliber. Advanced colon cancer may be associated with weight loss, fatigue, jaundice, or abdominal mass. However, early colon cancer, while still potentially curable, may present only with altered bowel habits. The patient should be questioned about the character of the stool. Black stool or *melena* suggests a proximal intestinal lesion. Blood mixed in with stool suggests colonic bleeding, whereas blood on the outside of the stool suggests distal colonic and rectal disease. Blood on the toilet paper only suggests perirectal disease. Examples are rectal fissure, hemorrhoids, or, less commonly, prolapsed rectal polyps. Pellet-shaped stools are seen with IBS, dehydration, inadequate diet, or ignoring the urge to defecate.

Pain is another important symptom. Nonspecific discomfort suggests colonic spasm, deep-seated disease, or psychogenic pain. Such discomfort can be seen with the spasm of IBS, diverticulitis, or the intermittent obstruction of a colon cancer. Rectal burning or anal pain is seen with hemorrhoids, rectal fissures, proctitis, or rectal prolapse. Acute, severe abdominal pain in the setting of constipation suggests a surgical emergency, and the physical examination will be most revealing. This acute abdomen may be the result of conditions such as intestinal infarction, colonic volvulus, strangulated hernia, or bowel obstruction by adhesions, tumor, or polyps.

Additional symptoms may reflect other possible etiologies. Constipation in the presence of thickened skin, cold intolerance, and fatigue suggest hypothyroidism. In the presence of fatigue, muscle weakness, and the use of diuretics, constipation suggests hypokalemia. Constipation, in the presence of hypertension, confusion, and peptic ulcers, suggests hypercalcemia.

Once the spectrum of symptoms is clear, explore the setting under which symptoms began. How long have symptoms been present and why does the patient now seek help? How has the constipation affected lifestyle and what has been done to relieve the symptoms? Questioning should address diet and specifically estimate fiber content and fluid intake. Identify events that occurred around the onset of symptoms, whether dietary, environmental, or psychosocial. Was there an anniversary of a major loss (e.g., a friend, loved one, or job)? Did activity patterns change, precluding a set time of the day available for bowel movements? These explorations again are most successful in the context of open-ended questions that encourage the patients to speak, thereby acknowledging the legitimacy of the concern. An example: "Often bowel habits are affected by changes in events, life-style, or diet. Has anything like that happened to you?"

The final aspect of this section is medication use. Medications that commonly cause constipation are listed in Table 14-6. Patients may have been self-medicating with laxatives or enemas for long periods of time before seeking evaluation. Look for the use of types of enemas or laxatives, as well as other OTC drugs.

Historical concerns that need to be sought are past medical history, family history, and psychosocial history. A past medical history may reveal prior surgery, which may predispose to the development of adhesions. There may be a history of colon cancer, polyps, or diseases that can cause stricture, such as syphilis, tuberculosis, radiation therapy, colitis, or proctitis. The patient may have had a history of hemorrhoid surgery, or neurologic disease resulting in sensory or motor deficits of the sacral nerve roots that

are involved in defecation. Metabolic diseases that predispose to constipation like hyperparathyroidism, hypothyroidism, or diabetes mellitus may be present. Finally, assess childhood bowel habits.

Family history is also important since colon cancer, some colonic polyp syndromes, and pelvic cancers may have a hereditary component. Certainly the knowledge of a parent's colon cancer may shape the concern of a patient regarding change in bowel habits. As always, asking a patient what he thinks caused the problem is appropriate.

The psychosocial history can double check the impact of life events on a particular patient's bowel habits. Soliciting support systems, gains of illness, coping patterns, as well as reviewing life events and past evaluation of this problem, provides insights for the provider of what issues may be under the surface. It is impressive that major psychosocial factors often are found to be involved in symptomatology in addition to coexistent anatomical disease. It is in this light that the comprehensive history, employing a bio-

TABLE 14-6
COMMON DRUGS CAUSING CONSTIPATION

DRUGS USED FOR DIAGNOSTIC TESTING	DRUGS USED FOR PSYCHIATRIC DISORDERS	ANTACIDS	DRUGS USED FOR NEUROLOGIC DISORDERS	ANALGESICS	ANTICHOLINERGICS
Barium sulfate	Tricyclic antidepressants Chlorpromazine/ phenothiazines Monoamine oxidase inhibitors Phenobarbital	Calcium carbonate Aluminum hydroxide Bismuth	Anticonvulsants (diphenylhydantoin) Antiparkinsonian drugs (L-dopa)	Opiates (codeine, meperidine hydrochloride, morphine, diphenoxylate) Antitussives (codeine, paregoric)	Atropine Scopolamine Propantheline bromide Belladonna

psychosocial approach, aids in definition, evaluation, and provision of the tools needed to establish individualized treatment plans for patients.

PHYSICAL EXAMINATION

The physical examination provides valuable information in the further assessment of a constipated patient. The general inspection can show evidence of weight loss, cachexia, and malnutrition, suggesting cancer, depression, or inadequate nutritional intake. The patient may have a goiter or a thyroidectomy scar, along with slowed reflexes and coarse skin suggesting hypothyroidism. Observe expression and nonverbal activity for signs of depression or anxiety, or for signs of toxic illness such as fever, chills, or pain. As mentioned earlier, a thoroughly performed abdominal examination is crucial. A tender abdomen with guarding, rigidity, or rebound tenderness with absent bowel sounds suggests an acute process requiring immediate surgical consultation. Surgical scars suggest a history of surgery. An enlarged liver with jaundice suggests the possibility of metastatic disease. A mass suggests structural disease. A tender, palpable sigmoid bowel in a patient with pellet-shaped stools suggests IBS.

The rectal examination is a *mandatory* part of the physical examination, complete with Hemoccult slide testing. First the anus is inspected. Rectal fissures, prolapsing, external hemorrhoids, or blood may be seen. The anal sphincter is palpated for laxity or stricture. A gloved finger inserted into the rectum can ascertain the amount of stool in the rectum. A full rectum suggests sensory deficit from nerve damage or chronic failure to heed the urge to defecate . Absence of stool suggests the possibility of a more proximal obstruction or of laxative abuse. Pellet-shaped stools suggest IBS, dehydration, or inattention to the need to defecate. In addition, rectal polyps, adenomas, or carcinomas may be palpated. A stool sample can then be examined for blood or mucus.

The remainder of a thorough examination is performed. Pertinent aspects are evidence of sensory or motor neurologic deficits, retinal fundoscopic changes of diabetes mellitus, diminished pulses (suggesting peripheral vascular disease), and hyporeflexia (suggesting hypothyroidism).

LABORATORY TESTS

Testing for blood is best done with Hemoccult slides. False-positive tests may be seen in those who have been drinking alcohol or using medication that can cause gastritis. Examples are aspirin, indomethacin, or other nonsteroidal anti-inflammatory drugs. False positives are also seen if the diet contains red meat, rutabagas, turnips, or horse-radish. False-negative test results are seen with use of vitamin C or low-fiber diets. In Hemoccult testing, the most reliable results are obtained with a high-fiber diet free of red meat, medications, and alcohol for 3 days before testing. On the fourth day, two stool samples are taken from each of three consecutive bowel movements. These samples are placed on Hemoccult slides and tested within 3 days of collection. The presence of blood in the stool, collected in this manner from a patient of any age, demands a more thorough evaluation. Never accept hemorrhoids in such a situation as a sufficient reason for the presence of blood.

Besides Hemoccult testing, the laboratory tests used in the evaluation of constipation are the same as those used in diarrhea suspected to be of colonic origin. In consultation with an internist or gastroenterologist, standard first steps are sigmoidoscopy and an air contrast barium enema. Most structural defects are identified using these techniques. If blood has been found and the results of these two tests are negative, fiberoptic colonoscopy is performed. When metabolic disease is suspected, fasting plasma glucose, T_3, T_4, serum calcium, and potassium levels are sufficient diagnostic measures.

In summary, keep in mind a number of concepts when evaluating patients. First, in patients over age 45, sigmoidoscopy and barium enema must be performed in patients who describe constipation. Consider the possibility of concurrent malignancy, perhaps clouded by psychosocial problems. In patients under 45, in whom the incidence of cancer is much lower, further diagnostic testing may be postponed while other problems are being reviewed. In general, the risks of Hemoccult testing, sigmoidoscopy, and barium enema are small, and the risks of not identifying an occult malignancy are large. Therefore, in cases in which recovery is not prompt, referral for these procedures is warranted.

Second, in elderly patients, a response to diet therapy does not exclude the need to search for underlying structural defects. Again, diagnostic testing is warranted if the patient chooses.

Third, stools found positive for presence of blood should not be discounted in the face of hemorrhoidal disease. Here again, referral for diagnostic testing is warranted to exclude structural disease.

Finally, concurrent psychosocial stressors and nutritional problems are critical to identify and explore. The nurse is well-suited to elicit this component of the problem, whether it is the major aspect or a small part of the problem. In such a condition, then, the quality of the health team has a major impact on the quality of care delivered, as well as the patient's perception of the humaneness of the care.

NURSING DIAGNOSIS

Diagnoses should describe the response of the whole person to constipation. Because the essence of nursing is to manage the response to a disorder, it is mandatory to document what the response has been. (Only general categories of diagnosis are presented and are boldface for easy reference.)

Alteration in bowel function: constipation (as defined by small volume stools passed twice weekly). The parenthetical expression is a hypothetical patient's definition of constipation.

At risk for presence of colorectal disease (Family or personal history of colorectal cancer, polyps, other cancer, positive hemoccult screening, 45 years of age or older, low-fiber diet)

Document specific risk factors. This activity is a priority. If any risk factors are present, refer the patient to the physician for further diagnostic investigation.

Effects of constipation on activities of daily living is diagnosed by specifically inquiring into mobility and avoidance of activities. In our experience, mobility is affected less with constipation than with diarrhea. However, some people described planning vacations in only familiar settings, stating that strange toilet facilities contribute to difficulty with bowel habits. One patient timed departures from a cottage to home so that there would be no need to stop at public restrooms. This same person stated that during periods of constipation with accompanying bloating, she stayed home and avoided all but essential activities.

Bloating that accompanies constipation often causes people to change the way in which they dress. These differences may be subtle and go unnoticed by others. Unless the provider specifically asks directed questions, adaptations will not be discovered. Alteration in dress or grooming usually results in the patient's wearing looser fitting garments. When changes are necessary, changes in body image often follow. Patients frequently say that they feel fat, ugly or "like a balloon" when they note abdominal distention. Role function may be changed when sexuality or comfort is affected by bloating or constipation.

The status of factors influencing normal bowel function is often impaired. Reduction in normal exercise levels can cause constipation from altered muscle tone or inadequate stress-relieving activity. Travel often leads to changes in fluid intake and habit or ritual changes, especially postponement of the urge to defecate. The latter is a major factor in perpetuating constipation. Diet, in the form of a usual 24-hour pattern, is often low in fiber in constipated persons. Finally, the use of drugs, especially laxatives, is a major factor in the development of long-standing constipation. The vicious cycle of difficulty with stool passage, leading to laxative use, and resulting in diarrhea followed by more constipation, develops. Over time, laxatives reduce intestinal muscle tone, thus impairing propulsive functions of the colon. Do not assume that laxative use occurs only in the older person. Clinical laxative abuse may be present with any constipated person, regardless of age. Family toileting habits and expectations of regularity seem most predictive of excessive laxative use.

Information about bowel function is evaluated as adequate or inadequate for self-care. Many people believe that it is "normal" to defecate daily, although the range of bowel elimination is probably twice daily to three times weekly. The factors discussed in the previous paragraph are all part of the knowledge that the nurse should evaluate.

Associated **discomfort** in the abdomen or rectal area should be documented. Note gas production, even if not always painful.

The person's **concern or anxiety** about constipation and the **symptom meaning** are essential diagnoses. When shared, it is often possible for the provider to address anxiety directly and thus provide for anxiety reduction. **Stressful events and coping repertoire** may have impact on constipation. Look for less obvious stressors like multiple life changes and developmental issues. Note whether diagnosed stress is situational or maturational. Constipation is a common companion of depression. Assess patients for flatness of affect, lethargy, fatigue, and other depressive expressions. Ask them specifically if they feel "numb" or sad. If the answer is affirmative, referral for further psychiatric evaluation may be appropriate. If the patient states suicidal or homicidal intent, immediate psychiatric referral is mandatory. As part of assessment of **support systems**, the response of significant others to constipation is helpful. Patients with long-standing constipation often relate that families joke about the problem. Patients may feel disregarded when others do not think the problem is serious.

Document the patient's **level of readiness** to take remedial action. Additionally, identify **potential barriers to adherence** to the management plan. As noted in previous discussion, cultural, financial and communication elements can impede outcomes. **Secondary gain** is a diagnosis the provider makes when it becomes apparent that the constipation appears to be meeting other needs or allowing the person to avoid threatening events.

MANAGEMENT

Goals of management and appropriate related strategies will be discussed. In cases where management is similar to that already presented in the diarrhea section, the reader will be referred to that area.

Goal Restore normal elimination pattern, evidenced by passage of formed, bulky stool without discomfort.

Goal Enhance information level about normal bowel function, evidenced by patient or significant other verbal statements.

Goal Improve status of factors influencing bowel function, evidenced by: 1½ hrs exercise weekly; 2000–3000 ml fluids in 24 hours; maintenance of toileting 20 minutes after meals and attending urge to defecate, high-fiber diet containing 6 to 10 g fiber/24 hr, and avoidance of laxatives or constipating drugs.

Strategies Information relevant to normal bowel function has already been discussed. Again, attention to principles of learning is also appropriate. Exercise and hydration remain important issues. The major influence of stool consistency in normal adults is fiber in the diet. The major types of fiber and the rationale for its use have been noted in the introduction to this chapter. In clinical practice, the role of fiber should be clearly emphasized. After explaining why fiber is important, it is helpful to give the patient specific written instructions to follow. Our regimen breaks down foods into lists: breads/cereals, fruits, vegetables, and so forth. Common foods from each group are listed along with their amount of fiber content in grams. In this way, patients can select foods to their taste and add up their daily fiber intake. For example, 1 cup of broccoli contains about 1.5 g fiber, 1 cup of zucchini about 1.4 g and cabbage 0.8 g.[18] Patients are advised to begin with their normal diet pattern. To this, they choose one list of foods and select one high-fiber entry. Additional servings of other similar foods are added every 2 to 3 days. Each week a new list is added and the same pattern continues. At the end of 4 to 6 weeks, the goal of 6 to 10 g fiber daily should have been attained.[8] People often experience bloating and gaseousness when adding fiber and should be warned to expect these sensations. Encourage them to persist because the symptoms usually resolve within a week or two. Sometimes more than 6 to 10 g fiber will be needed to control symptoms.

If patients do not wish to use extensive diet manipulation, unprocessed wheat bran or miller's bran can be used instead. Unprocessed bran absorbs eight times its weight in water. It is tasteless and can be added to usual foods without changing flavor. Patients may use it over cereal, on toast, or added to salad, meat loaf, cakes, muffins, or bread. It adds very few calories and is inexpensive. One teaspoon of bran yields about 1 g of fiber. As with other fiber, some distention and flatulence occurs initially but often resolves within several weeks. The initial doses of bran should be 1 teaspoon or less for several days, increasing by 1/2 teaspoon until the 6 to 10 g goal has been reached.[25] It is vital to take at least 3 liters of fluid daily with the added fiber.

There are a number of excellent cookbooks that discuss fiber, include lists of fiber content, and suggest recipes. Two that we have found helpful are Jean Jones' *Fabulous Fiber Cookbook* and Barbara Kraus' *Guide to Fiber in Foods*. Table 14-7 shows a few foods with their fiber content.

If patients are willing, a diet diary is a helpful way to keep track of response to new foods (see the Sample Diary entry). Patients who keep these records for several weeks usually learn a great deal about their food habits. Record-keeping also facilitates adherence. When patients return to the office for follow-up visits, we request that they bring their diaries along for review by provider and patient. Review can be facilitated simply by asking the patient what has been learned from the diary. We also suggest that patients

Sample Diet Diary Showing Response to Foods

DATE/TIME	FOOD/AMOUNT	RESPONSE	STOOL PATTERN
August 8 9:00 AM	1 cup strawberries 1 slice wheat toast 1 tsp miller's bran with jelly 1 egg	No pain	Formed, easily passed

keep records of exercise, visualization, or any other new life-style activities they are practicing. Rewards for accomplishment of mutually set goals are negotiated. Contract writing is another helpful strategy.

Toileting habits that appear to be most relevant to constipation relate to timing of defecation and utilization of the gastrocolic response. It is helpful if people use the toilet 20 minutes after eating breakfast. The urge to defecate should not be ignored; the longer that stool remains in the colon, the more water is absorbed from it, and the more difficult it is to pass. To take advantage of body mechanics and position discussed earlier, avoid the use of the bedpan whenever possible. In the hospital, privacy and control of odor and noise will facilitate defecation. If using the bathroom is not possible, a bedside commode is preferable to a bedpan.

TABLE 14-7
EXAMPLES OF FOODS
WITH THEIR FIBER CONTENT

FOOD	FIBER CONTENT (g)
Carrots, 1 medium	1.0
Dandelion greens, 1 cup	1.6
Eggplant, 1 cup	1.8
Tomatoes, 1 cup	1.2
All bran cereal, 1/2 cup	2.4
Beans, 1/2 cup	1.4
Oatmeal, 1/2 cup	.2
Peanuts, 10	.4
Filberts, 5	1.2

Medications to establish easily passed, bulky stools include miller's bran. Adsorptive products like Metamucil are helpful and can be taken up to three times daily. This product should be taken with a full 8 oz of fluid to enhance its hydrophilic properties. Stool softeners are used perhaps too extensively. We prefer bulking agents because the stool softener can make stool pasty in consistency and does not add to its bulk so that it may not be easier to pass.

Goal Information about risk factors, and the need for further screening, evidenced by patient verbal statements about these factors and patient's informed decision about screening.

Goal Support for the level of readiness to take remediation, including diagnostic studies, evidenced by patient's verbal statements of perceived risk/benefit of testing and completion of diagnostic studies.

Strategies If any risk factors are present, inform the patient of what they are. Physician management is necessary to determine further medical diagnosis. Patients are usually at least concerned when informed about risks. The nurse's role at this point is to facilitate understanding of the risk and proposed testing, to support the decision-making process, and to facilitate anxiety expression.

Goal Reduce discomfort, evidenced by verbal statements of the patient and body language that indicates absence of pain.

Strategies Measures to reduce abdominal cramping include local heat and ambulation to facilitate passage of gas. If unable to walk, have the patient try rotating positions beginning from lying on the right side to lying on the back, then lying on the left side every 5 to 10 minutes. Movement of the legs as well as sitting also favors gas passage. Placement of a rectal tube for 20 minutes will allow expulsion of gas already in the rectum. Cramping with constipation can be quite sharp and alarming to patients. Reassuring the patient that it will not last can reduce some anxiety. Some patients relate that distracting activities or a prone position with a pillow under the abdomen sometimes brings about a measure of relief.

Goal   Reduced anxiety about constipation, evidenced by verbal statements, calm facial expression, and absence of agitated body language,

Goal   Effective coping repertoire, evidenced by verbal statements of reduced perceived stress and regular practice of negotiated activity.

Goal   Return to usual activities of daily living, evidenced by verbal statements of the patient or significant other.

Strategies   Principles of stress management have been briefly discussed earlier in this chapter and those also apply here. There are also many helpful texts on the subject. Several techniques are used extensively in our clinical practice. If patients are willing, request them to keep a symptom diary. Data recorded include discomfort sensations felt, stool pattern, date, time of onset and relief, food eaten, and events of daily life. Review the diary with the patient and look for patterns and relationships. Symptom episodes often are related to issues involving anger expression or stressful events. Sometimes it is unclear why symptoms develop. During these times, the person is informed that it is not always possible to know why symptoms

begin. Encourage the patient to use the symptoms as a message from the body that it needs care and to implement those measures chosen in the treatment plan. Keeping a diary makes the patient a partner in health care and enhances feelings of control over what is often a long-term, frustrating problem.

When the nurse suspects that social reinforcement of bowel symptoms (secondary gain) is occurring, it is best not to confront this pattern directly. Management should have two goals: reduction of gratification for illness and substitution of other behaviors that produce rewards instead of illness. Whitehead and Schuster suggest that the provider acknowledges that the patient has a physical dysfunction that will persist for some time.[36] They challenge their patients to see how much can be accomplished in spite of discomfort and remind people that remaining active, not focusing on the problem, can lessen discomfort. Patients are encouraged to talk about symptoms only to the provider. Some patients find symptom diaries a useful modality to communicate their concerns. Others respond to an instruction to focus on their bowel symptoms for a specific period every day. We are careful to listen actively to these concerns while simultaneously rewarding activities accomplished "in spite of" symptomatic difficulties. These strategies are not uniformly successful but are offered as alternatives for use in situations when pervasive focusing on symptoms is frustrating to patient, family, and provider. Another strategy used extensively with patients is that of relaxation exercises with visualization. Rationale for this modality has been discussed by Lang.[23]

Goal   Reduce barriers to adherence, evidenced by patient verbal statements that the regimen is being followed.

Strategies   Discussion presented earlier in the chapter applies here as well.

SUMMARY

We hope that the reader has gained some helpful information about the symptoms of constipation and diarrhea. Our intent has been to view these alterations as symptomatic of underlying physiologic or pathological events with multiple causative factors. Our bias has been to present a specific way of interacting with patients, which gives information about the response of the whole person to altered bowel function, supports individual self-care activities, and enhances comprehensive, accurate, caring nursing management.

REFERENCES

1. Abbey J: Digestive Disorders in the Aged. In Burnside J (ed): Nursing and the Aged. New York, McGraw–Hill, 1976
2. Almy TP: Wrestling with the irritable colon. Med Clin North Am 62:203, 1978
3. Almy TP: Therapeutic strategy in stress-related digestive disorders. Clin Gastroenterol 6:709, 1977
4. Almy TP: Experimental studies on the irritable colon. Am J Med 10:60, 1951
5. Bartlett J: Postantibiotic diarrhea. Practical Gastroenterology 4:23, 1980
6. Bayless T, Rosenberg I, Walker W: When you suspect lactase intolerance. Patient Care 14:136, July 15, 1980
7. Bond J. Levitt M: Gaseousness and intestinal gas. Med Clin North Am 62:155, 1978
8. Burkitt D, Meisner P: How to manage constipation with a high fiber diet. Geriatrics 34:33, 1979
9. Chang B: Evaluation of health care professionals in facilitating self care: Review of the literature and a conceptual model. Advances in Nursing Science 3:43, 1980
10. Connell AM, Helten HC, Irvine G et al: Variation of bowel habit in two population samples. Br Med J 2:1095, 1965
11. DuPont HL, Hernick RB: Clinical approach to infectious diarrheas. Medicine 52:265, 1976
12. Field M, Fordtran JS, Schultz SQ (eds): Secretory Diarrhea. Bethesda, American Physiological Society, 1980
13. Glaser JP, Engel GL: Psychodynamics, psychophysiology and gastrointestinal symptomatology. Clin Gastroenterol 6:507, 1977
14. Grand R, Ulshen M: Diarrhea in childhood and adolescence. Practical Gastroenterology 4:9, 1980
15. Greenbaum DS: Intestinal gas in normal subjects and patients with IBS. Practical Gastroenterology 3:26, 1979
16. Guyton AC: Textbook of Medical Physiology. Philadelphia, WB Saunders, 1981
17. Halpern A et al: The straining forces of bowel function. Angiology 11:426, 1960
18. Jones J: Fabulous Fiber Cookbook. San Francisco, 101 Publications, 1977
19. Joseph L: Self Care and the nursing process. Nurs Clin North Am 15:131, 1980
20. Khare R: Ritual practice and pollution in relation to domestic sanitation. In Landes D (ed): Culture, Disease and Healing: Studies in Medical Anthropology. New York, MacMillan & Co, 1977
21. Kim M, Moritz D (ed): Classification of nursing diagnosis. Proceedings of the Third and Fourth National Conferences. New York, McGraw–Hill, 1982
22. Kirsner J: The irritable bowel syndrome. A clinical review and ethical considerations. Arch Intern Med 141:635, 1981.
23. Lang P et al: Emotional imagery: Conceptual structure and patterns of somatovisceral response. Psychophysiology 17:179, 1980
24. Latimer P: Psychophysiologic disorders: A critical appraisal of concept and theory illustrated with reference to the irritable bowel syndrome. Psychol Med 9:71, 1979
25. Mayer A: The Fiber Factor. Emmaus, PA, Rodale Press, 1976
26. MacCara ME: The uses and abuses of laxatives. CMA Journal 126:780, 1982
27. National Center for Health Statistics. Acute conditions: Incidence and associated disability United States 1977–1978. Vital and Health Statistics, Series 13: Data from the National Health Survey, no. 56. DHHS Publication No. PHS82-1717 Hyattsville, MD, National Center for Health Statistics, 1981.
28. Paul B: The role of beliefs and custom in sanitation programs. In Landy D (ed): Culture, Disease and Healing: Studies in Medical Anthropology. New York, MacMillan & Co, 1977
29. Orem D: Nursing: Concepts of Practice. New York, McGraw–Hill, 1971
30. Rees W: Treatment of IBS and peppermint oil. Br Med J 2: 835, 1979
31. Ritchie JA: Pain from distention of the pelvic colon

by inflating a balloon in the irritable bowel syndrome. Gut 14:125, 1973

32. Rodman M: Diarrhea: Think twice before giving medications. RN 43:73, 1980

33. Shaw PK et al: A community wide outbreak of giardiasis with evidence of transmission by a municipal water supply. Ann Intern Med 87:426, 1977

34. Silver B, Blanchard E: Biofeedback and relaxation training in the treatment of psychophysiologic disorders. J Behav Med 1:217, 1978

35. Snape WJ et al: Colonic myoelectric activity in the irritable bowel syndrome. Gastroenterology 70:326, 1976

36. Whitehead W, Schuster M: Psychological management of the irritable bowel syndrome. Practical Gastroenterology 3:32, 1979

37. Wolf S: The digestive system in psychosomatic perspective. Psychosomatics 19:720, 1978

BIBLIOGRAPHY

Antonovsky A: Health, Stress and Coping. San Francisco, Jossey–Bass Publishers, 1979

Berk JE (ed): Gastrointestinal Gas. New York, New York Academy of Sciences, 1968

Blacklow NL, Cukor G: Viral Gastroenteritis. N Engl J Med 304:397, 1981

Bry A: Visualization: Directing the Movies of Your Mind. New York, Barnes & Noble Books, 1978

Jones J: Fabulous Fiber Cookbook. San Francisco, 101 Publications, 1977

Kraus B: Guide to Fiber in Foods. New York, New American Library, 1975

MacCara ME: The uses and abuses of laxatives. Can Med Assoc J 126:780, 1982

McCaffrey M: Nursing Management of the Patient with Pain. New York, JB Lippincott, 1979

Pelletier KR: Mind As Healer, Mind As Slayer. New York, Dell Publishing, 1977

Plotkin GR, Kluge RM, Waldman RH: Gastroenteritis: Etiology, pathophysiology and clinical manipulations. Medicine 58:95, 1979

Samuels M, Samuels N: See With the Mind's Eye: The History, Techniques and Uses of Visualization. New York, Random House, 1975

Sherlock P, Lipin M, Winawer SJ: The prevention of colon cancer. Am J Med 68:917–931, 1980

Spiro HM: Clinical Gastroenterology. New York, MacMillan & Co, 1977

15 | Nausea, Vomiting, and Dehydration

Elizabeth M. Nolan

Nausea and vomiting are associated with numerous diseases, medications, and psychological states. Borison and Wang point out that vomiting may follow simple overeating or may signal approaching death.[4] When one considers the distress that nausea and vomiting cause patients, the fact that the symptoms can be incapacitating, the interference with an otherwise therapeutic treatment, and other factors, it becomes more apparent why there is a need to better understand these symptoms. Because nausea and vomiting occur so frequently and under such varied conditions, nurses in most specialty areas often are called upon to help patients manage these symptoms and to observe these patients for signs of dehydration.

It is beyond the scope of this chapter to describe every known cause or treatment for nausea and vomiting. Instead, the focus is on the most likely causes or categories of causes. The discussion of dehydration is limited to its description as a sequela of nausea and vomiting.

DEFINITIONS

Nausea: A subjective unpleasant sensation that vomiting is imminent; usually referred to the back of the throat, the stomach, or the epigastrium[19]

Vomiting: The forceful expulsion of gastrointestinal contents through the mouth[4]

Retching: The labored, rhythmic respiratory activity that usually precedes or accompanies vomiting[4]

Regurgitation: The return of solids or foods to the mouth from the stomach. It is usually not accompanied by nausea or abdominal diaphragmatic muscular contraction; it is associated with gastroesophageal sphincter incompetence (hiatal hernia) or peptic ulcer[19]

Waterbrash: A term used to describe regurgitation. It is common in infants due to incomplete development of the lower esophageal sphincter[29]

Dehydration: An abnormal depletion of body fluids

HISTORICAL PERSPECTIVE

The stimulus for learning about these symptoms has come from various sources. When air travel became more popular and available, the need to develop treatments for air sickness arose, quite possibly for economic reasons. If one could ensure a comfortable experience, one might encourage larger numbers of travelers. In times of war, a cure for motion sickness had implications for defense because the symptoms could weaken or incapacitate a fighting man.[4] In recent years, the increased development and use of chemotherapeutic agents has necessitated a further look at the mechanisms related to nausea and vomiting. Drugs that are effective for milder forms of nausea and vomiting have not been totally effective in abolishing these symptoms in the patient receiving cancer chemotherapy. Several authors note that the progress seen in the development of cancer chemotherapeutic agents has not been paralleled by the development of effective antiemetic agents.[34,40] In fact, 76% of the research on effective antiemetic agents has been done in the past 4 years.[26] During the Columbia space shuttle's first operational flight, planned extravehicular activity was cancelled when the astronaut developed nausea or space sickness. Because 50% of all travelers in zero gravity experience space sickness, possible causes and treatment will be studied during future missions.[6]

MECHANISMS OF NAUSEA, VOMITING, AND DEHYDRATION

NORMAL MOVEMENT OF FOOD

Before discussing the mechanism involved in nausea and vomiting, we will review the mechanics of the passage of food from the mouth to the stomach. The unidirectional flow of food and fluids from the mouth forward through the pharynx, the esophagus, stomach, and small intestine allows digestion and absorption of fluids and nutrients to occur.[36] When vomiting occurs, this process is disrupted.

Swallowing is the first process involved

in this mechanism. Swallowing is an all-or-none phenomenon, a reflex coordinated by the swallowing center in the medulla. It involves coordination of numerous muscles that move the food forward and prevent backward flow. It is initiated when the tongue forces the contents from the back of the mouth into the pharynx; once it has begun, it cannot be stopped voluntarily. Pressure receptors in the pharynx are stimulated by the bolus of food and afferent impulses are sent to the swallowing center in the medulla (Fig. 15-1A). As food moves toward the pharynx, the soft palate rises, preventing backward flow into the nasopharynx. Additionally, the medulla inhibits respiration, closing the glottis, so that food does not enter the trachea (Fig. 15-1B). As the food is pushed further into the pharynx, it (the food) tilts the epiglottis backward so that the epiglottis covers the already closed glottis (Fig. 15-1C). Skeletal muscles in the upper portion of the esophagus contract to open the hypopharyngeal sphincter and permit entry of the bolus of food into the esophagus (Fig. 15-1D). Waves of contraction, *peristaltic waves*, move the food down the esophagus into the stomach. The gastroesophageal sphincter, the last 4 centimeters of the esophagus, relaxes as peristaltic waves begin and allows food to enter the stomach. Normally the gastroesophageal sphincter is contracted, preventing gastric contents from entering the esophagus. The muscles in the antrum of the stomach are thicker and more powerful than those in the fundus (body) of the stomach. (Fig. 15-1E). It is the contractile activity of these muscles that empties the stomach of food. The stomach empties at a rate proportional to the volume of material in it at any given time. Additionally, the chemical composition and the amount of chyme in the duodenum are important factors that control gastric emptying. For example, fat in the duodenum is the most potent stimulus for the inhibition of gastric

Soft palate · Tongue · Glottis · Trachea · Esophagus · Pharynx · Epiglottis · Hypopharyngeal sphincter

Esophagus · Pyloric sphincter · Duodenum · Antrum · Fundus · Body

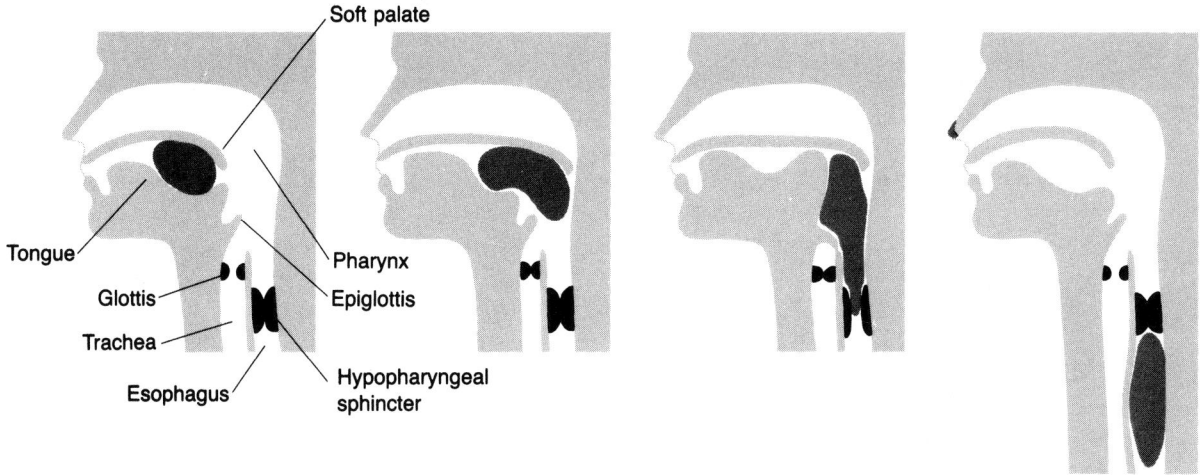

FIG. 15-1 *The movement of a bolus of food from the mouth to the stomach. (Vander AJ, Sherman JH, Luciano DS: Human Physiology: The Mechanisms of Body Function. Copyright © 1970, 1975 by McGraw–Hill. Used with the permission of the McGraw–Hill Book Co.)*

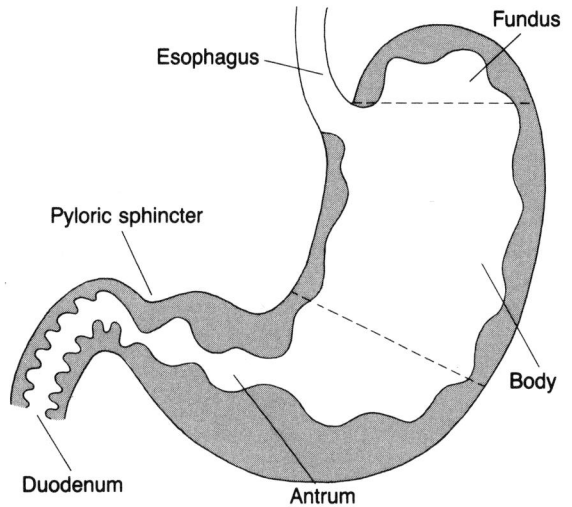

motility. This allows more time for digestion and absorption.

NAUSEA AND VOMITING

Nausea and vomiting can occur separately but quite commonly occur together and thus often are considered together.[19] Nausea usually precedes vomiting; in fact, vomiting may relieve the symptom of nausea.

Nausea

Nausea is the conscious recognition of subconscious excitation in an area of the medulla either closely associated with or part of the vomiting center (VC). Because nausea does not always accompany vomiting, it is believed that only certain areas of the VC are associated with the sensation of nausea.[13]

The mechanism of nausea is poorly understood. Nausea may be associated with certain intestinal activities or may be a response to the stimuli that induce vomiting. Nausea is frequently accompanied by a generalized contraction of the descending duodenum regardless of the cause. This contraction is seen even after transection of the midbrain or transection of the splanchnic nerves. Changes in the gastrointestinal tract have been observed to occur before the sensation of nausea.[4]

There are gastrointestinal disorders in which vomiting does not occur but in which nausea is a symptom, for example, disorders of the esophagus and small intestine. Stimuli associated with the onset of nausea include irritation of the gastrointestinal tract by distention of the duodenum or lower intestine, impulses originating in the lower brain associated with motion sickness, and impulses from the cerebral cortex that initiate vomiting. Nausea can result from increased tension on the gastric and intestinal walls induced by distention of the lower wall of the esophagus.[18] Nauseating odors can cause the lower border of the stomach to distend 1 or 2 inches, perhaps owing to sudden relaxation of abdominal muscles.[15] The stretch on esophageal and gastric walls causes tension on nerve endings; passage of a peristaltic wave that relieves tension on the nerve fibers in the esophageal wall may relieve nausea. This may be a reason that persons are encouraged to take a deep breath when they feel nauseated.

Vomiting

Vomiting reverses the normal unidirectional flow of food and fluids. It may be preceded or accompanied by signs of sympathetic nervous activity such as tachycardia, tachypnea, sweating, salivation, pallor, and dilated pupils.[11,22] The actual act of vomiting involves several phases or steps. Initially the glottis closes, preventing aspiration of vomitus into the trachea. The breath is held in midinspiration. The soft palate rises, increasing intra-abdominal pressure because the chest is held in a fixed position. The esophagus and cardiac sphincters relax, allowing stomach contents to enter the esophagus; next, reverse peristalsis begins and the gastric contents are ejected.[10] As is swallowing, the act of vomiting is a coordinated event.

Descriptions of the vomiting act are not always consistent in describing the sequence of events. Lumsden and Holden noted that patients became nauseated and vomited during barium studies and documented the events associated with these symptoms (Fig. 15-2).[25]

Vomiting, a reflex response integrated in the medulla oblongata, is under the control of two functionally distinct medullary centers: the emetic center or VC, and the chemoreceptor trigger zone (CTZ). These centers lie close to each other, near the brain stem centers that regulate vasomotor and autonomic functions.[25] These are schematically represented in Figure 15-3. The VC is in the reticular formation of the medulla, at the level of the olivary nuclei; it controls and integrates the actual act of vomiting. Stimuli to the VC come from three major sources: 1) the periphery (the intestinal tract and other parts of the body); 2) the CTZ; and 3) the higher cortical centers, including the labyrinth apparatus (Fig. 15-4). Other afferent impulses presumably reach the VC from the limbic system and the diencephalon, because emetic responses to emotionally charged situations such as nauseating odors or sickening sights are known to occur.[10,19]

The CTZ is also located in the medulla, near the area postrema; by itself, the CTZ is incapable of mediating the act of vomiting. When the CTZ is activated, efferent impulses go to the VC, which initiates the act of vom-

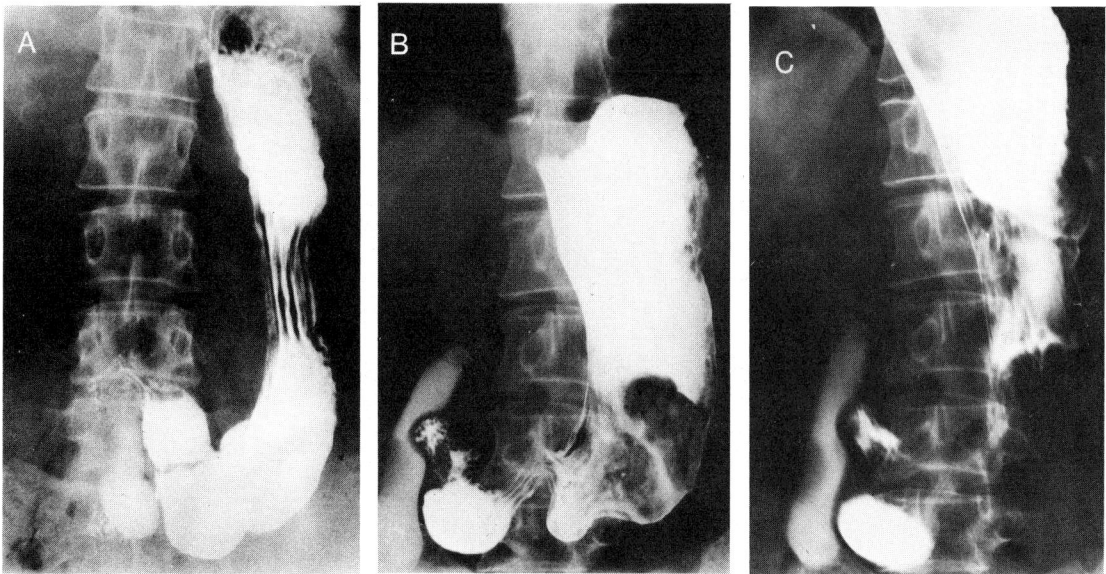

FIG. 15-2 Radiographic findings observed during a barium study demonstrate events that occur in the gastrointestinal tract during nausea, retching, and vomiting. (A) The patient was experiencing nausea but had not yet begun to retch or vomit. The duodenal bulb is distended with barium and the stomach has not yet begun to contract. (B) The patient had begun to retch. The duodenal bulb is empty, and its contents seem to have backed up into the stomach; the proximal part of the gastric antrum is tightly contracted, and there has been a shift of barium from the lower part to the upper part of the stomach. There is an assumption that this reflux occurs during nausea, while the stomach is inactive and its tone reduced. This has been observed on a number of occasions. (C) The patient was vomiting; the cardia has elevated and is opened widely; barium is forced from the stomach into the esophagus. In the lower part of the stomach, there is a long, contracted segment. It is usually observed that the opening of the cardia coincides with the cessation of retching and the occurrence of vomiting. (Lumsden K, Holden WS: The act of vomiting in man. Gut 10:173–179, 1969.)

FIG. 15-3 Schematic representations of vomiting control centers in the medulla oblongata. (Key: CTZ, chemoreceptor trigger zone; EC, emetic center; IV, fourth ventricle; VIII, vestibular nerve; X, vagus nerve.) (A) shows a Cross-sectional representation; (B) a longitudinal representation. (Redrawn from Siegel LJ, Longo DL: The control of chemotherapy-induced emesis. Ann Int Med 95:352–359, 1981)

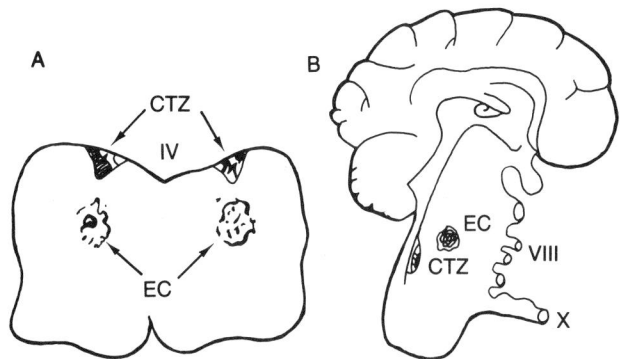

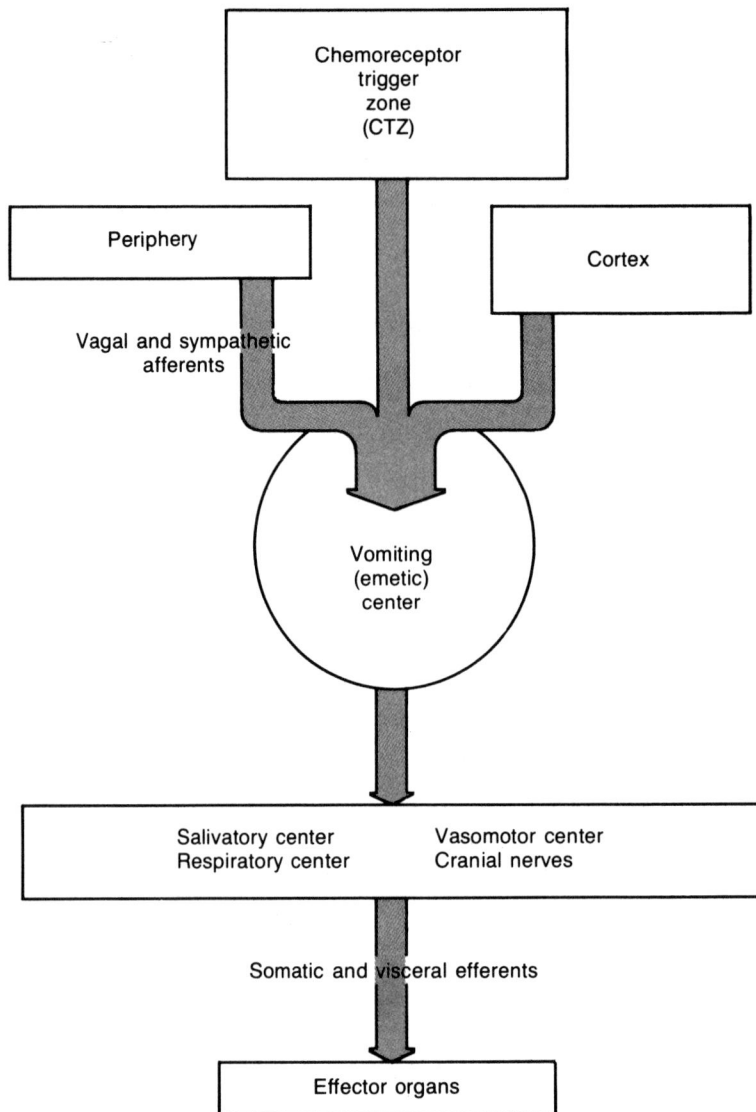

FIG. 15-4 *Schematic representation of reflex pathways for vomiting. Vomiting can be triggered at one (or more) sites: the chemoreceptor trigger zone (CTZ), the pharynx and gastrointestinal tract (periphery), and supramedullary loci (cortex). Afferent impulses from the three trigger sites are integrated at the medullary emetic center. When the vomiting threshold is exceeded, the emetic center programs the vomiting act through the neighboring medullary control centers and somatic and visceral efferent nerves. (Redrawn after Seigel LJ, Longo DL: The control of chemotherapy-induced emesis. Ann Intern Med 1981, 95:352–359)*

iting. Many stimuli, for example, apomorphine, digitalis, antibiotics, alcohol, ergot alkaloids, cytotoxic agents, inhalation anesthetics, and radiation are known to activate the CTZ.[41] Some phenothiazide derivatives are believed to antagonize the effects of the above-mentioned drugs on the CTZ, and are used as antiemetic agents.[15]

Important efferent pathways in vomiting are phrenic, spinal, and visceral efferent nerves, which innervate the diaphragm, abdominal musculature, and stomach and esophagus respectively.[15]

DEHYDRATION

In addition to the discomfort to the patient caused by nausea and vomiting, the losses of fluid and electrolytes can result in dehydration. In many cases, the body's normal regulatory mechanisms are sufficient to adapt to fluid losses such as those that occur with nausea and vomiting. However, with prolonged or severe losses, metabolic alkalosis or metabolic acidosis can occur.[32,36,37]

Normal Fluid Balance

Water comprises about 60% of a human's body weight. Intracellular fluid, about 40% of body weight, contains potassium as the major ion. Extracellular fluid is distributed as *interstitial fluid,* bathing the cells (18% of body weight); and as plasma, the dynamic fluid component of blood, which carries oxygen and nutrients to the cell (2% of body weight). Sodium is the major ion of extracellular fluid, which also has a greater concentration of the chloride ion than does intracellular fluid. Regulation of fluid occurs through the renal regulation of water, sodium, and potassium, as well as through the mechanism of thirst. Water and sodium also are lost normally through the skin and the gastrointestinal tract, albeit in small amounts. When vomiting is severe, the losses from the gastrointestinal tract become significant.

Body sodium and water are primarily regulated through the control of the renal excretion of these substances. Chloride, sodium, and water are freely filterable at the glomerulus and all but 1% are reabsorbed as they pass through the tubule. The reabsorption of sodium from the tubule is an active process, requiring energy. Chloride and water passively diffuse from the tubule to the capillary; reabsorption of both are dependent on the active reabsorption of sodium.

Although water reabsorption is dependent on sodium reabsorption, water excretion is not dependent on sodium excretion. It is possible to excrete large volumes of water without loss of sodium. A factor that affects the amount of water reabsorption is the antidiuretic hormone (ADH) synthesized by the hypothalamus. When there is a hypovolemic state, decreased atrial pressure may cause decreased firing of baroreceptors, which stimulates ADH synthesis and release. Increased permeability of the renal tubules results; this facilitates the reabsorption of water so that less fluid is excreted. Subsequently, vascular fluid volume is restored.

When a deficit in body sodium occurs, less sodium is excreted by the kidneys. This is accomplished by increasing the amount of sodium reabsorbed, or decreasing the amount of sodium filtered. In conditions in which there is decreased plasma volume, cardiac preload decreases; stroke volume, cardiac output, and arterial blood pressure eventually fall. In response to the decrease in arterial pressure, the renal arteries constrict due to the increased activity of the renal sympathetic nerves. The glomerular filtration rate (GFR) decreases, less sodium is filtered, and subsequently less is excreted.

In a normal person, the regulatory mechanisms are so effective that sodium balance will vary less than 2%, even in the presence of dietary changes in sodium intake or in losses due to vomiting, sweating, or diarrhea.

Except in cases of vomiting or diarrhea, potassium (K^+) losses are usually minimal. Like sodium and chloride, potassium is freely filterable at the glomerulus; however, only potassium is secreted by the renal tubules. The kidneys are able to excrete more potassium than they filter through the glomerulus.

The renal tubular secretion of K^+ regulates the serum K^+ concentration. The concentration of K^+ in the renal tubular cells is believed to be an important factor. When K^+ intake is high, the concentration in the tubule is high. Therefore, more K^+ is secreted into the lumen and excreted. When the serum K^+ is low, less of it is secreted into the lumen and excreted into the urine, thus reestablishing its normal levels. Low levels of the potassium ion in the extracellular fluid also stimulate the adrenal cortex to decrease secretion of aldosterone, so that potassium excretion decreases and excretion of sodium is facilitated.

In addition to maintaining a balance of water, sodium, and potassium, the kidneys regulate the extracellular hydrogen ion concentration, which helps to maintain a normal pH, acid–base balance. The kidneys accomplish this through the carbon dioxide–bicarbonate buffer system. The kidneys regulate bicarbonate concentration by varying its reabsorption into the plasma or by adding new bicarbonate to the plasma. Normally very little bicarbonate is excreted, and the urine is slightly acid. When the plasma level of the hydrogen ion is reduced, as in alkalosis, the kidneys can reestablish equilibrium and a normal pH by increasing the amount of bicarbonate excreted in the urine.

The result is a decrease in plasma bicarbonate and an increase in hydrogen ions.

Likewise, when the level of hydrogen ions is increased, as in acidosis, the kidneys reabsorb all the filtered bicarbonate, and also produce bicarbonate ions and add them to the plasma. The increase in the level of bicarbonate offsets the increased level of hydrogen ions and reestablishes equilibrium.

Regulatory mechanisms can be effective in maintaining homeostasis even when there is vomiting, diarrhea, or other fluid-depleting states. However, when losses are profound, as occurs with persistent vomiting, and when fluid intake ceases or is markedly reduced, normal mechanisms may fail. Metabolic alkalosis or metabolic acidosis may ensue. Although alkalosis is more likely to occur in vomiting, one should not overlook the possibility that the patient can be in an acidotic state (explained in the following sections).

Metabolic Alkalosis

Metabolic alkalosis results from losses of hydrogen ions and chloride ions. With profound vomiting, 1 to 2 liters of gastric fluid can be lost per day, and large amounts of hydrogen and chloride ions are lost. As the hydrogen ion concentration in the blood falls, the kidneys limit the reabsorption of the bicarbonate ion, excreting it in the urine to reestablish a normal pH. Initially this is effective in reversing alkalosis; over several days, however, the mechanism can break down and the alkalosis can become profound.

With severe vomiting, the kidneys must adjust not only to a loss of hydrogen and chloride ions, but also to losses of fluid, sodium, and potassium ions. Fluid loss causes a decrease in plasma volume, ultimately resulting in a decreased GFR. As the GFR diminishes, less sodium is filtered, decreasing the amount of sodium available for reabsorption. When there is a persistent metabolic alkalosis and salt depletion occurs, the kidneys will be unable to compensate for the alkalotic state. The sodium deficit will not only stimulate sodium reabsorption but also hydrogen ion secretion; this makes the alkalosis worse. Salt depletion stimulates the secretion of aldosterone, which will help to conserve sodium and excrete potassium. The hypokalemia seen with vomiting is usually due not to the gastric losses, but to secondary hyperaldosteronism and to an increased filtered load of bicarbonate. As described earlier, low levels of potassium in the renal tubules will stimulate the secretion of potassium, which prevents the compensatory excretion of bicarbonate.

Clinical signs and symptoms and laboratory findings seen in metabolic alkalosis are listed in Table 15-1.

Metabolic Acidosis

Metabolic acidosis results from the loss of bicarbonate, which lowers the plasma pH and plasma bicarbonate composition. Gastric contents are acidic; therefore losses that occur in vomiting result in an alkalotic state. However, the intestinal secretions of pancreatic juice and bile are alkaline, and vomiting these fluids results in the loss of bicarbonate. In some cases of vomiting, there is reflux of small intestine contents into the stomach before emesis. When alkaline losses exceed acidic losses, metabolic acidosis will result.

When bicarbonate ions are lost along with chloride ions, the kidney needs to increase the level of plasma bicarbonate to restore the normal pH. Less bicarbonate will be filtered, and therefore fewer hydrogen ions need to be secreted to reabsorb bicarbonate. Additionally, the kidney will reabsorb all fil-

---

TABLE 15-1
A COMPARISON OF CLINICAL FINDINGS IN METABOLIC ALKALOSIS
AND METABOLIC ACIDOSIS

CLINICAL FINDINGS	ALKALOSIS	ACIDOSIS
Urine pH	>7	<6
Plasma pH	>7.45	<7.35
Plasma bicarbonate	>24 mEq/liter	<24 mEq/liter
pCO_2	>40 mm Hg	<40 mm Hg
Serum sodium	Decreased	Decreased
Serum potassium	Decreased	Decreased
Serum chloride	Decreased	Decreased
Signs and symptoms	Shallow, slow respirations	Deep rapid respirations
	Cyanosis and hypoxia	(Kussmaul's sign)
	Irregular pulse	Restlessness
	Uncooperative	Stupor
	Irritable	Coma
	Tetany	Weakness
	Muscle cramps	General malaise
	Paresthesia	Headache
		Flushed skin

tered bicarbonate and contribute new bicarbonate to the plasma.

Table 15-1 contains signs and symptoms as well as laboratory findings seen in metabolic acidosis.

Thirst

An initial method to compensate for fluid loss is for the person to increase oral intake. The sensation of thirst is the stimulus to increase fluid intake. Thirst is stimulated by a decrease in extracellular volume and a higher plasma osmolarity, the same changes that trigger the production of ADH. A dry mouth and throat commonly stimulate a sensation of thirst; usually the person then drinks an amount sufficient to replace the lost fluid. A person will cease drinking even before the fluid has been absorbed from the stomach into the vasculature.[4,36] Such mechanisms are often effective in replacing losses. However, when nausea and vomiting occur, a person may consciously or unconciously decrease fluid intake. Even though the person may desire fluid, it is avoided to alleviate the nausea and vomiting. In these states, the renal mechanisms predominate, and thirst has a minor role in fluid regulation.

CAUSES OF NAUSEA AND VOMITING

> "Tis profitable for man that his stomach should nauseate and reject things that have a loathsome taste or smell"[11]
> Boyle R., 1686

Nausea and vomiting are common signs of organic and functional disorders but the precise mechanism by which they occur in each condition is not well understood. Though the previous quotation suggests a useful function for these symptoms, there is no apparent useful function for nausea and vomiting in many of the conditions in which they occur.

The causes of nausea and vomiting may be *pathogenic*, related to a disease process such as intestinal obstruction; *iatrogenic*, related to the treatment of a disease, such as cancer chemotherapy; or *psychogenic*, related to a psychological state such as the sight of a repulsive scene.

Conditions associated with the occurrence of nausea and vomiting are numerous. The listing in the accompanying chart is not intended to be all-inclusive but rather a compilation of some potential causes of these symptoms.

Acute Inflammatory or Infectious Diseases

Nausea and vomiting commonly occur in acute inflammatory and infectious diseases. They are seen not only with inflammation and infection of the gastrointestinal tract, such as appendicitis and gastroenteritis, but also in numerous systemic infections such as pyelonephritis. Children with fevers often have nausea and vomiting.[19]

Gastrointestinal Disorders

In many gastrointestinal disorders, there is local distention and the mechanism that causes nausea and vomiting is believed due to stimulation of afferent impulses, which are sent to the VC.

Reflux esophagitis, achalasia, and hiatal hernia are associated more with regurgitation than with vomiting. A patient is unlikely to distinguish between these signs and may present with the latter complaint. In reflux esophagitis, acid regurgitation and other symptoms will be brought on by any condition that increases intra-abdominal pressure (e.g., lying down). These symptoms may awaken a sleeping patient. Seventy percent of patients with achalasia note regurgitation several hours after a meal. Nausea is not present, and the symptoms recur when the

Conditions Associated with Nausea and Vomiting

PATHOGENIC

Acute systemic infections
  Pyelonephritis
Fever, especially in young children
Viral, bacterial, or parasitic infections of the GI
    tract
  Viral hepatitis
  Appendicitis
  Peritonitis
  Pancreatitis
Acute or chronic indigestion
  Irritating GI contents
  Irritated GI tract
CNS disorders
  Disorders of the labyrinth apparatus and its
    central connections
  Meniere's syndrome
  Labyrinthitis
Increased ICP
  Neoplasms (medullablastoma)
  Hydrocephalus
Vascular disorders
  Migraine headaches

Cardiac disorders
  Acute myocardial infarction, especially in-
    ferior wall
  Chronic right-sided heart failure
Endocrine disorders
  Diabetic acidosis
  Adrenal insufficiency
  Pregnancy (morning sickness, hyperemesis
    gravidarum, toxemia)
  Thyrotoxicosis

IATROGENIC

Side-effects or toxic effects of pharmacologic
    agents
  Inhalation anesthetics
  Cardiac glycosides
  Opiates
  Cytotoxic agents
Alcohol
Radiation

PSYCHOGENIC

Anorexia nervosa, bulimarexia
Noxious stimuli (odors, sights, tastes, sounds,
    thoughts)

patient assumes a recumbent position. A sudden, choking sensation may awaken the patient. Sleeping with the head of the bed elevated may relieve the symptoms. With hiatal hernia, regurgitation without vomiting is seen; these signs usually accompany or follow severe heartburn.

Patients with uncomplicated peptic ulcer disease (PUD) do not commonly have nausea and vomiting. These symptoms seem to occur more frequently when the ulcer is in the pylorus or the antrum, rather than in the body of the stomach, or when there are complications of PUD. Borison and Wang found that distention of the pouches of the gastric fundus never resulted in emesis, whereas distention of pyloric pouches with pressures of 30 to 35 mm Hg always resulted in vom-

iting, regardless of the substance used to cause the distention—water, acids, alkalis, or a milk solution. The location of the distention appeared to be the critical factor. In ulcers, swelling and edema at the site can be sufficiently extreme to cause gastric stasis; stenosis may occur in the duodenum or the pylorus. Vomiting that occurs with stasis is potentially serious, because with stasis there is increased gastric secretion and greater delay in the stomach contents reaching the small intestine.[4] Electrolyte depletion may be quite severe. Some patients with PUD note relief of their pain and nausea following vomiting, even with nonobstructive ulcers. Vomiting or regurgitation of gastric juices may occur with pyloric or duodenal ulcers; this typically occurs at night and may awaken a patient from sleep. As a rule, patients with PUD are not anorexic; when vomiting occurs, it is usually an early symptom of pyloric obstruction. Anorexia is seen with gastritis and cancer. With cancer, the lesion may obstruct the gastrointestinal tract, and vomiting or regurgitation may occur.[12]

Severe nausea and vomiting are prominent symptoms of acute gastritis; vomiting may be also noted in chronic gastritis.[12]

Cholecystitis causes distention of the gallbladder and the biliary passages; the severity of symptoms appears to be related to the degree of distention and the structure involved. For example, distention of the ducts results in worse nausea and vomiting than does distention of the gallbladder.

Nausea, vomiting, and anorexia occur in the early stages of hepatitis, even before the patient becomes icteric. These symptoms also occur in patients with hepatic tumors. In cirrhosis, these symptoms are believed due to venous congestion of the gastrointestinal tract.

Acute and chronic pancreatitis also causes nausea and vomiting. In acute pancreatitis, they occur after the onset of pain, which is the major symptom. Initially, vomiting may relieve the pain, but continued vomiting increases ductal pressure, causing the reflux of bile into the pancreatic ducts and further feelings of distress. Nausea and vomiting in chronic pancreatitis usually accompany the attack of pain.[12]

Cardiac Disorders

Vomiting may occur at the time of a myocardial infarction (MI), especially inferior wall infarction and in congestive heart failure (CHF).[1] It is hypothesized that at the time of the MI, local irritation of the diaphragm is related to the onset of vomiting. The arrhythmogenic effects of electrolyte disturbances

that can result from vomiting, and the retching that accompanies vomiting is a concern in the patient with an MI. A state of fluid depletion may be missed in a patient with an acute MI because clinicians often are more attuned to the risk of fluid overload in these patients. The anorexia, nausea, and vomiting that accompany CHF are attributed to passive congestion, resulting in congestion of the gastrointestinal tract, but may be also due to digitalis toxicity.[17] It has been suggested that nausea appears more commonly with tachycardia, whereas retching occurs more commonly with bradycardia.[4]

Central Nervous System Disorders

When the total incidence of vomiting is considered, the central nervous system (CNS) lesions represent a small proportion of the causes; because of this, CNS lesions may be overlooked, while other causes of vomiting are sought.

Vomiting associated with CNS lesions often is characterized as being projectile and without the warning symptom of nausea. Although there is a tendency to attribute vomiting accompanied by nausea to disorders of the gastrointestinal tract, most intracranial lesions that produce vomiting also produce nausea.[28]

Central neurologic lesions that can produce vomiting are those involving the vestibular nuclei or their projections; those impinging on the floor of the fourth ventricle, such as a medullablastoma or ependymoma; or those producing brain stem compression due to increased intracranial pressure (IIP). Early morning vomiting is common with medullablastoma. Children with craniopharyngiomas often complain of headaches and vomiting as early symptoms.[28,38]

Migraine headaches, acute meningitis, and Meniere's syndrome are often associated with nausea and vomiting. In Meniere's syndrome, attacks of severe vertigo usually are accompanied by nausea and frequently by severe vomiting.

Endocrine Disorders

Vomiting associated with conditions such as adrenal insufficiency, diabetic ketoacidosis, thyrotoxicosis, and pregnancy is believed to be due to stimulation of the CTZ.[3]

Adrenal Insufficiency It is not clear whether gastrointestinal symptoms are the result of adrenal insufficiency or whether they precipitate an episode of adrenal insufficiency. In chronic adrenal insufficiency, anorexia slowly progresses to mild nausea in about 90% of patients. This may have serious consequences if the nausea prevents the patient from taking the necessary medications.

Nausea and vomiting are prominent signs of acute adrenal insufficiency. Anorexia, which occurs in virtually all patients, is followed by nausea and vomiting in 50% of patients. Shortly after vomiting occurs, the blood pressure, already low, plummets. In this condition, there is a decrease in mineral corticoids, and one would expect to see hyperkalemia; however, as the vomiting progresses, the potassium level does not increase.

Diabetes Nausea and vomiting have been described as early harbingers of diabetic ketoacidosis (DKA). However, even if the symptoms are not due to DKA, they may lead to DKA when intake diminishes and electrolyte and fluid losses increase.

Vomiting also occurs in diabetes due to the loss of gastric tone that is seen in gastric stasis, a complication of diabetes.

Thyrotoxicosis Although thyrotoxicosis is seen less frequently today, due to advances in diagnosis and treatment of hyperthyroidism, this cause of vomiting may be overlooked, especially when vomiting is the sole clinical sign. Several case studies describe patients in whom treatment was delayed because vomiting was not considered a sign of thyroid disease. Once treatment was initiated, vomiting ceased.[31]

Pregnancy Vomiting associated with pregnancy is thought to be due to stimulation of the CTZ. Several types of vomiting have been associated with pregnancy: morning sickness, hyperemesis gravidarum, vomiting due to causes other than pregnancy, and vomiting in late pregnancy.[2]

Morning Sickness Most pregnant women have nausea and vomiting early in their pregnancy, although nausea occurs more commonly than vomiting. In fact, there is some suggestion that among women with these symptoms, there are fewer perinatal deaths.[16] These symptoms occur less frequently in women who smoke and drink alcohol during their pregnancy.

Morning sickness can occur even before the first missed menstrual period and can alert the woman to the fact that she may be pregnant. It is not uncommon to vomit once or twice a day, but more frequent vomiting is cause for concern. Nausea and vomiting often occur upon arising but can occur any time during the day. Women who work at night and sleep during the day will have symptoms upon arising in the afternoon, rather than in the early morning. In some women, the symptoms are more acute when they are tired or when they are preparing food. Although the symptoms are uncomfortable, the woman is usually able to maintain a normal intake and avoid weight loss. Symptoms usually subside by about the end of the third month.

Hyperemesis Gravidarum Hyperemesis gravidarum, seen in about 1% to 5% of all pregnant women, is a condition in which there is severe vomiting and a high potential for dehydration and weight loss. The symptoms can be severe enough to necessitate hospitalization for fluid and electrolyte replacement.

Vomiting Due to Other Causes Vomiting may be attributed to the condition of pregnancy, when in fact there is an underlying treatable cause. The incidence of urinary tract infections is sufficiently high in pregnant women to warrant consideration of this cause. Flu, appendicitis, and cholecystitis can also explain these symptoms in the pregnant woman. Bowel obstructions and cerebral tumors have been missed when nausea and vomiting were attributed to threatened abortion or premature labor.

Vomiting in Late Pregnancy In late pregnancy, vomiting has been linked to liver disease and preeclampsia, as well as the conditions described in the previous sections. Intrahepatic cholestasis, characterized by jaundice and vomiting, can occur, and tends to recur in subsequent pregnancies. It can also occur in women taking oral contraceptives. Vomiting also is associated with acute fatty infiltration of the liver, which is associated with tetracycline therapy, especially when administered in high doses and late in pregnancy. The prognosis is poor for the mother and the fetus, since liver failure develops rapidly.

No definite mechanisms have been found to explain the frequent occurrence of nausea and vomiting in pregnancy. There are efforts to identify the physiological changes that activate the vomiting center. Since the use of medications to alleviate these symptoms is limited, due to concerns of teratogenicity, a clearer understanding of causal mechanisms might facilitate identification of effective treatments for the prevention or relief of these symptoms.

Some of the changes that occur with pregnancy may help to explain possible causes. During pregnancy, smooth muscle tone in the gastrointestinal tract decreases, the cardiac sphincter relaxes, and stomach emptying is delayed.

Recent studies focus on the hormonal changes of pregnancy that might explain these symptoms. Although it has not been established as a causative agent, human chorionic gonadotrophin (HCG) reaches its highest levels at the same time as the incidence of nausea and vomiting peaks. In conditions in which HCG levels are high, such as twin pregnancies and hydatidiform moles, the symptoms of nausea and vomiting are more severe. Estrogen levels may play a role in the causation of these symptoms. Estrogen levels increase rapidly during early pregnancy; also, persons having taken exogenous estrogen (e.g., oral contraceptives) often report nausea.

There is also a view that nausea and vomiting of early pregnancy result from a systemic reaction to decreased glucose levels as glucose is utilized in great quantities by the growing fetus. This may be the reason that a carbohydrate snack often relieves the symptoms.

Psychological factors have been viewed as significant to the occurrence of these symptoms.[2,15] However, physiological causes are supported by the observation that the symptoms occur even before the woman knows she is pregnant.

Iatrogenic Causes

Medications Nausea and vomiting are common side-effects of many medications. Nausea and vomiting are not allergic reactions, but may be major symptoms of drug toxicity. These symptoms occur with both oral and parenteral medication. Drugs are categorized by the degree to which they cause these symptoms, that is, as mild, moderate, or severe emetic agents. Although cytotoxic agents are associated with severe vomiting, they too can be grouped into these categories. Local irritation of the gastrointestinal tract and central effects on the CTZ are probably the etiology of nausea and vomiting. When the CTZ is ablated, an emetic substance may no longer cause vomiting. Drugs known to block the CTZ will be effective antiemetic agents in some instances but ineffective in other cases. Drugs cause vomiting by peripheral pathways as well, stimulating the VC by way of visceral afferent nerves, often from the pharynx and gastrointestinal tract.[4]

Medications that cause nausea and vomiting can sometimes be withdrawn and another agent substituted when the symptoms cause discomfort to the patient. In the case of cancer chemotherapy, the side-effects usually are considered less worrisome than the patient outcome without these drugs; thus, the medications are continued although the patient may experience severe nausea and vomiting. Skeletal fractures and esophageal tears have been reported in cancer patients with severe vomiting.[11,40] Because the severe nausea and vomiting has received such widespread attention, and because many patients are unwilling to suffer through the symptoms, no matter how ominous the outcome, there has been increased emphasis on the relief of these symptoms by oncologists in recent years. According to one author, the resulting psychological trauma may be serious enough to cause some patients to refuse further therapy.[26]

Postoperative Vomiting Approximately 30% to 40% of all surgical patients develop nausea and vomiting.[12] This may be due to local irritation from anesthetic gases, deep levels of anesthesia, or direct stimulation of the VC. Initially, vomiting empties the stomach of mucus and saliva swallowed during surgery and may subside after this occurs. In some patients, vomiting persists postoperatively, possibly due to medullary ischemia, prolonged hypotension, or aftereffects of the anesthetic agents. It can occur with intestinal obstruction such as paralytic ileus. Vomiting can cause tension on suture lines, increasing the risk of dehiscence or evisceration. It can also increase the amount of pain and discomfort of the postoperative patient.

Surgery is a stressful experience for most patients; there are concerns related to the risks of the procedure, the anticipated pain and discomfort afterwards, and the possible outcome of the procedure as in the case of an exploratory surgery. As Dumas demonstrated in a study of surgical patients, preoperative fears can affect the incidence of postoperative vomiting.[8]

Motion Sickness

Labyrinth stimulation appears to be the primary factor in the etiology of motion sickness, which can occur with air, sea, or even motor travel. The CTZ is the direct pathway of the vestibular reflex concerned with motion sickness. Following ablation of the CTZ, animals are no longer susceptible to the emetic effects of swinging motion. A labyrinthectomy or sectioning of the eighth cranial nerve eliminates the emetic response to motion.[4]

Psychogenic Vomiting

Noxious sights, smells, tastes, and sounds, as well as stressful events, are known to cause vomiting. Supramedullary centers are believed to act on the VC to induce vomiting. These types of events are not likely to result in profound or persistent vomiting, as they tend to be isolated events that a person can consciously or unconsciously avoid in the future.

A problematic cause of vomiting is self-induced vomiting, which can be a mild-to-serious condition. Although there is a possible role for cerebral, pituitary, and hypothalamic factors in the etiology of self-induced vomiting, there is strong support for the view that is psychogenic in origin.[27] In early Roman times, self-induced vomiting was primarily a male phenomenon; today, it is almost exclusively female. There is little doubt that the emphasis our society places on thinness, especially for women, has a role in the cause of this present-day phenomenon. Clothing styles accentuate the value of thinness, but there is an abundance of food and drink available, and food has a strong social and psychological significance.[23,24]

The use of vomiting and purging as a measure of weight control is believed to be quite prevalent among women from late teens through the early twenties; some experts believe it is quite common among apparently well-adjusted people who are striving to maintain a desirable body weight. Because of the desirability of thinness, the weight point set by persons is lower than what one would biologically expect, and therefore great control must be exerted to achieve and maintain this low weight. During periods of stress or relaxation, the self-control wavers, and the person will often overeat rather than eat a normal amount.[14]

Bulimia nervosa (BN), or *bulimarexia*, is a condition characterized by a ravenous appetite and intake of food, a desire to avoid fattening foods, and a morbid fear of becoming fat. BN may be a type of anorexia nervosa (AN) in which food intake is severely restricted, or it may be a separate phenomenon. Much discussion and research is being done on both of these conditions.[23,24]

Two types of anorexia nervosa patients have been described: food restrictors and patients with BN. The food restrictors are seen by some to be compulsive persons, able to exert a great degree of control over their behavior. They are more often seen as perfectionists by their parents than are persons with BN. Behaviors not seen in food restrictors are often seen with BN: impulsive behavior such as kleptomania, feelings of depression and guilt, anxiety, somatic concerns, sexual activity, suicide attempts, substance abuse, and self-mutilation.[20]

However, most patients who self-induce vomiting do not have AN; most have either a normal or slightly lower than normal body weight. Nevertheless, this behavior is not benign. Dental caries occurs due to erosion of tooth enamel in chronic vomiting. Painless enlargement of the parotid glands is frequently seen, although the causal mechanism is unclear. Menstrual irregularities, including amenorrhea, are seen, particularly when there is a radical dietary change. Pyle noted that 77% of women who self-induced vomiting had at least one episode of amenorrhea lasting 3 months or longer.[30] Abrasions and callous formation may be seen on the knuckles because of the person's using the fingers to induce vomiting. Weakness may be noted in patients who are hypokalemic or dehydrated.[23,24]

Although self-induced vomiting is a growing health care problem, persons with this behavior are unlikely to present with a complaint of vomiting. The secrecy surrounding this behavior makes obtaining good epidemiological data difficult.

In a study of 1000 women who admitted to self-induced vomiting, Fairburn categorized the 620 respondents as either anorectics (3%) or bulimics (83%). Most bulimics self-induced vomiting at least daily for an average duration of 4.5 years, and had a normal body weight; half had menstrual irregularities. Self-induced vomiting occurred more frequently than eating binges. Secrecy was characteristic; 39% maintained total secrecy and 47% said fewer than four people knew about their behavior. In fact, among women who reported having stopped the behavior, many did so only after their behavior had become known to others.[9]

NURSING ASSESSMENT

Patients who present with one or all of the symptoms of nausea, vomiting, and dehydration need a thorough assessment to determine not only the underlying cause but also the degree to which they are tolerating the symptoms, both physiologically and psychologically.

SUBJECTIVE DATA

When a patient reports nausea or vomiting, the initial focus is on these symptoms. Although it is less likely that a patient will report dehydration, the nurse should keep this problem in mind when obtaining the history.

The dimensions of symptoms that are a useful framework for eliciting data follow.

Quality and Intensity

How does the patient describe the sensation? It it constant or intermittent? Have the patient describe the emesis. Note color, presence of blood, bile. Certain characteristics of emesis may point to the etiology, such as a black color that may indicate bleeding, or a fecal odor that may indicate peritonitis.

Quantity

How much is the person vomiting? Is the person retching without any fluid or electrolyte losses? How often does it occur? If it is intermittent, how frequently does it occur during the day? How long does the sensation of nausea last? Does the person vomit once or several times with each episode?

Chronology

When did the vomiting or nausea first occur and how long has it been present? How long has the person been unable to take fluids? Does it occur before, during, or after meals?

Setting

Where is the patient when the symptom occurs and what is he doing? Does it occur when the person lies down after dinner, during the night, or in the morning?

Alleviating and Aggravating Factors

What, if anything, relieves the symptom and what makes it worse? Some patients report relief of nausea by vomiting; some patients find movement makes nausea worse.

Associated Symptoms

Has the patient noted other symptoms associated with nausea and vomiting, such as decreased urination, fever, sweating, diarrhea, dizziness, irregular pulse, abdominal pain, jaundice, or headache?

Table 15-2 outlines some possible conditions associated with various symptoms.

PAST HISTORY

Once data is obtained about the symptom, the nurse should obtain data about the patient's recent and past health. This may reveal the cause of the symptoms and can help to assess the degree of risk that the symptoms present to the patient. Nausea and vomiting in a healthy 20-year-old are less worrisome than in a 20-year-old person with insulin-dependent diabetes.

One can often elicit data about recent and past health by asking about systems such as kidney, stomach, and heart disease, or by asking about categories of disease such as

(Text continues on page 392)

TABLE 15–2
DIMENSIONS OF SYMPTOMS OF NAUSEA AND VOMITING

DIMENSION	SEEN IN
Quality	
Emesis has	
Mucus	
Small amount	Gastritis
Large amount	Gastric carcinoma
Hydrochloric acid	
Free	Gastric ulcer
Absent	Gastric malignancy
Odor	
Fecal	Peritonitis
	Lower intestinal obstruction
	Gastrocolic fistula
Penetrating	Hydrochloric acid in emesis
Bile	Prolonged vomiting
	Obstruction below the ampulla of Vater
Blood	Coagulation disturbance
	Esophageal varices
	Ulcer
	Bleeding in the esophagus, stomach, or duodenum
Regurgitation without emesis	Hiatal hernia
	Cancer of esophagus
Projectile vomiting	CNS lesion
Projectile vomiting without bile	Pyloric obstruction
Chronology	
Vomiting occurs	
Early morning	Alcoholic gastritis
	Medullablastoma
Morning	Uremia
	Hyperemesis gravidarum
Shortly after eating	Pylorospasm
	Anorexia/bulimia nervosa
	Gastritis
	Hiatal hernia
4–6 hr after eating	Pyloric obstruction
	Gastric retention due to diabetic gastric atony
After the onset of pain	Pancreatitis
Night	Reflux esophagitis
	Achalasia
Aggravating Factors	
Activity that increases intra-abdominal pressure (bending, lifting, stooping, coughing)	Reflux esophagitis
	Hiatal hernia

TABLE 15–2   (continued)
DIMENSIONS OF SYMPTOMS OF NAUSEA AND VOMITING

DIMENSION	*SEEN IN*
Aggravating Factors	
Diet	
Indiscretions	Achalasia
Rapid eating	Achalasia
Fatigue	Morning sickness
	Hyperemesis gravidarum
Pregnancy	Achalasia
Preparing a meal	Morning sickness
	Hyperemesis gravidarum
Stress	Achalasia
Upper respiratory infections	Achalasia
Alleviating Factors	
Nausea relieved by vomiting	Gastric ulcer
Associated Signs and Symptoms	
Fatigue	Biliary carcinoma
	Early cirrhosis
	Hepatitis
	Hepatic carcinoma
Fever	Crohn's disease
	Ulcerative colitis
Low-grade fever	Cholecystitis
	Acute pancreatitis
	Hepatic carcinoma
GI Symptoms	
Ascites	Cirrhosis
Constipation	Bowel obstruction
	Cirrhosis
	Hepatic carcinoma
Diarrhea	Crohn's disease
	Ulcerative colitis
	Cirrhosis
	Hepatic carcinoma
Dysphagia	Achalasia (tolerates fluids better than solids)
	Cancer esophagus (tolerates solids better than fluids)
Food intolerance	Cholecystitis
Foul breath	Cancer esophagus
Hiccups	Cancer esophagus
Pain	Achalasia
	Acute gastritis
	Peptic ulcer
	Cholecystitis
	Cholelithiasis
	Biliary cancer

(continued)

TABLE 15–2 (continued)
DIMENSIONS OF SYMPTOMS OF NAUSEA AND VOMITING

DIMENSION	SEEN IN
Associated Signs and Symptoms	
Pain	
	Acute pancreatitis
	Chronic pancreatitis
	Pancreatic cancer
	Hepatic cancer
	Crohn's disease
	Bowel obstruction
	Myocardial infarction
Skin conditions	
Jaundice	Biliary carcinoma
	Pancreatic carcinoma
	Hepatitis
	Cirrhosis
	Hepatic carcinoma
Bleeding skin and mucous membranes	Biliary carcinoma
Spider lesions	Cirrhosis
Ecchymosis	Hepatic carcinoma
Weight loss	Biliary carcinoma
	Cirrhosis (often masked by fluid retention)

childhood diseases, tumors, and infections. If the woman or young girl is postmenarche with a recent onset of nausea and vomiting, assess the date of her last menstrual period. If the vomiting is due to pregnancy, treatment alternatives are limited because of their potential teratogenic effects on the fetus.

A medication history from the patient may help to identify an underlying disease that is either causing the symptoms or that makes them cause for concern; also, the drugs themselves may cause the symptoms.

PSYCHOSOCIAL DATA

Psychological factors include the response to illness, coping strategies, and the values of the person. Explore the family relationships, including spouse, parent, child, siblings, and significant others. Identify the supports available to the person. Older persons who live alone may be at a higher risk to develop problems when they are weakened by an episode of nausea and vomiting. Consider the role of environmental factors in the onset of the symptoms. A hospitalized patient may share a room with a patient with a tracheostomy, a colostomy, or a patient with a loose, productive cough who leaves his sputum in plain sight. Although the sights, sounds, and odors are usual for personnel, they can cause a patient some discomfort, including nausea and vomiting.

Identify the age of the person, because very young children and very old adults are more prone to develop dehydration.

OBJECTIVE DATA

The subjective data guide the nurse in determining the necessary depth of the physical examination.

Consideration of the person's general appearance provides an overall view of the physical condition and the psychological state. Is the person alert, or dull and listless? Is the person well nourished or cachectic? Does the person appear calm or jittery? Is the person well-groomed or slovenly? For example, several days growth of beard on a man may indicate that he has been too weak to shave.

Obtain vital signs on all persons; this includes blood pressure, heart and respiratory rate, and temperature. Other basic data are weight pattern, especially recent changes, and intake and output. When there is an index of suspicion that hypovolemia is present, assess for signs of dehydration, metabolic alkalosis, and acidosis. The dehydrated patient may have signs and symptoms of thirst, dryness of tongue, oliguria, a high urine specific gravity, decreased tissue turgor, elevated BUN, tachycardia, fever, mental confusion, and sunken eyeballs. Signs and symptoms may be related to the degree of dehydration (Table 15-3). The examination also should include assessment of the abdomen, skin, hair, head, motor, and neurologic states. Increased intracranial pressure (IIP) may be present in a patient who is vomiting; therefore, signs of IIP should be kept in mind during the physical examination. Table 15-4 lists physical examination findings and conditions in which they are seen.

LABORATORY DATA

When laboratory data are available, they can be checked to determine whether abnormalities indicate causes or results of nausea and vomiting. Biochemistry values such as serum glucose and electrolytes (Table 15-1); hematological values such as hemoglobin, hemotocrit and white blood cell count; and coagulation values, such as clotting and prothrombin time, may be informative. Drug levels may indicate toxicity as a cause of the symptoms.

NURSING DIAGNOSIS

Once the data base is completed, there are two important questions for the nurse to consider:

1. Are the symptoms self-limiting or do they present a problem for the patient?
2. How likely is it that the symptoms represent an underlying condition that needs medical diagnosis and treatment?

Both questions are important as they will aid in a decision regarding medical referral. In the first case, a patient may not be concerned about vomiting because he has vomited in the past; however, if the patient is a recently diagnosed insulin-dependent diabetic, the nurse realizes that symptoms have serious implications for the patient. Another patient may develop these symptoms when he has stage fright and may be incapacitated by them; although the nurse appreciates that they are self-limiting and that the person is unlikely to become dehydrated, she recognizes their significance in that they may be affecting the person's career and livelihood and that a solution or cure of the problem is important to the person. In the second case, regardless of the nature of the nausea and vomiting, self-limiting or incapacitating, a patient with an underlying disorder needs to have an evaluation, not just symptomatic treatment.

(*Text continues on page 396*)

TABLE 15–3

SYMPTOMS RELATING TO PERCENT LOSS OF TOTAL BODY FLUID

LOSS OF TOTAL BODY FLUID (%)	SYMPTOM OR CLINICAL MANIFESTATIONS	REFERENCE
1%	Thirst	Bell et al, 1976 and Pflaum, 1979
1%–2%	Thirst	Kleeman and Fichman, 1967
2%–4%	Thirst	Shoemaker and Walker, 1970
Mild–moderate dehydration	Dryness of tongue	
	Scanty or decreased urine output	
	High urine specific gravity	
2.5%–5.0% Due to diarrhea	Skin turgor time of 0.5 sec	Kleeman and Fichman, 1967
3-liter fluid loss in patients weighing 50–130 kg (110–286 lb) (2%–6%)	Furrowed tongue Decreased turgidity of skin Increased thirst Elevated BUN	Lapides et al, 1965
5%–8%	Fatigue Increased pulse Elevated temperature Deterioration of mental processes	Pflaum, 1979
5%–8% Due to diarrhea	Skin turgor time of 1.0–2.5 sec	Kleeman and Fichman, 1935
6% *Serious dehydration*	Elevated BUN Blood concentrated Protein, casts, and erythrocytes excreted in the urine	Coller and Maddock, 1935
6%–10%	Skin turgor time of 0.5–1.0 sec	Kleeman and Fichman, 1967
8%–10% *Severe dehydration*	Loss of skin turgor Sunken eyeballs Profound depression Anuria	Shoemaker and Walker, 1970
10%	10% increase in hematocrit	Lindeman and Papper, 1975
11%–15%	Delirium Deafness Kidney failure	Pflaum, 1979
10%–20%	Death	Bell et al, 1976

(From Carpenter LC: Hydration and symptom distress during cancer chemotherapy. Master's thesis, unpublished, University of Michigan, 1983)

TABLE 15–4
ASSESSMENT AND CLINICAL FINDINGS IN THE PATIENT WHO IS VOMITING

AREA	ASSESS FOR	SEEN IN
Vital Signs		
Heart rate	Tachycardia	Infection
		Hypovolemia
		Heart failure
		Hyponatremia
	Bradycardia	IIP
	Other arrhythmias	Metabolic alkalosis
		Hypokalemia
Blood pressure	Hypotension	Hypovolemia; adrenal insufficiency
	Hypertension	IIP
	Widening pulse pressure	IIP
Respirations	Increased rate and depth (Kussmaul's sign)	Metabolic acidosis
	Shallow, slow (apnea)	Metabolic alkalosis
	Change in pattern	IIP
Fever		Infections
		IIP
Weight	Gain	Heart failure
		Pregnancy
	Loss	Dehydration
		Anorexia nervosa
Intake and output	Oliguria	Dehydration
		Hyponatremia
	Polyuria	Diabetes
	Decreased specific gravity	Hyponatremia
Abdomen	Distention	Dehydration
		Pregnancy
		Gastric dilatation in metabolic acidosis
		Bowel obstruction
	Rebound tenderness	Appendicitis
		Pancreatitis
		Peritonitis
		Cholecystitis
	Fluid wave of ascites	Cirrhosis
		Right ventricular failure
	Tumors or masses	Hepatic or gastric tumors
	Hyperactive bowel sounds	Crohn's disease
	Upper abdominal tenderness without muscle rigidity	Pancreatitis
	Hypoactive bowel sounds	Obstruction of the small bowel

(continued)

TABLE 15–4 (continued)
ASSESSMENT AND CLINICAL FINDINGS IN THE PATIENT WHO IS VOMITING

AREA	ASSESS FOR	SEEN IN
Integument		
Skin	Jaundice	Hepatitis
		Obstruction of the liver
	Pigmentation	Adrenal insufficiency
	Decreased turgor	Fluid volume depletion
	Dry skin and mucous membranes	Fluid volume depletion
	Flushed	Metabolic acidosis
	Fingerprinting on sternum	Hyponatremia
Hair distribution	Alopecia	Decreased nutritional intake (anorexia nervosa, cancer)
Head and neck	Bulging ear drums	Otitis media
	Stiff neck	Meningitis
	Jugular venous filling	
	Decreased	Hypovolemia
	Increased	Heart failure
Motor/Neurologic	Muscle weakness	Hypokalemia
	Hyporeflexia	Hypokalemia
	Muscle twitching/seizures	Hyponatremia
	Nystagmus	Meniere's syndrome
	Hearing loss	Meniere's syndrome
	Sluggish pupil reaction	Trauma
	Pupillary dilatation	IIP
	Papilledema	IIP
	Staggering gait	IIP
	Hemiparesis, hemiplegia	IIP
	Anxious, agitated, fatigued	Dehydration
	Cerebral disturbances	Metabolic alkalosis
	Coma	
	Delirium	
	Restlessness, coma	Metabolic acidosis

When the symptoms are of short duration, less than 1 week since onset, and the patient is without symptoms of fluid depletion or pathogenic conditions, the nurse may manage the patient symptomatically, keeping in mind situations that necessitate physician referral. Examples of such patients are those who have the flu, gastroenteritis, or those who are pregnant. There is no easy formula to determine when to refer a patient to a physician versus when to observe him and provide nursing measures. Generally, because of the numerous and various etiologies of these symptoms, medical referral or consultation is indicated in most cases of nausea and vomiting, since early treatment can prevent the occurrence of serious fluid and electrolyte problems.[37]

Several diagnoses taken from the National Conference Group for Classification of

Nursing Diagnosis can be used to describe the needs or problems of patients who have nausea and vomiting:[21]

Fluid volume deficit, potential
Fluid volume deficit, actual
Nutrition, alteration in: Less than body requirements
Nutritional deficit (specify)

Fluid Volume Deficit, Potential

The patient who is nauseated and vomiting is losing fluid and may be limiting oral intake. However, the regulatory mechanisms described in the section of dehydration are usually quite effective in adjusting to fluid losses. Thus in many cases, rather than being actually fluid depleted, the patient is at risk for fluid volume deficit. Factors that increase the risk of fluid volume deficit must be considered in caring for patients with these symptoms:

Extremes of age: The very old and the very young are more prone to dehydration.
Body temperature: Metabolic needs increase with fever.
Resources available for fluid intake: An infant is dependent on others for fluid access and intake.
The patient's knowledge that he is at risk for fluid depletion.
The use of medication that may accelerate dehydration (e.g., diuretics).

Fluid Volume Deficit, Actual

The diagnosis of *actual fluid volume deficit* is defined as decreased circulatory volume due to active loss of body fluid. When this occurs, the nurse refers the patient for medical evaluation.

The defining characteristics of this diagnosis include the following:

Decreased urinary output
Concentrated urine
Output greater than intake
Sudden weight loss
Decreased venous filling
Hemoconcentration
Decreased serum sodium

Hypotension, thirst, increased pulse, decreased skin turgor, decreased pulse volume/pressure, a change in mental state, increased body temperature, and weakness also may be present.

The nurse, having collected subjective and objective data in assessing the patient, can validate the diagnosis by reviewing the defining characteristics.

Alteration In Nutrition: Less Than Body Requirements or Nutritional Deficit

The diagnosis of *alteration in nutrition* is defined as insufficient intake of nutrients to meet metabolic needs. The defining characteristics include:

Loss of weight, with adequate food intake
20% or more under ideal body weight
Aversion to eating
Satiety immediately after ingesting food
Reported inadequate food intake, less than minimum daily requirements
Diarrhea or steatorrhea
Pale conjunctiva and mucous membranes
Excessive loss of hair
Lack of information, misconception about minimal daily requirements

The etiology of this problem can stem from a knowledge deficit, anorexia, an emotional disturbance, or the inability to ingest or digest food or absorb nutrients due to biological, psychological, or economic factors.

Other Considerations

The nurse must consider the degree to which the symptoms are causing the patient discomfort and anxiety. In the case of the patient who is receiving cancer chemotherapy, the mechanism to replace fluid and electrolytes may be in place and the cause of the symptoms may be known; however, the symptoms may be intolerable to the patient. The nurse must address such needs in her plan of care.

Among other considerations are harm to patients aside from potential and actual fluid depletion. Postoperative vomiting may be self-limiting, but following certain ophthalmology procedures, no vomiting or retching is desired since the actual act of vomiting may increase pressure and traumatize the eye. Similarly, in other types of surgeries, the act of vomiting, more than the effects of vomiting, places the patient at risk for strain on the operative area, with resultant bleeding and wound dehiscence or evisceration. In such cases, even if the patient feels he can tolerate the discomfort, and even if fluid depletion is unlikely, the nurse needs to notify the physician.

MANAGEMENT

Though diagnosis and treatment of the underlying causes of nausea and vomiting are important, relief of the discomfort and prevention and treatment of serious fluid and electrolyte disorders are immediate goals.

Management of symptoms includes medication therapy, fluid replacement and dietary modification, environmental and comfort measures to alter stimuli, and psychological support. In many cases, the symptoms are self-limiting and the patient manages them independently.

MEDICATION THERAPY

Medication has been the major focus of therapy in reduction or alleviating nausea and vomiting. One stimulus to understand the physiology of nausea and vomiting has been

the need for the development of effective antiemetic therapy. As described earlier, not all emetic agents cause vomiting by the same mechanism. Some cause vomiting through the stimulation of the CTZ; others stimulate afferent impulses that activate the VC and cause vomiting. It is believed that in some situations, the VC is stimulated by more than one pathway. It may be that in an infectious gastrointestinal disease, afferent impulses from the gastrointestinal tract stimulate the VC to induce nausea and vomiting, and the toxins released into the bloodstream reach the CTZ, which triggers the VC to induce vomiting. Antiemetic medications have specific mechanisms of action; some drugs may be effective agents to relieve symptoms resulting from CTZ stimulation but may be ineffective in relieving the symptoms when they result from peripheral stimulation of the VC. The present view regarding antiemetic medications is that the type of medication should be matched to the causative agent.[41]

Several categories of drugs have been used as antiemetic therapy. These include antihistamines, anticholinergics, butyrophenones, phenothiazines, and corticosteroids.[35,41]

Antihistamines

Antihistamines may work directly on or near the VC. Conditions in which these drugs have been effective are motion sickness; Meniere's syndrome; myocardial infarction; or mucosal irritation of the gastrointestinal tract due to viral or bacterial infections, or following the ingestion of irritants; viral hepatitis and mechanical dilation of the gastrointestinal tract. These agents are not effective in alleviating nausea and vomiting related to cancer chemotherapy. Side-effects include sedation and anticholinergic effects. The sedative effect may be helpful in the bedridden patient but may be worrisome in the ambulatory patient engaging in activities that require mental alertness. Examples of these drugs are meclizine (Antivert), diphenhydramine (Benadryl), hydroxyzine (Atarax), dimenhydrinate (Dramamine), doxylamine with pyridoxine (Bendectin), and trimethobenzamide (Tigan).[35]

Dopamine Antagonists

Phenothiazines are believed to work at or near the CTZ, blocking a portion of the zone. The phenothiazines have been effective in alleviating nausea and vomiting associated with drugs (antibiotics, cytotoxic agents, alcohol, ergots, opiates, and the inhalation anesthetics), diabetic acidosis, and radiation sickness. The phenothiazines have been described as the only class of drugs that have shown efficacy and safety in large numbers of cancer patients. Unfortunately, certain cytotoxic drugs are strongly emetic agents, and phenothiazines have not been effective in treating the associated nausea and vomiting.

Side-effects reported include sedation, hypotension and orthostatic hypotension, and extrapyramidal symptoms that are more severe in the aged and in small children.

Examples of phenothiazines used as antiemetic agents are chlorpromazine (Thorazine), prochlorperazine (Compazine), perphenazine (Trilafon), and trifluoperazine (Stelazine).

Butyrophenones Like phenothiazines, butyrophenones are dopamine antagonists, potent inhibitors of the CTZ. In uncontrolled trials, they have been shown to be effective in combating nausea and vomiting associated with potent emetic agents such as cisplatin, doxorubicin, and mechlorethamine. They have minimal effects on the respiratory and cardiovascular systems. Side-effects reported are sedation, and agitation and restlessness. Extrapyramidal symptoms occur less frequently with butyrophenones than with phenothiazines.

Examples of butyrophenones are haloperidol (Haldol) and droperidol.

Metoclopramide Metoclopramide, a procainamide derivative, is being used with cancer patients. It accelerates gastric emptying and inhibits gastric relaxation, an initial step in the vomiting act. It has both central and peripheral actions. In adults, 10% have CNS effects such as sedation; dizziness and faintness are less common, and extrapyramidal effects are infrequent. In children, the CNS toxicities are more common and may be exacerbated when phenothiazines are used concomitantly.

Miscellaneous

Corticosteroids Corticosteroids such as dexamethasone and methylprednisone relieve the nausea and vomiting associated with potent emetic agents. Corticosteroids exert an antiemetic effect through inhibition of prostaglandin synthesis. One drawback to their use is the concern that these agents may stimulate tumor growth. However, some experts believe that a few boluses of steroids with chemotherapy are unlikely to cause such effects. Toxicities have been transient and not life-threatening.

Other Agents Agents including cannabinoids, tetrahydrocannabinol (THC), and nabalone, recently have received widespread attention from the media for the relief of nausea and vomiting associated with cancer chemotherapy. Most studies report that THC is effective in relieving symptoms associated with the potent emetic agents.[26] Younger patients appear to fare better with these agents than do older patients, especially those who have never taken them before. While less than 2% of younger patients have to withdraw from the drug because of toxicities, such as severe dysphorias, hallucinations, or syncope, up to 35% of older patients experience these toxicities.

FLUID REPLACEMENTS AND DIETARY MODIFICATIONS

If the patient is able to tolerate oral fluids, these can be given. However, oral fluids may stimulate further vomiting; when this occurs, not only does the patient lose the fluid taken in, but also gastric juices rich in electrolytes, which makes the fluid and electrolyte problems more severe. To prevent this, initially fluids should be given in small amounts.

Dietary modifications are helpful in the management of nausea and vomiting. If the patient can tolerate them, small amounts of fluids with dry carbohydrates can be given; spicy and greasy foods are usually withheld. Patients with nausea can often tolerate dry carbohydrates. Small sips of fluid can be tried about 2 hours following the last episode of vomiting. The diet is advanced according to the person's tolerance. Scogna found that dietary modifications were not particularly effective in reducing nausea and vomiting associated with cancer chemotherapy.[34] Radiation therapy patients, however, seemed to do better when they ate a substantial meal before the treatment, and then limited themselves to light meals for the remainder of the day.[38] Given noted that patients seem to tolerate the foods that they crave. She also described "sick foods," foods that patients associate with illness, and she suggested that these foods may trigger symptoms in some patients.[12] Small feedings are advocated to relieve the nausea and vomiting associated with heart failure and morning sickness. In the latter case, dry carbohydrates (e.g., crackers) are specifically advised.

When parenteral fluid and electrolyte replacement is necessary, the physician prescribes fluids and additives, based on the patient's laboratory data, the previous fluid and electrolyte losses, and volume of losses that are anticipated over the next 24 hours.

ENVIRONMENTAL AND COMFORT MEASURES

Minimize stimuli that can influence the occurrence of nausea and vomiting. Mouth care and oral hygiene can remove noxious tastes. Because water is odorless and tasteless, it may be preferable to mouthwash. Patients may not wish to brush their teeth, remove their dentures, or gargle, as this may gag them and exacerbate symptoms.

A clean environment is optimal. Airing the room can be helpful, because odors, even ones usually considered pleasant, can be offensive to the patient. Removing emesis promptly from the area is important; a clean emesis basin should be within reach although not necessarily within sight to avoid its becoming a cue to vomiting. The sight of a gastric tube exiting a patient's nose or the smell of certain foods (e.g., spaghetti) may trigger symptoms. Although nurses are accustomed to the sights, smells, and sounds of the hospital, many patients are not. Consider the total environment when trying to eliminate noxious stimuli. In some cases, another room arrangement may be necessary.

Rest and reduction of activity may alleviate symptoms, particularly in patients who find that motion increases the severity of nausea.

Because the pregnant woman is limited in treatment choices, it is important to counsel her and significant others regarding symptom relief. As food preparation and fatigue are known to trigger symptoms, the use of ready prepared foods and the shifting of household responsibilities may be needed to alleviate the symptoms.

PSYCHOLOGICAL SUPPORT

Staying with the patient during a period of nausea and vomiting is not only a safety measure, but also provides support and comfort. A positive attitude on the part of the clinician is advocated by some to alleviate the symptoms.[33] In contrast, in Welch's study of radiation therapy patients, it was found that such an approach was not favored by patients, who preferred acknowledgment and concern for their symptoms.[39] Scogna found that although cancer patients valued support when they had their symptoms, only 12% of patients reported receiving it from the staff; 62% derived support from their family members.[34]

To provide support, determine first what the patient's needs are and then meet these needs. Not only is no one therapy 100% effective in alleviating nausea and vomiting in every patient, but the efficacy of many of the nursing measures, such as alteration of environment, diet, and activity, is determined by the nature of the patient's response to them. The nurse assists the patient in controlling or regulating these factors, and is guided by the patient's response.

Support groups for persons with BN may be helpful. Women's groups have been effective with some persons, by raising their consciousness about the role of women and the risks of self-destructive behavior. Information about resources and support groups may be obtained by writing to these groups:

National Anorexic Aid Society
P.O. Box 229461
Columbus, Ohio 43229

or

American Anorexia Nervosa Association
133 Cedar Lane
Teaneck, New Jersey 07666

The management of nausea and vomiting has long been a concern of nurses. In a significant clinical research study done in the early 1960s, Dumas and Leonard demonstrated that nursing interventions could reduce the incidence of postoperative vomiting.[8] Dumas noted that others had observed that anxious patients seemed to vomit no matter what treatment they received postoperatively, whereas calmer patients in the same situation vomited less frequently. While acknowledging the chemical and physiological factors related to postoperative vomiting, Dumas focused on psychological factors, preparing patients preoperatively for the stressful experience of surgery. Before surgery, she met with patients, talking with them to determine whether they were anxious, and if so, the nature of their anxiety. Lastly, she asked what might be done to relieve their stress. This interaction, plus usual preoperative care, was the experimental treatment; usual preoperative care alone was the control treatment. After surgery, the incidence of vomiting was 50% in the control group; but only 10% of the experimental group vomited. The conclusion reached was that relief of preoperative distress reduced the incidence of postoperative vomiting.[7]

Dumas demonstrated that helping patients to explore the underlying causes of anxiety could alleviate postoperative vomiting. The role of anxiety in cancer chemotherapy is also being explored, since it is known that some patients vomit in anticipation of the administration of chemotherapy.[5] It may be that a deliberative nursing intervention to reduce anxiety may decrease the incidence of vomiting in these patients as well.

PATIENT EDUCATION

Because nausea and vomiting occur in such varied circumstances, it can be difficult for patients to determine when they ought to be concerned about them. Patients need to know what the potential effects are, what situations need further evaluation, and what they can do to minimize problems associated with the symptoms.

Medications taken for relief of nausea and vomiting often have sedation as a side-effect. Patients must be cautioned about the use of both prescribed and over-the-counter (OTC) antiemetics so that they take them safely.

Patient education may help persons with BN. Although education alone will not eliminate the behavior, many bulimics do not appreciate that self-induced vomiting can be harmful. Knowledge of the possible consequences of such behavior is essential. Self-help groups mentioned earlier provide educational materials and resources on this topic.

IMPLICATIONS FOR RESEARCH

Many of the nursing measures advocated for the relief or amelioration of nausea and vomiting are based on experience. For example, patients who report nausea are encouraged to take slow, deep breaths. One wonders whether this is done as a patient distractor or whether changes in intra-abdominal pressure may alter VC stimulation and actually block vomiting. Research is needed to identify effective psychosocial measures to help control nausea and vomiting and to determine nursing interventions to reduce stress and anxiety, which aggravate the symptoms. Research also is needed to determine whether psychosocial interventions potentiate the effectiveness of medication therapy.

SUMMARY

The symptoms of nausea and vomiting and the potential for dehydration are seen in patients with acute and chronic illness as well as in otherwise healthy people. The effects vary from slight discomfort to severe fluid and electrolyte disturbances. Nurses caring for persons with symptoms need to be cognizant of the problems that may develop when these symptoms persist or when the underlying causes of these symptoms are not explored. Ongoing assessment is one of the most important measures the nurse can provide the patient, especially when it facilitates prevention of further problems. Additionally, support for safety and comfort to minimize or relieve symptoms is valuable.

REFERENCES

1. Ahmed SS, Gupta RC, Brancato RR: Significance of nausea and vomiting during acute myocardial infarction. Am Heart J 95, No. 5:671–672, 1978
2. Biggs JSC: Vomiting in pregnancy: Causes and management. Drugs 9, No. 4:299–306, 1975
3. Bondy PD, Rosenberg LE: Metabolic Control and Disease, 8th ed. Philadelphia, WB Saunders, 1980
4. Borison HC, Wang SC: Physiology and pharmacology of vomiting. Pharmacol Rev 5:193–234, 1953
5. Chang JC: Nausea and vomiting in cancer patients: An expression of psychological mechanisms? Psych 22, No. 8: 707–709, 1981
6. Drydock for a Used Spaceship. Time Nov 29: 81, 1982
7. Dumas, RG: Psychological preparation for surgery. Am J Nurs 63, No. 8:52–55, 1963
8. Dumas RG, Leonard RC: The effect of nursing on the incidence of postoperative vomiting. Nurs Res 12, No. 1:12–15, 1953
9. Fairburn CG, Cooper PJ: Self-induced vomiting and bulimia nervosa: An undetected problem. Br Med J 284:1153–1155, 1982
10. Ganong WF: Review of Medical Physiology, 10th ed. Los Altos, CA, Lange Med Publishing, 1981
11. Gibbs D: Diseases of the alimentary system: Nausea and vomiting. Br Med J 2:1489–1492, 1976
12. Given BA, Simons SG: Gastroenterology in Clinical Nursing, 3rd ed. St. Louis, CV Mosby, 1979
13. Guyton AC: Textbook of Medical Physiology, 6th ed. Philadelphia, WB Saunders, 1981
14. Hawkins RC, Clement PF: Development and con-

struct validation of a self-report increase of binge-eating tendencies. Addict Behav 5, No. 3:219–226, 1980

15. Hightower JR, Janowitz HD: In Brobeck JR (ed): Best and Taylor's Physiological Basis of Medical Practice, 10th ed. Baltimore, Williams & Wilkins, 1979

16. Huff PS: Safety of drug therapy for nausea and vomiting of pregnancy. J Fam Pract 11, No. 6:969–970, 1980

17. Hurst JW, et al: The Heart Arteries and Veins, 4th ed. New York, McGraw–Hill, 1978

18. Ingelfinger FJ, Moss, RE: The activity of the descending duodenum during nausea. Am J Physiol 136:561–566, 1942

19. Isselbacher KJ: In Isselbacher KJ, Adams RD, Braunwald E et al (eds): Harrison's Principles of Internal Medicine, 9th ed. New York, McGraw–Hill, 1980

20. Katz JL, Sitnick T: Anorexia nervosa and bulimia. Arch Gen Psychiatry 39, No. 4:487–489, 1982

21. Kim MJ, Moritz DA (eds): Classification of Nursing Diagnosis: Proceedings of the Third and Fourth National Conferences. New York, McGraw–Hill, 1982

22. Kinney MR et al (eds): AACN's Clinical Reference to Critical Care Nursing. New York, McGraw–Hill, 1981

23. Lucas AR: Bulimia and vomiting syndrome. NY State J Med, 82, No. 3:390–399, 1982

24. Lucas AR: Pigging out? JAMA 247, No. 1:82, 1982

25. Lumsden K, Holden WS: The act of vomiting in man. Gut 10:173–179, 1969

26. Meyer M: Physiology and treatment of chemotherapy-induced nausea and vomiting. The Michigan Drug Letter 1, No. 6:1982

27. Minuchin S, Rosman BL, Baker L: Psychosomatic Families Anorexia Nervosa in Context. Cambridge, MA, Harvard University Press, 1978

28. Plum R, Posner JF: The Diagnosis of Stupor and Coma, 3rd ed. Philadelphia, FA Davis, 1980

29. Price SA, Wilson LB: Pathophysiology, Clinical Concepts of Disease Processes, 2nd ed. New York, McGraw–Hill, 1982

30. Pyle RL, Mitchell JE, Eckert ED: Bulimia: A report of 34 cases. J Clin Psych 42, No. 2:60–64, 1981

31. Rosenthal FD, Jones C, Lewis S: Thyrotoxic vomiting. Br Med J 2:209–211, 1976

32. Schrier RW: Renal and Electrolyte Disorders, 2nd ed. Boston, Little, Brown & Co, 1980

33. Schrier AM, Lavenia J: Nutritional management of radiation therapy patients. Nurs Clin North Am 12, No. 1:173–182, 1977

34. Scogna DM, Smalley RV: Chemotherapy-induced nausea and vomiting. Am J Nurs 79, No. 9:1562–1564, 1979

35. Seigel LJ, Longo DL: The control of chemotherapy-induced emesis. Ann Intern Med 95:352–359, 1981

36. Vander AJ, Sherman JH, Luciano DS: Human Physiology, 2nd ed. New York, McGraw–Hill, 1975

37. Vander AJ: Renal Physiology, 2nd ed. New York, McGraw–Hill, 1980

38. Vick NA: Grinker's Neurology, 7th ed. Springfield, IL, Charles C Thomas, 1976

39. Welch DA: Assessment of nausea and vomiting in cancer patients undergoing external beam radiotherapy. Can Nurs 3, No. 5:365, 1980

40. Whitehead VM: Cancer treatment needs better antiemetics. N Engl J Med 293:199–200, 1975

41. Wyman JB, Wick MR: The vomiting patient. Am Fam Physician 21, No. 2:139–143, 1980

16

Urinary Incontinence

Susan De Rosa

Urinary incontinence is an embarrassing and frustrating problem for the patient, the family, and the nurse. It has an impact on the person's social, emotional, and physical well-being and self-concept. This chapter is concerned with urinary incontinence in the adult and its prevention, assessment, and management.

Although incontinence is not limited to a specific age group, it is most common in the adult population. There is a general tendency for the prevalence and severity of incontinence to increase with age. Overall, more women than men have a problem with incontinence and the majority of them are living in the community.[20]

For many reasons, accurate statistics on the incidence of urinary incontinence are difficult to obtain. First, little research has been done on this problem. Second, the silence of those who suffer with urinary incontinence has hindered progress in research and management. Many do not seek help because they perceive incontinence as an inevitable aspect of aging or a problem that can not be reversed. They are embarrassed about losing control of a body function and are therefore reluctant to talk about it. Third, urinary incontinence has always been a frustrating and time-consuming problem for nurses. The focus of nursing care has been on preventing or minimizing the sequelae of incontinence rather than assessing and managing the problem. Nursing education has suggested methods of good skin care, padding of furniture and patient, and toileting procedures. This information has certainly helped to alleviate some of the social and physical side-effects, but it has not alleviated the problem. Finally, the number of people who have a problem with urinary incontinence has been difficult to determine because there has been a lack of agreement in its definition. The complexity of determining the cause of incontinence has also been a deterrent in both definition and diagnosis.

INCONTINENCE DEFINED

It is generally accepted that urinary incontinence is a symptom rather than a disease. *Incontinence* has commonly been described as a situation in which urine is passed at an inappropriate time and in an inappropriate place. Hald's definition clearly identifies the physical and social ramifications of incontinence: "Urinary incontinence is a condition characterized by involuntary escape of urine from the lower urinary tract in a degree that imposes a social or hygienically unacceptable situation upon the individual."[9]

IMPACT OF INCONTINENCE

Urinary incontinence evokes a variety of emotions and responses in people. The loss of urine at the wrong time and in the wrong place can be devastating to the person's self-esteem and body image. Embarrassment is common and incontinence may dramatically change a person's behavior and life-style. Most people tend to deal with the problem by wearing some type of protective padding made of cloth or paper. This method is ineffective, though, because the odor, the discomfort of dampness, and irritation to the skin still remain. Some people exhibit an almost obsessive need to be clean. Many avoid certain social situations or travel opportunities, fearing that their problem will be discovered by others.

The family of the incontinent person may react in a variety of ways. The precautionary methods they take to avoid soiling of their furniture, for example, may be perceived by the incontinent person as insulting or as a method of dealing with a seemingly unsolvable problem. The family may exclude the incontinent person from some social events if toilet facilities are not convenient, or the family may be always watchful and questioning to avoid "accidents."

Open communication of the problem is necessary to avoid misinterpretation. Wells and Brink have stated that the common phrases, "the roof is leaking" and "I spilled some of my water," are comments that may be made by the incontinent person and suggest a lack of directness.[16] Nurses have a similar problem with confronting the problem directly. "You seem to be having problems with your plumbing," they may say, hoping to make light of the real issue. People do not feel comfortable talking about matters dealing with excretion, and therefore attempt to keep the problem to themselves as long as possible. The hesitation to discuss incontinence is a problem for both the patient and the nurse.

MECHANISMS OF URINARY INCONTINENCE

NORMAL ANATOMY AND PHYSIOLOGY OF THE LOWER URINARY TRACT

The lower urinary tract consists of the bladder and the urethra (see Fig. 16-1). The bladder acts as a reservoir and is normally able to accommodate 350 ml to 400 ml of fluid. It consists of the trigone area and the detrusor muscle. The *trigone area* is at the base of the bladder. Through this area the ureters and the urethra open. The *detrusor muscle* is the smooth muscle of the bladder wall. The urethra, or bladder outlet, a narrow tube through which the urine exits, consists of an internal and an external sphincter, both of which normally are contracted. The intravesical (bladder) pressure is low and does not increase greatly until the bladder contains more than 150 ml of urine. The function of the bladder outlet is to maintain a pressure that is higher than the intravesical pressure, which helps to maintain continence.

Bladder and urethral function is controlled by the parasympathetic pathways at

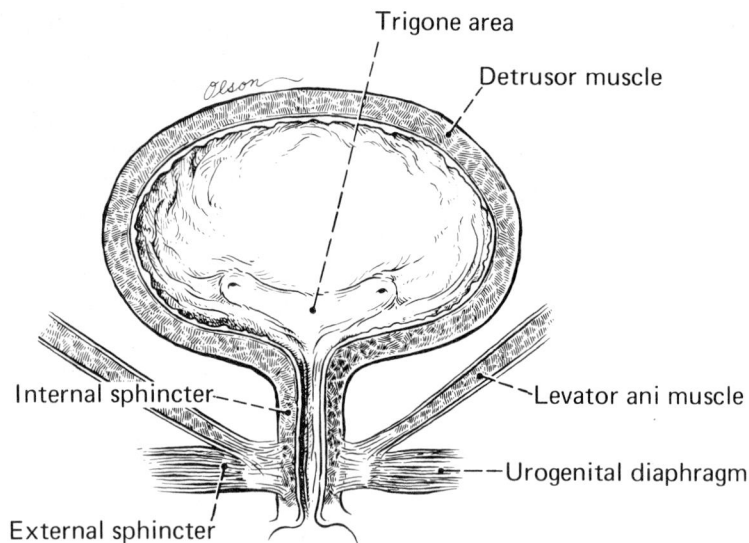

FIG. 16-1   *The urinary bladder.*

the level of S_2, S_3, and S_4.[12] The frequency of the impulses from the bladder wall to the spinal cord are related to the degree to which the detrusor muscle is passively stretched by the urine within the bladder.[12]

THE MICTURITION PROCESS

Normal expulsion of urine from the bladder is under both voluntary and involuntary control. The micturition process involves signals being sent through the parasympathetic nervous system to the reflex center located at S_2, S_3, and S_4, and up to the cerebral cortex. Centers that facilitate and inhibit micturition are located in both the brain stem and the cerebral cortex. Those in the cerebral cortex are primarily inhibitory in nature.

When the bladder fills to approximately 150 ml to 200 ml, the intravesical pressure suddenly increases and the urge to void becomes conscious. The stretching of the bladder wall causes afferent impulses to be sent by way of the parasympathetic nerves to the spinal cord, which initiates the spinal reflex.

The spinal reflex causes contraction of the detrusor muscle and relaxation of the internal sphincter. The relaxation of the external sphincter is controlled by the higher centers in the cerebral cortex. The spinal reflex can be inhibited voluntarily for a limited amount of time, which permits voiding to occur at an acceptable time and place. However, the urge to void will occur more frequently and be more intense. When conditions are satisfactory, the external sphincter is consciously relaxed, the bladder contracts, urine is released, and the intravesical pressure returns to normal.

POSSIBLE CAUSES OF URINARY INCONTINENCE

There is no universal agreement on the classification of the causes of incontinence. Table 16-1 presents several different classification systems discussed in the research literature.

The complexity of determining the etiology of incontinence cannot be overstated. Physiological and psychological factors are

TABLE 16-1
CLASSIFICATIONS OF INCONTINENCE

Researcher	Categories	Types of Classifications
Hald (1975)	Neurogenic, psychological, gynecological, overflow, congenital	Eclectic
Brocklehurst (1976)	Disorders of pelvic diaphragm, urethra and bladder outlet, bladder, neurologic control of micturition	Anatomic
Bates et al (1976)	Stress, urge, reflex, and overflow incontinence	Physiological
Resnick and Rowe (1982)	Temporary or fixed incontinence	Eclectic
Other	Severity: Number of incontinent episodes per day or amount of urine passed during an incontinent episode	Graded

not mutually exclusive, nor can the influence of medications and environment be ignored. Once identified, most underlying causes of urinary incontinence can be eliminated and the problem resolved. The physical causes, psychological factors, factors related to medications, and environmental factors will be considered separately within this section.

Physical Causes

Physiologically, urinary incontinence in the adult can be caused by impairment of neurologic control causing a neurogenic bladder, dysfunction of the bladder or of the urethra, fecal impaction or prostatic enlargement, alteration of the pelvic diaphragm, or metabolic abnormalities.

Impairment of Neurologic Control Impairment of the nerve pathway to the bladder causes various types of a neurogenic bladder. Brocklehurst classifies the neurogenic bladder into four groups: the autonomous, the reflex, the atonic, and the uninhibited; the latter two are the most common. The level at which the central nervous system (CNS) is disrupted determines the par-

ticular type of neurogenic bladder (Fig. 16-2).[6]

"The autonomous neurogenic bladder occurs when the bladder centre in the sacral cord is destroyed and the bladder is completely decentralized."[6] The person with an *autonomous* neurogenic bladder will be incontinent because he feels no conscious sensation to void, and there is irregular reflex activity. The irregular reflex activity is because of the loss of the micturition reflex. Damage to the lower portion of the spinal cord due to trauma or congenital abnormalities may cause this problem.

A *reflex* neurogenic bladder occurs when the person suffers damage to the spinal cord between the cortical and the sacral bladder centers. The person becomes incontinent because he feels no sensation of bladder distention and loses the ability to inhibit reflex contraction. Some paraplegics who have this problem are able to stimulate bladder contractions by using manual techniques within the second, third, and fourth sacral dermatomes.[6]

The *atonic* neurogenic bladder caused by damage to the posterior nerve roots leads

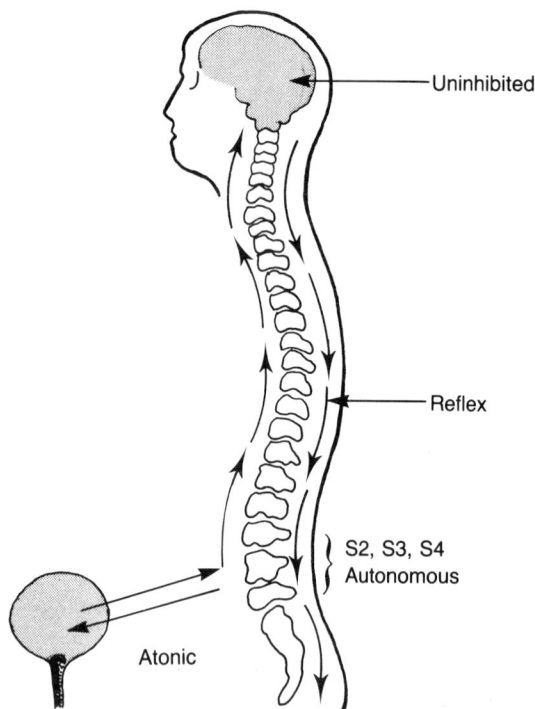

FIG. 16-2 *Physiological centers of urine control and types of neurogenic bladder.*

to retention with overflow incontinence. Overflow incontinence occurs when there is a high volume of urine, and the intravesicular pressure is greater than the urethral pressure. In this situation the person retains voluntary control but loses sensation of bladder distention. The condition is common to people with diabetic neuropathy.[6]

The fourth type of neurogenic bladder is the *uninhibited,* in which the bladder center within the patient's cerebral cortex is damaged. The person's ability to inhibit urination is lost and he has only a limited sensation of bladder distention. People with this type of dysfunction are not necessarily incontinent but may suffer from urgency. There is little time between sensation to void and the uninhibited contraction.[6] The impact

of this on behavior is obvious. People who have suffered a cerebral vascular accident (CVA) or who have Parkinson's disease may experience this type of bladder dysfunction. Deconditioning of the voiding reflex can result in incontinence through self-induced or iatrogenic causes. A cycle of frequent voidings and low bladder volume reduces bladder capacity and increases bladder wall thickness to potentiate incontinent episodes. Iatrogenic causes include placing a patient on the toilet after the incontinence episode or using uncomfortable equipment to make him continent.[17]

Dysfunction of the Bladder or Urethra Another possible cause of urinary incontinence is dysfunction of the bladder or urethra. This occurs because of an acute cystitis or a urinary tract infection that leads to bladder irritation. The irritation may increase bladder contractibility, causing subsequent loss of urine control. A carcinoma also may cause this dysfunction by obstruction.

Fecal Impaction and Prostatic Enlargement Two common causes of urinary incontinence are fecal impaction and prostatic enlargement. The impacted stool or an enlarged prostate will compress the urethra, so that urine is retained until the bladder distends to cause overflow incontinence.

Alteration in the Pelvic Diaphragm An alteration in the pelvic diaphragm occurs when the pubococcygeus and levator ani muscles are weak. Stress incontinence is a common sequela to this alteration. It can occur when the urethra is shortened as the patient assumes an upright position. Most often it occurs because of a rise in intra-abdominal pressure that increases the intravesical pressure. This rise in pressure may originate from sneezing, coughing, or laughing. There is no detrusor activity but the intravesical pressure exceeds the urethral pressure and a small amount of urine is released. A uterine prolapse, cystocele, or rectocele may contribute to incontinence but they do not necessarily cause the problem.

Metabolic Abnormalities During a work-up for incontinence, consider metabolic abnormalities that increase urinary flow. The common conditions of hypokalemia, hypercalemia, and hyperglycemia cause an increase in urinary output that can aggravate incontinence.

Psychological Factors

The cerebral deterioration that occurs with dementia may precipitate incontinence and should be considered as a neurologic problem rather than an emotional one. Incontinence that occurs in a person with dementia may or may not be a result of the dementia. Therefore, the usual procedure for diagnosis of incontinence is necessary for these patients. Often a treatable underlying cause can be identified. Most of the psychological factors that contribute to incontinence are temporary ones. An acute confusional state caused by a physical problem, such as an upper respiratory or urinary tract infection or anemia, may render the person unaware of the need to void. Once the person becomes cognizant of the situation, the problem is resolved.

Sutherland states that the psychological causes of incontinence include regression, dependency, rebellion, insecurity, attention-seeking, disturbance of conditioned reflexes, and sensory deprivation.[15] Many of these can be viewed as the person's attempt to adapt to a stressful situation. For example, regression and dependency are closely related because they are used as defense mechanisms to return to an earlier stage of development that is relatively less stressful. The incontinence evolves as a symptom of the childhood need to be taken care of and the need to be useful.

Often the symptoms or behaviors will be exacerbated if the person perceives the caretaker as negative or disgusted with him. The nurse or family may object to the amount of time the patient requires, or may be repulsed by the type of care required. Handling urine-soaked clothing, providing personal hygiene for another, and accepting the loss of control of elimination by an adult can be overwhelming. Typically, the nurse focuses her attention on the "chore" or the cleaning up rather than discussing the problem with the person. Everyone involved shares a sense of hopelessness.

Factors Related to Medications

Drug-related incontinence in the elderly is common because of the number of prescription and over-the-counter (OTC) drugs used by this age group. Diuretics increase urine volume within a few hours and may precipitate incontinence because of the frequency and urgency to void. The use of sedatives or hypnotics may cause a spurious episode of incontinence because of drug-induced drowsiness and a decrease in the person's awareness of his need to void. Some antidepressants and sympathomimetic drugs have a secondary effect on bladder function and may cause urinary retention or urgency.

Environmental Factors

Environmental factors can be an important determinant of whether a person is continent or incontinent. Environmental barriers are numerous and ubiquitous in the home, in public buildings, and in institutions. The distance to a toilet facility, the accessibility, the privacy allowed, and the knowledge of toilet location all are important factors.

NURSING ASSESSMENT

The nursing assessment of the incontinent person contains both subjective and objective data. Through the patient's history, the nurse assesses the health problem and identifies the patient's responses to changes in health status and patterns of living.

SUBJECTIVE DATA

It is important to know the meaning that incontinence has for each patient. Incontinence may signify a physical deterioration due to aging, a reason for institutionalization, or a possibility of surgery. The accompanying sample symptom analysis format is a means of collecting the subjective data. It is not all-inclusive but does provide an initial data base.

Questions 1 and 2   A determination of the date of onset of incontinence can help the nurse to assess whether this is an acute or chronic condition. The person may be able to put the date of onset in better perspective by associating it with an important event in his life. It is usually a social involvement that makes the problem noticeable. If incontinence has been a long-standing problem, the diagnosis will be more difficult to make and the adaptation in life-style may be well-established.

Question 3   The possible cause of the problem as perceived by the patient helps the nurse to assess the person's attitude toward the problem. This encourages discussion, assessment of the patient's understanding of the problem, and the development of rapport with the nurse. The nurse also may find that the response to this question elicits information about changes in prescribed medication use or home remedies.

Question 4   A determination of the frequency and amount of urine passed, a description of what happens, and an estimation of when incontinence occurs is essential for an assessment of the problem, but also helps in the evaluation of treatment. Asking if such activities as coughing, sneezing, or laughing cause incontinence may suggest a diagnosis of stress incontinence. Specific documentation of the voiding pattern will be discussed later.

Questions 5 and 6   The distance and the availability of toilet facilities may act as barriers to continence. Distance may be a problem if the patient has short warning time of the need to void or has a low energy level

---

Symptom Analysis for Urinary Incontinence

1. When did you first notice that you had trouble controlling your urine?
2. Did the problem come on slowly or suddenly?
3. What do you think caused the problem?
4. Description of the pattern
   a. Describe what happens when you become incontinent.
   b. When does it usually occur?
   c. How often do you urinate with control during the day? Amount each time?
   d. How often are you incontinent during the day? Amount?
   e. How often do you urinate with control at night? Amount?

   f. How often are you incontinent at night? Amount?
   g. Do you pass urine when coughing, sneezing, or laughing?
5. Were toilet facilities available when you had the urge to void?
6. Have you been able to continue with your normal activities?
7. How have you tried to deal with the problem of incontinence (*i.e.,* padding, OTC medications, fluid restriction)?
8. What is your average fluid intake?
9. Do you have hesitancy in initiating a stream, decreased force of stream, urinary frequency, or nocturia?

and is unable to get to a toilet. Toilet facilities in public areas are often difficult to find, difficult to gain access to, or limited to employee use. A change in normal activities may indicate a need for assistance to return to a previous life-style. Questions 5 and 6 provide the nurse with information about the environment and its influence on the patient's behavior.

Question 7 The patient's attempt to correct the problem is specifically addressed in question 7. Specific information about medications, devices, or exercises that the patient may be using must be clearly documented.

Question 8 Fluid intake is considered for both proper hydration and bladder elimination. Poor urinary output or bladder stasis are situations that create an environment conducive to bacterial growth.

Question 9 Question 9 is directed toward prostate enlargement as the cause of the incontinence. Further investigation is necessary beyond the subjective data.

In addition to a symptom analysis, a complete medication history of both prescription and nonprescription medications would be appropriate. Document other pertinent data about past medical and surgical problems. Significant problems that may be a cause of incontinence are urinary tract infection, prostatic hypertrophy, CVA, vesicovaginal fistula, spinal injury or tumor, previous surgery of the bladder, prostate, or pelvic floor, and pregnancy.

OBJECTIVE DATA: FEMALE

The physical examination of women should be based primarily on inspection and palpation. The external genitalia should be inspected by spreading the labia. The urethral meatus is usually midline and visible. In the older woman the urethral meatus may be very near the vagina or within the vaginal orifice due to the relaxed pelvic musculature. Abnormalities that should be referred include polyps, inflammation (may indicate a possible urethritis), or a caruncle (a small vascular growth), all of which can cause discomfort during voiding, but not necessarily incontinence.

The vaginal introitus should be a moist, vertical slit with regular or irregular edges. Investigate any inflammation, profuse vaginal discharge, lesions, or mucosal tissue bulging into or through the vagina. In postmenopausal women a decrease in vaginal secretions because of a decrease in estrogen should be expected. Before completing the inspection, the nurse should have the women bear down and note any urine leakage or vaginal bulging.[5] The rise in intra-abdominal pressure may cause the urine leakage and the vaginal bulging may reveal a cystocele, a rectocele, or uterine prolapse. An internal vaginal inspection can be done but is not necessary. Take a culture of any abnormal discharge.

The urethral meatus may be palpated to determine tenderness and any discharge. This is done by inserting a gloved finger into the vagina and stroking the interior vaginal wall toward the opening. Palpate the lateral and posterior areas of the vaginal introitus for tenderness, discharge, and bulging. Check the strength of the pelvic musculature by having the women squeeze the examiner's finger, which is in the vagina, with her pelvic muscles. Any amount of pressure on the examiner's finger should be considered normal and suggest some muscle tone.

OBJECTIVE DATA: MALE

The assessment for the male patient includes palpation of the prostate gland, in addition to the inspection of the urethral meatus. The prostate is normally smooth, firm, and about 1½ inches in diameter. Investigate variations. Because the prostate surrounds the urethra and bladder neck, prostatic hypertrophy causes urethral obstruction, producing hesitancy in initiating a stream, urinary frequency, a diminished force of the stream, and possibly nocturia.

PARACLINICAL DATA

After the collection of subjective and objective data, the diagnostic work-up begins. The nurse should work with the physician or other specialist to avoid duplication or unnecessary waste of time and services. The complexity of determining the cause of incontinence is facilitated by a team approach in diagnosis.

Laboratory tests include a urinalysis with culture to assess urinary tract infection, and a metabolic survey of the serum levels of glucose, calcium, and potassium.

A variety of radiological and urodynamic studies are used to diagnose the suspected etiology of incontinence. The studies most often used and the appropriate nursing intervention are listed below.

Cystography

Cystography is a radiographic study done to visualize the structure and the filling of the bladder. It helps to differentiate between a neurogenic and a non-neurogenic cause. Radiopaque dye (250–300 ml) is injected into the bladder through a urethral catheter. X-rays are taken and the table on which the patient is lying may be tilted to note the effect of postural change on bladder function. If a micturition cystogram is needed, the catheter is withdrawn, the patient voids, and x-rays are taken during this time. Clear liquids the day of the procedure and voiding immedi-

ately before the test are recommended. After the procedure is complete the patient should void to prevent bladder distention.

Cystometry

Cystometry helps to differentiate among the various types of neurogenic bladder conditions. During this process, a manometer is attached to a catheter, which is inserted into the bladder through the urethra. The pressure/volume relationship of the bladder is measured during both the filling and the emptying phases. Residual urine is measured before the test. Fluid enters the bladder through the catheter at a specified rate per minute. Pressure changes are charted against the volume instilled. At the end of the procedure, the person is asked to void. Contraction of the detrusor muscle indicates an intact nervous pathway. No specific nursing interventions are required.

Cystoscopy

Cystoscopy allows direct visualization of the bladder and the urethra by the insertion of a lighted telescopic tube through the urethra. Bladder capacity and abnormalities can be visualized. Oral fluid intake is increased before the procedure so that urine can be collected during the procedure. A local anesthesia is typically used. Because hematuria and sepsis are possible complications of this procedure, the nurse should assess the vital signs and record urine output, color, and amount for 24 hours following the procedure or recommend the patient observe for changes in the urine or fever at home.

Urethral Pressure Profile

Urethral pressure profile measures urethral and intravesical pressures with a double lumen, pressure-measuring catheter. Urethral pressures are taken at several levels of bladder fullness. The profile is used to identify whether urethral dysfunction is a cause of incontinence.

NURSING DIAGNOSIS

The primary nursing diagnosis for a person with incontinence would be stated as **alteration in urinary elimination: incontinence.** The medical diagnosis, together with the nursing assessment, determines the specific goals and plans for each type of incontinence. **Alteration in self-image related to incontinence** is an important nursing diagnosis to consider since it relates to the psychological well-being of the patient. The nursing diagnosis should include conclusive statements based on the data that put the specific needs of a patient in perspective.

Is the Incontinence Temporary or Fixed? *Temporary* incontinence refers to health changes that are short-term and reversible. *Fixed* incontinence refers to a chronic incontinence, usually with a neurologic dysfunction as its origin.[14] The nurse's awareness of whether the problem is temporary or fixed will help to determine the goals. The medical etiology should be the source for an answer to this question. The approach to a fixed problem may involve more preparation and planning to promote compliance to the proposed regimen.

Does the Incontinent Person Believe There is a Problem? Health promotion begins with a person's belief that there is a problem and that there is a perceived need for knowledge to resolve the problem. Active participation by the patient in the treatment regimen is important.

What Supports (Staff or Family) Are Available to the Incontinent Person? The complexity of the problem dictates the need for continuity of support for the incontinent person.

What is the Mental Status of the Incontinent Person? This question is a global one and is used to identify the extent of the person's ability to understand and participate in the plan of care. Adams suggests three groups of patients who will require a difference in approach:[1]

- *Patients who are mentally clear and willing to cooperate in the efforts to regain continence control.* Change in the environment, medications or bladder retraining may be all that is necessary.
- *Patients who are mentally clouded for a transient reason.* If the person has been continent before an acute illness (e.g., a high fever with delirium) or injury, he has a good chance of recovery with implementation of a well-developed plan.
- *Patients whose continence is beyond their control.* The reason may be physical (inoperable neoplasm) or mental (end-stage dementia). Any patient needs to be encouraged to be as self-reliant as possible.

What Are the Facilitators and Barriers to a Successful Goal Attainment? To decrease the opportunities for failure, it is important to identify facilitators and barriers to successful goal attainment. These factors include, for example, environment, support, physical condition, and psychological factors.

MANAGEMENT

Management of the incontinent person requires a great investment of time, energy, and resources by all involved. Incontinence is not exclusively a medical problem, nor a nursing one, but a team problem that must include the patient and family in planning the management program. According to Bartol,

> Psychological etiology, psychological responses to incontinence, and the psychodynamics of caregiver's reactions are the initial issues to be raised through inservice education with staff and as part of general health education with family members.[2]

EVALUATION OF PROVIDER'S ATTITUDES

The nurse should reflect on her attitude toward the incontinent person and identify her usual pattern of intervention. Willington suggests typical reactions of the caregiver to an incontinent person.[18] A nurse is trained to suppress a feeling of disgust; however, the nurse feels guilty because of this feeling and overcompensates by being overly permissive. The common practice of padding the person or the furniture with several layers of material is an example of how nurses deal with the problem. Often the nurse will pad all the beds "just in case," which suggests that the nurse expects the individual to be incontinent and sanctions it. A vicious psychological cycle can be initiated. The nurse who works in a situation in which there are many incontinent persons may experience a decrease in job satisfaction because of the time and energy expended without positive results. After the nurse evaluates her feelings and usual interventions for incontinent patients, she may be overwhelmed by the actual number of incontinent persons. For the nurse who works with many incontinent persons, she should select one or two to work with at a time to develop a continence regimen. This will help to concentrate effort and promote continuity of assessment and planning for the incontinent person. It should also improve the nurse's sense of accomplishment.

PATIENT-CENTERED EDUCATION

A consistent approach and reinforcement of behavior is necessary. If the person is living in the community, there must be a mechanism of contact with the person and the family to evaluate the plan's effectiveness, make appropriate changes, and provide adequate praise. When working in an institution, all caregivers need to use the care plan and provide the same support and reinforcement that is given to others.

Bladder Retraining

One form of patient-centered education is bladder retraining. The purpose of bladder retraining is to develop habits. The retraining may be used for many patients who have uninhibited bladder incontinence. The approaches can vary; however, Willington suggests the following guidelines for any retraining plan.[19]

1. The sequence of conditioning stimuli should be consistent and any inhibiting stimuli should be avoided.
2. A full bladder is a requisite.
3. Before the retraining program, assess the fluid intake pattern, the voiding pattern, and the patient's behavior around each voiding episode.

Because retraining focuses on a reflex activity, consider both conditioning and inhibiting stimuli. Sitting on a toilet seat in the correct position with the appropriate clothing removed would be conditioning stimuli. Privacy is also an important factor. The lack of one or more of these conditioning stimuli produces an inhibitory effect. The behavior exhibited before an incontinence episode may include restlessness, crying, or increased verbalization.[8] A 5-day record of incontinence and continence episodes is helpful in obtaining this information. Figure 16-3 is an example of an incontinence record. Additional notation may include bowel evacuation, and whether a commode or urinal is used instead of a toilet.

Documentation can be used as reference for the nurse and as reinforcement for the patient. Use the record to adjust the time for toileting to avoid an incontinence episode.

Encourage the patient to use the toilet 30 minutes before he or she is usually incontinent. If this is unsuccessful, readjust the schedule. When the patient is continent for 2 hours, increase the time between voidings by 30 minutes each day until a 3- to 4-hour voiding pattern evolves.[7] The expected outcome of the retraining program would be four voidings per day and no incidence of inconti-

FIG. 16-3 *Incontinence chart.*

Date			
Time	Fluid intake	Continent or incontinent	Behavior
12 am			
2 am			
4 am			
6 am			
8 am			
10 am			
12 noon			
2 pm			
4 pm			
6 pm			
8 pm			
10 pm			

nence. If incontinence has been a problem at night, the patient should be awakened at the appropriate intervals. There will be a disruption in sleep until an appropriate pattern is achieved. The attitude of the nurse and the patient can be a major factor in success because of the typically long period of time (often several weeks) for change to occur.

Pelvic Floor Exercises

Stress incontinence is a problem for women of all ages. Sometimes exercise of the pelvic floor muscles will alleviate or minimize the problem. A typical exercise regimen involves

1. Sitting or standing, without tensing other muscles, the patient tenses the area around the anus. This affects the posterior muscles of the pelvic floor.
2. While passing urine, the patient stops the flow and then restarts it. This affects the anterior muscles of the pelvic floor.

By doing these preliminary steps, the patient is able to identify which muscles are affected. Patients may do the exercises while sitting or standing and at any time; watching television, riding in a car, and waiting in line can be convenient times for them. The patient is asked to tighten the pelvic floor muscles slowly and then slowly release them. This should be done four times every hour for at least 3 months.[11] This exercise regimen can also be taught as a preventive measure.

Inducing Voiding

Many researchers have suggested the icing and brushing technique to induce voiding.[4,16] This technique is applicable to patients who experience incontinence because of retention. The technique is based on the principle that sensory receptors can be stimulated by external forces (icing and brushing) that are strong enough to initiate the micturition reflex.

The method of icing and brushing is as follows:

1. Using a cloth-covered ice cube with an exposed side, stroke the skin from the iliac crest to the groin area. Repeat every 3 seconds for 30 seconds (the skin may appear to be slightly red).
2. If the skin is wet, blot dry.
3. Brush rapidly and lightly over the same area for 30 seconds at 3-second intervals.

To provide even stimulation during brushing, a battery-powered, hand-held portable fan replaced with a soft brush can be used. If the procedure is successful, the patient should be able to void within 30 minutes. If the technique is ineffective, it may be tried again before an alternate method is attempted. Results from this process are usually evident within 1 to 2 weeks.

ENVIRONMENTAL FACTORS

Toilet Distance

Assess the patient's normal daily activities first. If the patient has difficulty holding urine for a particular distance, provide suggestions. For a patient with an upstairs bathroom in the house, the nurse might recommend a portable commode during the day. The institutionalized patient should be moved to a room closer to the toilet facilities. The patient who is frequently out of the house should be aware of the location of toilet facilities before the need to void arises. Safety is of particular importance at night. To maintain nocturnal continence furniture should be situated so as to provide a clear pathway to the bathrooms. Lights should be left on for clear visibility.

Many of the following suggestions have been found useful particularly for the care of elderly persons. However, the nurse may find these suggestions applicable to a patient of any age.

Furniture

Attention should be given to both beds and chairs. Ideally, the patient's feet should touch the floor when he sits on the side of the bed. If the bed is appreciably lower or higher, the person may need assistance getting into and out of it. Waiting for assistance increases the amount of time between sensation to void and voiding and therefore increases the incidence of incontinence. The nurse should check the depth and height of chairs normally used by the patient to identify their practicality. Chairs with arms are preferable to those without because the patient can use the arms for additional leverage.

Clothing

Encouraging the patient to wear normal clothing promotes the expectation that continence is possible. Full or wrap-around skirts can be both practical and stylish. Elastic or Velcro waistbands make removal of pants quick and easy. Incontinent persons often use protective pads and garments to prevent odor and protect furniture. Cost, skin condition, and availability of cleaning or disposal should be taken into consideration before using the product. Individual preferences and comfort should be priorities. Disposable adult briefs, briefs with disposable liners, and washable undergarments are available in most areas. For women who experience occasional dribbling, the use of sanitary pads is sufficient. The amount of urine expelled at an inappropriate time helps to determine whether to use a pad or a brief. In one of the few studies of this problem, Beber compared the comments of incontinent nursing home residents who used a disposable brief with those who had the usual care regi-

men (which included bedding and clothing changes and disposable bed pads.)[3] There was no statistical significance in comments about skin condition. Staff observed an increase in activity and mobility in a large number of persons who used the briefs. (However, some patients objected to the idea and considered it infantile. A few felt that there was no difference in the quality of life.)

Other Devices

The portable commode, with a toilet-shaped seat and a collecting unit, can be used at the bedside or in some convenient area. This device is available with a padded seat that can be placed over the toilet seat, converting it into a functional piece of furniture when not used as a commode. Of similar design is the portable chair with wheels, which has a toilet-shaped seat and can be used to transport the patient to a toilet. The chair fits over the toilet and there is no need for transfer within the toilet facilities. Bedpans and urinals are used for persons who are unable to transfer to a toilet. They should not be used just as a matter of convenience.

Protective furniture pads usually consist of an absorbent layer and a waterproof sheet on the bottom. The quality and price of these products will vary.

Catheters are a last resort in the management of incontinence. The incidence of a urinary tract infection associated with indwelling catheter use warrants careful consideration of this technique. If a catheter is used, it should be only for a short time to allow the skin to heal. The only acceptable external collection device is for males, the condom catheter. A pliable sheath is applied to the penis, secured by foam-backed tape and is connected to a collecting device. The sheath should be changed at least once a day and the penis should be monitored for edema and excoriation.

COMMUNITY RESOURCES

The nurse should be knowledgeable about the resources in the community. Resources include agencies that have contact with a population of incontinent people, and that may have developed a cadre of persons with expertise in the care regimen (*i.e.,* home health agencies or the Visiting Nurse service), and urology specialists. Medical supply companies should be contacted to obtain a list of appropriate products available, and a cost comparison of these made.

PHYSIOLOGICAL FACTORS

Hydration

The patient who suffers incontinence for the first time often attempts to correct the problem by restricting his fluid intake. He believes that less fluid leads to less urine to expel, better control, and less chance for incontinence. However, dilution of urine helps to "prevent urinary stasis and subsequent urinary infection and calculi formation."[10] Over time, recurrent bladder infections will cause changes in the bladder that lead to a lower capacity and change the voiding reflex. The nurse should encourage a fluid intake of 2000 ml to 2500 ml each day. Limit fluid intake in the evening to decrease the disruption of sleep. A physical problem such as congestive heart failure may limit the fluid intake, and in this situation an appropriate plan should be developed.

Bowel Regularity

Constipation and impaction can cause urinary retention because of the pressure of a full bowel on the urethra. Attention to hydration, proper nutrition, and regular evacuation will help to decrease the problem of constipation. Bowel regimens need to be developed by the nurse with the patient. Often

an increase in fiber content of the diet is the most effective method of preventing constipation. (For more information the reader is referred to Chap. 14.)

MEDICAL MANAGEMENT

Surgery and drug therapy may be used as interventions for the various types of incontinence. Electronic stimulation devices are being studied, primarily in Britain. This alternate intervention is used with persons who have stress incontinence or lower motor neuron dysfunction.

Surgical procedures to correct stress incontinence include urethral suspension and urethral lengthening.[13] The urethral suspension returns the bladder neck and the urethra to the normal retropubic position and the lengthening (usually done at the same time) positions the urethra so that shortening cannot occur when the woman assumes the upright position.

For men, a prostatectomy usually aids in correcting the problem of urinary retention and overflow. However, some patients continue to suffer from incontinence postprostatectomy. Surgical interventions for the problem may include urethral reconstruction, urethral compression, or implantable incontinence devices.[13] Urethral reconstruction may involve decreasing the diameter of the bladder neck and urethra or constructing a new bladder neck from the anterior bladder wall. Urethral compression is accomplished by implanting a gel-filled cushion over the bulbous urethra. Variations in pressure applied to the urethra are accomplished by postoperative withdrawal or injection of gel into the cushion by means of a transperineal needle.[13] There can be fistula formation and pain with this method. Implantable incontinence devices, such as electrical stimulation devices, are in the experimental stage. Implantable devices have the benefit of being controlled by the patient. However, the mechanical failure and the fibrosis or infection that may occur outweigh its widespread utilization. Urethral reconstruction is the most common form of treatment.

Before drug therapy is implemented, the nature of the problem must be determined. When appropriate, drug therapy may be used in conjunction with other interventions.

Anticholinergic drugs such as propantheline (Pro-Banthine), and oxybutynin (Ditropan) are commonly used to suppress the hyperactivity of patients with uninhibited and reflex bladders. These drugs inhibit the action of acetylcholine and therefore decrease the frequency of uninhibited contractions. This decrease in contractions will be followed by an increase in bladder capacity. Note any side-effects, such as constipation, dry mouth, and restlessness. Anticholinergics are contraindicated in patients with glaucoma.

Patients with urinary retention due to insufficient detrusor contractions may benefit from a cholinergic agent, such as bethanecol (Urecholine). This type of drug increases the tone and contractility of the bladder and encourages bladder emptying. Side-effects include hypotension, abdominal cramps, and urinary urgency. Cholinergics are contraindicated for persons with urinary tract obstruction, Parkinson's disease, chronic obstructive pulmonary disease, cardiac disease, or acute inflammatory diseases of the gastrointestinal tract.

SUMMARY

Urinary incontinence is a frustrating but manageable problem. In the majority of cases there is a treatable cause that is identified through a thorough diagnostic work-up. The team approach, with maximum support to the incontinent person and caregiver, will improve the chances for successful goal attainment. Assessment of physical, psychological, and environmental factors should be completed before any implementation of the treatment regimen. Finally, adequate time should be allowed for both intervention and evaluation.

REFERENCES

1. Adams G: Essentials of Geriatric Medicine. New York, Oxford University Press, 1977
2. Bartol M: Psychosocial aspects of incontinence in the aged person. In Burnside I (ed): Psychosocial Nursing Care of the Aged, 2nd ed. New York, McGraw–Hill, 1980
3. Beber, C: Freedom for the incontinent. Am J Nurs 80:483–484, 1980
4. Bergstrom N: Ice Application to induce voiding. Am J Nurs 69:283–285, 1969
5. Brink C: Assessing the problem. Geriatr Nurs 1:241-245, 1980
6. Brocklehurst J, Hanley T: Geriatric medicine for students. New York, Churchill–Livingstone, 1976
7. Clay E: Habit retraining. Geriatr Nurs 1:252–254, 1980
8. Demmerle B, Bartol M: Nursing care for the incontinent person. Geriatr Nurs 1:246–250, 1980
9. Hald T: Problems of urinary incontinence. In Caldwell K (ed): Urinary Incontinence. New York, Grune & Stratton, 1975
10. Johnson J: Rehabilitative aspects of neurologic bladder dysfunction. Nurs Clin North Am 15:293–307, 1980
11. Mandelstam D: Special techniques: Strengthening pelvic floor muscles. Geriatr Nurs 1:251–254, 1980
12. Malvern J: The mechanism of continence. In Stanton S, Tanagho E (eds): Surgery of Female Incontinence. New York, Springer–Verlag, 1980
13. Merrill D: Surgical treatment of urinary incontinence. In Caldwell K (ed): Urinary Incontinence. New York, Grune & Stratton, 1975
14. Resnick N, Rowe J: Urinary incontinence in the elderly. In Rowe J, Besdine R (eds): Health and Disease in Old Age. Boston, Little, Brown & Co, 1982
15. Sutherland S: The psychology of incontinence. In

Willington FL (ed): Incontinence in the Elderly. New York, Academic Press, 1976

16. Wells T, Brink C: Urinary continence: Assessment and management. In Burnside I (ed): Nursing and the Aged, 2nd ed. New York, McGraw–Hill, 1981
17. Williams M, Pannill F: Urinary incontinence in the elderly. Ann Intern Med 97:895–907, 1982
18. Willington R: Psychological and psychogenic aspects (Incontinence 3). Nurs Times 71:422–423, Mar 13, 1975
19. Willington F: Training and retraining for incontinence (Incontinence 5). Nurs Times 71:500–503, Mar 27, 1975
20. Yarnell J, Leger A: The prevalence, severity, and factors associated with urinary incontinence in a random sample of the elderly. Age Ageing 8:81–87, 1979

BIBLIOGRAPHY

Agate J: The Practice of Geriatrics, 2nd ed. Springfield, IL, Charles C Thomas, 1970

Bates P, Bradley W, Glen E, et al: The standardization of terminology of lower urinary tract function. J Urol 121:551–554, 1979

Brocklehurst J: Management of the uninhibited neurogenic bladder. In Willington FL (ed): Incontinence in the Elderly. New York, Academic Press, 1976

Brocklehurst J, Fry J, Griffiths L et al: Dysuria in old age. J Am Geriatr Soc 197:582–592, 1971

Calder J: The nursing of incontinence. In Willington FL (ed): Incontinence in the Elderly. New York, Academic Press, 1976

Chapman W, Bulger R, Cutler R et al: The Urinary System. Philadelphia, WB Saunders, 1973

Coni N, Davison W, Webster S: Lecture Notes on Geriatrics. London, Blackwell Scientific Publications, 1977

Eastwood H: Urodynamic studies in the management of urinary incontinence in the elderly. Age Ageing 8:41–45, 1979

Edwards L: Mechanical and other devices. In Caldwell K (ed): Urinary Incontinence, New York, Grune & Stratton, 1975

Field M: Urinary incontinence in the elderly: An overview. In Stilwell E (ed): Readings in Gerontological Nursing. Thorofare, New Jersey, Charles B Slack, 1980

Finkbeiner A, Bissada N: Drug therapy for lower urinary tract dysfunction. Urologic Clin North Am 7:3–15, 1980

Glen E: Stress incontinence: The turning tide. In Cantor E (ed): Female Urinary Stress Incontinence. Springfield, IL, Charles C Thomas, 1979

Hodgkinson C: Abnormalities of female bladder function and urinary control. In State W (ed): Disorders of the Female Urethra and Urinary Incontinence. Baltimore, Williams & Wilkins, 1978

Lapides J: Physiology of the urinary sphincter and its relationship to operations for stress incontinence. In Slate W (ed): Disorders of the Female Urethra and Urinary Incontinence. Baltimore, Williams & Wilkins, 1978

Rowan D, Glen E: Clinical investigation and evaluation of urinary incontinence. In Cantor E (ed): Female Urinary Stress Incontinence. Springfield, IL, Charles C Thomas, 1979

Specht J, Cordes A: Incontinence. In Carnevali D, Patrick M (eds): Nursing Management for the Elderly. New York, JB Lippincott, 1979

Thompson J, Bowers A: Clinical Manual of Health Assessment. St. Louis, CV Mosby, 1980

Wells T: Promoting urine control in older adults. Geriatr Nurs 1:236–240, 1980

Wells T, Brink C: Helpful equipment. Geriatr Nurs 1:264–269, 1980

Willington F: Management of urinary incontinence. In Caldwell K (ed): Urinary Incontinence. New York, Grune & Stratton, 1975

Willington F: Problems in the aetiology of urinary incontinence (Incontinence 2). Nurs Times 71:378–381, Mar 6, 1975

Willington F: The nursing component in diagnosis and treatment. (Incontinence 4). Nurs Times 71:464–467, Mar 20, 1975

17

Dyspnea and Cough

Mary Niemeyer

Dyspnea and cough are common manifestations of respiratory system dysfunction. Although cough may be ignored or passed off as a nuisance, dyspnea usually is responded to quickly as a potentially serious problem. Whether they occur in the outpatient clinic or hospital, each can be a puzzling problem or signal of impending emergency.

Prompt assessment, accurate diagnosis, appropriate treatment of the underlying cause, and evaluation of the treatment process and patient outcomes are essential to restoring the patient to a state of optimal functional ability.

Dyspnea

INTRODUCTION

DEFINITION

Dyspnea is a symptom, a sensation felt by the patient that can be defined as difficult, labored, uncomfortable breathing. The unique characteristic of dyspnea is that it is *subjec-* *tive*. It is perceived and interpreted solely by the patient. When the patient complains of dyspnea, or "shortness of breath," one thing is certain: the patient is aware of having difficulty breathing. Because dyspnea is a subjective sensation, it can not be equated with any objective sign. It may be absent in the face of apparently labored, abnormally rapid, or deep breathing. Or it may be present in a patient who appears to be breathing normally.

Dyspnea should not be confused with hyperventilation, tachypnea, or hyperpnea, all of which can be seen or measured clinically by the practitioner.

Dyspnea is a symptom that usually prompts a patient to seek attention from a health care professional. Inability to breathe is a distressing event that alarms the patient and often, those around him. The patient's reaction to dyspnea may vary from the realization of the sensation (usually after some exertion or strenuous exercise), to anxiety, fear, and panic. The severity of the symptom depends not only on the degree of respiratory embarrassment, but also on other circumstances, such as physical condition and mental–emotional status.

Studies have shown no consistent relation between physiological variables and the experience of dyspnea.[1,16] Dyspnea may depend in part on past conditioning experiences.

Patient awareness of dyspnea does not necessarily mean the presence of a disease process. Everyone experiences dyspnea on occasion, especially with physical effort. On the other hand, a patient with a respiratory disease may not report dyspnea unless asked specifically. Such patients are so accustomed to "shortness of breath" or "not enough air" that they do not consider it unusual unless there is a significant change.

Dyspnea is a common symptom associated with cardiopulmonary disease. Patients' reports vary, but generally they complain of "not getting enough air," or "discomfort in the chest." The degree of dyspnea can not be measured accurately with pulmonary function tests or blood gases.[9] Some people experience considerable dyspnea with minimal structural changes in the cardiopulmonary system, whereas others report no dyspnea in the presence of severe structural changes.

MECHANISMS OF DYSPNEA

There have been many theories proposed as to the physiological abnormalities that cause dyspnea; however, none have been identified or accepted as the sole explanation of this disturbing clinical symptom. Generally, it is recognized that dyspnea represents an imbalance between ventilatory demand and ventilatory capacity.

One theory, proposed by Campbell and Howell, is the *length–tension appropriateness concept*, which states that the discomfort or awareness of difficult breathing is felt by the person when he senses an unexpected or inappropriate relationship between the size of the breath taken (*length* of the respiratory muscles) and the force required to produce it (*tension* of the stretch receptors).[10]

Regardless of the exact mechanism, dyspnea represents an increase in the work of breathing. The patient may have an awareness of the need to increase ventilation or realize the need to use the respiratory muscles more forcefully. Dyspnea is essentially the result of the same factors, whether in the normal person, the cardiac patient climbing stairs, or the patient with chronic lung disease subjected to the stress of activity.

Most of the causes of dyspnea can be traced to disorders of the respiratory and cardiac systems (Table 17-1). A variety of other causes, including vascular diseases, psychoemotional states, and metabolic dysfunction, also have been identified.[1,7,9,10,11,15,16]

DISORDERS OF THE RESPIRATORY SYSTEM THAT CAN CAUSE DYSPNEA

Dyspnea is caused by disorders of the respiratory system that are the result of obstruction to air flow (*obstructive disorders*), or resistance to chest wall or lung movement (*restrictive disorders*). Dyspnea most probably is related to increased work of breathing and decreased oxygen available for tissue metabolism.

Obstructive disorders include chronic obstructive pulmonary disease (COPD), infection, and tumor. COPD (asthma, chronic bronchitis, and emphysema) results in decreased ventilation and therefore decreased oxygen available for gas exchange. The result is an increased work of breathing as the body attempts to maintain normal functioning. Airway obstruction also may occur acutely as the result of the inflammation and edema of airways associated with an upper respiratory

TABLE 17-1
CAUSES OF DYSPNEA

DISORDERS OF THE RESPIRATORY SYSTEM	DISORDERS OF THE CARDIOVASCULAR SYSTEM	PSYCHOGENIC DYSPNEA	OTHER CAUSES
Obstructive disorders	Left ventricular failure	Acute and chronic anxiety	Anemia
Bronchitis	Mitral stenosis	Preexisting mental disorders	High altitude
Emphysema	Aortic insufficiency	Patient perception of signs	Smoking
Asthma	Pericardial effusion/tamponade	or symptoms	Metabolic disorders
Neoplasm	Cardiac arrhythmia	Fear of dyspnea	Diabetes Mellitus
Restrictive disorders	Pulmonary hypertension	Fear of treatment	Uremia
Lung rigidity	Pulmonary emboli	Psychogenic hyperventilation	Hepatic insufficiency
Pulmonary edema			
Collagen disease			
Pulmonary fibrosis			
Neuromuscular disorders			
Myasthenia gravis			
Guillain–Barré Syndrome			
Decreased chest–wall movement			
Pain			
Obesity			
Pregnancy			
Ascites			
Reduced lung volume			
Pleural effusion			
Pneumothorax			
Hemothorax			

infection. Dyspnea in this case is transient, limited to the acute episode. Similarly, upper airway infection or inflammation can be superimposed on a chronic respiratory obstruction, resulting in acute exacerbation of stable chronic symptoms.

A neoplasm occurring in an airway or compressing an airway by its presence in adjacent tissue can result in significant obstruction to airflow. The extent of respiratory embarrassment and therefore the presence and severity of dyspnea will be related to the underlying level of pulmonary function. In someone with chronic pulmonary dysfunction, obstructive or restrictive, the impact on overall functioning would be greater than in someone whose respiratory function is within normal limits.

Restrictive lung disorders that can cause dyspnea are those that increase lung rigidity, alter respiratory muscle function, decrease the bellows action of the chest, or decrease effective lung volume. Lung stiffness accompanies collagen disorders, such as lupus erythematosus and scleroderma. Diffuse interstitial fibrosis also reduces the normal elasticity of the lung, since fibrotic tissue replaces normal cells of the alveoli and respiratory bronchioles.

A more commonly occurring cause of lung stiffness is the presence of water at the alveolocapillary membrane, as in congestive heart failure. The resulting decrease in compliance can increase the work of breathing markedly as the amount of available oxygen in the blood is reduced.

The cardinal effect of neuromuscular disorders on the respiratory muscles is decreased strength of muscle contraction and therefore decreased ventilation. In the presence of myasthenia gravis, normal ventilatory function may be interrupted by episodes of severe muscle weakness. The paralysis associated with Guillain–Barré

syndrome diminishes respiratory muscle function similarly.

A less common neuromuscular cause of decreased ventilation is the permanent disruption of nerve impulses to the muscles of respiration. Spinal poliomyelitis and high spinal cord injuries are two examples. In such patients, dyspnea may be increased acutely by upper respiratory infection.

Normal bellows function, without accompanying lung parenchymal disease, may be decreased substantially by processes that affect the chest wall and diaphragm. Chest pain can reduce normal ventilatory activity significantly. Pleuritic chest pain is usually localized and can be aggravated by yawning, coughing, and sneezing. Muscular chest pain is caused most often by muscular strain, fractured ribs, or trauma. The chest pain that accompanies myocardial ischemia can also reduce ventilatory bellows action greatly and result in dyspnea. Ascites and pregnancy also can limit diaphragmatic excursion and produce decreased ventilation. Severe obesity may reduce bellows function by limiting chest wall excursion, since the sheer weight of the chest exceeds muscle strength.

Loss of lung volume can easily precipitate dyspnea because the demand for oxygen exceeds the supply provided by the remaining lung. Pneumothorax or collapse of ventilated lung tissue can reduce the amount of available oxygen. Similarly, compression of lung tissue by fluid, as with pleural effusion or hemothorax, can cause dyspnea.

DISORDERS OF THE CARDIOVASCULAR SYSTEM THAT CAN CAUSE DYSPNEA

Dyspnea in the presence of cardiovascular disorders is usually the result of reduction of pulmonary compliance, which increases the work of breathing. Cardiac failure, resulting in engorgement of the pulmonary capillary bed, is the primary factor in reduced pulmonary compliance. Fluid in the interstitial and alveolar spaces impairs gas exchange, especially oxygen, thereby increasing ventilatory demand. The severity of dyspnea depends on the degree of left-sided failure and, in fact dyspnea may occur with strenuous exertion, during the performance of activities of daily living, or at rest, depending on the degree of cardiac failure.

In mitral stenosis the same rise in pulmonary capillary pressure and subsequent engorgement is seen, but without an increase in ventricular pressure. Dyspnea on exertion is often an early symptom and may become the dominant complaint as the mitral valve narrows and atrial pressure rises. There are other cardiac disorders that are much less common causes of dyspnea. One disorder is acute paroxysmal cardiac arrhythmia, occurring during periods of effort. Such an arrhythmia may be associated with impaired ventricular performance or, in the elderly patient, with preexisting heart disease.

Dyspnea is commonly found in patients with primary pulmonary hypertension or pulmonary hypertension resulting from repeated episodes of pulmonary emboli. The exact stimulus for dyspnea is unclear. Similarly, the mechanism of dyspnea in cardiac tamponade is unknown.

Dyspnea frequently occurs in patients who have both respiratory and cardiac disease. The presence of other signs and symptoms, along with a specific history, will facilitate differentiation of the primary mechanism.

PSYCHOGENIC DYSPNEA

Dyspnea may accompany psychogenic disorders and emotional stress, both transient and chronic. However, the patient may be unaware of any relationship of his dyspnea to disturbances in his emotional well-being. Dyspnea also may be provoked by physiological or psychological stress. Once dyspnea is sensed, the patient's emotional response to it may aggravate the original stress situation and perpetuate the dyspnea.

Both acute and chronic anxiety states may cause a patient to complain of dyspnea. For example, a patient may state that he experiences dyspnea while sitting or resting at the end of a particularly discouraging day, when not engaged in a task requiring direct effort. Or the patient may complain of having trouble breathing when carrying out usual tasks. Normal breathing may be interspersed with deep sighing respirations. Associated with such dyspnea may be other symptoms, such as excessive tiredness and fatigability, palpitations, and general irritability.

Fatigue and cardiorespiratory insufficiency may be related to a variety of life situations in otherwise generally healthy people. A person who feels dejected and discouraged may approach tasks awkwardly, so that muscular-energy consumption increases at the same time that cardiopulmonary efficiency is at a low level. Similarly, extreme weakness (physical deconditioning) from prolonged bed rest or enforced immobility may aggravate dyspnea.

Psychogenic hyperventilation can be a most dramatic event. The patient breathes as forcefully and rapidly as he can and continues until the sensorium becomes dulled as a result of the alkalosis. Normal respiration is then restored. Psychogenic dyspnea may also depend on mental disposition. The patient's perception of his symptoms and his disease process may promote dyspnea. Similarly, interpretation or misinterpretation of explanations, instruction, and symptoms may contribute to breathlessness. Fear surrounding a particular procedure or event may provoke an episode of dyspnea. On the other hand, fear of recurring dyspnea may precipitate the cycle of fear and decreasing physical activity often seen in patients with chronic lung disease.

A common complaint related to dyspnea is a disturbance in the normal breathing rhythm. The patient feels that he cannot get a deep breath or that he is not getting enough air. He reports a heaviness in the chest. To correct this, he inhales a forceful deep breath, giving the respiratory pattern a sighing character. Such "sighing respirations" may be an isolated occurrence or accompany a stressful event or encounter.

OTHER CAUSES OF DYSPNEA

Dyspnea on exertion is a common symptom in patients with a hemoglobin concentration of 7 mg/dl or less, particularly when such an anemia is acutely produced. Such patients usually have increased ventilation; however, the exact mechanism for this kind of dyspnea is unknown.

Certain environmental factors also influence dyspnea, of which high altitude is the most common. Heights of over 6000 feet may produce dyspnea on exertion in normal people.

A most important environmental exposure is smoking. Smoking can aggravate several of the obstructive or restrictive disorders previously mentioned, and thereby contribute to dyspnea.

Disturbances of metabolism, such as diabetes mellitus, that cause an increase in oxidative processes, also may cause dyspnea. Similarly, accumulation of waste products may stimulate increased respiratory activity and cause dyspnea, as in the case of uremia or hepatic insufficiency.

NURSING ASSESSMENT

Management of the patient with dyspnea begins with careful determination of pertinent subjective and objective data.[1,4,5,7,9,10,16] Such assessment is crucial to developing a plan with specific, individualized outcomes.

SUBJECTIVE DATA

Description of the Complaint

Have the patient describe the sensation in his own words.

Onset: Chronology

Determine when the dyspnea began and the course that it has followed. Recent events and the presence of other symptoms may facilitate understanding of the underlying pathologic process(es).

When did the patient first experience dyspnea? Was it during a bout with a cold or influenza 3 weeks ago? Has the onset been so insidious that the patient cannot recall clearly the first symptoms?

Is the dyspnea always the same or has it gotten worse over time? Have there been periods of time when the severity of dyspnea was less, followed by times when it seemed more severe? Are such variations associated with the seasons, or other recurring patterns?

Does the patient attribute shortness of breath to age? Statements such as, "I'm getting older and can't do what I used to," or "I always take an elevator now" are indications of this.

Setting: Precipitating Factors

Have the patient describe 1) where he is, 2) what he is doing, and 3) with whom or what when the dyspnea is experienced.

Does the onset of dyspnea or an increase

in severity occur with lifting, shoveling, during sleep, or only after several minutes of strenuous exercise or jogging? Exercise may cause dyspnea in a normal person. Similarly, a person with a respiratory handicap may be free of dyspnea only when at rest.

Is dyspnea more likely to occur when the patient is alone, or in a crowded space?

Looking at each of these factors assists the nurse in understanding the nature of dyspnea in the particular patient, how life activities influence the dyspnea, and how the dyspnea influences the patient's life.

What is the patient's smoking history? Cigarette smoking is usually found in patients with chronic bronchitis and emphysema, most of whom experience dyspnea or a sensation of breathlessness.

Associated Symptoms

Rarely, if ever, will dyspnea be the only symptom. Most probably it will occur as part of a symptom complex, such as ankle edema, fatigue, weight gain, and cough. Does the patient report a "smoker's cough," a history of chronic bronchitis, or sputum production? Does the patient complain of leg or calf pain, or the sudden onset of chest pain? Is there associated dizziness, numbness or tingling around the mouth, or changes in mentation?

Determine if other influenza or cold symptoms are usually present, (e.g., sore throat, cough, fever, runny nose, generalized malaise) along with an increase in dyspnea. This symptom complex is common in patients with underlying chronic lung disease, especially bronchitis and emphysema.

The patient may report an abdominal complaint, such as distention immediately after eating, that accompanies the shortness of breath. Such patients may have chronic respiratory disease, so that pressure on the diaphragm causes respiratory discomfort.

Aggravating Factors

Identify activities or physiological processes that increase the severity of the dyspnea. Has there been a recent change in sputum thickness or amount? Has the patient recently begun working in a different environment?

Determine if the patient has recently experienced significant decrease in activity, such as bed rest because of illness or injury. Or does the patient's sedentary life-style preclude even normal exercise and activity?

Determine whether the patient uses any respiratory therapy equipment. Contaminated equipment is an excellent medium for growth of bacteria, especially Pseudomonas. The patient may report recurrence of upper respiratory symptoms (dyspnea) soon after treatment of an acute episode, suggesting reinfection from organisms in equipment tubing.

Alleviating Factors

What treatment methods does the patient usually employ? Does rest relieve the dyspnea? How long must the patient rest before the symptom subsides? Has the amount of needed rest increased?

Have the patient recall changes in activities made to accommodate the dyspnea (e.g., always taking an elevator rather than stairs, using a golf cart rather than walking, taking the car even for short excursions).

Does the patient sleep in a chair to avoid episodes of dyspnea, or to relieve onset of dyspnea after several hours of sleep?

Clearing the airways of accumulated secretions may reduce the amount of dyspnea. Does the patient cough upon first arising? How much sputum is raised? What is its color and its consistency? Is this pattern repeated after a nap or rest period?

What medications relieve the dyspnea?

Are these taken as prescribed by a physician to treat specific episodes of illness? Are over-the-counter (OTC) medications used, in addition to regularly prescribed medications? Even taken as the manufacturer directs, such medications can interfere with a prescribed treatment regimen. Determine not only the names of all medications, but also the pattern of use. The potential for abuse of inhaled medications is significant and may result in increased severity of dyspnea.

Also important in determining the nature of reported dyspnea is any family history of cardiopulmonary diseases. The familial tendency for coronary artery disease is well-known. The incidence of congestive heart failure or myocardial dysfunction also is recognized. Family history is also important in identifying patients with an allergic background or those with predisposing factors such as alpha$_1$-antitrypsin deficiency. There may be a strong family history of COPD, without the genetic predisposition.

OBJECTIVE DATA

Physical Examination: Inspection and Observation

Determine respiratory rate, rhythm, depth. How much effort does the patient appear to expend when breathing at rest?

What position does the patient assume? A position that enables the patient to raise the shoulder girdle to increase ventilation suggests respiratory insufficiency. In fact, the patient may find that resting his elbows on some surface to elevate the shoulder girdle relieves shortness of breath and restores comfortable breathing. What is the resting pulse rate? How long after exercise does the pulse return to normal resting rate?

Assess the patient's general appearance. Does facial expression suggest anxiety, fatigue, or depression? Does the patient use pursed-lip breathing? Patients with emphysema many times find this technique relieves shortness of breath.

Determine general muscle mass and strength. Lack of physical conditioning may make even a simple task a chore that precipitates shortness of breath. Decreased strength of major muscle groups may be associated with prolonged bedrest and inactivity.

Is there ankle or pedal edema?

Inspect the thorax. Is there an increase in the anteroposterior diameter suggesting COPD? Is there deformity of the rib cage such as kyphosis or scoliosis, or scars from surgery or trauma that might restrict ventilation or cause discomfort with deep breathing?

When the patient takes a deep breath, is chest movement symmetrical, or does one side move less, or not at all? Is there use of either the intercostal or sternocleidomastoid muscles as accessory muscles of ventilation?

Is the patient obese, so that movement of the chest wall is inhibited by its sheer weight?

Is there leg or calf pain or tenderness that might suggest thrombophlebitis and possible pulmonary embolus as a cause of dyspnea?

Palpation

Is there pain or tenderness over a portion of the chest wall? Chest wall discomfort can cause a patient to splint, especially with deep breaths. Is the pain over a rib or muscle? Muscle spasm can occur with strenuous exercise or severe coughing.

Percussion

Percussion of the chest may reveal areas of dullness over less ventilated lung areas. The area may be confined to one segment of one lobe or may involve the lower lobes of both lungs. Percussion will assist in localizing the area and determining the extent of involvement. A dull or flat sound is often heard over areas of atelectasis and pneumonia. Pleural effusion will cause a flat sound. Hyperresonance is associated with emphysema.

Auscultation of the Chest

Listen for breath sounds. Are the breath sounds decreased in any area? How extensive is the change? Is it a small segment of one base? Or are the sounds decreased or absent over a major portion of one lung?

Are there bronchial breath sounds over any area? Again, what portion of the lung is involved?

Determine if adventitious breath sounds (rales, rhonchi, and wheezes) are present. Are the rales audible only at the end of inspiration or throughout the inspiratory cycle? Rales are often present with pneumonia or interstitial fluid in the lungs. In pneumonia, rales are localized or scattered; in pulmonary edema rales are usually basilar. Are rhonchi present during the latter portion of expiration or throughout the respiratory cycle? Do the rhonchi clear after the patient coughs vigorously? Rhonchi are found typically with bronchitis. Determine not only the presence of rales and rhonchi, but also the intensity of the sounds.

Is wheezing audible? Again, localize the sound to determine the extent of involvement.

Is there prolongation of forced expiration, which can be timed while auscultating over the trachea (normally 3 seconds or less).

PARACLINICAL DATA

A sputum culture or Gram's stain may determine the presence of an intrapulmonary infection such as bronchitis or pneumonia.

Results of a recent chest x-ray may reveal pneumonia or an interstitial process. Increased cardiac size may be present. Similarly, the results of an electrocardiogram (ECG) may reveal a variety of disorders, from silent myocardial infarction to left ventricular hypertrophy.

A complete blood count may reveal an anemia or a hematologic disease such as leukemia. Polycythemia may be associated with advanced COPD.

Results of pulmonary function studies can be useful in determining the amount of airway obstruction and its reversibility.

NURSING DIAGNOSIS

Analysis of assessment data will guide diagnosis in one of two directions (Table 17-2). Dyspnea may be occurring in the presence of the patient's usual, stable state, or the dyspnea may be a new symptom or a significant increase in severity in the patient's usual stable state.

DYSPNEA IN THE PRESENCE OF THE PATIENT'S USUAL STATE

The patient may report that although he is able to participate in his usual daily activities, dyspnea is present occasionally, sometimes, or most of the time. Such patients may express concern that the symptom persists or ask for ways to minimize its occurrence.

Dyspnea Related to Exertion in Usual State of Health

Dyspnea can occur in the healthy patient whose life-style includes little or no regular exercise. When confronted with activity that requires exertion, he experiences dyspnea that is frustrating and tends to restrict his willingness to pursue that activity, whether climbing a flight of stairs or playing a game of tennis. The patient may express concern,

TABLE 17-2
DIAGNOSIS OF DYSPNEA AND COUGH

DIAGNOSIS	
Symptom occurs in the presence of usual stable state	Symptom is new or has increased in severity from a stable state
(Patient frustrated, discouraged by symptom and impact of symptom on functional ability)	(Patient alarmed by symptom, unable to attain or maintain usual level of function)

DIAGNOSIS OF DYSPNEA			
Dyspnea related to exertion in usual state of health	Dyspnea related to stable, chronic disorder	Onset of dyspnea related to: Pulmonary disorder Cardiovascular Disorder Other cause	Increased dyspnea related to acute exacerbation of symptoms of underlying disease related to: Infectious process Myocardial dysfunction Other cause

DIAGNOSIS OF COUGH			
Cough to clear airways: Usual accumulation of secretions or response to an irritant	Cough related to need to maintain airway patency in the presence of chronic sputum production	Onset of cough related to disease process or presence of irritant	Increased cough frequency and effort related to difficulty clearing secretions

frustration, or annoyance with the symptom, seeking advice or direction for ways to cope with it.

Dyspnea Related to a Stable, Chronic Disorder

Dyspnea is experienced as a way of life because of chronic pulmonary or cardiac disease. Such patients learn that dyspnea accompanies many or most daily activities. The severity of the dyspnea may remain fairly constant, but is persistent and unending. Such patients may become tired and discouraged by the chronicity of their symptom, expressing a desire for some type of relief.

Dyspnea as a New Symptom or an Increase in Severity in a Stable Condition

The patient may report dyspnea as the only symptom. It may occur along with one or more other symptoms, and he may be alarmed or frightened. Such patients are anxious for an explanation of why the dyspnea occurs and are seeking relief from its presence.

Dyspnea as a New Symptom   The onset of dyspnea in the patient who is normally asymptomatic usually is accompanied by considerable concern and determination to eliminate its cause. In fact, the anxiety that accompanies the dyspnea may contribute to its severity, heightening the patient's awareness and response to the dyspnea.

Increased Dyspnea Related to Acute Exacerbation of Symptoms of an Underlying Disease The patient with chronic pulmonary or cardiac disease may experience an exacerbation of the underlying symptoms of the disease, including dyspnea. Such a patient may report that the dyspnea is more severe than usual, that more time is needed to recover from physical activity, and that the current severity of the symptom restricts usual activity patterns in a new way.

MANAGEMENT

The goal of management of dyspnea is to promote the optimal level of patient functioning, one in which dyspnea is controlled, minimized, or eliminated. The plan of care is often multidisciplinary, recognizing the need for nursing intervention, along with medical management of the disease process, and assistance from other disciplines.[2,8,11,12]

MANAGEMENT OF DYSPNEA IN THE PRESENCE OF THE PATIENT'S USUAL STATE

Dyspnea Related to Exertion in a Usual State of Health

The patient in a usual state of health who experiences dyspnea during exercise or strenuous activity may need assistance in setting realistic goals. A regimen of age-appropriate, physical conditioning exercises can promote gradual increase in strength and endurance, and reduce the occurrence of dyspnea. With the current interest in physical activity, opportunities to become involved in a "shape-up" program are numer-

ous, whether it is a jog around the block or membership at a spa. Indeed, some may see dyspnea on exertion as a sign of increasing endurance or a badge of survival.

Dyspnea Related to Stable, Chronic Disorder

Patients with chronic lung or heart disease, who experience dyspnea as a way of life, can lead productive and satisfying lives with a regular program of care.

Medications Patients with chronic dyspnea first of all may need to follow a medical regimen to control reversible airway obstruction. Control and elimination of dyspnea and cough may be achieved through the use of specific medication. Most patients do not mind taking medications because with them they find relief from their symptoms. A common problem, however, is omission of a dose because of forgetfulness or confusion. The patient may need assistance in developing a strategy to ensure that the medication schedule is followed.

Bronchodilators   An important part of the treatment of the patient who has reversible airway obstruction are bronchodilators. When essentially irreversible bronchial obstruction is present, the benefits of bronchodilator therapy are minimal.

The two basic types of bronchodilators are: 1) sympathomimetic or adrenergic drugs, and 2) the methylxanthines or theophylline-type drugs. The *sympathomimetic* drugs stimulate the beta-adrenergic receptors, especially $beta_2$, to produce bronchodilation. These drugs can be given orally, subcutaneously, by nebulization, or in combination. Cartridge nebulizers are especially convenient and easy to use. The effectiveness depends however on the patient's neuromuscular coordination and ability to 1) exhale completely; 2) coordinate inhaling the medication with the beginning of a deep inspiration; 3) hold the breath for 3 to 4 seconds at the end of maximum inspiration; and 4) to exhale slowly through pursed lips.

The *methylxanthines* are absorbed readily by the oral route and therefore are easy and convenient to take. Gastrointestinal irritation can be minimized by taking the drug with milk and crackers, or with a meal.

Self-Help Techniques   Two techniques that may help control and minimize dyspnea are diaphragmatic breathing and pursed-lip breathing. Diaphragmatic breathing assists the patient to take deeper breaths, for more efficient ventilation. The patient is encouraged to breathe in slowly through the nose while keeping one hand in the "V" of the ribs, just below the xiphoid process, so that he is more aware of achieving the deepest breath possible.

After reaching maximum inhalation, the patient relaxes and exhales passively through pursed lips. Exhalation should be twice as long as inhalation and a quiet maneuver. Forced exhalation could trigger uncontrolled coughing. The patient will feel the upper abdomen move in as exhalation proceeds.

When he is using diaphragmatic breathing, the patient should relax his shoulders and neck. The upper chest should remain still. This assures that the bulk of ventilation occurs because of diaphragmatic motion, rather than the less efficient muscles of the shoulder girdle. Diaphragmatic breathing can be used with relaxation techniqes and with controlled coughing techniques.

Pursed-lip breathing is exhalation through pursed lips so that back pressure is created to keep airways open and promote more complete exhalation. It can also facilitate removal of secretions from the tracheobronchial tree. The patient inhales through the nose and exhales slowly and quietly through pursed lips. A forced exhalation can contribute to airway closure and negate the effect of the pursed-lip maneuver. Pursed-lip breathing can be used with diaphragmatic breathing and is a good way to make the patient more aware of slowing the respiratory rate and achieving more complete exhalation.

Physical Conditioning   A critical goal of management is to improve the patient's exercise tolerance. Through a program of regular activities and exercise, the patient can be assisted to participate comfortably in activities of daily living. Through physical activity and training to build exercise tolerance, patients may return to daily activities without severe shortness of breath and, most important, feeling better and more confident about themselves. Intensive programs, including efforts to improve exercise tolerance and reduce the work of breathing, are available in many settings. Many times the results of pulmonary function tests do not show significant improvement; however, improvement in the patient's sense of well-being and feelings of greater self-worth may be well worth the effort.

Patients with dyspnea related to a stable, chronic disorder may benefit greatly from a program that encourages walking, simple exercises, and relaxation techniques, and discourages a sedentary existence in either chair or bed. Incorporating controlled breathing and rest periods into a pattern of activity can enhance functional ability greatly.

Nutrition   Whenever dyspnea accompanies a chronic disease state such as emphysema or congestive heart failure, adequate nutritional intake becomes a focus of management. Adequate energy to carry out normal activities, to participate in social interactions, and to feel good about oneself depends in part on proper diet.

The patient may be experiencing problems with anorexia, epigastric distress, shortness of breath after eating, weight loss, or loss of energy. Attention to nutritional status may minimize or eliminate such complaints.

If a dietitian is available, the patient may be referred to her; however, the nurse should be prepared to provide information and guidance in proper food selection. A modified pattern of intake (six small meals) may be indicated. High-calorie, high-protein supplements may be appropriate. Use of less salt, more fruits and vegetables, substitution of fish for red meat all may be appropriate recommendations, depending on the patient's underlying condition.

Psychoemotional Counseling and Support Because dyspnea can be such a frightening symptom, most patients and families need time to talk about how they feel, and how to deal with fears and anxiety. Whether with one patient or with a group, the nurse can guide discussion to greater awareness of the cause of the symptom, and reinforce ways of controlling it.

Fear of dyspnea may reduce significantly the patient's ability to engage in physical activities, and therefore the ability to pursue or maintain social contacts. The patient and his family may be assisted to deal with this fear through education about the reason for the dyspnea, instructions on pursed-lip and diaphragmatic breathing, and relaxation techniques. Although it is not sufficient to tell the patient to use "mind over matter" in attaining a breathing pattern to minimize dyspnea, he should however believe in his own role in controlling it.

Some patients and families may find that a self-help group helps them to deal with the frustrations of chronic symptoms or disease. The opportunity to express such feelings and to share with those who have similar concerns can be an important source of support and encouragement.

Patient and Family Education Patient education plays a critical role in management of the patient with chronic dyspnea. Patient and family members need to know that dyspnea is a symptom of difficult breathing. It does not cause the difficulty, nor is the feeling harmful in itself. Dyspnea does not make lung or heart disease worse.

The patient should know that some dyspnea may be good, that some dyspnea can indicate exercise to tolerance, which is always a goal, especially in the presence of chronic heart and lung disease.

MANAGEMENT OF DYSPNEA THAT OCCURS AS A NEW SYMPTOM

Onset of Dyspnea

When dyspnea is a new symptom, management will be directed at treating the underlying cause and restoring the patient's usual state of health.

Severe or acute dyspnea can be frightening for the nurse and the patient. To be most effective, the nurse must have a plan of care in mind, be aware of his or her own reactions to the severe respiratory distress, and calmly and efficiently carry out clinical actions designed to provide relief for the patient. Such actions may also include attention to the family, who may become alarmed at seeing a member in such acute distress.

Several activities need to be carried out for the acutely dyspneic patient:

Maintain a clear airway. If the secretions are a problem, assist the patient to cough or initiate suction of the upper airway to maintain clear airways.

Allow the patient to assume a position that is most comfortable for breathing. The patient may want his elbows propped on a table or other surface. Or he may need to lean forward to promote optimum ventilation and assist in clearing secretions.

Encourage the patient to practice controlled diaphragmatic breathing, if he is familiar with the procedure. (This is not, however, the time to teach the technique.)

Anticipate the need to initiate oxygen or bronchodilator therapy. There may be a standard protocol or procedure to begin such therapy; otherwise, the patient will need to be referred to a physician.

Stay with the patient as much as possible. Maintain a calm, positive approach. A quiet and reassuring manner will assist the patient to begin to relax. It may have a similar effect on the family. A cool, calm environment is a critical aspect of treatment.

Conserve the patient's energy for work of breathing. Anticipate needs. Avoid requiring the patient to talk or move more than is minimally necessary.

Avoid the use of tranquilizers or sedatives. Pursue activities and treatments directed at the cause of the dyspneic attack.

Monitor respiratory rate and effort continuously, evaluating the patient's response to treatment. Lack of response to initial treatment may indicate the need for more aggressive therapy.

Increased Dyspnea Related to Acute Exacerbation of Symptoms of an Underlying Disease

The patient with chronic respiratory or cardiac disease may report an increase in the severity of dyspnea while on an established treatment schedule. Examine all aspects of the treatment regimen to determine adherence to such things as medication schedules, exercise prescriptions, and nutritional intake. It may be that one or more aspects of the

regimen is being neglected—a bronchodilator taken b.i.d. rather than the prescribed q.i.d., heart medication taken p.r.n. rather than every day. Tightening or "fine-tuning" an existing program may promote relief of the dyspnea. The patient very well may need support and encouragement to carry out the program in its entirety.

If the current treatment regimen is no longer providing symptom control or an acute process is evident (respiratory infection, cardiac failure), definitive (i.e., medical) treatment will need to be initiated. Anticipate the need to teach the patient about new medication or other modifications of the present treatment regimen.

Cough

Cough is an explosive expiratory maneuver that helps to protect the tracheobronchial tree from the entry of foreign substances or the accumulation of bronchopulmonary secretions. Normally, a cough is taken for granted; however, habitual cough is not a normal phenomenon and deserves careful assessment and appropriate intervention. Cough is a critical part of the normal airway clearance mechanism. It is a back-up to the mucociliary elevator. In most persons, cough is acute and self-limiting, as in the presence of an acute upper respiratory infection. Cough that is chronic and persistent usually is due to chronic bronchitis or other chronic respiratory disorders.

MECHANISMS OF COUGH

Each cough involves a reflex arc that begins with irritation of a receptor in the respiratory tract. Once started, it proceeds in a fixed pattern from receptor to central "cough center" to expiratory musculature.[4]

There are three phases to the cough mechanism. First, there is a deep inspiration that permits rapid entry of large amounts of air into the lungs. Next is the compressive phase, which begins with closure of the glottis and active contraction of the expiratory muscles. The result is an increase in intrathoracic pressure sufficient to produce the flow rates necessary for effective cough.

It is during the third, expiratory phase that the function of the cough is carried out with the coordinated movements of the glottis, respiratory muscles, and tracheobronchial tree. When the glottis opens, there is explosive release of the trapped intrathoracic air. The muscles of the thorax and abdomen further contract to maintain high pressures and therefore high flow.

The significance of thoracic and abdominal muscle contraction in producing an effective cough can be seen in patients with a tracheotomy or vocal cord paralysis. Such patients can cough quite effectively despite the inability to achieve glottic closure.

With the combination of high intrathoracic pressures and high flow, secretions are removed first from the larger airways. With successive coughs they are moved from the smaller bronchi into the larger ones. After another deep breath and series of coughs, the secretions, even from small airways, can be eliminated.

Not every cough is effective, however. There are many pathologic conditions that lead to an ineffective cough by interfering with the inspiratory or expiratory phases of cough, or both.[4] Pain, weakness, or central nervous system (CNS) depression can limit inspiratory and expiratory efforts. COPDs are characterized by reduced expiratory flow rates and, therefore, expiratory cough effort. Similarly, an endobronchial lesion, foreign

body, bronchospasm, or secretions can also reduce expiratory effort.

CAUSES OF COUGH

Cough can be produced by a multiplicity of disorders in a variety of anatomical locations.[4,6] Environmental irritants may cause cough by irritating receptors in the larynx, trachea, or bronchi. Smoking, by far the most common offender, produces chronic, persistent cough in two ways. As a bronchial irritant, it triggers the cough reflex directly. More importantly, it can produce inflammatory changes and large amounts of secretions that stimulate receptors in the trachea and bronchi. Cigarette smokers who inhale have a higher prevalence of cough than either pipe smokers or cigar smokers. One study of over 200 persons with chronic cough who stopped smoking showed that 77% reported eventual complete disappearance of cough, with 17% noting considerable improvement.[4]

Inhalation of allergens is a common cause of cough in asthma. In this case, cough frequently is associated with wheezing and dyspnea. Allergens also may produce cough by stimulating receptors outside the respiratory tract. Irritants to the nose may stimulate cough alone, or, more commonly, sneeze and cough.

Receptors in the trachea and bronchi may be stimulated by aspiration from pharyngeal or gastrointestinal disorders, an infectious disorder, or mass lesion. Indeed, cough occurs in 70% to 90% of patients with bronchogenic carcinoma sometime during the course of their disease.[4]

Disorders of the upper respiratory tract (nose, pharynx, and paranasal sinuses), external auditory canal, and eardrum produce cough by stimulating receptors outside the lower respiratory tract. Similarly, cough receptors may be triggered by disorders of the diaphragm, pleura, pericardium, and stomach.

By far the most common cause of transient cough is the common cold. Chronic cough, on the other hand, may be the result of allergic rhinitis, chronic sinusitis, nasal polyps, enlarged adenoids, or infected tonsils.

Somewhat common in children and adolescents is the psychogenic cough "tic." In adults, psychogenic cough may cause severe paroxysms of cough that last for hours and produce physical exhaustion.

NURSING ASSESSMENT

Although cough is a common occurrence of everyday living, constant cough warrants investigation. Frequent or persistent coughing may be a sign of serious respiratory disease.[3,12,13]

SUBJECTIVE DATA

Description of the Complaint

Have the patient describe the character of the cough. Is it a constant hacking due to throat irritation? Does cough occur upon arising? Does it disturb sleep?

Chronology: Onset

Determine the onset and course of the cough, identifying day, month, or year as closely as possible. A chronic cough is any cough that persists for a month or longer—even if it occurs only upon arising or lying down at the end of the day. Determine if the cough has been stable or if there has been a pattern to the severity of the symptom.

Setting: Precipitating Factors

Determine the factors that induce the cough. By far the most common factor is smoking, although the patient may not identify it as

such. Determine whether a particular environment stimulates the cough—the dust in a work setting or the fumes of a cleaning agent. Does cold air precipitate coughing? Does the cough vary with changes in the seasons? If so, what is that pattern?

Associated Symptoms

Determine if the cough is the solitary complaint or if other symptoms are present. Are there signs of an upper respiratory infection, an allergic response, or chest pain? Is there associated dyspnea and fatigue? Has there been recent weight loss?

Is the cough productive or nonproductive? What is the color, consistency, and amount of sputum? Has there been a recent change that might suggest an infectious process?

Are the episodes of coughing associated with eating or drinking, especially fluids? Is there gastric distention or nausea?

Alleviating Factors

What actions relieve the severity or frequency of the cough (e.g., leaving a dusty environment, using air conditioning or a furnace filter to remove particles in the air)?

Do coughing and deep-breathing techniques assist in removing secretions and thereby reduce coughing episodes?

Determine the medications that the patient uses. Are they prescription drugs such as a bronchodilator or antibiotic? Has he tried OTC medications? (If so, which ones and with what frequency?)

OBJECTIVE DATA

Observation and Inspection

Ask the patient to cough voluntarily and note the character of the cough. Is the cough wet, coarse, brassy, or self-propagating? Such characteristics often are associated with the productive cough of tracheobronchial disease. Is the cough more of a throat-clearing maneuver, as in post-nasal drip?

Inspect the sputum for color, consistency, and amount. Observe the amount of effort required to clear secretions from the airways. Does the patient accomplish this with minimal effort, or does he become fatigued or dyspneic?

Palpation

Identify or locate areas of chest wall tenderness associated with forceful coughing. Determine if the pain represents muscle spasm or fatigue. Rib fractures with excessive coughing are possible, but rare.

Percussion

Dullness on percussion may assist in localizing areas of consolidation and retained secretions.

Auscultation

In the presence of a productive cough, auscultate lung fields to evaluate cough effectiveness or the patient's ability to clear secretions. Many times rhonchi will clear with deep coughing.

Paraclinical Data

Laboratory data may be useful to confirm a specific diagnosis. A sputum culture or Gram's stain may reveal an infectious process. A complete blood count may be helpful in differentiating an allergic disorder from an infectious process.

Data from a chest x-ray may suggest either a pulmonary or cardiac disorder as the cause of the cough.

NURSING DIAGNOSIS

Cough can be analyzed in the same fashion as dyspnea (see Table 17-2). For the patient in a usual, stable state, coughing occurs as part of

the normal protective act, clearing the tracheobronchial tree of mucus and irritants. On the other hand, cough may represent a new symptom or a significant increase in frequency or effort in a patient's usual, stable state.

COUGH IN THE PRESENCE OF THE PATIENT'S USUAL STATE

Cough Related to Usual Airway Clearance

The healthy patient probably will be unaware of any cough activity. Processes of airway clearance will be unnoticed, except for an occasional cough to clear water, food, or an irritant.

Cough Related to the Need to Maintain Airway Patency in the Presence of Chronic Sputum Production

The patient with stable COPD will consciously use effective coughing techniques to facilitate airway clearance. Such patients can maintain their usual state in the presence of chronic disease, through regular and meticulous attention to airway clearance techniques.

COUGH AS A NEW SYMPTOM OR INCREASE IN SEVERITY FROM A STABLE STATE

Onset of Cough Related to Disease Process or Presence of Irritant

For the healthy person, the onset of a cough usually accompanies a transient upper respiratory infection and is self-limiting, or, the cough may signal the presence of or accompany other pulmonary and nonpulmonary disorders.

Those who smoke may be truly unaware of their cough or dismiss it as unimportant.

In a purely clinical sense, such patients experience chronic cough. For the patient, however, to acknowledge or become aware of the symptom is a new experience that requires that patient to reevaluate what he considers his usual "healthy" state.

Increased Cough Frequency and Effort with Difficulty Clearing Secretions

Determine whether there is significant increase in cough frequency and sputum production in the patient with stable chronic disease. Such changes almost always accompany exacerbation of the symptoms of the underlying disease because of an infectious process. The presence of dyspnea, cough, and sputum production may represent a serious threat to the patient's ability to carry out activities of daily living.

MANAGEMENT

Management of cough is designed to ensure optimal clearance of the airways, whether the cough is a spontaneous, reflex maneuver or part of a bronchial hygiene program. Many nursing interventions aim at decreasing the symptom, increasing the patient's ability to tolerate the symptom, and assisting him to use cough to the best advantage.[3,6,12,13]

COUGH THAT OCCURS IN THE PRESENCE OF THE USUAL STABLE STATE

The cough may go unnoticed, be dismissed as a minor irritation, or be part of an overall program of pulmonary hygiene.

Cough Related to Usual Airway Clearance

Because cough is a normal, protective reflex in healthy people, clinical management usually does not become an issue. Cough that accompanies strenuous exertion or other activity usually has a readily identifiable source, that can be avoided, eliminated, or tolerated briefly. Cough associated with the hyperventilation and transient pharyngeal and tracheobronchial irritation of vigorous activity can be relieved with rest and a drink of water or other soothing liquid. Leaving a close, smoke-filled room may relieve cough associated with that source of irritation. Under these circumstances, cough is a natural event and a part of the normal protective mechanism of the lung.

Cough Related to Need to Maintain Airway Patency in the Presence of Chronic Sputum Production

Management of cough in the patient with chronic sputum is designed to promote effective airway clearance while minimizing the effort and nuisance of cough activity.

Teaching or reinforcing coughing techniques may seem mundane and time-consuming, but ultimately may save the time and money of additional health care. Controlled coughing depends on the patient taking as deep a breath as possible. After inhaling a slow, deep breath through the nose, the patient should cough two or three times in a row, without breathing between the coughs. The patient should then relax, inhale, and exhale fully at least three times before repeating the cough sequence. The goal is controlled coughing to clear secretions. Forceful, violent coughing may precipitate uncontrolled coughing and collapse of small airways.

The patient may be able to keep secretions thinner, and therefore easier to raise, by drinking at least 2 liters of fluid a day, unless this is contraindicated medically.

Although usually reserved for inpatient treatment, postural drainage and percussion, along with effective, controlled coughing, may assist the patient to maintain clear airways in the presence of chronic sputum production.

Stress the importance of the need for the patient to monitor sputum for signs of infection. Increase or decrease in amount, or change of color of sputum to green or yellow, usually indicates the presence of an infectious process. The patient should be able to describe when to contact a health care professional for suspected infection. If the patient is given a prescription for an antibiotic, be sure he knows to start the medication when symptoms of respiratory infection (e.g., sore throat, change in sputum amount or color, fever, and malaise) develop.

COUGH AS A NEW SYMPTOM OR INCREASE IN SEVERITY FROM A STABLE STATE

A goal of management is to control, minimize, or eliminate cough and restore the patient's usual state of health.

Onset of Cough Related to Disease Process or Presence of an Irritant

Onset of cough frequently is related to upper respiratory infection. In most patients the cough will be self-limiting and can be treated with soothing liquids, rest, and saline gargle. Avoid cough suppressants, except in the presence of a nonproductive, irritative cough.

The patient with a severe upper respiratory infection, with frequent cough and sputum production, may be amenable to consider the need to stop smoking. The best cough suppressant in this case is removal of that which causes it.

Effective coughing, which clears the airways with the least amount of patient effort, is the goal when the cough is productive. Inspect the sputum for color, consistency, and amount for signs of infection. The presence of yellow or green sputum almost always indicates an acute infectious process. Anticipate starting the patient on antibiotic therapy by established protocol or referral to a physician. It is essential that the patient understand not only the name, dose, and side-effects of the medication, but also the length of time the medication should be taken. Inadequate treatment of an upper respiratory infection can result in reinfection, and significantly, exacerbation of symptoms of COPD.

Onset of cough also may signal the presence of a disease such as lung cancer or tuberculosis. Patients may need information and support while undergoing the diagnostic process to medical diagnosis.

Increased Cough Frequency and Effort Related to Difficulty Clearing Secretions

Difficulty clearing secretions because of ineffective cough or increased amount and thickness of secretions can result in increased cough frequency and effort. Patients with chronic lung or heart disease may experience exacerbation of symptoms such as dyspnea, fatigue, and activity intolerance when confronted with such increased work to clear airways. Similarly, patients with chest pain, chest wall deformity, and neurologic dysfunction may be unable to clear secretions adequately in the presence of an upper respiratory infection. Such patients need prompt meticulous attention to airway clearance.

A program of bronchial hygiene may include postural drainage, chest percussion, humidity therapy, inhaled bronchodilator therapy, or airway suctioning.

Postural drainage is a technique that promotes removal of secretions by taking advantage of gravity. Various upright, head-down, and side-to-side positions are used to

---

facilitate removal of secretions. The positions selected are based on chest assessment of the location of the secretions. The head-down position may not be tolerated by the dyspneic patient. The patient should use controlled coughing in the sitting position and at the end of the postural drainage treatment.

Percussion of the chest during postural drainage may help loosen mucus plugs. The cupped hand is used to "clap" the chest while the patient takes deep breaths in the drainage position. Controlled coughing is used in the same way as with postural drainage. Potentially the greatest benefit from a bronchial hygiene program is obtained by delivering the inhaled bronchodilator and humidity *before* instituting postural drainage techniques.

The energy required to participate in bronchial hygiene techniques can be considerable. Careful assessment of the patient's tolerance of activities of daily living as well as treatment activities is necessary so that maximum benefit is gained from airway clearance techniques.

A worthy goal is to capitalize on effective deep-breathing and coughing activities to minimize uncontrolled, exhausting coughing episodes.

EVALUATION OF THE MANAGEMENT OF DYSPNEA AND COUGH

Management of dyspnea and cough should be accompanied by on-going evaluation of the patient's progress, if possible, and final determination of the effects of treatment. Such evaluation activities can guide future care of a patient or group of patients, and justify nursing intervention to patients, the institution, or regulatory agencies, and third-party payers.

It may be appropriate to document certain aspects of the care process; that is, that the patient was taught diaphragmatic breathing, that a prescription was given, or that the patient was referred to a particular physician.

Determine the patient's response to the treatment plan. For instance, documentation such as "reports that episodes of dyspnea have resolved" and "describes increased participation in activities of daily living" indicate positive outcomes of therapy.

Regular documentation of patient care, especially patient progress toward identified outcomes, provides evidence of the quality of that care. Such objective data become the basis for continuing or modifying the plan of care, and more importantly, for promoting individualized care delivery. The method of evaluation is not as important as the commitment to making certain that it occurs.

SUMMARY

Dyspnea and cough are common symptoms reported by patients with a variety of underlying disorders. Both can be fatiguing, embarrassing, inconvenient, and otherwise bothersome.

Knowledge of the usual pathophysiological mechanisms of dyspnea and cough can guide careful assessment and diagnosis of the patient's specific health care problem. Management should reflect careful selection of nursing interventions that address the particular care needs. Ongoing and terminal evaluation will reveal the extent to which an optimal level of functioning was achieved by the patient with either or both symptoms.

REFERENCES

1. Banyai AL, Levine ER: Dyspnea: Diagnosis and treatment. Philadelphia, FA Davis, 1963
2. Bartow RE: Coping with emphysema: A field study. Respiratory Care 24:913,1979

3. Hietpas BG, Roth RD, Jensen WM: Huff coughing and airway patency. Respiratory Care 24:710, 1979
4. Irwin RS, Rosen MJ, Braman SS: Cough: A comprehensive review. Arch Intern Med 137:1186, 1977
5. Harrison BDW: Breathlessness. Br J Hosp Med 19, No. 2:112, 1978
6. Lagerson J: The cough—its effectiveness depends on you. Respiratory Care 24:142, 1979
7. Luisada AA: The differential diagnosis of dyspnea. Hosp Med 38:45, 1975
8. MacDonnell RJ: Suggestions for establishment of pulmonary rehabilitation programs. Respiratory Care 26:966, 1981
9. Moser KM: Evaluation of the dyspneic patient. In Shibel EM, Mosers KM (eds): Respiratory Emergencies. St. Louis, CB Mosby, 1977
10. Rapaport E: Dyspnea, pathophysiology and differential diagnosis. Prog Cardiovasc Dis 13:532, 1971
11. Rifas EM: Dyspnea. Nursing 80, 10:34, 1980
12. Smith SJ: Clinical Assessment of the Pulmonary Patient. In Traver GA (ed): Respiratory Nursing. New York, John Wiley & Sons, 1982
13. Traver GA: Patients with ineffective airway clearance. In Traver GA: Respiratory Nursing. New York, John Wiley & Sons, 1982
14. Webber–Jones JE, Bryant MK: Over-the-counter bronchodilators. Nurs 80, 10:34, 1980
15. Whitelaw WA: The respiratory pump. In Guenter CA, Welch MH (eds): Pulmonary Medicine, 2nd ed. Philadelphia, JB Lippincott, 1982
16. Zelechowski GP: Physiological and Psychological Implications of Dyspnea. Respiratory Therapy: 7:18, 1977

BIBLIOGRAPHY

Chronic obstructive pulmonary disease, 5th ed. New York, American Lung Association, 1981

Comroe JH: Physiology of respiration, 2nd ed., p. 259–263. Chicago, Year Book Medical Publishers, 1974

Harper RW: A guide to respiratory care. Philadelphia, JB Lippincott, 1981

Luckman J, Sorenson KC: Medical–Surgical Nursing, 2nd ed. Philadelphia, WB Saunders, 1980

Moeckly M, Kile M: The psychosocial assessment. In Traver GA (ed): Respiratory Nursing. New York, John Wiley & Sons, 1982

Moeckly M, Kile M: Caring intervention. In Traver, GA: Respiratory Nursing. New York, John Wiley & Sons, 1982

18

Allergy

E. Suzanne McAuliffe

Allergy is a common yet difficult health problem that nurses manage in a variety of settings. Ten percent to twenty percent of the population is affected by allergies. The exact causes of allergies are not known. Various theories have been put forth to explain why certain people react strongly to some substances whereas others do not react at all. Even the pathology of the allergic reaction is poorly understood and is under current investigation.

There seems to be a genetic predisposition to allergies. If one parent has allergies of a genetic basis, each child has a 50% chance of developing an allergy. Heredity also may determine the type of allergy and the substance to which the person is allergic. Allergic sensitivities also can be acquired across the placenta during prenatal life.

Even though heredity and congenital environment play an important part in development of allergies, the critical factor is the contact between the person and the allergy-producing substance. If a person who is at risk for developing an allergy is in contact with various substances, and factors such as psychological or physical stress are introduced, it may upset the person's homeostatic balance and lead to an allergic response.

The *allergic response* is a variation or exaggerated response of the body's normally efficient immune system. The immune system functions to protect the person from invasion by harmful internal and external forces. The allergic response is an overreaction of the immune system to a usually harmless substance, for example, plant pollens and animal danders, and that response is potentially harmful to the host.

DEFINITIONS

Several definitions are necessary to provide a common understanding of the language and concepts of the allergic response. The word *allergy* describes a hypersensitive state initiated by a substance that is usually innocuous to most people. The *hypersensitive state* is acquired through an initial exposure (defined as *sensitization* to a specific substance) with subsequent reexposure to that substance producing an altered or exaggerated allergic reaction. Although the term *hypersensitivity* is preferred by some allergists, most people use the terms *allergy* and *hypersensitivity* interchangeably.

Substances that can cause an allergic reaction are usually proteins and are called *allergens.* Some nonprotein allergens are found among plant oils and nonprotein drugs. Allergens are presented to the body's immune system by inhalation (plant pollens), ingestion (food, drugs), skin contact (soaps, plants), infection (bacteria, viruses) and injection (insect venom, drugs). In addition to external allergens, the body can also react to its own tissue when that tissue has been altered physically or chemically. This form of allergy to one's own tissues or organs, *autoallergens,* plays an important role in development of autoimmune diseases.

The term *allergen* frequently is used synonomously with the term *antigen.* An *antigen* is a substance capable of stimulating the immune response. The distinction is that an antigen (or *immunogen*) typically initiates the immune response in most people, whereas an allergen initiates an atypical immune or allergic response in a person previously sensitized to the normally harmless substance.

The body responds to antigens by producing cells and antibodies that recognize and help to eliminate or neutralize the antigens. *Antibodies* are protein substances synthesized by the body, and are found in the gamma globulin portion of serum. There are five major classes of antibodies, called *immunoglobulins.* Each of the five immunoglobulin classes is named by using a letter and an abbreviation for the word immunoglobulin (Ig). These classes are: IgG, IgM, IgA, IgD, and IgE. Each immunoglobulin has a specific role in the immune and allergic responses of the person.

The term *atopy* is used interchangeably with the terms *hypersensitivity* or *allergy.* Technically, the term *atopy* refers to an allergic reaction that involves the specific immunoglobulin, IgE. Atopic people are those who respond to allergens by producing large amounts of IgE and who suffer the effects of

an immediate, exaggerated allergic response. The atopic reaction is also called an *anaphylactic reaction* and can range from a mild local reaction at the site of contact with the allergen, to a systemic response that can rapidly progress to shock and death.

The nature and magnitude of the allergic response of the person to a foreign substance or protein depends on many factors. The specific type of allergen, the concentration of the allergen, the route or site of presentation, the type of antibody involved, the type of tissue or organ affected, toxic substances released by the allergic reaction, and local or systemic responses to the reaction all play important roles in each allergic response. These factors, in combination with the genetic, congenital, physical, and psychological states of the individual, determine the response to a potential allergen.

There are various ways of classifying and describing allergic responses. Gell and Coombs developed a classic framework for explaining and describing allergic reactions.[1] The four categories are

Type I: Anaphylactic or immediate hypersensitivity
Type II: Cytotoxic reactions
Type III: Immune complex mediated reactions
Type IV: Delayed hypersensitivity

The Gell and Coombs' framework is used as an organizing structure throughout this chapter and will be described in more detail in the pathophysiology section.

LIMITATIONS

Allergies are a problem throughout life and can start even *in utero* (e.g., *erythroblastosis fetalis*). Infancy and early childhood are fraught with allergic episodes and substances. Sensitization frequently leads to lifelong allergy problems. The topic of childhood allergy will be mentioned only as it relates to adult allergy. We will focus primarily on the allergy problems of adults.

The field of allergy and its diagnosis and treatment is an area that lends itself to collaborative work between physicians and nurses. For the purposes of an adequate understanding of allergy and its treatment, the pathophysiological mechanisms, diagnosis, and management will be discussed, including medical as well as nursing responsibilities. The emphasis of this chapter, however, will be nursing implications and the collaborative nature of the health care team activities.

ADVERSE REACTIONS

Reactions that are adverse and exaggerated may be labeled idiosyncratic, intolerant or functional reactions. *Idiosyncratic reactions* are not clearly understood and are highly individualized reactions, in which the person experiences a qualitatively different reaction than would normally be expected to a food or a drug, based on an alteration in the way the person handles the substance. For example, the very young (or the very old) may become agitated with the administration of barbiturates, yet amphetamines serve to slow down the hyperactive child. There is no evidence of an immunologic basis for idiosyncratic reactions.

Intolerance refers to the undesirable toxic effects from substances well tolerated by the general population. Certain persons are extremely susceptible to expected side-effects of drugs. Examples include extreme, prolonged somnolence in response to antihistamines or sedatives, and unexpected agitation following a stimulant such as caffeine. There is no evidence of involvement of the immune system or an allergic response in these intolerant episodes.

Functional reactions usually involve an exaggerated response of the autonomic nervous system. For example, vasomotor congestion and rhinitis can occur in response to cold, fumes, or cigarette smoke. An exaggerated gastrocolic reflex can cause gas and cramping, leading to gastrointestinal motility that may mimic allergic symptoms but are without involvement of the immune system and are truly functional.

Nonimmunologic adverse reactions occur in isolated persons and are distinguished from allergic reactions by the lack of antibodies or sensitized cells of the usual immune or allergic response. The underlying mechanisms have not been well defined but account for many hospital admissions and 15% of reactions of patients receiving drug therapy. Many of these adverse reactions are the results of side-effects, overdosage, or combinations of a number of drugs. Without an immunologic component of the exaggerated reaction, an attempt is made to explain the adverse reaction through the terms idiosyncratic, intolerant, or functional reaction.

MECHANISMS OF ALLERGIES

The immune system assists the person in the complex process of adapting to the environment. Environmental chemicals, viruses, bacteria, fungi, and parasites greatly affect a person's responses and sensitivities to substances in one's surroundings. Variables, such as genetic predisposition, age, and state of health also affect the individual's immune status. Poor health, early childhood, and old age are all conditions that decrease the effectiveness of the immune response and lead to an increased risk of infection.

The immune process not only serves to protect the person from external threats (i.e., microorganisms), but from potential internal threats as well. In addition to eliminating or neutralizing harmful substances, the immune system assists in the regulation of abnormal cellular growth (tumor cells) and the removal of senescent cells through cellular metabolism.

Deficiencies in the immune system can lead to poor or inadequate immune responses, as in the case of immunodeficient diseases. Abnormalities in the immune system can lead to immunity to one's own cells, autoimmune diseases, or to exaggerated responses such as allergy and hypersensitivity to usually noninjurious substances.

IMMUNE SYSTEM ORGANS AND FUNCTIONS

Many cells, tissues, and organs are involved in the complex activities of the immune response (Fig. 18-1). The bone marrow, thymus gland, lymph nodes, spleen, and gut-associated tissues (tonsils, appendix, and Peyer's patches of the small intestine) are the major organs and tissues involved in the immune processes of mammals. The bone marrow forms the basic cell (*stem cell*) from which the specific cells of the immune process mature and develop, or differentiate. Stem cells then differentiate into lymphocytes and other cells. The thymus gland, located in the mediastinum, helps to develop fully immunocompetent cells called *T cells*. The thymus also secretes many hormones and eliminates lymphocytes that might react against the person's own cells. *Lymph nodes* are specialized tissue found throughout the body, which localize and attempt to prevent the spread of infection. Lymph nodes function as filters, housing a network of many types of lymphocytes through which the blood, other lymphocytes, and antigenic substances must pass. The *spleen* is a lymphoid organ in the abdomen that filters and processes lymphocytes and antigens in the blood. The gut-associated tissue may play a part in the differentiation of stem cells into B cells.

CELLS OF THE IMMUNE SYSTEM

The cells of the immune system include lymphocytes, phagocytic cells, basophils, and mast cells. Lymphocytes are divided mainly into the *B cells* (bursal) and *T cells* (thymic).

FIG. 18-1 *Cellular development in the immune system.*

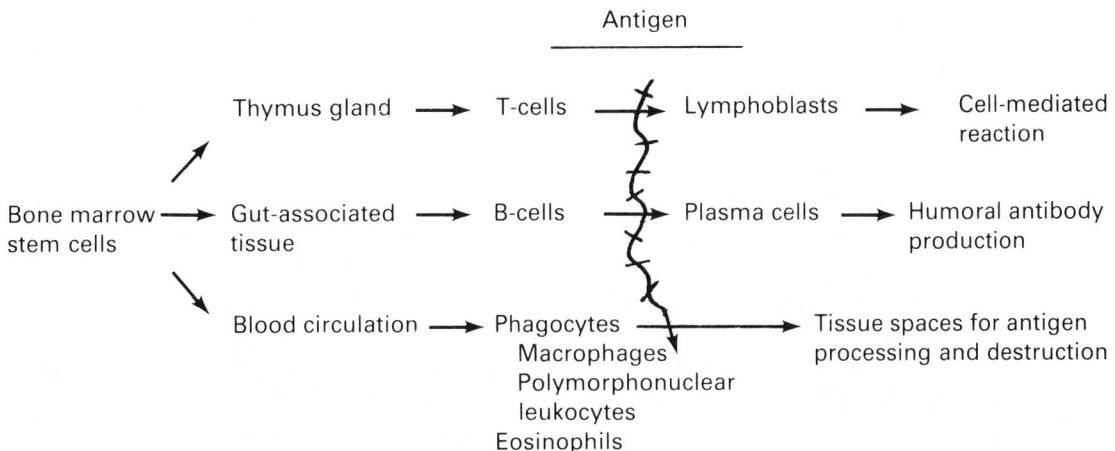

The B cells become plasma cells, which produce antibodies (immunoglobulins). The T cells may develop further into T-helper cells (T_H), T-suppressor cells (T_S), or T-killer cells (T_K). Sensitized T cells can react directly with an antigen without the assistance of immunoglobulins.

Phagocytes are produced in the bone marrow and travel in the blood to tissue spaces. The phagocytes pass through capillary walls in response to chemical factors released by the inflammatory process; these chemical factors that attract the phagocytes are called *chemotactic factors*. Specific phagocytes such as macrophages, polymorphonuclear leukocytes, and eosinophils play slightly different yet interrelated roles in antigen engulfment and removal.

Basophils are found in the bloodstream, mast cells are found in tissue cells. When these cells are sensitized or changed by contact with an antigen, they release chemical substances such as histamine, serotonin, heparin, acetylcholine, and the slow-reacting substances of anaphylaxis. These chemical substances have a significant effect on the blood vessels and on the inflammatory response, causing many of the symptoms and discomforts associated with inflammation.

IMMUNE PROCESSES

The stem cells of the bone marrow are released into the bloodstream, some are processed by the thymus (T cells) and some by gut-associated tissues (B cells). These cells migrate to the lymph nodes, spleen, and gut-associated tissue, where they proliferate, differentiate, and mature in response to antigen stimulation. There are four different immune processes that can be activated by the immune response: humoral immunity, cell-mediated immunity, phagocytic immunity, and the complement system.

Humoral Immunity

Humoral immunity is mediated or controlled by antibodies and involves antigen–antibody reactions. B cells are responsible for the humoral immune response, which is mediated or controlled by antibodies. B cells are transformed into plasma cells that produce the antibodies (immunoglobulins). Structure and function of the immunoglobulins help to identify the site of activity and role in the immune process of each immunoglobulin (Table 18-1).

The most abundant immunoglobulin, IgG is found in the blood and extravascular spaces, diffuses easily into body tissue, and facilitates elimination of antigens. This is the only immunoglobulin that crosses the placenta and can provide protection to the fetus. Viruses and gram-positive organisms are particularly susceptible to IgG.

IgM plays a major role in the early humoral response. This immunoglobulin has the largest molecular size and is similar to IgG in function. IgM is effective against bacteria and stimulates macrophage ingestion of antigens.

IgA is the primary immunoglobulin of all mucosal surfaces and is present in all seromucous secretions (i.e., saliva, tears, respiratory, and gastrointestinal tract). The exact physiological function of IgA is not known, but it is thought to play a significant role in the body's first line of defense at the mucosal level.

IgD and IgE are present normally in small quantities; their function is also not well understood. They are found in the mucosa of respiratory and gastrointestinal tracts and are thought to be responsible for control of parasites and are involved in many allergic reactions. Although IgD has not been identified with a particular function, IgE has been found to mediate hypersensitivity and atopic reactions (i.e., dermatitis and asthma).

TABLE 18-1
IMMUNOGLOBULINS

IMMUNOGLOBULIN	BODY SITE	ACTIVITIES
IgG	Internal body fluids (extravascular)	Combats microorganisms and toxins in secondary immune response. Crosses placenta
IgA	Seromucous secretions and serum	Defends mucous membranes against microorganisms
IgM	Bloodstream	Defends against bacteria and infection in early humoral response
IgD	Small amounts in serum	Not well understood
IgE	Normally small amounts in serum	Combats parasitic and fungal infections. Atopic allergic reactions

Cell-Mediated Immunity

Cell-mediated immunity is responsible for host defense against viruses, fungi, tumor antigens, and intracellular organisms. T cells are responsible for cell-mediated immunity. In contrast to the antigen–antibody reaction of the humoral response, cell-mediated immunity occurs through immunocompetent T cells reacting in direct cell-to-cell contact, or by T cell production of soluble factors called *lymphokines*, which aid in the immunologic process. For example, lymphokines attract phagocytes, inhibit cell growth, and interfere with viral reproduction. The macrophage also plays an important part in cell-mediated immunity. Functions of the macrophage include processing antigen, phagocytosis, activating T cells, and responding to lymphokines.

Phagocytic Immunity

Phagocytes engulf and destroy foreign material as their contribution to host defense. Without phagocytes, there would be an increased occurrence of infection.

Complement System

The complement system is composed of 17 plasma proteins that are activated in sequence during specific kinds of immune responses. Complement proteins amplify the host defenses by assisting with phagocytosis, chemotaxis (attraction of specific chemicals), and cytolysis (cell breakdown). The complement system also can be activated by certain cells (*i.e.*, bacteria) and some immunoglobulins, allowing for host protection before the humoral (antibody) response has had a chance to start. Because of the role the complement system plays in releasing chemical substances from cells, the effects of many allergic responses are due to activation of this system.

IMMUNE RESPONSE

When an antigen enters the body through the skin and mucosal surfaces of the respiratory and gastrointestinal tracts, the local lymph nodes are the site of antibody production. If the antigen enters the bloodstream directly (e.g., by injection), the spleen is the usual site of antibody production. In both situations, the antigen may continue to stimulate both the regional and central lymphoid tissue, the lymph nodes, and spleen respectively. Upon contact with lymphoid tissue, the antigen is processed by the macrophages (phagocytes). This processing serves to present the antigen to certain lymphocytes that will then react with the antigen. This reaction causes an increase in the number of certain lymphocytes and stimulates B cells to become antibody-producing plasma cells. The T cells may function as "helper cells" for B-cell functions. These activities cause the lymph nodes to become engorged with lymphocytes, to enlarge, and to start antibody production. The plasma cells within the lymph nodes secrete antibodies into the circulatory system for disseminated host defense.

The antigen–antibody complexes form a union and then either agglutinate (clump) or precipitate. Gradually, the antigen–antibody complexes are phagocytized and catabolized by the body.

The process, from initial antigen contact to production of antibodies, can take 5 to 7 days during the initial, primary response. During the initial immune response, certain lymphocytes become "memory" lymphocytes and retain the ability to respond to the specific antigen upon reexposure. The successive contacts with the antigen provide for a more rapid, increased response than the initial response. The memory function of the lymphocytes also provides a systemic immune response because the lymphocytes and antibodies circulate throughout the body. No matter where the second antigenic contact occurs, the immune system can respond because of the memory capability of the system.

The antigen–antibody reaction is specific, yet reversible, with factors such as pH,

temperature, and concentration greatly affecting the reaction. *Specificity* is the ability of the antibodies to react only with a specific antigen or with a substance that has virtually identical molecular structure to the antigen. The immune response occurs in the normally functioning immune system and small amounts of antibodies are constantly present in each person. Immunity also can be acquired artificially by immunizations.

Usually, the immune response is directed against foreign materials and not against the body's own cells. The body has the ability to recognize its own tissues and proteins and can become tolerant to substances occurring naturally in the environment. Thus, the immune system is normally protective, preserving the integrity and health of the person.

ALLERGIC RESPONSE

There is a vast range of antigens and foreign substances, from pollen to perfume, that can elicit an allergic response. The allergic response is an exaggerated, altered response of the immune system. These altered responses can cause tissue injury to the host. The classification of these harmful immune reactions by Gell and Coombs provides a useful way of organizing allergic reactions (Fig. 18-2).[1]

Type I: Anaphylactic or Immediate Hypersensitivity Reactions

Type I reactions are mediated by IgE antibodies fixed to the surfaces of mast cells. This reaction requires an initial contact between the antigen and the surfaces of mast cells and basophils, where the IgE antibodies are made and widely circulated throughout the body. When the antigen is subsequently reintroduced, the bridging interaction of the antigen with the IgE antibody on the mast cell causes the release of chemicals within

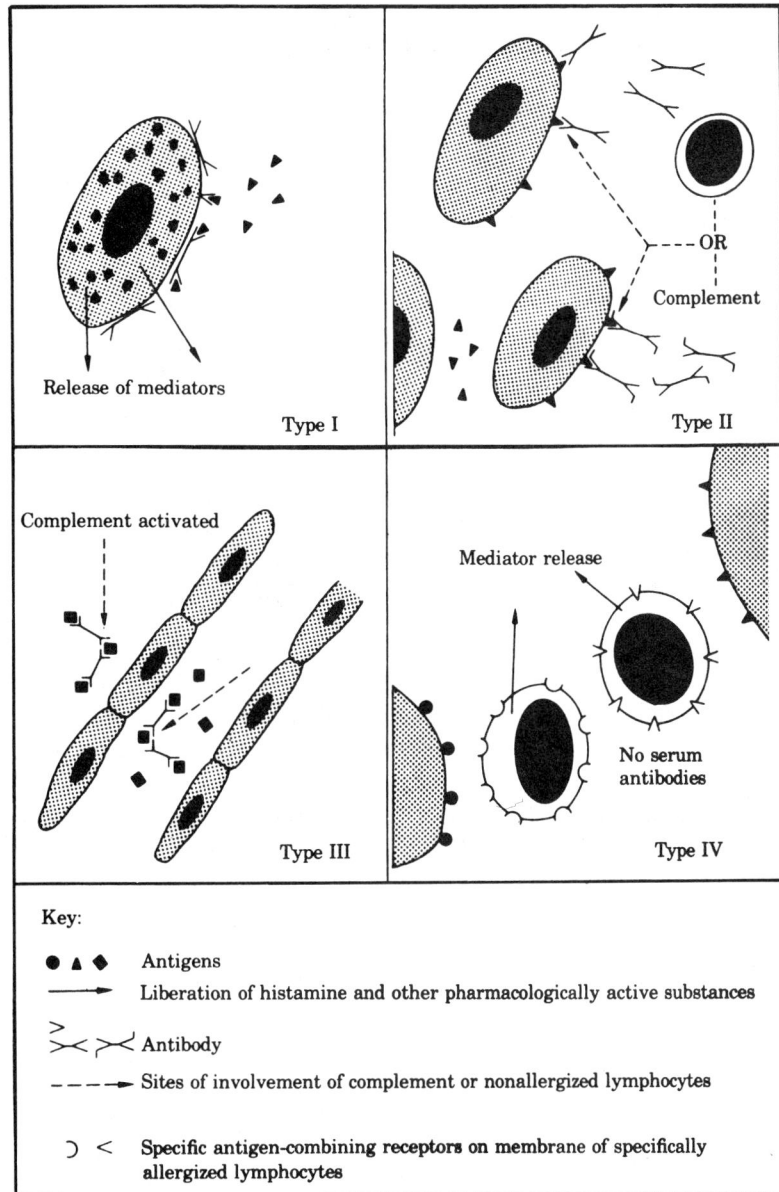

FIG. 18-2 *Classification of allergic reactions. (Hobart MJ, McConnell I (eds): Classification of Allergic Reactions, Appendix A, in The Immune System: A Course on the Molecular and Cellular Basis of Immunity. Oxford, Blackwell, 1975)*

Figure labels:
Release of mediators — Type I
OR — Complement — Type II
Complement activated — Type III
Mediator release — No serum antibodies — Type IV

Key:
● ▲ ◆   Antigens
———►   Liberation of histamine and other pharmacologically active substances
＞＜ ＞＜   Antibody
— — —►   Sites of involvement of complement or nonallergized lymphocytes
⊃ ＜   Specific antigen-combining receptors on membrane of specifically allergized lymphocytes

granules of the mast cell. Through a series of enzymatic steps initiated by the antigen–antibody union, the basophils and mast cells discharge their intracellular collection of

granules, a process called *degranulation*. After a few days, the mast cells recover from the degranulation process and function normally again. It is the degranulation process that releases the chemicals within the cell granules. These chemical mediators are

Histamine, the slow-reacting substance of anaphylaxis (SRSA)
Eosinophil chemotactic factor of anaphylaxis (ECF-A)
Neutrophil chemotactic factor of anaphylaxis (NCF-A)
Platelet-activating factor (PAF)
Heparin
Other chemically active substances

These chemical mediators are responsible for the inflammatory responses, such as muscle constriction, increased capillary permeability, dilation of venules, increased production and secretion of mucus, and attraction of lymphocytes. Specific biological activities of the chemical mediators are listed in Table 18-2.

The anaphylactic reactions may be small and localized, like itching and watering of the nose and eyes, if the dose of the antigen is small. Larger doses of antigens or intra-venous introductions into the previously sensitized person can result in a severe systemic reaction, such as hives or respiratory distress due to massive release of chemical mediators from basophils and mast cells.

Normally, all people have small amounts of IgE within their bodies. As was mentioned previously, IgE is the antibody formed in response to parasitic infections. Some individuals and families form the IgE antibodies in response to many naturally occurring substances like grasses, weed pollens, animal dander, house dust, mold spores, drugs, and insect venoms. It is not understood why certain people respond to substances usually tolerated by the general population.

Type II: Cytotoxic Reactions

The cytotoxic reactions involve circulating IgG and IgM antibodies, which bind with an antigen that is bound to the surface of a cell. The antigen–antibody union accelerates

TABLE 18-2
CHEMICAL MEDIATORS

CHEMICAL	ACTION
Histamine	Causes vasodilation Increases vascular permeability Constricts visceral and bronchial smooth muscle Increases respiratory gland mucus production Causes itching
Slow reacting substance of anaphylaxis (SRSA)	Constricts bronchial smooth muscle Causes vasodilation
Eosinophil chemotactic factor of anaphylaxis (ECF-A)	Attracts eosinophils to site of antigen–antibody reaction
Neutrophil chemotactic factor of anaphylaxis (NCF-A)	Attracts neutrophils
Platelet-activating factor (PAF)	Clumps and degranulates platelets
Heparin	Anticoagulant

phagocytosis or may activate the complement system that *lyses*, or kills the antigen-bound cell. If the antigen is bound to a bacterium, the immune system has performed beneficially; if the antigen has bound to one of the host's cells, then cellular destruction can be harmful to the host. In transfusion reactions or drug-induced hemolytic anemia, the red blood cells or drugs attached to the red blood cells are considered foreign by host antibodies. The antigen–antibody union activates the complement system, and the red blood cells are damaged or destroyed. The cellular contents are released into the bloodstream, creating the symptoms of hemoglobinemia, hemoglobinuria, and fever.

In contrast to mast cell and basophil degranulation, in which the cell remains alive and functioning, type II reactions result in destruction of the cells to which the antigens are bound.

Type III: Immune Complex Reactions

Type III reactions involve the development of immune complexes when antigens bind directly to antibodies. Usually, IgG is the antibody involved. These immune complexes usually are cleared from the system by phagocytosis; however, when sufficient quantities of antigen are present, the antigen–antibody immune complexes precipitate into various parts of the microvasculature of the kidney, skin, and joints. There may be sufficient quantities of immune complexes and complement proteins to activate the complement system and produce an inflammatory response. The inflammatory response produces local edema, vasculitis, and local tissue injury. Examples of this type of immune complex reaction are serum sickness, some types of nephritis, and certain types of bacterial endocarditis. It is important to note that the tissues that are injured because of immune complex deposition are not necessarily the tissues involved in the immune response. Specific sites such as the joints and kidneys are affected with immune complex precipitants by chance. Unlike other types of allergic response, this reaction can occur with the initial contact of an allergen if the dose is large enough and a large number of immune complexes are formed.

Type IV: Delayed Hypersensitivity

Type IV reactions are mediated by sensitized T cells. The T cells unite directly with the antigen and require 24 to 72 hours to reach maximal effectiveness. The antigen causes the sensitized T cells to release lymphokines that cause local inflammatory reactions, such as edema, redness, and tissue injury. The skin-test reaction of a person exposed to tuberculosis (TB) is the result of sensitized T cells interacting with the TB antigen and causing induration, redness, or necrosis of the test site after 24 to 72 hours. Allergic contact dermatitis is another example of a delayed cell-mediated response. The antigen on the skin interacts with the protein of the skin, causing sensitization of T cells, which then interact with the antigen in the skin. The cells of the skin are then damaged by the lymphokines released during the reaction, as demonstrated by reactions to poison ivy, certain metals, and cosmetics.

The type IV response is the body's main defense against mycobacteria, fungi, viruses, neoplasms, and transplanted tissues.

The Gell and Coombs classification is a useful way to classify and understand complex physiological activities. The four categories explain the majority of allergic reactions, although many details of the specific mechanisms are still in the investigational stage. There are also some reactions that defy explanation and do not fit neatly into a particular category. Advances in knowledge about allergic reactions require totally different approaches and explanations for these complex processes. Some scientists feel that the Gell and Coombs classification is too simple and insufficient to explain all the subtleties, but it is useful as a basic understanding of the various allergic reactions.

LATE PHASE REACTIONS

There has been recent documentation of what is termed a *late phase allergic reaction* (LPR), which is an immediate inflammatory reaction (1 to 15 min) followed by a later inflammatory response at 6 to 48 hours. Both immediate and late reactions are the result of mast cell degranulation and are not dependent on complement activation or immunoglobulin deposition. The late phase reactions can occur in skin, airways, and wherever there are mast cells. Clinically, the immediate wheal and flare (smooth, red raised area) of a skin test can progress to a LPR or erythema, induration, warmth, itching, and burning. The lungs manifest an immediate response of bronchospasm, edema, and mucus production, which may progress to a LPR of bronchospasm, mucus secretion, and inflammation.

The implications of LPR for practice are extremely important. The health caregiver needs to be aware of the type of allergic response occurring, and if the response involves mast cell degranulation, the possibility of a LPR exists. In addition, research studies indicate that the LPR is difficult to treat and is not as responsive to some commonly used drugs that are effective against immediate allergic reactions. Avoidance of a LPR seems to be preventive therapy with steroids. The steroids can alter the course of the inflammatory response and prevent the symptoms and distress of a LPR.

SOURCES OF ALLERGENS

One of the crucial components of the diagnostic work up of allergic disease is the determination of the allergen as well as its source. Some of the common sources include common airborne and environmental agents, drugs, foods, insect venoms, pathogens, and blood transfusions.

Airborne and Environmental

The air around us contains a large number of large and complex particles that can initiate an allergic reaction. Pollens (male reproductive structures of seed-producing plants) of weeds, grasses, and trees are common allergens. Most pollens are shed in the morning, but winds stir up pollen concentrations in the afternoon and early evening. Winds carry pollens for many miles, accounting for high pollen levels in urban areas.

Molds are common components of house dust and live in damp basements, bathrooms, humidifiers, vaporizers, soiled upholstery, food and garbage containers. Mold allergy symptoms are usually sporadic, since exposure and mold growth vary. High growth periods are during warm, moist summer and fall seasons (fallen leaves). Geographic prevalence of molds includes all areas except locales with subfreezing temperatures, high altitudes, or arid climates.

Animal dander (skin scales) is a common allergen that can lead to sensitization. The most common sources are dogs, cats, and fur or feathers used for stuffing pillows and furniture. Dander can accumulate in a house or other enclosed space and is easily disseminated by heating systems.

House dust is a composite of many airborne allergens, such as animal dander, indoor molds, vegetable fiber, food particles, insect parts, algae, and human dander. The amount of indoor particles depends upon the numbers of sources and the amount of circulating air that may dilute the concentration of particles. House-dust mites live on animal dander and are a common allergen found in mattresses, stuffed furniture, rugs, and pillows. The mite population peaks in September and October. Any part of the mite, whether dead or alive, is a potential allergen to a sensitized person.

Climate and air pollution affect the precipitation of allergic symptoms, particularly in those persons with respiratory hypersensitivity and symptoms. Sudden temperature changes, high humidity, and drops in barometric pressure can precipitate an asthma attack. Industrial pollutants, automobile emissions, and perfumes contain substances irritating to normal respiratory mucosa and can aggravate or initiate symptoms in a sensitive, asthmatic airway. Although tobacco smoke similarly acts as an irritant that can precipitate an allergic episode, it is unclear whether there is a true allergic response to tobacco smoke. Other irritants that can precipitate an IgE hypersensitivity reaction include chemicals (formaldehyde, kerosene, gasoline), wood smoke, and cooking odors.

Drugs

Drugs are small molecules called *haptens* that do not have antigenic properties by themselves. To initiate an allergic response, the drug hapten must combine with a carrier molecule, forming an allergen. Drug allergies are not dose-related and provoke a specific allergic response through antibody formation or sensitization of lymphocytes. As we discussed previously, many drug reactions are really side-effects, or toxic or idiosyncratic reactions. True drug allergies are rare, occurring in a small percentage of the population.

For drug allergy to exist there must be sensitization by exposure. Initial exposure usually does not produce a reaction and is followed by a latent period, with no ill effects caused by the drug. Allergic symptoms appear and recur on each subsequent drug administration. Symptoms usually dissipate 3 to 5 days after the drug is stopped. If a type I allergic reaction is involved, development of systemic anaphylaxis, particularly for injected drugs, is a concern. Drugs most commonly implicated in allergic reactions are the penicillins and sulfonamides.

Aspirin is frequently the cause of adverse reactions, but only rarely the cause of a true allergic reaction. There is an increased susceptibility to adverse aspirin reactions in people with allergic asthma and rhinitis. Similarly, local anesthetics frequently are known to cause toxic effects, but rarely a true allergic response. Radiographic contrast materials (dyes) create reactions, some of them disastrous, in 5% to 8% of the population. These reactions have not been demonstrated to be IgE-immediate hypersensitivity reactions, but an anaphylaxislike (anaphylactoid) response to nonimmune release of chemical mediators.

Insulin can create local and systemic allergic reactions. Local reactions (swelling, itching, pain) develop within a few weeks of the initiation of insulin therapy and resolve without treatment in weeks. Large local reactions may progress to a systemic reaction (urticaria or anaphylaxis). These usually appear when insulin therapy has been restarted, after a period of time without it.

Food

Any food can cause an allergic reaction, but raw foods are more allergenic than cooked foods. Some food additives and dyes also create adverse, sometimes allergic, reactions. Foods may cross-react and foods of similar food families (i.e., grains) may contain similar allergenic characteristics. Vomiting, diarrhea, bloating, and gastrointestinal pain are commonly found symptoms with a variety of disorders, not just food allergy. Infectious, metabolic, toxic, functional, and emotional causes need to be investigated carefully and ruled out in the diagnosis of food allergy.

Insects

Insect sting allergy (*Hymenoptera sensitivity*) can occur in people with no history of atopy. The allergic responses range from mild local reactions to fatal systemic responses. Most people react to an insect bite or sting with a sharp pain and reddening of the site, which resolves in 24 hours. An allergic reaction is usually large and contains IgE antibodies. A local reaction may progress to a systemic reaction merely from the toxic histaminelike substances in the insect venom. Systemic reactions may be limited to urticaria, or, within an hour of the sting, may progress rapidly to a severe systemic anaphylactic reaction. Delayed reactions (serum sickness, vasculitis, neurologic reactions, and coagulation disturbances) can occur hours to weeks after the sting. Secondary infections can complicate a sting reaction if the stinger is contaminated. Insect habitats and life cycles account for geographic and seasonal variations in exposure. Personal habits (*i.e.,* bright clothing, perfumes, outdoor hobbies) can increase exposure to and attract stinging and biting insects.

Miscellaneous Sources

Exposure to certain sensitizing agents can lead to a type IV delayed hypersensitivity reaction. Plants (poison ivy), metals and their salts (nickel), and chemicals in rubber compounds, drugs, cosmetics, perfumes, and dyes are the most common sources of allergic contact dermatitis.

Certain microorganisms and pathogens, in addition to initiating an immune response, also sensitize a person and lead to an allergic response to the pathogen. Occasionally, an individual also develops antibodies to their own cells, creating an autoallergic or autoimmune response. Any foreign protein or substance has the capability of sensitizing a susceptible person and creating an allergic reaction.

PSYCHOSOCIAL ASPECTS

The psychosocial aspects associated with allergy are as varied and complex as the allergic responses themselves. With a chronic allergic condition that persists over an extended period of time, the person deals with similar problems elicited by any chronic illness, as well as the pains and discomforts from the actual allergic reactions. In addition, the diagnosis and treatment regimens for allergies are often uncomfortable and may occur over long periods of time.

Chronic allergy can cause one to withdraw, become concerned about oneself, and lose interest in others. Areas of bodily concerns can become magnified when senses become heightened and distorted by focusing on an actual or potential allergic response. Once a person is not healthy physically, he is frequently exempt from certain roles and responsibilities. As activities are altered, social roles may change, potentially leading to altered self-esteem. A person who has the burden of a chronic health problem may be unable to perform activities in the usual manner and may suffer the psychological and physical deprivation of his usual lifestyle. Altered life-styles affect significant others as well, further stressing the allergic person.

The allergy itself or changes in life-style may lead to a myriad of reactions, from anxiety to anger or denial. Anxiety is a normal reaction to stress and may manifest itself physiologically or psychologically. The body's reactions to mild anxiety are viewed as beneficial because they promote learning and the ability to function; however, mild, moderate, or severe anxiety in the presence of a physiological stressor such as an allergic reaction may exaggerate or increase the distress and injury caused by the allergic reaction. For example, an allergic response in the respiratory tract can cause bronchospasm and dyspnea. Anxiety related to this allergic reaction and the dyspnea itself may increase the respiratory rate and the sensation of air hunger. The faster the person breathes, the more air is trapped behind the constricted airways, and the more short of breath the person becomes, creating a vicious cycle.

Anger is a normal reaction borne of frustration and is also a way of coping with anxiety. Anger can cause others to withdraw or fight back, creating situations that only increase a person's stress and anxiety. Anger may be displayed to persons or things that are not the real cause of the person's threat or fear. The angry person may exhibit hostile behavior toward the health caregiver or significant others. Alienation of these people will serve only to isolate and further threaten the person, rather than removing the cause of the anger.

Another method of coping with a threat is to deny the existence or severity of the problem. Denial protects the person from the reality of the situation. A small amount of denial is considered healthy and appropriate at times. However, total denial can lead to lack of acknowledgment of a health problem and failure to follow treatment regimens. Because much of allergy control and treatment depends on the person's awareness and responsibility for action, denial could be a major, even life-threatening problem in the allergic person.

The concept of body image merits consideration in view of the physical changes many allergic reactions elicit. *Body image* is a person's perception of his physical self based on internal and environmental sensations and experiences (see Chap. 4). Perceptions of a distorted, ugly, or undesirable body image are stress-producing because of the societal value placed on physical health and beauty. Many allergic reactions cause skin changes, rashes, swelling, and physical limitations due to pain. The actual or potential threat of the unwanted physical manifestations of the allergic response is a source of great concern to many allergic persons.

Although the problem of chronic allergy may consist of a series of acute yet reversible episodes, many people live with continuous allergic reactions. Adaptation to a chronic health problem is a long, continuous process. The severity of the reaction, the disability created by the reaction, and the person's personality, coping styles, and previous life experiences all assist the person with a successful adaptation.

Some people experience allergic reactions that are severe enough to be life-threatening. The fear created by a threat to life magnifies the reactions and behaviors of the person with a chronic, usually reversible problem. The health caregiver must consider the extreme fear the person experiences, and view the person's behavior and coping mechanisms from this perspective.

Other variables that may aggravate further the delicate balance of physical and psychological well-being are related to the diagnosis and treatment of allergies. Identification of a specific allergen is difficult and not accomplished in some instances. If an allergen or group of possible allergens is identified, then the person must avoid them. Avoidance of common, naturally occurring substances is not always easy or possible. The treatment plan may require frequent, ongoing medication administration. The medication may have unpleasant side-effects or may not eliminate the symptoms of the allergic response. There are also risks associated with some of the drug and treatment plans.

Economic factors are significant in the diagnosis and treatment of allergy. The diagnosis may involve a large number of costly and time-consuming tests. Expenses mount from drug therapy, ongoing immunizations, changes in the home and work environment to eliminate the allergen, time lost from work and responsibilities due to allergic symptoms or the effects of treatment, and frequent medical or emergency care required for exacerbations of allergic symptoms. The economic demands can be a major source of stress in the household of an allergic person.

EMOTION AND ALLERGY

The acknowledgment of a relationship between mind and body has been gradually gaining credibility and acceptance; however, the terms describing the mind–body relationship frequently are used synonomously with words that carry a negative tone. "Psychosomatic" and "psychogenic" can degenerate to "neurotic," "malingering," or "hypochondriasis." The fact that a psychological or emotional stress can trigger a physiological allergic response is poorly described and not well understood. The delicate balance between psychological and physiological functioning can be upset by stress, such as job or money worries, increasing a person's susceptibility to allergic symptoms without additional exposure to the allergen. Chronic anxieties and worries intensify existing allergic responses and symptoms. The lack of a specific physiological explanation for these phenomena frequently has resulted in negative attitudes toward people susceptible to such interactions. The perception that "it's

all in your head" or "you bring this on yourself" can strain relationships and cause anger and withdrawal from a person who has already succumbed to the effects of stress. The nurse can help the person to identify sources of stress and suggest methods of coping with stress to help prevent aggravation of an allergic response. Most importantly, the nurse needs to accept the psychological triggering mechanism of stress and to convey a positive attitude toward the person, encouraging others to avoid negativism and to adopt a supportive approach in dealing with the person.

CLINICAL MANIFESTATIONS OF ALLERGIES

Allergic Rhinitis

Some of the most common complaints arise from allergic rhinitis, resulting from exposure to a specific antigen. Rhinitis, an inflammation of the mucous membranes inside the nose, is characterized by sneezing and a stuffy, itchy, watery nose. The area affected is red, congested, swollen, and may be tender. Some people also complain of itching of the throat or palate. Mucus drainage may lead to frequent throat clearing, a cough, or hoarseness. Additional complaints of headache, pain over sinus areas, and recurrent epistaxis may be manifestations of allergic rhinitis.

Allergic rhinitis may be seasonal, or continuous throughout the year, depending on the particular allergen. Seasonal allergens (e.g., pollen) and perennial allergens (e.g., house dust) are airborne and initiate an allergic response in atopic persons. Once a person is sensitized to the allergen, either by ingestion or inhalation, recurrent contact with the allergen causes a type I allergic reaction characterized by antigenic interaction with IgE-fixed mast cells, mast cell degranulation, chemical mediator release, local inflammation, and the symptoms of allergic rhinitis. Allergic rhinitis can lead to complications such as sinusitis, recurrent ear infections, or nasal polyps.

Rhinitis can also be caused by nonallergic mechanisms such as infections, excessive use of nasal sprays, certain endocrine states (pregnancy), cerebrospinal (CSF) leaks, foreign body irritation, and nonspecific or idiopathic causes (vasomotor rhinitis).

Conjunctivitis

Frequently, accompanying allergic rhinitis are symptoms of allergic *conjunctivitis*, in which the person complains of redness, swelling, tearing, and itching of one or both eyes. Photophobia and blurred vision may also occur. These symptoms are a direct result of IgE sensitization, antigen–antibody complexes, or delayed hypersensitivity reactions that result in inflammation and may lead to tissue injury without medical intervention. Allergic conjunctivitis may also persist in a chronic state, causing itching, dryness, blurring, and photophobia.

Asthma

Asthma is a reversible narrowing of the airways that diminishes airflow into and out of the lungs. The person usually describes unexplained episodes of dyspnea, chest tightness, wheezing, cough, sputum production, fatigue, exercise intolerance, frequent chest colds, or bronchitis. These attacks may occur at any time and last from 30 minutes to hours, sometimes taking days to resolve.

There are many causes of asthmatic attacks. A common way of classifying the causative factors is through the terms *extrinsic* and *intrinsic* asthma. *Extrinsic asthma* is triggered by an environmental allergen. *Intrinsic asthma* usually is initiated by nonallergic sources such as infection, exertion,

emotion, or nonspecific temperature and environmental changes. Many forms of asthma are provoked by a combination of the extrinsic and intrinsic factors.

The reactivity of the airways and lungs is initiated by IgE-sensitized cells, a type I immune response that results in the release of chemical mediators from mast cells and basophils. These chemicals can cause smooth muscle constriction, edema, and mucosal irritation of the airways. The vagus nerve is believed to be the neurogenic mediator by which the chemical substances act upon cells of the airways. In addition to the allergic response of the IgE-sensitized cells, there may be a deficiency of secretory IgA in asthmatics. Normal protection of the lungs by IgA from bacteria, viruses, and antigens may be disrupted. There is also an exaggerated hyperreactive release of chemical mediators and a hyperresponsiveness of bronchial smooth muscle cells in asthmatics that cannot be totally accounted for by an allergic response. Finally, there may be a component of autonomic dysfunction contributing to allergic asthma.

Hypersensitivity Pneumonitis

Hypersensitivity pneumonitis (extrinsic allergic alveolitis) is an allergic response to inhaled organic dusts, usually animal or vegetable. The person complains of fever, chills, dyspnea, and chest tightening. Chronic exposure to the allergen results in progressive dyspnea, decreased exercise tolerance, productive cough, weight loss, and signs of chronic pulmonary disease (i.e., wheezing, cyanosis, clubbing). The allergic mechanisms may involve IgE antibodies in the atopic person or a combination of type III and IV immune reactions. The type III immune complexes are probably formed by IgG and the antigen (e.g., parakeet protein) whereas the type IV reaction involves T cells sensitized to the antigen. Ten percent of the people with hypersensitivity pneumonitis also have allergic asthma. The asthmatic response (type I) is immediate and followed in 4 to 6 hours by the type III immune complex response of hypersensitivity pneumonitis.

Skin Lesions

The skin is frequently a source of allergic reactivity. Atopic and contact dermatitis are the results of two types of allergic mechanisms. Atopic dermatitis is a type I allergic reaction, although the exact pathological mechanism is not well understood. Atopic dermatitis can occur by itself, or in conjunction with other atopic disorders in all age groups. The person complains of chronic, recurrent inflammation of the skin, with itching as the primary symptom. The lesions may be a small single patch or more numerous, generalized patches. Common symptoms include lesions that burn, redden, and may become edematous, excoriated, and may weep, bleed, or become secondarily infected. Pain may be associated with secondary infection. Lesions resolve by drying followed by desquamation. Chronic allergic reactions may cause skin thickening, fissure formation, scaling, and hyperpigmentation. The person may complain of excessive dryness of the skin. Allergic flares are related to heat, sweating, harsh fabrics, scratching, or exposure to irritants.

Allergic contact dermatitis results from a delayed hypersensitivity or type IV reaction to an allergen. The sensitization phase takes 10 to 14 days. T cells sensitized by the antigen (e.g., perfume) disseminate throughout the body conferring sensitivity to the entire skin surface. Usually contact sensitivity remains for life. The cell and skin changes that occur are similar to those of atopic dermatitis, resulting in similar signs and symptoms. Cross-sensitization can occur between substances of similar chemical nature, leading to an allergic dermatitis reaction to many substances.

Photoallergic contact dermatitis is similar to allergic contact dermatitis, except that ultraviolet light from the sun or an artificial source in the presence of an allergen can cause an allergic response. Common sources of allergens are sulfa drugs and some sunscreens.

Urticaria and Angioedema

Other common signs of an allergic response are urticaria (hives) and angioedema (swelling). The person will describe reddened or pale raised areas that itch (urticaria). The hives may occur on any body part, including mucous membranes. The lesions appear and disappear over several hours to days.

The allergic mechanism that causes urticaria also causes angioedema, except that angioedema involves deeper tissues and more widespread swelling. Common areas of angioedema are lips, eyelids, cheeks, hands, feet, genitals, tongue, and mucous membranes. The swelling usually involves one area at a time and lasts 24 to 36 hours. Angioedema may appear in cycles of days or weeks.

There are many nonallergic causes of urticaria and angioedema. An allergic process is implicated if antigens, antibodies, or sensitized cells are identified. A type I immediate hypersensitivity allergic reaction is the most common cause of acute urticaria. Cutaneous mast cells with sensitized IgE degranulate in the course of systemic anaphylaxis or as the only symptom of immediate hypersensitivity. The most common antigens involved in type I urticaria and angioedema are foods, drugs, stinging insects, and animal danders. Urticaria and fever also can occur in type II cytotoxic reactions (e.g., transfusion reactions), and type III immune complex reactions (e.g., serum sickness).

Systemic Symptoms

Specific complaints of allergic reactions include gastrointestinal symptoms of pain, nausea, vomiting, and diarrhea. Other symptoms of allergy usually coexist with abdominal symptoms. True food allergy is clouded by the many causes of gastrointestinal distress that may not involve immune or allergic mechanisms.

Localized symptoms of enlarged lymph nodes or inflammatory responses to insect bites or medication may be indicative of an allergic reaction. Generalized systemic complaints of joint pains, rashes, peripheral neuritis causing temporary paralysis or even symptoms of cardiac or renal impairments also may be manifestations of an allergic reaction such as serum sickness.

Systemic anaphylactic reactions may occur rapidly. General complaints of anxiety, malaise, weakness, and an impending sense of doom may be early symptoms of a systemic anaphylactic reaction. Later complaints include symptoms of skin and nervous system irritation, respiratory distress, gastrointestinal distress, and cardiovascular decompensation. Systemic reactions may range from a mild reaction of numbness, tingling, itching, and fullness of the throat to frank respiratory distress, seizures, and cardiovascular collapse. Systemic reactions usually occur within 30 minutes of exposure to the antigen.

Localized anaphylactic reactions can cause severe symptoms and discomfort but are rarely as life-threatening as systemic reactions. The most common causes of anaphylaxis (type I immediate hypersensitivity reaction) are insect venoms and drugs.

NURSING ASSESSMENT

Assessment of an allergy-prone person is critical for accurate diagnosis and determination of the success of treatment.

SUBJECTIVE DATA

To obtain an accurate impression of the causes and effects of an allergic reaction, a detailed description of the person's complaints is critical. An allergy history form can facilitate completeness and organization of the information desired. The history form should include chief complaints, family history, medical history, environmental reactions, and an environmental survey.

The chief complaint or concern of the person is best described in his own words. Emphasis should be placed on eliciting as much information about each of the presenting symptoms as possible. The exact nature of the problem needs to be thoroughly described, with respect to onset, chronology, and predisposing factors. Reporting the severity and extent of symptoms, in addition to aggravating factors, aids in describing the allergic reaction. Important also are the physical, emotional, and environmental factors that either alleviate or exacerbate the allergic episode. Other associated symptoms, even though they may appear unrelated to the allergic response, are helpful in completing the assessment data base. Always include information regarding the current therapeutic regimen because many modalities may or may not be effective or may be subject to abuse in an attempt to alleviate the allergic symptoms. Most people will have a general idea what causes their problem as well as what helps to lessen or relieve their symptoms.

Because atopic (IgE-mediated) diseases
(Text continues on page 462)

Name _____

Age _____ Sex _____ Date _____

I. Chief complaint:

II. Present illness:

III. Collateral allergic symptoms:
   Eyes: Pruritus_____ Burning_____ Lacrimation_____
           Swelling_____ Injection_____ Discharge_____
   Ears: Pruritus_____ Fullness_____ Popping_____
           Frequent infections_____
   Nose: Sneezing_____ Rhinorrhea_____ Obstruction_____
           Pruritus_____ Mouth-breathing_____
           Purulent discharge_____
   Throat: Soreness_____ Postnasal discharge_____
           Palatal pruritus_____ Mucus in the morning_____
   Chest: Cough _____   Pain _____   Wheezing _____
           Sputum _____   Dyspnea _____
           Color _____   Rest _____
           Amount _____   Exertion _____
   Skin: Dermatitis _____   Eczema _____   Urticaria _____

IV. Family allergies:

V. Previous allergic treatment or testing:
   Prior skin testing:
   Drugs: Antihistamines   Improved _____   Unimproved _____
             Bronchodilators   Improved _____   Unimproved _____
             Nose drops   Improved _____   Unimproved _____
             Hyposensitization   Improved _____   Unimproved _____
                Duration _____
                Antigens _____
                Reactions _____
             Antibiotics   Improved _____   Unimproved _____
             Steroids   Improved _____   Unimproved _____

VI. Physical agents and habits:

                                      Bothered by:

   Tobacco for _____years   Alcohol _____   Air cond. _____
   Cigarettes _____packs/day Heat _____   Muggy weath. _____
   Cigars _____per day   Cold _____   Weath. chngs. _____
   Pipe _____per day   Perfumes _____   Chemicals _____
   Never smoked _____   Paints _____   Hair spray _____
   Bothered by smoke _____ Insecticides _____ Newspapers _____
                               Cosmetics _____

                                                        (Continued)

VII. When symptoms occur:
    Time and circumstances of 1st episode:
    Prior health:
    Course of illness over decades: progressing_____ regressing_____
    Time of year: Exact dates
      Perennial_____
      Seasonal_____
      Seasonally exacerbated _____
    Monthly variations (menses, occupation):
    Time of week (weekends vs weekdays):
    Time of day or night:
    After insect stings:

VIII. Where symptoms occur:
    Living where at onset:
    Living where since onset:
    Effect of vacation or major geographic change:
    Symptoms better indoors or outdoors:
    Effect of school or work:
    Effect of staying elsewhere nearby:
    Effect of hospitalization:
    Effect of specific environments:
    Do symptoms occur around:
      old leaves_____ hay_____ lakeside_____ barns_____
      summer homes_____ damp basement_____ dry attic_____
      lawnmowing_____ animals_____ other_____
    Do symptoms occur after eating:
      cheese_____ mushrooms_____ beer_____ melons_____
      bananas_____ fish_____ nuts_____ citrus fruits_____
      other foods (list) _____
    Home: city_____ rural_____
                house_____ age_____
                apartment_____ basement_____ damp_____ dry
                heating system_____
                pets (how long)_____ dog_____ cat_____ other_____

Bedroom:	Type	Age	*Living room*	Type	Age
Pillow	_____	_____	Rug	_____	_____
Mattress	_____	_____	Matting	_____	_____
Blankets	_____	_____	Furniture	_____	_____
Quilts	_____	_____			
Furniture	_____	_____			

    Anywhere in home symptoms are worse:_____

IX. What does patient think makes him worse: _____

X. Under what circumstances is he free of symptoms: _____

XI. Summary and additional comments:

Allergy assessment sheet (Patterson R: Allergic diseases. Philadelphia, J.B. Lippincott, 1972) have a high familial incidence, the allergy history of parents and other family members is important. A medical history will provide information about medical problems and previous allergic reactions that may aggravate or mimic allergic reactions (*i.e.*, abnormalities of the immune system).

The degree of distress or difficulty that an allergy presents is a decisive factor in the extent of evaluation and treatment.

OBJECTIVE DATA

Physical Examination

The physical examination is an essential component of the data-gathering process. Even though special attention is devoted to the site of the symptoms, a complete physical examination is necessary. Components of the physical examination that most frequently are involved in allergic disorders are presented here:

Skin   Observe the skin for urticaria, angioedema, and signs of an atopic (eczematous) disorder or allergic contact dermatitis. Skin changes may not be reported by the patient because of embarrassment or thoughts of diminished importance, requiring thorough skin observation by the examiner.

Eyes   Examine the conjunctiva for redness, edema, secretions, or watering. Funduscopic examinations may reveal cataracts that are often found in atopic disease. "Allergic shiners" may be present as the result of dark-pigmented skin under the eyes. The eyes are also a common site for angioedema.

Nose   The nose may have a transverse line across the top, the allergic crease, that forms as a result of chronic upward rubbing of the nose due to itching and drainage. (This gesture is more common in children and is termed the *allergic salute*.) Examine the interior of the nose for patency, secretions, pres-

ence of polyps or foreign bodies, and the condition of the mucosa, which is usually pale due to the edema of rhinitis. There may be sneezing and a profuse watery discharge. The nasal examination may be normal during a nonallergic period.

Mouth and Oropharynx   The mouth and oropharynx may look reddened and edematous in the presence of rhinitis.

Middle Ear and Sinuses   The middle ear and sinuses should be examined as sources of secondary complications of allergic reactions (*i.e.*, otitis media and sinusitis).

Chest   Use the usual techniques of inspection, palpation, percussion and auscultation to determine any unusual findings. The chest may be normal during intervals between allergic episodes. Abnormal findings may include the changes of chronic lung disease from repeated asthma attacks or hypersensitivity pneumonitis (*i.e.*, a barrel chest, reflecting an increased anterioposterior thoracic diameter). During an allergic attack, physical examination may reveal labored breathing, use of accessory muscles, a prolonged phase of expiration, wheezing, decreased breath sounds, and cough with tenacious mucus.

Musculoskeletal   Observe the joints for the edema and tenderness that accompany some of the immune complex (type III) allergic reactions.

Other systems may yield abnormalities specific to the allergic response, such as lymphadenopathy or neurologic changes. Most abnormal findings appear during the allergic reaction and disappear upon resolution of the episode.

Paraclinical Data

The results of laboratory tests are used to aid in the diagnosis of an allergic disorder. In combination with information elicited by the history and physical examination, laboratory tests can strengthen a diagnosis, but by themselves do not make a diagnosis. In addition, laboratory tests also may aid in evaluating the effectiveness of therapy.

Blood Studies A complete blood count (c.b.c.) is usually normal except with infection and during increased catecholamine output. Eosinophilia of 5% to 15% is suggestive of atopic disease. Smears of nasal and conjunctival secretions and sputum of atopic people usually contain eosinophils. During an allergic reaction eosinophils predominate in these secretions.

Total serum IgE levels help to determine whether a disease is allergic in nature. High levels of serum IgE have been found to correlate positively with allergy, but a normal IgE level does not rule out an allergic reaction. Atopic dermatitis and respiratory symptoms usually correlate with a highly elevated serum IgE.

The paper radioimmunosorbent test (PRIST) is designed to quantitate the total amount of IgE in blood serum. The test involves the use of radioactive anti-IgE^{125} globulin, which combines with IgE of a person's blood sample, giving a radioactivity reading that is indicative of the amount of IgE in the blood. A nonradioactive test (ELISA) performs in the same manner without the use of a radioactive substance. The results of these tests are interpreted according to the established laboratory's methods and established normal ranges because these ranges vary from laboratory to laboratory. Results are also age-related because IgE levels increase from birth to age ten.

The serum radioallergosorbent test (RAST) measures allergen-specific IgE. The allergen and person's serum are combined. Radioactive anti-IgE^{125} globulin is added and the amount of allergen-specific IgE is determined by the radioactivity count. RAST has the following advantages: objectivity, which can be used to evaluate cross-reactivities of allergens; it involves no patient risk; it can be used if the skin is unsuitable for skin testing (due to disease, age, or medication); stable antigens; it can help standardize allergy extracts; and it can be used if specific allergens are not locally available. Disadvantages of RAST include the cost, the delay in results, the requirement of radioactive isotopes, and less sensitivity than in skin testing.

Confirmatory Tests Skin tests are the most commonly used mechanism for determining offending allergens. The introduction of an allergen into the skin is a simple and effective way of determining atopy to specific antigens. Skin tests are performed by the scratch, prick, and intradermal techniques. Skin responses of swelling and redness (wheal and flare) are correlated to the allergens. Allergens are presented as crude extracts of pollen, dust, foods, animal danders, and other allergy-producing substances. There is little to no standardization of the extracts. Most extracts contain the allergen to be tested in varying amounts, as well as a number of other potential allergens. The skin tests usually are performed as a battery of tests with a number of possible allergens tested simultaneously. The determination of the allergens to be tested is based on the person's history and allergens common to the person's environment.

Skin testing is indicated if there is a suspicion that specific allergens are producing allergic reactions. Precautions are necessary when skin testing is undertaken because allergen introduction could precipitate a massive or systemic allergic reaction. Testing should not be done during an allergic episode. Emergency treatment materials and a physician should be immediately available.

The tests themselves are performed using diluents of allergen extracts and a control (i.e., sterile saline). The prick technique is performed by dropping the diluent on the skin and pricking the skin to allow introduction of the antigen below the barrier level of the skin. A scratch test involves placement of the extract onto a superficial scratch. The intradermal or intracutaneous method is accomplished by injection of the diluent in between the layers of the skin. Although the intradermal method is one hundred times more sensitive than the scratch method, it is also more difficult to administer and carries a greater risk of an adverse reaction. The scratch or prick test may be done first, followed by intradermal testing of questionable or positive allergens. If the number of allergens is five or under and the reactions are limited, the skin-testing series may be completed in one visit.

The back and upper arms are the most common sites of skin testing. The actual size of the wheal and the dilution of the allergy extract are taken into account in determining positive tests and specific allergens. Both false-positive and false-negative reactions can occur due to improper administration or loss of potency of the extracts. Before skin testing, the person is instructed not to take medications that may interfere with the skin reactions (i.e., antihistamines).

Provocative testing involves the direct administration of the allergen in a diluent on the nasal, conjunctival, or respiratory mucosa. A positive reaction elicits allergic symptoms. This usually is used in conjunction with skin testing to validate equivocal or positive skin tests further. The provocative test is limited to one test antigen at a time and is contraindicated in people with a history of anaphylaxis, urticaria, angioedema, or acute bronchospasm.

Challenge tests involve exposing or "challenging" the person to increasing doses of a suspected antigen. This test is frequently used with suspected food allergies. The aller-

gic food is eliminated from the diet for 2 to 3 weeks, and then the person is given increasing doses of the suspected food and control substances in capsules or hidden in other foods. Allergic symptoms help to confirm the diagnosis.

Patch testing is used to determine the allergen responsible for contact dermatitis. The history, physical findings, and substances known to be common sensitizers are used in selecting contact irritants to patch test. If a large number of substances are to be tested, the back is the site of testing. The irritants are applied directly to the skin in a diluent or in solid form, covered with gauze, paper, and adhesive. The tests are read after 48 hours using a scale of one plus (mild erythema) to four plus (erythema, papules, and vesicles). Delayed hypersensitivity results can be read in 72 hours. Burning or itching test sites should be removed immediately and washed with soap and water. As with other testing procedures, care should be taken to use appropriate testing materials and to avoid patients with active allergic symptoms, or an anti-allergy medication.

X-ray examinations of the chest are used to evaluate allergic respiratory disease. X-ray examinations are also used to evaluate other symptomatic areas such as sinuses or the gastrointestinal tract. Pulmonary function studies and spirometry are useful for diagnostic purposes as well as evaluation of therapy of respiratory allergy symptoms.

Because serum IgE levels are elevated with parasitic infection, stool specimens for ova and parasites may be needed. Urinalysis, serum chemistries, and erythrocyte sedimentation rate are normal in atopic persons, and abnormal values may indicate an alternative or infectious diagnosis.

All testing modalities are considered against the background of a thorough history and physical examination to confirm a diagnosis of allergy. No testing techniques are currently definitive or sufficient to establish a diagnosis of allergy by themselves.

NURSING DIAGNOSIS

The history and physical examination are performed by a physician, nurse, or other health care professional trained in these skills. The physician orders the blood studies, allergy testing, and miscellaneous laboratory studies. The nurse aids in diagnosis through performance of skin, provocative, and patch testing. The results of tests are interpreted by both physician and nurse, and a prescription for allergy treatment is ordered by the physician. The prescription for treatment is recommended and discussed with the person and a treatment program established.

ALLERGY RELATED TO A SPECIFIC ANTIGEN

The assessment data provide the history of symptoms and environmental information required to initiate the diagnostic work-up for the offending allergen(s). The diagnosis of the etiology is the responsibility of the physician. Some of the common sources include common airborne and environmental agents, drugs, foods, insect venoms, pathogens, and blood transfusions. A complete discussion of these was presented previously.

SEVERITY OF SYMPTOMS

A nursing diagnosis should be made in regard to the severity of symptoms. Examples include the local reactions of rash and swelling because of a bee sting, or the more severe systemic reaction of bronchospasm and shortness of breath related to a bee sting. The acuity of the current symptoms will determine if immediate intervention is necessary.

LEVEL OF READINESS OF PATIENT FOR THERAPY

The readiness of the patient depends on how symptomatic he is and how intolerant the symptoms are. Diagnosis and treatment of allergic symptoms proceed depending on the person's desire to prevent or alter the allergic reaction. Examples include, "Patient unwilling to undergo desensitization owing to fear of injections," and "Patient receptive to intensive therapy related to hay fever symptoms."

PSYCHOSOCIAL IMPACT

Nursing diagnoses should be made regarding the effect of the allergy on the patient's lifestyle, family relationships, body image, and emotional state. Examples include "altered role functions related to withdrawal response to the allergy," "denial of possibility of systemic reaction occurring from a bee sting."

MANAGEMENT

GOALS

The goals of allergy treatment are

- To identify the allergen(s)
- To control or alleviate allergic symptoms
- To prevent allergic attacks
- To prevent permanent damage or complications of allergic reactions
- To minimize potential adverse effects of allergy treatment.

This section deals primarily with the treatment and prevention of allergic reactions and their complications.

ALLERGEN AVOIDANCE

The primary treatment for allergic conditions is the avoidance or removal of the allergen from the person's environment. Although this seems obvious, it is very difficult to accomplish. First, it demands that the allergen be identified. This in itself is a tedious and at times an imprecise process. Although certain suspected allergens may be confirmed, the person may experience allergic symptoms from unidentified allergens simultaneously. Some of the allergy testing may strongly suggest specific allergens but may not really confirm the diagnosis. The allergy tests themselves may cause reactions (redness, swelling, pain) that mimic or cloud the allergic response. Once the allergen has been tentatively identified, however, attempts to avoid the allergen can be made.

Actual avoidance is not always feasible or practical. Airborne and environmental factors are difficult to avoid totally. A change in geographic location may be recommended, but often this is unrealistic and prohibitively expensive for most people. A more realistic approach to some of the more pervasive and plentiful allergens is to reduce the amount of exposure. Pollen exposure can be reduced by avoiding rural settings during peak pollen seasons. Face masks that filter airborne particles can be worn outdoors during peak seasons or when the person is engaged in activities that necessitate exposure to allergens (i.e., raking leaves, gardening, mowing the lawn). Exposure to airborne allergens can be reduced by using air conditioners, keeping building and car windows closed, and using extra filters on forced-air heating systems. Air conditioners are usually helpful but may stir up dust and spread other allergens if the air conditioner or environment is not clean.

House dust can be controlled by regular vacuuming and damp dusting, which stirs less dust than sweeping and dry dusting. Removal of overstuffed furniture, rugs, drapes, and knickknacks will reduce collection sources of house dust significantly. Everything should be washable: sheets, blankets, and curtains. Mattresses and pillows can be encased in plastic with attention to the stuffing material. Dacron and new synthetic materials are preferable to feathers and old, reused stuffing materials.

Humidity, usually 35% to 50%, can prevent drying and irritation of airways; unfortunately, high or low humidity can aggravate breathing difficulties. Dehumidifiers and humidifiers can disseminate dust, molds, and spores if not properly cleaned and maintained. Air filters come in a variety of types and can be beneficial for environmental particle reduction. The effectiveness, convenience, and expense need to be considered before purchasing an air filter.

Animal dander may require removal of the pet and thorough cleaning of the house. Allergy to a house pet can create a great deal of emotional difficulty and stress in a household. Sensitization to a long-time family pet can occur, causing many people to live with their allergy rather than give up the animal. Sometimes scrupulous cleaning and keeping the pet out of bedrooms help keep the allergic symptoms tolerable.

Mold control is achieved by removal of house plants, dehumidification, cleaning of mold growth areas, and the use of fungicides. Humidity in excess of 60% enhances mold growth. Fungicides are effective if used regularly, either by fumigating or by direct application. Fumigation fumes can be irritating to the allergic person and should be dissipated by proper ventilation.

Smoke and odor control are necessary for the allergic person. The allergy sufferer should avoid insect sprays, deodorizers, perfumes, and fireplaces. Lids should be kept on cooking pots and exhaust fans used to disperse cooking fumes. Cigarette smoke aggravates asthmatic symptoms, increases the number of respiratory infections, and should not be allowed in the presence of the allergic person. Air pollution is a pervasive problem, particularly in urban areas. Staying indoors, avoiding excessive activity, and leaving the polluted area temporarily may help control allergic episodes.

Allergy-producing contactants, such as plants, chemicals, and metals found in the house or work environment, need to be avoided. Contact can be reduced by special equipment, protective clothing, and special cleaning. If contact is made, the skin should be washed immediately with soap and tepid running water. Dressings, soaks, and ointments may be useful for chronic skin allergies. Work environments may need to be changed if exposure to a contactant cannot be avoided.

Drug allergies can be prevented by avoidance of drugs known to cause adverse reactions. Previous drug reactions may precipitate cross-reactions between similar drugs (e.g., penicillin and cephalosporins). A thorough history is essential to obtain drug sensitivities and alert the health care team to potential allergic and adverse reactions. If a current medication is thought to be the cause of a reaction, ideally, the drug should be discontinued. However, if the drug is essential to patient management, the nurse should alert the physician to the potential or actual adverse reaction and a decision will be made whether to discontinue the drug. Cessation of a drug that is causing severe symptoms should be called to the immediate attention of the physician. Mild or nonthreatening symptoms may be treated while the drug is continued, based on a physician's decision and orders.

Transfusion reactions can be reduced by adequate typing and crossmatching of blood, careful checking of blood labels (correct blood type, unexpired blood), flushing IV tubing with isotonic saline, and close monitoring of the patient, especially for the initial 15 minutes, and then throughout the blood administration. Symptoms of a reaction require the nurse to stop the transfusion immediately, keep the IV line patent, notify the physician at once, check vital signs, save the blood, and carry out routines of the particular institution.

Avoidance or elimination of a particular or cross-reacting food is the treatment for a food allergy. A variety of food-elimination diets are available and some can be complex. Sometimes a food hypersensitivity is "outgrown" or becomes tolerated, especially in children. Exposure to the allergy-producing food should be done slowly and carefully, and should not be considered if the allergic response was anaphylaxis.

Educate people with allergies to insect bites or stings about the characteristics and habitats of the particular insect. Systemic reactions will require drug therapy and knowledge about the particular drugs and their use. Treat local reactions by removing the stinger, cleansing the area with soap and water, and applying ice. If a sting site is on a limb, systemic venom spread can sometimes be slowed by application of a tourniquet proximal to the site. Pharmacologic intervention may be required (discussed in the next section).

PHARMACOLOGIC THERAPY

In conjunction with other forms of allergy treatment, medication frequently is prescribed to prevent, control, or alleviate allergic symptoms. Antihistamines are commonly prescribed because they counteract the effects of histamine by competing with histamine for specific cell-surface receptors. Antihistamines, however, are most effective in preventing rather than neutralizing the effects of histamine and are therefore more efficient if used preventatively. Allergic problems that respond well to antihistamines are rhinitis, acute urticaria, anaphylaxis, drug reactions, mild transfusion reactions, and contact dermatitis. Symptomatic relief ranges from alleviation of sneezing and rhinorrhea to reduction of rash and itching. Antihistamines usually are prescribed in combination with other drugs. Common side-effects include sedation, somnolence, dry mouth, dizziness, and irritability. Potentiation of the drug's effects can occur with alcohol, barbiturates, or tranquilizers. Choice of antihistamines usually is based upon the medication's side-effects and the person's tolerance. One of the more commonly used antihistamines is diphenhydramine hydrochloride (Benadryl).

Sympathomimetic or adrenergic drugs simulate the actions of the sympathetic nervous system. Stimulation of receptors on the surfaces of muscles causes constriction of smooth muscle in skin, intestines and mucous membranes, dilatation of the bronchi, and cardiac stimulation. These drugs are effective in providing temporary relief of the symptoms of rhinitis (decongestion) and in the treatment of asthma (bronchodilatation). For the treatment of rhinitis, a topical preparation (e.g., nose drops, sprays) is more effective than oral preparations. Unfortunately, nasal administration frequently is abused, and such overusage can cause a rebound congestion, dryness, and chronic swelling of the nasal mucosa. Systemic preparations are recommended for chronic rhinitis if medication will be necessary for more than 5 days. Decongestants should be used with caution in people with thyroid disease, hypertension, diabetes, heart disease, or in people using tricyclic antidepressants.

Adrenergic drugs are also commonly used in the treatment of asthma. The most well-known of this group of drugs are epinephrine and ephedrine. The routes of administration are primarily by subcutaneous injection, aerosol, nebulization, and some oral preparations. Side-effects include nervousness, irritability, tremors, tachycardia, nausea, and vomiting. As with decongestants, symptomatic relief is dramatic and there is a tendency to overuse these agents, especially the inhaler form. Asthmatics with hypertension, thyroid disorders, and cardiac disease need to pay special attention to specific drug selection and side-effects. Usually, systemic side-effects are less with the inhaled preparations. Epinephrine is available in a kit for home usage for the person with severe allergic reactions.

In addition to these sympathomimetic drugs, theophylline has become one of the cornerstone medications used for the management of acute and chronic asthma. Theophylline provides bronchodilatation by smooth muscle relaxation. There are many forms and preparations of theophylline available for oral and intravenous use. It is well absorbed from the gastrointestinal tract and is readily available to body tissues. The dose is usually dependent on age and lean body weight and is therefore individually determined. Toxic effects include agitation, gastrointestinal distress, tachycardia, arrhythmias, and grand mal seizures.

Cromolyn sodium (Intal), effective as a prophylactic treatment of allergic reactions, acts by preventing the degranulation of mast cells, avoiding release of histamine and the subsequent type I response. Cromolyn also may inhibit late-phase reactions (LPRs) that are precipitated by degranulation of mast cells. Treatment of asthma, rhinitis, conjunctivitis, and gastrointestinal disorders is achieved by direct application of cromolyn on the target organ before allergen exposure.

Cromolyn preparations can be administered by inhaler, nasal spray, eye drops, and capsule. The nasal spray and eye drops are not available in the United States (pending FDA approval); however, they are used in Great Britain with success. Cromolyn is the treatment of choice for seasonal asthma, animal-induced asthma, and food allergies. Cromolyn is poorly absorbed by the body in all forms and may be most effective because of a mechanical blocking of the allergic response. The preventive action of cromolyn needs to be emphasized because it is ineffective as treatment for an acute attack. Side-effects, ranging from hypersensitivity reactions, nausea and vomiting, and respiratory irritation from inhalation of the powder have been reported in very few people.

Corticosteroids are useful in allergy treatment because of their anti-inflammatory actions. Owing to serious side-effects (e.g., masking symptoms of infection, excessive weight gain, osteoporosis, gastritis, hypertension, psychosis, glucose intolerance, adrenal suppression), steroids are used judiciously. States of acute asthma, anaphylaxis, and exfoliative dermatitis are potentially life-threatening and warrant steroid use. Limited or chronic allergic reactions that cause severe discomfort or are not responding to other forms of therapy also may require steroids for a short duration. Patients with previous steroid administration, especially for long periods of time, may require repeat treatment during acute allergic episodes. The risks and discomfort of the allergy must be weighed against the adverse effects of the steroids. Treatment with steroids is accomplished with the lowest possible dose that controls symptoms, short-acting preparations, limited duration of steroid therapy (5–7 days), and tapering doses of long-term, high-dose therapy. If prolonged therapy is required, intermittent, alternate-day doses of steroids are administered. Steroids usually are administered as a single dose in the morning to avoid adrenal suppression. Preparations for oral, injectable or intravenous, inhalation, and topical administration are available. Nasal spray preparations have been associated with abuse and complications but are still recommended for careful use in alleviation of rhinitis symptoms. Steroids are also suggested as the treatment of choice in preventing LPRs. Patients must be watched closely for response to treatment as well as adverse affects of the steroids.

IMMUNE THERAPY

Immune therapy, also known as hyposensitization or desensitization, is successful against allergic symptoms such as rhinitis and asthma due to identified pollens, molds, house dust, animal danders, insect venoms, and foods. Through multiple subcutaneous injections of gradually increasing concentrations of the allergen, the body is immunized against the allergen. The immunization occurs through the stimulation of IgG-blocking antibodies produced by repeated exposure to the allergen in the injection. The IgG antibodies bind more easily with the allergen, thus avoiding the antigen/IgE-mediated mast cell degranulation reaction. There also seems to be a suppression of specific IgE-antibody production against the allergen thought to be mediated by T-suppressor cells sensitized by the repeated injections. Immunotherapy does not cure the allergy, and it is performed in conjunction with other treatment methods, such as allergen avoidance.

Desensitization can cause a systemic response if carried out when the person is symptomatic or during the person's allergic season. The injections usually are begun 3 months before the peak allergy season to prevent seasonal allergic symptoms. Perennial therapy is administered throughout the year and provides longer lasting results than seasonal therapy alone for relief from chronic allergy symptoms.

The starting dose and subsequent doses are determined by each patient's response. The allergens are administered every 4 to 7 days in increasing doses until a maximal maintenance dose is established. Higher doses of allergen offer better relief from symptoms. Injections of the maintenance dose are given weekly for 3 to 4 months and gradually progress to a 4-to 6-week interval between injections. Maximum improvement of symptoms occurs between 1 and 2 years. If no relief of symptoms is achieved after 2 years, the desensitization program is stopped. If relief is obtained, immunotherapy may be stopped or continued for another year or two to avoid relapse of allergic symptoms. Relapses may occur around 6 to 12 months after cessation of injections, requiring further immunotherapy or other treatment methods if the symptoms do not respond to retreatment.

During the densensitization treatment regimen the person is observed for 20 to 30 minutes after the injection in case there is a systemic reaction. Swelling usually occurs at the site of the injection, but a large local swelling demands evaluation of the next dose by the physician to prevent a possible systemic reaction.

Severe reactions to the injections usually occur within 20 to 60 minutes. Treat wheals greater than 2 cm with an ice pack, oral antihistamines, notification of the physician, and documentation on the person's record. A systemic reaction is heralded by anxiety, restlessness, flushing, urticaria, itching, angioedema, bronchospasm, laryngeal edema, progressing to cardiac and respiratory arrest. Because of the life-threatening nature of a systemic reaction, a physician must always be immediately available and emergency equipment and drugs ready for immediate use.

If multiple allergens are administered, no more than three or four are mixed in one injection. Allergens causing severe local reactions should not be mixed with other allergens.

ALLERGY EMERGENCIES

Most allergic reactions, although annoying and uncomfortable, are not life-threatening. In extreme cases, however, severe allergic reactions may progress quickly to shock and death if intervention does not occur quickly. Although anaphylaxis is the most familiar allergic emergency, acute asthma, status asthmaticus, exfoliative dermatitis, and angioedema of the head and neck can also lead quickly to emergent situations.

The most common causes of systemic anaphylaxis are drugs (penicillin, aspirin, horse serum), allergen extracts, blood products, insect venoms, radiopaque dyes, shellfish, and peanuts. The treatment of the anaphylactic reaction is dictated by the severity of the reaction. Immediate action is extremely important in reversing the process and preventing a cardiorespiratory arrest. Stay with the person and try to remain calm and reassuring. Evaluation of cardiac and respiratory status will determine whether the airway is patent and whether cardiopulmonary resuscitation needs to be started. Simultaneously, call for assistance, in particular a physician. Epinephrine is given immediately, orally for mild reactions, intramuscularly or intravenously (slowly) for severe reactions. The physician may order the site of the allergen (i.e., bite) infiltrated with epinephrine. A tourniquet above and ice pack on the site may slow the spread of the allergen. Establish an intravenous line for administration of drugs and fluids. Diphenhydramine hydrochloride is given intramuscularly or intravenously (over 5 to 10 minutes) and then continued orally for at least 48 hours.

Severe bronchospasm may require administration of oxygen by mask or nasal catheter and aminophylline intravenously, either continuously or bolus (over 15 to 20 minutes). Hypotension requires fluid administration and vasopressor support (i.e., dopamine, levarterenol, metaraminol). Steroids do not help in the acute phase of anaphylaxis, but are started early for moderate, severe, or prolonged anaphylaxis. An initial intravenous dose of steroids is followed by a maintenance dosage (any appropriate route) every 6 hours for 2 to 3 days.

Death from systemic anaphylaxis usually occurs within the first 30 minutes. Recovery from anaphylaxis usually is complete but may require medical support for several hours to days. Repeated exposure to the allergen leads to more rapid, severe reactions. One key to anaphylaxis treatment is prevention. Careful history-taking, awareness of other sensitivities and allergies, avoidance of parenteral medication administration, skin testing before administering vaccines, patient education, carrying epinephrine kits, and use of identification tags (e.g., Med-Alert) for allergic people may save a life or prevent a severe anaphylactic reaction.

Acute asthma can compromise the well-being of the person. If the asthma attack is severe and is not alleviated by routine therapy, it will require immediate medical attention. Treatment of acute asthma includes oxygen administration, epinephrine, nebulized bronchodilators, intravenous aminophylline, and Sus-Phrine (a long-acting preparation of epinephrine) for rebound bronchospasm. Failure to respond to the above treatment may lead to status asthmaticus, an asthmatic crisis characterized by severe and continuous aggravation of asthmatic symptoms, exhaustion, shock, ventilatory collapse, and failure. Status asthmaticus requires hospitalization and intensive medical care. Treatment includes the above measures for severe asthma, and, in addition, vigorous hydration, sodium bicarbonate if acidemia exists, (pH equal to or < 7.2) vigorous pulmonary toilet, steroids, isoproterenol by nebulizer and intravenously, antibiotics if appropriate, and rarely, intubation with mechanical ventilation. There is a 1% to 3% mortality rate associated with status asthmaticus. Determination of precipitating factors and follow-up care are critical in preventing a recurrence of a life-threatening asthma attack.

An allergic reaction involving the entire skin surface is called exfoliative dermatitis, or erythroderma. The reaction may be erythema, or an actual sloughing of layers of the skin. Because of the extensive involvement of the body surface areas, there may be severe impairment of cutaneous function. Temperature regulation and protection from microorganisms are compromised, and protein and fluid loss occur. Exfoliative dermatitis has the potential to be life-threatening especially in the compromised host. Short-course systemic and topical steroids may be used in addition to other support measures such as fluids and antibiotics. Exfoliative dermatitis can occur in response to many precipitating factors. In allergic disease, the most common causes are from direct allergen contact with the skin or systemic response to an allergen such as a drug.

Angioedema of the head and neck constitutes a potentially life-threatening situation requiring immediate medical attention. Edema of the neck can progress until airway obstruction occurs, requiring intubation or tracheostomy. Any edematous response in the head area must be watched closely and treated with routine measures (i.e., antihistamines, sympathomimetic drugs), to avoid airway obstruction and respiratory distress.

In an acute allergic situation, prompt action is necessary to avoid worsening of symptoms. Initial measures of epinephrine administration can be performed by the trained person whether a family member, friend, technician, nurse, or physician. Medical attention should be sought immediately for allergic symptoms that worsen and cause distress; the cessation of such allergic responses is the key to preventing a life-threatening situation.

PSYCHOSOCIAL INTERVENTIONS

Emotional stress, fatigue, infection, air pollutions and weather changes can influence whether a person will respond to an allergen one day and not the next. All of these factors, in combination with the amount of allergen the body can handle, become the "allergic load." The delicate balance of internal and external environment can be tipped by increasing any one of the above factors, causing the person to have allergic symptoms for different reasons on different days. Sometimes the allergic load can be decreased by avoiding nonallergic factors (e.g., stress) to help make symptoms manageable.

The success of identification, avoidance, and treatment of allergy depends on the person's knowledge about and management of the allergy. Changes in environment, eating habits, work routines, and life-style are not easy to accomplish. Helping the person to identify the cause and effect of the allergic response, as well as having him thoroughly understand the treatment regimen, will increase participation in the allergy management program. The person has ultimate control over the prevention and alleviation of reactions to known allergens. The educational needs of allergic individuals are to provide a clear understanding of the condition and treatment, when to seek immediate help, how to know when the current treatment is no longer effective, how to achieve maximum relief of symptoms, and how to maintain optimal overall health. Failure of

allergy treatment is sometimes a failure to involve, educate, and support the allergic patient and family. Involvement of the patient must occur from the initial assessment and diagnosis through the interventions, and finally through the ongoing evaluation of the therapy.

The nurse plays a critical role in involving the person in his care and in coordinating the efforts of other members of the health care team. The nurse, as the person who frequently performs or assists with the initial history and physical examination, assists with and performs many diagnostic studies (e.g., skin testing), educates the person about allergy treatment plans (e.g., environmental controls and avoidance), and assists with evaluation of therapy, is in an optimal position to assess the entire process and ongoing needs of the patient. Psychiatric or social service referrals may be needed to help with family or individual crises in response to the chronic and acute nature of allergy. The emotional component of allergy may be a source of conflict or aggravating factor in a person's allergic load. Altered lifestyles can produce stress for the patient and family. Stress-reducing measures, such as counseling, relaxation techniques, and biofeedback may help to reduce or control allergy symptoms. Social service support for financial considerations may be necessary in view of the expense of environmental alterations and controls, special diets, medications, and medical bills.

A dietitian may need to help the person and family to plan elimination diets for diagnostic and therapeutic allergy control. Altered eating patterns may require ongoing support and creative input, particularly in the face of severely restricted diets.

The public health or visiting nurse may be consulted to aid in diagnostic determination of allergens in the environment, to assist with environmental and avoidance controls, to evaluate treatment effectiveness, and for follow-up for acute exacerbations of allergic episodes. The support and assistance in the home may be crucial to the person's successful management of the allergy.

Nurses are in a key position to coordinate the efforts of the health care team, to support and educate the patient and family, and to provide life-support measures in emergency situations. Nurses must be aware of actual and potential allergic situations in all areas of practice. Communicate any history or suspicion of allergy to health care colleagues, document it on the person's record, and inform him.

CONCLUSION

The mechanisms involving who develops allergies and why people develop allergies are poorly understood. Perhaps understanding allergy acquisition would lead to preventing development of allergies in high-risk and general populations.

Research is continuing to investigate the exact pathophysiological mechanism behind the allergic response in an effort eventually to intervene more effectively. Ongoing research is necessary to develop more refined and safer means of diagnosing allergies. Treatment and prevention of atopic allergies will be furthered with the development of therapy that specifically inhibits IgE production and mast cell degranulation. So much has happened in the last decade with respect to the understanding, diagnosing, and treatment of allergies, that this decade promises to bring further exciting and useful advances for allergy sufferers.

REFERENCES

1. Gell PG, Coombs RR: Clinical Aspects of Immunology. Philadelphia, FA Davis, 1977

BIBLIOGRAPHY

ARTICLES

Bielan B: Honing your assessment skills: What that rash really means. RN 42:58, Feb 1979

Bielan B: If it's wet, dry it; If it's dry, wet it. Occup Health Saf 47:32, Sep–Oct 1978

Capel L: Rhinitis and its management. Nurs Mirror 20:Sep 8, 1977

Description of allergic contacts. Hollister Stier Laboratories (Division of Cutter Laboratories)

Elpern EH: Asthma update: Pathophysiology and treatment. Heart Lung 9:655, July–Aug 1980

Fink J: Immunologic lung diseases. Hosp Pract 16:53, May 1981

Fruth R: Anaphylaxis and drug reactions, guidelines for detection and care. Heart Lung 9:66, July/Aug 1980

Harmon AL, Harmon DC: Anaphylaxis: Sudden death anytime. Nurs 80, 19:40, Oct 1980

Iveson–Iveson J: Silent sufferers. Nurs Mirror 151:38, Nov 27, 1980

Karr R: Mechanisms of immune injury. Chest 78(Suppl):388, Aug 1980

Maiman LA, Green LW, Gibson G et al: Education for self treatment by adult asthmatics. JAMA 241:1919, May 4, 1979

Mazow JB, Grant JA, Jackson D: Type I hypersensitivity and anaphylaxis from insect stings. Heart Lung 10:133, Jan/Feb 1981

Mullarkey M, Webb DR (eds): Symposium on clinical allergy. Med Clin North Am 65:1, Sep 1981

Parker C: Food allergies. Am J Nurs 80:262, Feb 1980

Pearson LB: Contact dermatitis as a clinical entity for the nurse practitioner. Nurse Pract 2:27, Mar/Apr 1977

Reactions to "x-ray dye": Different treatment for different types. Nurs Drug Alert 4:67, Jul 1980

Richerson HB: Immunology of the respiratory system. Basics of RD 2:1, May 1974

Rodman MJ: The drug interactions we all overlook, cold, allergy, and cough remedies. RN 1981, 44:36, Feb 1981

Salvaggio J: Diagnosis and management of hypersensitivity pneumonitis. Hosp Pract 15:93, Nov 1980

Stordy BJ, Hubbard R: When the body takes a stand. Nurs Mirror 150(Suppl):i, Mar 6, 1980

Sudden death during hyposensitization. Nurse Drug Alert 7:Jan 5, 1981

Walsh C: Please don't pluck the poison ivy. Am J Nurs 78:408 Mar 1978

Wardell G: Allergic conjunctivitis. Nurs Mirror 145:21, Sept 8, 1977

BOOKS

Albanese JA, Bond T: Drug Interactions, Basic Principles and Clinical Problems. New York, McGraw–Hill, 1978

Brunner LS, Suddarth DS: Textbook of Medical–Surgical Nursing. Philadelphia, JB Lippincott, 1980

Beyers M, Dudas S: The Clinical Practice of Medical Surgical Nursing. Boston, Little, Brown & Co, 1977

Frazier CA: Current Therapy of Allergy. Flushing, NY, Medical Examination Publishing, 1974

Gell PG, Coombs RR: Clinical Aspects of Immunology. Philadelphia, FA Davis, 1977

Gershwin ME, Nagy SM (eds): Evaluation and Management of Allergic and Asthmatic diseases. New York, Grune & Stratton, 1979

Lawlor G, Fischer T, eds: Manual of Allergy and Immunotherapy. Boston, Little, Brown & Co, 1981

Luckman J, Sorensen KC: Medical–Surgical Nursing: A Psychophysiologic Approach. Philadelphia, WB Saunders Co, 1974

Patterson R (ed): Allergic Diseases, Diagnosis and Management. Philadelphia, JB Lippincott, 1972

Price SA, Wilson LM: Pathophysiology: Clinical Concepts of Processes. New York, McGraw–Hill, 1978

Rodman MJ, Smith D: Pharmacology and Drug Therapy in Nursing. Philadelphia, JB Lippincott, 1974

Roitt I: Essential Immunology. Oxford Blackwell Scientific Publications, 1979

Scope Monograph on Immunology. Kalamazoo, Upjohn, 1972

AGENCY

University of Michigan Allergy Clinic, University Hospital, Ann Arbor, Michigan

UNPUBLISHED MATERIAL

Kaliner MA: Late phase allergic reactions. Lecture presented at the University of Michigan Medical School Department of Postgraduate Medicine and Health Professions Education, Advances in Internal Medicine. Ann Arbor, University of Michigan, May 1982

19

Obesity

Margaret M. Jacobs
Wilma Geels

SCOPE OF THE PROBLEM

Obesity is one of the most common health problems in America today. Estimates of the extent of the problem vary widely, because of the differing definitions of obesity. Bray, a well-known researcher on obesity, estimates that 10 to 50 million Americans are obese.[3] Using even the most conservative number of 10 million, obesity constitutes a major public health problem. It is associated with a variety of diseases that together account for 15% to 20% of the mortality rate.

The problem of obesity has been the subject of extensive study in recent years and as a result, there has been a large increase in knowledge about many of the factors related to obesity. Both the professional and the lay literature on obesity have become voluminous and at times confusing. Research findings are sometimes contradictory, and the more the topic is studied, the greater its complexity has become. Although there may be little consensus among researchers about many aspects of obesity, there is agreement that it is not a uniform condition. No one theory or finding has been accepted as *the* explanation for the development of obesity.

Some of the confusing and contradictory research findings are a result of the heterogeneity of the studies' subjects. Findings that are based on a population studied by a psychiatrist, for example, are likely to show a higher incidence of emotional and psychiatric symptoms in obese people than would a study done by an internist. Most of the studies are based on populations of patients who have sought help for their problem. Obese people who are healthy and who are not under treatment for their obesity, either by professionals or self-help groups, are less likely to be studied because their identities are not known to researchers.

Although the common denominator of all obese people is an imbalance between caloric intake and energy expenditure, the numerous and diverse factors that result in excess caloric intake mean that the often-heard advice to "go on a diet" is simplistic and ineffective. Factors related to the development of obesity, its assessment, and management will be the focus of this chapter. For a more detailed discussion of the problem, the reader is referred to Bray's *Obesity in America*, Powers' *Obesity: The Regulation of Weight*, and Bruch's *Eating Disorders*.

DEFINITION

The terms *overweight* and *obesity* often are used interchangeably, but they are not synonymous. *Obesity* is the condition of having an abnormally high proportion of body weight as fat. *Overweight* is the state of weighing more than average for one's height and age. Obese people usually are also overweight, but it is possible to be overweight without being obese. A football player, for example, may weigh more than the height/weight table says he should, but most of his weight is muscle, not fat. He may, in fact, be underfat. The obese person's excess weight is in the form of fat. (We will use the terms *overweight* and *obesity* interchangeably in this chapter to indicate excess weight and body fat.)

MECHANISMS OF OBESITY

MEASUREMENT OF OBESITY

Measurement of the degree of obesity is imprecise because direct measurement of the body's fat content is not possible in live human beings. Jean Mayer, the well-known nutritionist, has described a number of "unscientific" methods that can be used by the lay person to measure fatness: the mirror test, the pinch test, and the ruler test.[13] The *mirror test* is simple observation. When a person looks at himself in the mirror and he looks overweight, he probably is. The *pinch test* is done by lifting up a fold of skin and subcutaneous fat from one of three places: the back of the upper arm, the side of the lower chest, or the abdomen. The skinfold is then double thickness. If this fold is much greater than 1 inch, there is excessive fatness. A third method is the *ruler test*. When one is lying on one's back, the surface of the abdomen between the ribs and the front of the pelvis

should be either flat or slightly concave, and a ruler placed along the midline of the body should touch both the ribs and the pelvic area. If it does not, (and there is no other explanation, e.g., pregnancy), the person is considered obese.

More precise measurements of body fat require techniques and equipment not readily available to nurses. The first is the measurement of the body density, which is determined from the *specific gravity*, or the weight of the body both in and out of water. Once the person's weight is determined both in and out of water, it is possible to calculate the percentage of body weight that is fat, because fat is lighter than water and other tissues are heavier than water. Because of the equipment required for this technique, it is used mainly for research purposes.

Another method of measuring body fat is done by quantitating the amount of potassium in the body, which indirectly is a measure of cell mass. This and other dilutional methods are used primarily in research.

The degree of overweight is more easily calculated from either a height/weight table or by body mass index. Height/weight tables have been used for many years. These tables consist of three classes of frame size and ranges of weight, rather than a single figure. One of the main deficiencies of these tables is that there is no definition given of "frame size" and thus it is left up to the person to decide whether he is of small, medium, or large frame (Table 19-1). Body mass index, another method of measuring obesity, is determined by dividing the weight (*wt*) by the height (*ht*) squared (wt/ht^2) and can be obtained from a nomogram (Fig. 19-1). Using this method, overweight is defined as a body mass index between 24 and 30, and obesity as a body mass index of greater than 30.[2]

Skinfold measurement, obtained through the use of calipers, is a refinement of

TABLE 19-1
IDEAL WEIGHTS DERIVED FROM LIFE INSURANCE STATISTICS: 1983 METROPOLITAN HEIGHT AND WEIGHT TABLES*

MEN					WOMEN				
HEIGHT FEET	INCHES	SMALL FRAME	MEDIUM FRAME	LARGE FRAME	HEIGHT FEET	INCHES	SMALL FRAME	MEDIUM FRAME	LARGE FRAME
5	2	128–134	131–141	138–150	4	10	102–111	109–121	118–131
5	3	130–136	133–143	140–153	4	11	103–113	111–123	120–134
5	4	132–138	135–145	142–156	5	0	104–115	113–126	122–137
5	5	134–140	137–148	144–160	5	1	106–118	115–129	125–140
5	6	136–142	139–151	146–164	5	2	108–121	118–132	128–143
5	7	138–145	142–154	149–168	5	3	111–124	121–135	131–147
5	8	140–148	145–157	152–172	5	4	114–127	124–138	134–151
5	9	142–151	148–160	155–176	5	5	117–130	127–141	137–155
5	10	144–154	151–163	158–180	5	6	120–133	130–144	140–159
5	11	146–157	154–166	161–184	5	7	123–136	133–147	143–163
6	0	149–160	157–170	164–188	5	8	126–139	136–150	146–167
6	1	152–164	160–174	168–192	5	9	129–142	139–153	149–170
6	2	155–168	164–178	172–197	5	10	132–145	142–156	152–173
6	3	158–172	167–182	176–202	5	11	135–148	145–159	155–176
6	4	162–176	171–187	181–207	6	0	138–151	148–162	158–179

*Weights at ages 25–59 based on lowest mortality. Weight in pounds according to frame (in indoor clothing weighing 5 lbs. for men and 3 lbs. for women; shoes with 1″ heels).
(Revised Height/Weight Tables derived from life insurance statistics prepared by the Metropolitan Life Insurance Company: Men and women. Copyright 1983, Metropolitan Life Insurance Company.)

the pinch test described earlier. To obtain accurate data, skinfold measurements should be done on several areas of the body's surface. Skill in using the instrument must also be learned, so that results are reliable.

FACTORS RELATED TO THE DEVELOPMENT OF OBESITY

Numerous factors contribute to the development of obesity. Body type, socioeconomic class, cultural factors, age of onset, physical activity, environment, psychological factors, and genetic factors interact and contribute to the development of obesity.

Body type, or *somatotype*, has a genetic component and refers to the degree of round-ness (*endomorphy*), muscularity (*mesomorphy*), or tallness (*ectomorphy*) of the body. Most people are not exclusively in one category, but are likely to have more characteristics of one type than another. Although not all endomorphs are fat, the tendency to obesity is there. The mesomorph is more likely to be overweight (*i.e.*, have greater muscle mass) without being over fat.

Socioeconomic class is a strong predictor of obesity in the United States. In less affluent countries, there is a direct correlation between one's socioeconomic status and body weight. In contrast, in the United States there is an inverse correlation between socioeconomic status and body weight. As Powers has stated, "Only in an affluent country can

Weight
kg lb

Body
Mass
Index
(wt/(ht)²)

Height
cm in

Women

Men

Obese

Obese

Overweight

Overweight

Acceptable

Acceptable

© George A Bray 1978

To use this nomogram, place a ruler or straight edge between the body weight in kg or lb (without clothes), and the height in cm or in (without shoes). The body mass index is read from the middle of the scale and is in metric units. The normal limits are: a body mass index of 20–25 for males and 19–24 for females. Overweight is between the upper limits of normal body mass index and a body mass index of 30. Obesity is a body mass index greater than 30.

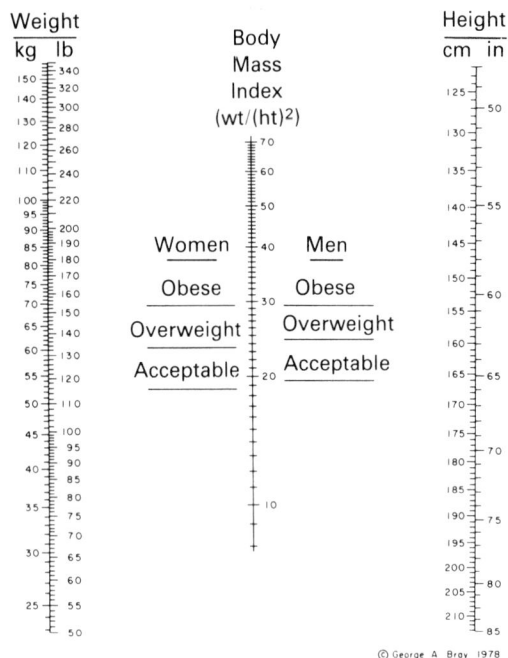

FIG. 19-1 *A nomogram for body mass index. (Bray GA: Definition, measurement and classification of the syndromes of obesity. Int J Obes 2:1–14, 1978)*

the poor be obese."[14] Inexpensive, high-calorie foods must be readily available for this to occur. In New York city a large study of both school children and adults found that at all ages the affluent are leaner and the poor are fatter.[7] Cultural pressure, especially among upper-class women, to maintain a fashionably slim figure is very strong. The poor, on the other hand, are not as likely to have either the time or money for expensive, fashionable clothing, nor does the fashion industry direct its advertising toward them.

Another determinant of obesity is age of onset. Obesity occurring in infancy, childhood, and adolescence tends to continue into adulthood. Adults who were obese as children usually are both fatter and more refractory to treatment than are those who become

obese as adults. One explanation for this finding is that people who were obese as infants have hypercellular obesity, rather than the hypertrophic form that is characteristic of adult onset obesity. The number of fat cells (*adipocytes*) a person has results from three periods in life during which new adipocytes are formed: 1) during the last trimester of fetal development, 2) during the first 6 months of infancy, and 3) at the time of puberty. Although the development of new fat cells is an ongoing process until approximately age 20, the greatest increase occurs during these three periods. Thus, the theory is that those people who become obese as adults do so by increasing the *size* of the adipocytes (*hypertrophic obesity*); whereas before that time, both the *number and size* of fat cells increase (*hypercellular obesity*). Once a new adipocyte is formed, it is always present. Therefore, the person with an increased number of fat cells may be able to lose weight only by starving them, presumably a much more difficult accomplishment than losing weight by decreasing the size of hypertrophied cells.

The tendency toward being overweight can begin as a result of infant feeding practices. The widespread use of infant formula, which is higher in calories than breast milk, and the early introduction of solid food into the diet, may give the infant far more calories than he needs for normal growth and development. Fat babies are not necessarily the healthiest babies; they may become fat adults with a lifelong weight problem.

Inactivity also can contribute to the development of obesity. Until recently, the relationship between physical activity and obesity was given little attention. The conventional wisdom was that exercise had little effect on body weight. That this belief was based on opinion, rather than research findings, did not make it any less popular. More recently, studies done by Mayer have shown that exercise is extremely important in weight control.[13] Mayer found that among people of normal weight there is a strong correlation between caloric intake and physical activity. As physical activity increases or decreases, so does caloric intake. This balance results in a stable weight. At both extremes, however, this correlation does not hold. With extreme inactivity, caloric intake increases. At the other extreme, the people who are very active physically no longer have an increased food intake; rather, their intake decreases, and they lose weight. Mayer studied infants, children, and adolescents, both obese and nonobese, and found that the obese persons were much less active than those of normal weight.

Modern labor-saving devices have decreased the need for people to be active physically. For most Americans (except farmers and others who engage in heavy physical labor) physical activity is not a regular part of the work day. Many Americans drive their cars to work, sit at a desk all day and in front of the television set at night. Exercise therefore must be planned on a regular basis if it is to be effective in weight control. The earlier in life this begins, the easier it is to maintain the habit. Physical activity is of great importance in both the prevention and treatment of obesity in people of all ages.

There is a variation in the occurrence of obesity between the sexes. More women than men are obese. In the age range of 20 to 74, 24% of women and 14% of men are overweight. Men are more likely to be 10% to 19% overweight, but there are more women who are 20% or more overweight. Women naturally have a greater percentage (20% to 25%) of their body weight as fat than do men (15% to 18%). It is believed that hazards to health are more likely for a person who is more than 20% overweight.[3]

As men and women age, their weight may remain stable, but a greater percentage of the weight becomes fat. Both older men and women have 50% more fat than they did as a youth. Exercise helps slow down this process, but it cannot retard it completely; therefore, as one gets older, one must decrease the number of calories taken in if one is to maintain a stable weight.

Psychological and emotional factors can play an important part in the development of obesity. There is no one personality type for all obese people; nor do all obese people have emotional problems. Powers estimates that one third of obese people have emotional problems, which is similar to the incidence among the nonobese.[14] One theory suggests that for some people obesity is a protective device against emotional instability. Some obese people, especially those who have been obese since adolescence, have a disturbance in body image. They tend to overestimate their size and use derogatory terms when referring to their bodies. (Body image disturbances are discussed in more detail in Chap. 4.)

At one time there was much controversy over whether genetics had a role in the development of obesity. Currently, agreement exists that genetics play a role; however, the relative importance of its role remains controversial. It is readily observable that there is a familial tendency toward obesity. Parents who are both obese are likely to have obese children, and lean parents tend to have lean children. Furthermore, according to Bray, 80% of obese persons had either one or both parents who were obese.[3]

Studies of identical twins raised together show that they have very similar weights. Similarity of body weights between identical twins raised apart is not as high, but it is higher than that for fraternal twins raised together. Furthermore, studies of adopted children show a low correlation of body weight between them and their parents, as distinct from genetic children and their parents, where the correlation is high. This suggests that there is a genetic component to body weight.[3]

REGULATION OF BODY WEIGHT: SET-POINT THEORY

Many studies have shown that a permanent loss of weight is very difficult, if not impossible, for most obese people to achieve, no matter what method is used to lose weight. The body's attempt to maintain a stable, although high, weight suggests the existence of a powerful regulatory mechanism. Experiments have been done in which normal-weight adult volunteers tried to increase their weight 25% by eating high-calorie meals. Most of them had great difficulty gaining this amount of weight, and when they did and the experiment ended, their weight promptly fell to previous levels.

Keesey points out that humans have a remarkably stable internal environment.[12] Blood pressure, temperature, pO_2, and blood pH are just a few parameters that are regulated within a very narrow range through homeostatic mechanisms. Although body weight varies greatly among different people (as other parameters do not), there is little variation within each person over time, whether at a normal or elevated level. This long-term stability of weight under widely varying environmental conditions may be possible because a set-point mechanism regulates body weight. The obese do not differ from people of normal weight in how they regulate their weight, but rather at what level it is done. Whether there is a set-point control mechanism has not been proven, but the available evidence suggests the presence of a central regulatory mechanism.

HEALTH CONSEQUENCES OF OBESITY

Obesity is hazardous to health in many ways. Some of the normal body functions are impaired by obesity. Ventilation, for example, is decreased, which leads to both increased carbon dioxide retention and a lowered oxygenation of arterial blood. This leads to a decrease in exercise tolerance, difficulty in breathing, and a higher incidence of respiratory infections.

Obesity is associated with an increased frequency of some diseases and aggravation of some other already existing diseases. One of the most important associations is that found between heart disease and obesity. Although obesity has not been shown to be a direct cause of heart disease, obese people do have a higher incidence of heart disease. When heart problems do occur, obesity aggravates the condition. There is a strong association between obesity and hypertension, and obesity and atherosclerosis, both of which lead to heart disease. Elevated cholesterol levels, which are more common in obesity, are important in the development of atherosclerosis. Fatty acid turnover is increased when adipose tissue is formed, which increases the synthesis and excretion of cholesterol. Weight reduction lowers cholesterol and triglyceride levels (also increased in obesity).

Hypertension is more common among obese people than among those of normal weight. The blood pressure of an obese, hypertensive person decreases as weight is lost.

Diabetes mellitus also can be caused or aggravated by obesity. Adult onset diabetes is much more prevalent among the obese. They have impaired carbohydrate metabolism because of an increased need for insulin. As weight is lost, however, the amount of insulin needed is decreased and sometimes may become unnecessary, especially if exercise is increased simultaneously.

Gallbladder disease occurs more frequently among obese people, probably because the obese person has a greater concentration of cholesterol in the bile, which may lead to gallstone formation. Whatever the disease condition, if surgical intervention is needed, the obese person has a greater risk of postoperative complications.

Obesity can also be hazardous to one's psychological health. Society discriminates against the obese, sees them as weak-willed, lazy, self-indulgent, or gluttonous. For the obese person who may already see himself as a failure, society's attitude only reinforces this negative self-image. If he has tried and failed to lose weight, his self-esteem is lowered, and if he has not even tried for fear of failure, the effect is often much the same. He may see his body as loathsome and undesirable and may avoid looking at himself in the mirror, shopping for clothes, or taking part in activities that require him to display his body.

America's emphasis on slimness as the ideal for everyone takes its toll on those who know they will never reach that ideal. Although there are some obese people who insist that "fat is beautiful" and are working to end discrimination against the obese and to enhance their self-esteem, the majority of overweight people are dissatisfied with their condition and their failure to lose weight. Dissatisfaction and concomitant feelings of powerlessness to change may lead to depression and a feeling of "what's the use." In turn, this leads to a search for some relief, however temporary, and relief often is found in food. Even as a person overeats, he may feel no hunger and very likely feels disgusted with himself. If food has been used from infancy onward as a satisfier of numerous needs, however, it will have powerful associations with comfort and pleasure.

The psychological effects of obesity are based mainly on the reports of the obese who seek treatment for their obesity. For those who are adjusted to their condition and never seek professional help, the psychological factors are not as well known. Therefore, one should be hesitant to generalize, but for the many coming for treatment, these psychological difficulties are important to consider in the management of their problem.

NURSING ASSESSMENT

The assessment of a patient's weight history provides the basis for helping that person manage his problem.

SUBJECTIVE DATA

Demographic Variables

Identify age, sex, marital status, race, employment status, economic status, and education level of the patient.

Patient's Weight History

Determine time and circumstances of the initial weight gain, episodes of large weight gains and current weight. Determine the patient's perception of his weight problem. How does he describe himself (obese, fat, chubby, a lot or a little overweight)? Identify past attempts to lose weight; the number of attempts, the amount of weight lost and regained, past emotional or physical reactions (e.g., depression, nervousness, irritability, weakness, nausea, fatigue) during or after the program. Obtain a diet diary, including what, how much, when, how often, where, and with whom the patient eats (see the sample Diet Diary form.) Assess the patient's mood before and after eating; ask about episodes of binge-eating or getting up at night to eat. Is the patient aware of his actual food intake? Evaluate how susceptible the patient is to environmental cues such as the time of day, availability of food, certain types of food, and the amount available. Identify who prepares meals and shops for food. Assess feelings of hunger and satiety. Determine the patient's activity level. Does he have a sedentary occupation? Does he exercise, walk, climb stairs, participate in sports? How often and how long does he exercise? Identify hobbies, recreational activities, and activities frequently engaged in that may be used as a substitute for eating. Identify participation in community activities, such as church or community organizations.

Motivation

Determine the patient's reasons for losing weight. Does he *want* to lose or does he feel he *should* lose weight? How much weight does he want to lose? At what weight does he feel best? Does he want to change eating and exercise habits (i.e., make a permanent change)? Does he perceive the program as a temporary change in life-style? Does he feel he has a solvable weight problem?

Emotional Assessment

Assess the patient's body image. How does he feel about himself and his appearance at his current weight? How does he feel about losing weight? Does he feel that reducing his weight will solve other problems, and if so, what problems? What are the patient's current circumstances? Is he currently under stress or undergoing any change in his life situation? Does the patient exhibit signs or symptoms of depression or anxiety? Is the patient emotionally stable? Does the patient feel that he can control his eating behavior? Does he feel that losing weight will result in approval from others? Identify any emotional or social barriers to losing weight. Weight loss can be perceived as a threat to the person, resulting in loss of love or increasing spouse jealousy, rather than as something positive. Identify the anticipated effect on the person's sexuality.

Family Weight History

Identify overweight relatives (siblings, parents, children, spouse). Identify who lives in the same household with the patient and their weight status. Assess the attitudes of the other family members, their degree of support or lack of support and the response of the patient to these attitudes. Determine possible effects of the program and actual weight loss on the family structure and on relationships with significant others.

Medical History

Identify any associated physical symptomatology (e.g., shortness of breath, constipation, skin problems, chest pain, headache,

Diet Diary

Time	Amount	Type of Food	Where Eaten	With Whom	Mood

and amenorrhea), associated disease (especially diabetes mellitus, hypertension, arthritis), cardiovascular risk factors, current medications, and allergies. Identify smoking or alcohol habits.

OBJECTIVE DATA

Physical Examination

Include weight, height, blood pressure, heart rate, and physical appearance (neat vs. disheveled).

Paraclinical Data

Fasting blood sugar, cholesterol and triglyceride levels (levels fall with weight loss), hematocrit (possible anemia in women who are dieting). Consider a stress test in patients over 40 years old to determine maximum heart rate and exercise tolerance before recommending an exercise program. These tests are expensive and require clinical judgment or consultation with a physician regarding whether the data is necessary.

NURSING DIAGNOSIS

DETERMINE THE DEGREE OF OBESITY

Using one of the methods to measure obesity, determine the amount that the patient is overweight. The body mass index is perhaps the easiest scientific method to use.[2] The patient can be categorized as overweight, obese, and obese to the degree that it is a potential health risk (See Fig. 19-1).

DETERMINE THE LIKELIHOOD OF SUCCESS

Researchers have identified characteristics common in people who succeed in losing weight.[15,16,18,19,22] People who lose weight have a meaningful reason for losing weight, which provides motivation to adhere to the reduction program. The patient's level of self-esteem does not predict success, but the degree to which social acceptance is important to a particular patient does influence success. Locus of control does not seem to affect the outcome, but the greater the patient's responsiveness to external nonfood stimuli (e.g., the time of day) as well as food related environmental stimuli, the more difficult it is to lose weight. Maintenance is easier if the environment is restricted in the number of cues that stimulate eating. The patient must believe the condition is reversible and not an inherent characteristic. Emotional stability is important: people under stress or who are emotionally unstable have a more difficult time losing weight. Most studies show that men lose weight more easily than women; those in a higher socioeconomic group and those who have adult onset obesity are more successful. The percentage of overweight affects the outcome. It is more difficult for the severely obese to lose weight than for those who are mildly obese. Accuracy in reporting intake and the extent of weight loss early in the treatment predict a person's success. People who have attempted to lose weight many times and failed or regained the lost weight have a smaller chance of succeeding. The skill and receptiveness of the therapist also affects success. The assessment data is evaluated in terms of these predictors of success. Use the resulting information to individualize the management plan.

DETERMINE THE LIKELIHOOD OF AN ADVERSE EMOTIONAL RESPONSE DURING OR FOLLOWING WEIGHT LOSS

The incidence of an adverse emotional reaction is high during treatment in an outpatient setting.[9,10] Patients can become irritable, weak, nauseated, depressed, or angry. The greater the calorie restriction and the longer the duration of treatment, the higher the incidence of such reactions. There seems to be a lower incidence of negative emotional and physical reactions when obesity is managed with behavioral modification techniques. The risk of negative reactions is higher in people with child onset obesity, severe obesity, and in those who previously had an adverse emotional response while losing weight. Patients with a high probability of adverse emotional responses should be monitored closely and may benefit from frequent contact for support.

DETERMINE THE GOAL OF MANAGEMENT

The management of obesity requires permanent changes in the patient's behavior and attitude. The patient needs to learn how to control his weight rather than to allow his weight to control him. The patient first takes control of the problem by deciding on a realistic goal. The goal may be to achieve ideal body weight, or to learn to live with obesity, or it may be somewhere between these two extremes. The goal should remain flexible, because it may require modification during the treatment period. The weight goal is specified with a numerical range (e.g., 130–135 lb), but short-term goals also may be beneficial in maintaining motivation. Short-term goals may include losing 1 to 2 lb/wk, changing one eating behavior at a time, or maintaining one's weight over a holiday. The management goal should include the loss of body fat through planned exercise, development of new eating patterns to facilitate weight maintenance, and promotion of a sense of physical and emotional well-being with a minimum of risks. A goal that is mutually agreed upon helps establish a collaborative effort between the nurse and patient, which facilitates achievement of that goal.

MANAGEMENT

The complexity of obesity as a health problem makes its management difficult. The literature is filled with studies documenting that of the small percentage of obese people who attempt to lose weight, most fail to lose a significant amount despite participation in systematic weight reduction programs. Attrition rates are high, and techniques to motivate patients to adhere to regimens are inadequate. Maintaining a normal weight is a major problem for those who do succeed in losing weight; most people regain the weight promptly and often gain more.

The management of obesity can be provided by one individual nurse or by a multidisciplinary approach. The setting, knowledge, and resources available influence the approach chosen. A nurse in the primary care setting or in the community may manage the patient herself, whereas the nurse in an inpatient setting may use other resources (dietitian, social worker, or psychologist in a coordinated team approach).

Management is based on the assumption that obesity is caused by habits of daily living that result in a greater intake of food than is needed for the person's level of energy expenditure.[18] The approaches discussed are directed at reducing food intake and increasing energy expenditure. The specific interventions selected should be directed at maximizing the patient's strengths and minimizing or eliminating deficits, thus developing a meaningful and realistic program. Use of strategies that are directed at long-term maintenance of desired eating habits and goal weight are important. Unfortunately, the effectiveness of these strategies on long-term maintenance is not clearly established in the literature. Techniques that strictly control the immediate environment (inpatient programs, camps) are effective for rapid weight loss, but not for maintenance after the person leaves that controlled setting. Patients do not learn how to alter eating behavior. Frequent contact with the therapist for guidance, counseling, and reinforcement facilitates weight loss. Initial visits should be weekly until the patient is following the program smoothly. Visits can then become biweekly and, after the goal weight is achieved, monthly, followed by a continual reduction in frequency over a 1-year to 2-year period. During the treatment the nurse should monitor weight, blood pressure, cholesterol and triglyceride levels if appropriate, and observe for negative emotional responses and physical responses such as constipation, flatulence, and orthostatic hypotension.

The research literature recommends the simultaneous use of more than one method. The overall program recommended is a multidimensional approach combining a calorie-restricted diet with behavior modification and exercise.[4,18,19] In addition to these three areas of management, use of support groups and medication can be considered. The chosen program should be safe and promote long-term change.

DIET

Body fat is lost when the food intake is less than the energy expenditure; 1 lb of fat is lost for each 3500 calorie deficit.[22] The initial loss of weight results from water and electrolyte loss and less content in the gastrointestinal tract. Water loss is remarkable in very low-carbohydrate and low-salt diets and can be responsible for fluctuations of weight while following a diet.

Characteristics of a "Good" Reducing Diet

Several characteristics constitute a "good" reducing diet.[5,16,22] The diet should be low in calories but free of side-effects (discussed later). It should satisfy all nutrient needs, be able to be followed for a long time and should facilitate retraining of eating habits so that its principles can be integrated into the patient's permanent life-style. It should prevent between-meal hunger, cause a minimum of fatigue, promote a sense of well-being, be easy to follow at home or in social settings, and be as close to the person's usual routine as possible. Fad diets should be considered with caution because they frequently do not meet these criteria.

Determining the Number of Calories

The caloric level of the diet depends on the patient's needs and rate of weight loss desired. A simple gross method to determine the number of calories required to lose weight is the following:[1] Determine basal caloric needs based on activity level of the patient. Multiply the patient's desired weight by 10 (e.g., $120 \times 10 = 1200$ kcal). Add calories needed for each level of activity:

1. For sedentary people, add (desired weight $\times$ 3), that is, $1200 + (120 \times 3) = 1560$ kcal = basal daily caloric need to maintain
2. For moderately active people, add (desired weight $\times$ 5), that is, $1200 + (120 \times 5) = 1800$ kcal
3. For strenuously active people, add (desired weight $\times$ 10), that is, $1200 + (120 \times 10) = 2400$ kcal

Reduce daily intake by 750 kcal to 1000 kcal below the basal caloric need to produce a weight loss of 2 to 2 ½ lb/wk. A reduction of 500 kcal will produce a weight loss of 1 lb/wk. The effect of these diets is based mainly on the number of calories, not the particular nutrients (i.e., carbohydrates).

Low-Calorie Diets

A diet in which the calorie intake is too low is often very difficult for a patient to follow.

Diets consisting of less than 1000 kcal can have side-effects resulting from a negative nitrogen balance. These diets also can be deficient in calcium. Liquid diets, one-item meals, or skipped meals inhibit re-education of eating habits.

200 Kcal to 400 Kcal Diet   This is recommended only for hospitalized patients. A vitamin supplement is required. It promotes rapid weight loss, decreased appetite, allows little time and decision-making for food selection since there is little variety and a great deal of monotony. Side-effects include postural hypotension, fatigue, menstrual irregularities, hair loss, cold intolerance, and constipation. Quick weight gain on refeeding is typical because eating patterns and behaviors are not changed.

Fasting   The weight loss that occurs as a result of fasting is at an approximate rate of 1 lb/day in a 300 lb subject over a two-month program.[6] Losses are greatest in the heaviest patients. Protein loss and lean body mass as well as fat loss is substantial. Side-effects are similar to the 200 kcal to 400 kcal diet. Nausea may be experienced because of ketosis. Serious side-effects have been noted with fasting of long duration, including death and psychosis. There is little success with maintenance following termination of the fast. There is no re-educative value to fasting. Short-term fasts of approximately 10 days' duration have fewer side-effects, promote initial rapid weight loss and, hence, can stimulate motivation. A short-term fast should be implemented in a hospital setting to ensure close monitoring for adverse effects.

Low-Carbohydrate Diet   The main advantage of a low-carbohydrate diet is that it provides satiety from the high protein and fat content. Ketosis is the main side-effect of a low-carbohydrate diet. Fifty grams of carbohydrate helps prevent ketosis, but one hundred grams is recommended if the diet is to be followed over a long period of time.[22] Caloric restriction seems to account for weight loss following the initial water weight loss. The diet may also be deficient in vitamins. It is not recommended for patients with gout or uric acid kidney stones because uric acid levels can be elevated. Fatigue and a low blood pressure are other side-effects, and if the diet is high in fat, it may increase the patient's risk of heart disease by elevating cholesterol and triglyceride levels. There is little re-educative value for changing long-term eating habits.

1000 Kcal to 1800 Kcal Diets   Setting a caloric restriction above 1000 kcal but 750 kcal to 1000 kcal below the patient's caloric needs allows more flexibility and variety in the diet. It necessitates re-education to learn how to choose food from a wide variety and to maintain a balanced diet while staying within the caloric restrictions. Learning this process can be difficult and frustrating for some people. Structuring the diet to limit choices can minimize this problem temporarily, but the need to learn how to exert control over choices remains.

Use of a food exchange list can be easier to follow than counting calories. One problem with food exchange lists is remembering what has already been eaten that day. Many people find keeping detailed daily diet diaries tedious. An alternative solution is keeping a checklist of daily allowed exchanges which can be faster and easier to use (Fig. 19-2). Accurate monitoring of intake is essential to ensure that caloric intake stays under the desired level.

The patient often needs assistance to follow the diet in social settings. Restaurant menu food choices that are consistent with his weight-loss goal need to be discussed. For example, the patient can choose clear soup or a fruit cup over creamed soup; baked or

	Mon.	Tue.	Wed.	Thurs.	Fri.	Sat.	Sun.
Fruit	( )	( )	( )	( )	( )	( )	( )
	( )	( )	( )	( )	( )	( )	( )
	( )	( )	( )	( )	( )	( )	( )
	( )	( )	( )	( )	( )	( )	( )
Bread	( )	( )	( )	( )	( )	( )	( )
	( )	( )	( )	( )	( )	( )	( )
	( )	( )	( )	( )	( )	( )	( )
	( )	( )	( )	( )	( )	( )	( )
	( )	( )	( )	( )	( )	( )	( )
Meat	( )	( )	( )	( )	( )	( )	( )
	( )	( )	( )	( )	( )	( )	( )
	( )	( )	( )	( )	( )	( )	( )
	( )	( )	( )	( )	( )	( )	( )
	( )	( )	( )	( )	( )	( )	( )
Vegetable (Restricted)	( )	( )	( )	( )	( )	( )	( )
	( )	( )	( )	( )	( )	( )	( )
Free Vegetables (As desired)	( )	( )	( )	( )	( )	( )	( )
Skim Milk	( )	( )	( )	( )	( )	( )	( )
	( )	( )	( )	( )	( )	( )	( )
Fat	( )	( )	( )	( )	( )	( )	( )
	( )	( )	( )	( )	( )	( )	( )
	( )	( )	( )	( )	( )	( )	( )

FIG. 19-2 *Twelve-hundred-calorie exchange checklist.*

broiled meat, turkey, fish, chicken, or veal over fried meat, casseroles, or creamed food; salad with oil and vinegar over french dressing; baked potato or vegetables without butter or sour cream over vegetables with cheese sauces; fruit, sherbert, plain angel food cake over pie, or cake and ice cream. These guidelines can be modified for social gatherings. Behavioral modification techniques in these situations are also helpful.

BEHAVIOR MODIFICATION

In addition to a diet program, the patient requires assistance in learning to exert control over the environment that affects his eating behavior. The patient needs to learn specific strategies to help him to manage the effect of people and specific situations on his eating patterns. These strategies can be loosely categorized as behavioral modification techniques and are described in depth by Stuart, Stunkard, and Coates.[4,17,18,19] The emphasis is on behavioral change rather than weight loss. The environment is manipulated to facilitate appropriate eating behavior and minimize or eliminate inappropriate eating behavior. Techniques that promote appropriate eating behavior are effective. Specific strategies used by a patient are based on his individual difficulties. Encourage the patient to identify strategies that may be helpful. Limit the number of strategies used at any one time to prevent the patient from feeling overwhelmed.

Increase the patient's awareness of his eating behaviors by analyzing his diet diary and other information regarding his weight history. Increasing the patient's awareness of his behaviors helps to decrease automatic eating. Identify behaviors that facilitate eating a proper amount and those that interfere with overeating. The patient should identify any forthcoming stress that may increase overeating and typical situations that influence between-meal eating. Strategies then can be devised to handle eating behavior during these situations. For example, the person can engage in an alternate enjoyable activity or call a friend at a time when he would normally eat. Methods to increase the patient's self-awareness on an ongoing basis include keeping a diet diary and weight chart.

Strategies to control events that precede eating to reduce environmental stimuli that trigger eating include the following:

- Increasing appropriate eating behavior
  Increase availability of low calorie food.
  Weekly meal planning to facilitate eating well-balanced low-calorie meals, reduce impulse eating, and guide shopping
  Shop for food on a full stomach, using a list.
  Prepare just enough food for one meal.

Keep food only for one meal in the kitchen.
Buy foods that require preparation.
Allow extra money to purchase proper foods.
- Decreasing inappropriate eating behavior
  Decrease availability of high-calorie food.
  Store foods in non-see-through containers.
  Do not hover over cooking foods or linger in the kitchen or at the table.
  At parties, sit away from snacks.
  Decide what to order before going to a restaurant.
  Avoid food deprivation before eating out.

Strategies that control the act of eating include the following:

- Increasing appropriate behavior
  Reduce size of portions.
  Measure food.
  Eat slowly by increasing chewing, replacing utensils on table between bites. These strategies also increase the enjoyment of eating and improve digestion.
  Premonitor: Write down what is about to be eaten.
  Save one item to eat later.
- Decreasing inappropriate behavior
  Eat in one place only.
  Discard leftovers.
  Leave some food on the plate.
  Eliminate other activities while eating. (If an activity is carried out while eating, then, at other times, the patient may want to eat while carrying out that activity.)
  Reduce stressful interactions at mealtime.
  Covert sensitization: Use of imagery to associate a desired high-calorie food with a negative event. (This technique has only a short-term effect.)
  Use small plates.

Strategies that have an impact on the consequence of eating:

- Positive reinforcement: Given by the patient himself or by the nurse. Abundant praise, rewards for achieving goals, hanging pictures of new clothes, and altering clothes are examples. Positive reinforcement should be given frequently.
- Adverse therapy: Using adverse stimuli has not been found to be successful.
- Contracts are found to affect short-term weight loss only during the time of treatment.
- Family involvement: Family members and significant others should be encouraged to provide praise only and should avoid offering food to facilitate the patient's success.
- Therapist support is an important factor in facilitating weight loss. In addition to positive reinforcement and facilitating problem-solving, the nurse should assist the patient in coping with any identified psychological stresses that may impede weight loss.

EXERCISE

Overweight people tend to be less active than normal weight people. Increasing energy expenditure does not affect weight loss significantly, but it does promote fat loss and increase lean body mass. It also promotes a feeling of well-being. It may also lower a person's set-point. It does not increase appetite. Hence, exercise is a good adjunct to a calorie-restricted diet. Exercise can be obtained through organized programs (e.g., Vic Tanny's), on one's own, or through increased general physical activity. Generally, before beginning a program, people over age 40 should have their exercise tolerance and cardiovascular risk factors evaluated. A maximum heart rate determination provides guidance for effective yet safe exercise levels.

Self-guided exercise programs should involve three phases; a 10-minute warm-up phase consisting of stretching exercises, a 20 to 30 minute minimum exercise period, and a 10-minute cool-down phase. For a more detailed discussion of exercise programs, the reader is referred to exercise literature. Most obese people can begin exercising safely by walking. Physical activity can be increased by incorporating it into the patient's daily routines (e.g., patients can park the car to necessitate walking, use stairs rather than an elevator).

SELF-HELP GROUPS

Self-help groups provide social support and pressure to follow the weight loss program. Some groups also provide behavioral re-education. These groups, like other programs, have high attrition rates. Examples of self-help groups include TOPS (Take Off Pounds Sensibly), Weight Watchers, and Overeaters Anonymous. Other groups, recently begun for people who have not been able to lose weight, try to help them live more comfortably with their obesity.

COMMERCIAL WEIGHT REDUCTION PROGRAMS

Commercial programs that charge a fee for their services have higher attrition rates than self-help groups, reaching as high as 70% at twelve weeks.[21] The methods used vary among clinics.

DRUG TREATMENT

Drug treatment of obesity consists of anorectic drugs used to depress appetite. These drugs may be useful for short-term weight loss, but the effect is transitory and does not promote long-term weight loss. A study by Stunkard showed a greater initial weight loss but a greater regain at 1 year follow-up. It also showed a negative effect on behavioral therapy when the methods were combined.[20] There are two classes of anorectic drugs, amphetamines and nonamphetamines (fenfluramine, mazindol, clortermine). The abuse potential of amphetamines because of central nervous system stimulation is great. Dependency is a problem and tolerance occurs (the effect is reduced over time). The nonamphetamines seem to have fewer adverse side-effects but minimal short-term efficacy. Overall, there is much controversy regarding the usefulness of these drugs in the treatment of obesity.

SURGERY

Surgical treatment of obesity to reduce the absorption ability of the intestines has been used as a last resort for severely obese patients refractory to other weight loss methods. The most common procedure is the jejunoileal bypass. This approach has severe side-effects, including diarrhea, poor absorption of fat-soluble vitamins, and electrolyte imbalances. There is a significant mortality risk with the procedure, as well as other organic complications involving the liver, kidney, and intestines. The gastric bypass has also been used for weight loss in the morbidly obese by limiting oral intake and producing early satiety. This procedure also is associated with serious complications occurring within a month postoperation, including death, obstruction, abscess, and ulcers. There seem to be fewer late complications than there are with the jejunoileal bypass. *Gastroplasty*, a modification of the gastric bypass, involves stapling of the stomach to form a small proximal pouch and a funnel connecting it to the distal stomach. It provides early satiety and avoids the metabolic complications of the small bowel bypass. However, the failure rate to produce weight loss varies from 43% to 53%.[11] The surgical approach is controversial because of the significant risks involved and the lack of objective analysis of its benefits in light of those risks.

SUMMARY

Obesity is a complex and poorly understood problem. Multiple factors contribute to its development, including body type, sex, socioeconomic level, age of onset, physiological factors, and psychological factors. Obesity can affect other health problems adversely, such as heart disease and diabetes mellitus. It also presents emotional, psychological, and social problems. Some of these factors are more important in some people and less so in others; hence the management of obesity is complex. There is little conclusive data that identify effective methods yielding long-term success. Future research should be directed toward methods that facilitate weight maintenance. A multidimensional approach incorporating a low-calorie diet, behavior modification, and exercise addresses the problems of high intake and low output. It also promotes re-education so that the patient controls his eating behavior rather than allowing his eating behavior and the environment to control him. The goal and the strategies chosen for the management of obesity should be individualized, based on the patient's strengths and the specific problems that aggravate his condition. No single treatment method is adequate for all people.

REFERENCES

1. Arky RA: Current principles of dietary therapy of diabetes mellitus. Med Clin North Am 62:655–662, 1978

2. Bray GA: Definition, measurement and classification of the syndromes of obesity. Int J Obes 2:1–14, 1978
3. Bray GA: Obesity. Disease-a-Month 26:1–85, 1979
4. Coates TJ, Thoresen CE: Treating obesity in children and adolescents: A review. Am J Public Health 68, No. 2:143–149, 1978
5. Debry G: Newer knowledge on the treatment of obesity. Bibl Nutr Dieta 26:44–59, 1978
6. Drenick EJ: Weight reduction by prolonged fasting. In Bray GA (ed): Obesity in Perspective. Publication No. NIH 75-708. Washington, DC, Department of Health, Education, and Welfare, 1975
7. Goldblatt PB, Moore NE, Stunkard AJ: Social factors in obesity. JAMA 192:1039–1044, 1965
8. Guggenheim FG: Approach to the patient with obesity. In Goroll AH, May LA, Mulley AG (eds): Primary Care Medicine: Office Evaluation and Management of the Adult Patient. Philadelphia, JB Lippincott, 1981
9. Hirsh J: The psychological consequences of obesity. In Bray, GA (ed): Obesity in Perspective. Publication No. NIH 75-708. Washington DC, Department of Health, Education, and Welfare, 1975
10. Jeffrey DB: Treatment outcome issues in obesity research. In Williams BJ et al. (eds): Obesity: Behavioral Approaches to Dietary Management. New York, Brunner/Mazel, 1976
11. Joffe SN: A Review: Surgery for morbid obesity. J Surg Res 33:74–88, 1982
12. Keesey R: A set-point analysis of the regulation of body weight. In Stunkard AJ (ed): Obesity. Philadelphia, WB Saunders, 1980
13. Mayer J: Overweight. Englewood Cliffs, NJ, Prentice–Hall, 1968
14. Powers PS: Obesity: The regulation of weight. Baltimore, Williams & Wilkins, 1980
15. Roden J et al: Predictors of successful weight loss in an outpatient obesity clinic. Int J Obes 1:79–87, 1977
16. Scott LW et al: Nutrition during weight loss. In Williams BJ (ed): Obesity: Behavioral Approaches to Dietary Management. New York, Brunner/Mazel, 1976
17. Stuart RB: Behavioral control of overeating. Behav Res Ther 5:357–365, 1967
18. Stuart RB: A three-dimensional program for the treatment of obesity. Behav Res Ther 9:177–186, 1971
19. Stunkard AJ: Behavioral treatment of obesity: The current status. Int J Obes 2:237–248, 1978
20. Stunkard AJ et al: Controlled trial of behavior therapy, pharmacotherapy, and their combination in the treatment of obesity. Lancet 2, No. 8203:1045–1047, 1980
21. Volkmar FP et al: High attrition rates in commercial weight reduction programs. Arch Int Med 141, No. 4:426–8, 1981
22. Young CM: Dietary treatment of obesity. In Bray GA (ed): Obesity In Perspective. Publication No. NIH 75-708. Washington DC, Department of Health, Education, and Welfare, 1975

BIBLIOGRAPHY

Abramson EE: Behavioral approaches to weight control: An updated review. Behav Res Ther 15:355–363, 1977

Ashby WA, Wilson GT: Behavior therapy for obesity: Booster sessions and long-term maintenance of weight loss. Behav Res Ther 15:451–463, 1977

Bray GA (ed): Obesity In Perspective. Publication No. NIH 75–708, Washington DC, Department of Health, Education and Welfare, 1975

Bray G: Obesity. Disease-a-Month, 26:1–25 October 1979

Bray G: Obesity in America: An Overview of the Second Fogarty International Center Conference on Obesity. Int J Obes 3:363–374, 1979

Bray G (ed): Obesity in America. Department of Health, Education, and Welfare. NIH Publication No. 80-359 Washington DC, Department of Health, Education and Welfare, 1980

Bruch H: Eating disorders. New York, Basic Books, 1973

Buckwalter JA, Herbst CA: Complications of gastric bypass for morbid obesity. Am J Surg 131, No. 1:55–60, Jan 1980

Croft C: Body image and obesity. Nurs Clin North Am 7:677–685, Dec 1972

Hall SM et al: Self and external management compared with psychotherapy in the control of obesity. Behav Res Ther 15:89–95, 1977

Howard AN: The historical development, efficacy and safety of very low-calorie diets. Int J Obes 5:195–208, 1981

Jones B: Weighty matters (unpublished paper). Ann Arbor, University of Michigan, 1979

Lutwak L, Coulston A: Activity and obesity. In Bray GA (ed): Obesity in Perspective. Publication No. NIH 75–708. Washington DC, Department of Health, Education, and Welfare, Washington DC, 1975

Wing RR, Jeffrey RW: Outpatient treatment of obesity: A comparison of methodology and clinical results. Int J Obes 3:261–279, 1979

Mahoney MJ, Mahoney K: Treatment of obesity: A clinical exploration. In Williams BJ et al (eds): Obesity: Behavioral Approach to Dietary Management. New York, Brunner/Mazel, 1976

McReynolds WT, Paulsen BK: Stimulus control as the behavioral basis of weight loss procedures. In Williams BJ et al (eds): Obesity: Behavioral approaches to dietary management. New York, Brunner/Mazel, 1976

Miller BK: Jejunoileal bypass: A drastic weight control measure. Am J Nurs 81:564–568, 1981

Mojzisik CM, Martin EW: Gastric partitioning: The latest surgical means to control morbid obesity. Am J Nurs 81:569–572, 1981

Overeaters Anonymous: A self-help group. Am J Nurs 81:560–563, 1981

Razensky RH, Bellack AS: Individual differences in self-reinforcement style and performance in self and therapist-controlled weight reduction programs. Behav Res Therapy 14:357–364, 1976

Samuel PD, Burland WC: Drug treatment of obesity. In Bray GA (ed): Obesity in Perspective. Publication No. NIH 75-708. Washington DC, Department of Health, Education, and Welfare, 1975

Stuart RB: Behavior control of overeating: A status report. In Bray GA (ed): Obesity in Perspective. Publication No. NIH 75–708. Washington, DC, Department of Health, Education, and Welfare, 1975

Stunkard AJ: Dieting and depression reexamined: A critical review of reports of untoward responses during weight reduction for obesity. Ann Int Med 81:526–533, 1974

Stunkard AJ: Presidential address, 1974: From explanation to action in psychosomatic medicine: The case of obesity. Psychosomatic Medicine 37, No. 3:195–235, May/June 1975

Vincent JP et al: Effect of deposit contracts and distractability on weight loss and maintenance. In Williams BJ et al (eds): Obesity: Behavioral Approaches to Dietary Management. New York, Brunner/Mazel, 1976

Williams BJ et al (ed): Obesity: Behavioral Approaches to Dietary Management. New York, Brunner/Mazel, 1976

Wing RR, Jeffrey RW: Out-patient treatment of obesity: A comparison of methodology and clinical results. Int J Obes 3:261–279, 1979

20

Menopause

Violet H. Barkauskas

Menopause is a benchmark in the lives of women. Physiologically it indicates a termination of reproductive capability; however, most women already have made a decision to terminate childbearing at an earlier age. Thus, the loss of reproductive ability is not in itself a major loss and is perceived by many as a benefit.

Menopause has a potent psychological impact because it indicates that the aging process is underway and that it is likely to accelerate. Although this perception is accurate, women can do much to maintain optimal physical and emotional health and functioning during the menopausal and postmenopausal periods. This chapter contains discussions of the physiology of menopause, the sequelae of resultant estrogen decline, the major health problems encountered during menopause, the indications and contraindications of estrogen replacement therapy, and the maintenance of postmenopausal health.

In this discussion, menopause is presented as a normal, developmental event, not as a deficiency disease. As with all developmental events, therefore, menopause needs to be understood and managed, not to be treated as a disease for the majority of women.

DEMOGRAPHY OF THE MENOPAUSE

The age at which menopause occurs normally is distributed with a mean of 51.4 years and a standard deviation of 3.8 years.[7] The onset of menopause does not appear to correlate with environmental factors, education, physical type, age at menarche, number of previous pregnancies, or age at last pregnancy. Women who have never been married and who are smokers experience menopause approximately 1 year earlier than the average.[7,9]

The health care of menopausal women is receiving increased attention for several reasons. Only in recent times have women had a life expectancy extending long beyond menopause. Whereas the life expectancy of women was approximately 50 years in the early 1900s, it is currently approximately 75 years. Thus, while the majority of women at the turn of the century lived only a short time after menopause, contemporary women are in the postmenopausal developmental stage for approximately one third of their lives.

Second, the discovery of synthetic estrogens provided what appeared to be an early, easy solution to the menopausal problems associated with estrogen decline. Large-dose, long-duration courses of estrogen were prescribed for many women until epidemiologic data demonstrated the detrimental sequelae of such therapy. Lastly, because of extended life expectancy in general, there is an increasing awareness and consideration of gerontology in all its aspects, especially factors relating to the general well-being and optimal functioning of older adults. The prevailing philosophy includes understanding the aging process for the purposes of working with it and fostering healthy development, rather than perceiving it negatively and pathologically, and consequently complicating it iatrogenically.

DEFINITIONS

The *climacteric* (from a Greek word, meaning "rung of a ladder") is a phase in a woman's life cycle; it is the transition from reproductive capacity to a nonreproductive stage. Climacteric is a general term without well-defined beginning and end points.

Menopause is determined retrospectively and refers specifically to the cessation of menstruation. It has occurred when no menstruation has been experienced for a full calendar year.

The terms *climacteric* and *perimenopause* are often used interchangeably. The *perimenopause* is characterized clinically by the shortening of menstrual cycle length, marked by menstrual irregularity that terminates ultimately in the permanent amenorrhea of menopause. The portion of the climacteric preceding menopause is termed the *premenopause* and the portion of the climacteric following menopause is termed the *postmenopause*.

Menopause may be artificial, premature, or natural. *Artificial menopause* is the abrupt termination of ovarian function by surgical castration or irradiation. *Premature menopause* is the cessation of ovarian function before age 40. *Natural menopause* is the result of decreased ovarian function because of the aging of the ovaries.

MECHANISMS OF MENOPAUSE

OVERALL PHYSIOLOGICAL MECHANISMS

Knowledge of the endocrinology and physiology of the climacteric is essential to the understanding and management of its symptoms and sequelae. The hormonal changes during the premenopause and postmenopause are summarized in Figure 20-1 and elaborated on in this section of the chapter.

The climacteric is characterized by increased levels of follicle-stimulating hormone (FSH), which cause changes in the hypothalamic–pituitary–ovarian feedback cycle. These changes result in cessation of ovulation and luteal function, and in decreased ovarian estrogen production.

The mechanism initiating climacteric endocrine changes is unknown. Depletion of ovarian oocytes was the central premise of early theories regarding menopause causation; however, more recent evidence suggests other possible mechanisms. One theory is that ovarian follicles produce a substance called *inhibin* that controls the amount of FSH, and that inhibin is proportional to the number of ovarian follicles. Thus, when the number of follicles is decreased, the amount of inhibin would decrease and the amount of FSH would increase. A second theory includes the hypersecretion of gonadotropin-releasing hormone (GnRH) or increased pituitary responsiveness to GnRH. Both of these

	Hormonal status	Ovarian status	Clinical signs/symptoms
Early premenopause	↑FSH →	rapid follicular →	shortened menstrual cycles (ovulatory cycles)
	↓ ↓Estrogen ↓		
Late premenopause	no LH → surge	no ovulation →	irregular cycles, with flooding due to hyperplasia
Menopause	↑FSH →	no responsive → follicles	menopause

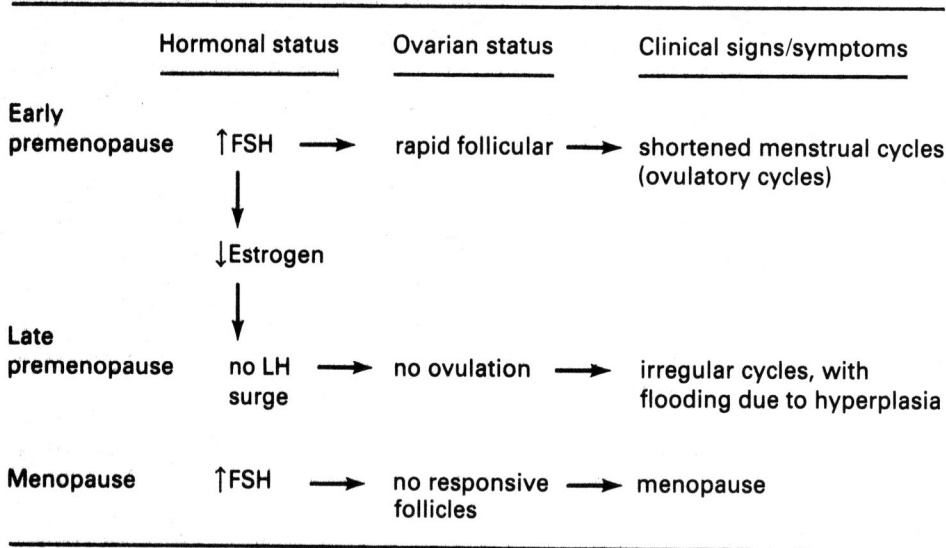

FIG. 20-1. *Relationships among hormonal status, ovarian status, and clinical signs and symptoms during the perimenopause. FSH, follicle stimulating hormone; LH, luteinizing hormone.*

mechanisms would result in increased levels of FSH.

Changes in ovarian function begin years before the menopause. In the late thirties and early forties, gradual rise in FSH and gradual decrease in serum estriol levels in both the follicular and luteal phases of the menstrual cycle can be measured. Increased amounts of FSH result in rapid follicular development, which is clinically noted as shortened menstrual cycles.

As the number of follicles decreases, estrogen production continues to fall. Eventually, estrogen is insufficient to induce a luteinizing hormone (LH) surge, and ovulation ceases or occurs irregularly. Clinically, irregular, anovulatory cycles with flooding (a sudden rapid gush of menstrual fluid because of uterine hyperplasia) are observed.

Variability in the menstrual cycle can occur as long as responsive follicles remain in the ovaries. Thus, variable cycles and con-

comitant signs and symptoms can occur for several years. Although the attrition of ovarian follicular units results in decreased estrogen levels, the postmenopausal woman is not totally depleted of estrogen. The ovarian stoma, adrenal cortex, and diet are remaining sources of estrogen and estrogen precursors. Metabolic conversion of estrogen precursors, primarily androstenedione, occur by means of aromatization in adipose tissue and the liver. Estrone is the product of the process, the efficiency of which increases with age and body weight and is enhanced by liver disease.

EFFECTS OF ESTROGEN DECLINE

Various changes in the body occur as sequelae of decreasing estrogen production. Early symptoms (e.g., hot flashes, sweating) can be attributed directly to estrogen decline and can be replicated in young women who have experienced oopherectomy. The causes of later symptoms, such as dry skin, are not directly attributable to estrogen decline, because of their temporal distance from the menopause and because of the complicating and complicated processes of aging. This section includes a discussion of physical events and changes believed to be related to estrogen decline.

Hot flashes and atrophic vaginitis definitely are related to estrogen decline and respond rapidly to estrogen therapy. Other problems that may be related to estrogen decline are atrophy of other genital and urinary tract organs, skin and hair changes, changes in breasts, coronary artery disease, increased serum lipids, and osteoporosis.

Hot Flashes

Hot flashes, with accompanying skin flushes and sweating, are the most common and most troublesome symptoms of menopause and are experienced by an estimated 75% to 85% of women. Hot flashes result from a not-well-understood syndrome termed *vasomotor instability*. They begin in the premenopausal period, peak around menopause, and usually cease 1 year to 2 years postmenopause, although they can continue longer.

Women's experiences with hot flashes vary widely. Some women do not experience them at all, whereas others may have many hot flashes within a 24-hour period.

Hot flashes are characterized by: 1) a sudden sensation of overwhelming warmth that is felt chiefly in the upper chest, neck, face, and forehead; 2) visible redness and perspiration in warm areas; and 3) brief duration.

Hot flashes characteristically begin with sensations of overwhelming heat occurring suddenly, spreading from the chest and up to the neck, face, or arms, and lasting for several seconds to a minute. They may occur many times in a 24-hour period. A hot flash may be accompanied by drenching perspiration, especially at night, and increased pulse and respiratory rates. Hot flashes are often provoked by a situation increasing body heat production, such as exercise, excitement, alcohol ingestion, eating, or excessive clothing or covering.

Physiologically, hot flashes are accompanied by an increase in skin temperature, but not in body temperature, and a transient tachycardia. Current research indicates a temporal relationship between the onset of a hot flash and a pulsate release of LH.[12] However, it is believed GnRH or hypothalamic neurotransmitters responsible for GnRH release, and not LH is the cause of hot flashes.

Changes in Genital Organs

Decrease in estrogen has various effects on the genital organs, because these organs are rich in estrogen receptors. Most of the genital organs undergo atrophic changes after the menopause. Many of these changes occur gradually during the decades after menopause and are exacerbated by aging; however, because many of these changes can be reversed by estrogen therapy, estrogen decline may be inferred to be at least a contributing factor.

The skin of the vulva undergoes atrophy and is prone to dystrophia and pruritus. The vulva appear dry, flaccid, flattened, and shriveled, conditions starting approximately a decade after the menopause.

The vaginal epithelium also displays atrophy and dryness. The vagina itself becomes narrowed and shortened because of an increase in submucosal connective tissue. These changes contribute to the clinical problems of atrophic vaginitis and dyspareunia. The postmenopausal cervix usually appears flat and small. The squamocolumnar junction of the cervix usually retreats into the endocervical canal. The cervical canal often becomes narrowed or stenotic. The uterus and any present uterine fibroids decrease in size and weight. The endometrial mucosa is usually thin and atrophic.

The ovaries begin to diminish in size at age 30 and the rate of diminution accelerates after age 60. The normal postmenopausal ovary is usually not palpable.

Changes in the Lower Urinary Tract

As with the tissues of the genital tract, estrogen decline is believed to also be, at least partially, responsible for the commonly observed atrophic changes of the urethra and bladder in postmenopausal women because changes sometimes can be reversed by estrogen therapy. The epithelium of the urethra and trigone of the bladder undergo thinning similar to that of the vaginal mucosa. The bladder sphincter also may lose tone, resulting in symptoms such as urgency, frequency, and incontinence.

Changes in the Skin

Decrease in estrogen is believed to affect thickness of the dermis and the number of mitoses. The thin dermis and accompanying loss of subcutaneous fat result in loss of elasticity and wrinkling. These changes are especially noticeable on the face and skin of the breasts.

Changes in the Breasts

In premenopause, the breasts may become tender and increase in size throughout the menstrual cycle because of the effects of unopposed estrogen in anovulatory cycles and because of the stimulation of pituitary hormones. During postmenopause, the breasts diminish in size and become increasingly flaccid owing to decrease in glandular tissue and increase in subcutaneous fat.

Coronary Artery Disease

The relationship between cardiovascular disease and menopause is still unclear. In nonsmoking premenopausal women, the incidence of coronary heart disease is rare; however, postmenopausally, male and female rates for cardiovascular disease are similar. An early menopause seems to increase the risk for coronary heart disease. After menopause, serum lipids also increase.

Osteoporosis

In women before age 40, the amount of bone formed equals the amount resorbed, resulting in a stable bone mass; after age 40, an imbalance in bone formation resorption results in a progressive loss of skeletal mass. Because loss of skeletal mass is thought to be a cause of osteoporosis, because skeletal mass loss and estrogen decline are initiated around the same time, and because osteoporosis is noted more frequently in women than men of comparable age, osteoporosis has been linked to estrogen deficiency.

Postmenopausal bone loss is a significant problem because of its associated morbidity and mortality. Hip fractures subsequent to falls are common in postmenopausal women and are associated with osteoporosis in 70% to 80% of the cases. One sixth of the patients with hip fractures die within 3 months of the injury because of complications associated with the injury.

SYMPTOMS AND PERCEPTIONS

The signs and symptoms of the climacteric can be divided into three categories: 1) those appearing before menopause, which indicate that hormonal changes have begun; 2) those in perimenopause, which indicate that menopause is near or which accompany the body's early adaptation after menopause; and 3) those appearing years after menopause, which are attributable both to estrogen deficiency as well as to aging.

In the decade before menopause, some women experience irregular menses, changes in menstrual flow (scant flow or flooding), and decreased fertility. These symptoms are probably because of the hormonal changes and resultant anovulatory cycles discussed in the previous section.

Neugarten and Kraines studied 460 women, aged 13 to 65, to determine the incidence of symptomatology frequently attributed to menopause and attitudes toward menopause itself.[13] The most commonly reported physical symptoms were hot flashes, sweats, aches, flooding, and paresthesias. This group did not report an increase in psychological and psychosomatic symptoms, but rather a significant decrease in such symptoms for women aged 55 to 64. Young women perceived menopause as a more significant event than middle-aged women. Responses to the worst aspect of menopause included not knowing what to expect (26%), discomfort and pain (19%), indication of aging (18%), loss of sexual enjoyment (4%), and not being able to have more children (4%). A large portion of women in the study (22%) replied that nothing bothered them about menopause.

Jaszmann studied 6,628 women to determine patterns for climacteric signs and symptoms.[7] This researcher noted an increase in the following symptoms during the premenopausal period: fatigue, headache, irritability, depression, and mental imbalance. After menopause, however, the incidence of these symptoms dropped to a lower level, lower than that for normally menstruating women. Hot flashes, aches in muscles, joints, and bones, perspiration, and paresthesia of the extremities occurred at menopause. Over 60% of respondents in this study complained of hot flashes. The one symptom that in-

creased during the postmenopause was insomnia. Jaszmann also discovered that late menarche, nulliparity, last pregnancy after age 40, higher income, higher level of education, and single marital status were characteristics of women with fewer menopausal complaints.

Bungay, Vessey, and McPherson studied the symptoms of approximately 1000 British men and women aged 30 to 64 to determine the influence of sex on the incidence of various complaints.[2] These researchers discovered that male and female age curves for the following symptoms were parallel: loss of appetite, crawling or tingling sensations in the skin, headache, difficulty with intercourse, indigestion, constipation, diarrhea, shortness of breath, coldness of hands and feet, skin and hair dryness, aching muscles, aching joints, feelings of panic and depression, and dysuria. At the time of menopause, women experienced flushing, night and day sweats, difficulty in making decisions, loss of confidence, anxiety, forgetfulness, difficulty in concentration, feelings of unworthiness, tiredness, dizzy spells, and palpitations. As in the Jaszmann study, the psychological symptoms peaked in premenopause, whereas flushes and sweats were most problematic during menopause. The symptoms of irritability, low backache, and aching breasts decreased after menopause.

As the previous studies indicate, hot flashes and sweats are major menopausal symptoms; however, findings regarding other physical symptoms and psychological complaints are inconsistent. After a review of midlife problems, Notman observed that a variety of symptoms have been attributed to menopausal changes, but that emerging data indicate that menopause does not appear to be responsible for most of the symptoms.[14] "Midlife stresses are the result of a combination of personal, family, social, and biological variables, with postmenopausal development an important phase."[14]

In a discussion of the psychosocial aspects of menopause, Severne recognized that climacteric symptoms are not only determined by the physiological changes in the organism, but are also greatly dependent upon their interaction with the social environment.[18] He speculated that the problematic menopause is largely generated by negative social attitudes toward aging in general and towards the aging female in particular:

> What is certain, in any case, is that the climacteric woman not only has to overcome the real difficulties of middle age and the menopause, but also has to cope with a whole gamut of prejudices and stereotypes which are associated with these events.[18]

The health care practitioner is not immune to prejudicial attitudes towards menopause. Self-understanding on the part of health care practitioners caring for menopausal women is an important prerequisite for objective, rational, holistic care. The practitioner managing the care of the premenopausal and menopausal woman has the difficult tasks of differentiating somatic from psychosomatic complaints and of differentiating hormonally related problems from those caused by other changes.

NURSING ASSESSMENT

A woman of perimenopausal age may see a health professional for reasons related or unrelated to menopause. Because menopause can be an important developmental milestone in a woman's life and because of the woman's need for anticipatory guidance regarding the facts and myths relating to this event, the author recommends that a menopausal health assessment be done for all premenopausal women to determine health problems and needs.

The areas of assessment discussed in this chapter are suggestions only, and relate specifically to menopausal health. In most cases, assessment must be expanded to understand adequately the additional health problems and needs of an individual patient. The following are recommended areas of assessment in the health history and physical examination.

SUBJECTIVE DATA

Present Illness

Determine the age at which symptoms began, if any are present. Obtain a description of the symptoms. Some practitioners find a checklist of symptoms with severity-rating options useful. The list of symptoms can include: hot flashes/flushes, drenching perspiration during day, night sweats, palpitations, vaginitis, painful intercourse, depression, tension, fatigue, headaches, insomnia, irritability, other. A severity-rating scale can include several options; for example, 0 = none, 1 = slight, 2 = moderate, and 3 = marked. Assess any disability regarding any symptoms present. Determine the patient's management of symptoms to date.

Complete Obstetrical and Gynecological Review of Systems

Obtain a description of menstrual cycles. Determine last menstrual period (LMP), last normal menstrual period (LNMP), contraceptive use, past genital surgery and problems, pregnancy history, and sexual activity.

Complete Past History and Medication Profile

If estrogen therapy is being considered, assess the following areas:

Breast cancer (or strong family history of breast cancer)
Genital cancer
Kidney disease
Cardiac problems
Liver disease
Hypertension
Diabetes
Breast disease
Thromboembolic disease

Psychosocial Assessment

For an asymptomatic, menstruating patient, assess the following:

Expectations regarding onset of menopause
Expectations regarding process of menopause
Feelings about menopause
Knowledge of menopause

For the symptomatic or postmenopausal patient, assess the following:

Feelings about menopause
Knowledge of menopause
Mechanisms of coping with menopausal changes

Developmental Assessment

Because menopause is a developmental event, an assessment of the patient's developmental status is important. If the woman has a husband or children, her satisfaction with her role as wife or mother, the quality of her relationship with her husband, her response to her children's increasing independence, and whether she is working or planning to work outside the home are determined. This helps the practitioner to understand the woman as a total person and the dynamics that may influence her perceptions of and coping with menopause.

For the single woman, knowledge of support systems, satisfaction with career or job, presence of any disappointments regarding absence of children, and life goals may yield important data for understanding the patient and choosing intervention alternatives.

Activities of Daily Living

Menopause occurs within, and the adaptation to it is facilitated or exacerbated by, the life habits and life-style of the premenopausal woman. Some menopausal problems may disrupt the woman's activities of daily living. Assessment of the woman's daily pattern, including health habits, rest, exercise, and diet, helps the practitioner to understand the meaning of menopausal events in the context of the woman's lifestyle and habits and provides a basis for considering the need or feasibility of interventions relating to activities of daily living.

OBJECTIVE DATA

Physical Examination

The physical examination should include data on the following:

Height and weight
Blood pressure
Thyroid examination
Cardiovascular system examination
Respiratory system examination
Breast examination
Lymph node examination
Abdominal examination
Pelvic examination
Musculoskeletal examination

Laboratory Tests

The following laboratory tests are recommended:

Pap smear with maturation index
Complete blood count (CBC)
Urinalysis
Mammogram

If estrogen therapy is being considered, the following tests may be done:

Endometrial biopsy
Liver function tests
Triglyceride level
Electrocardiogram (ECG)

NURSING DIAGNOSIS

DIAGNOSTIC PROCESS

For the perimenopausal woman, the diagnosis should include statements regarding the woman's physiological and psychological responses to menopause, as well as statements of any specific problems. The following steps should assist in organizing and summarizing data from the assessment.

Physiological Menopausal Status

Using information obtained in the assessment, estimate probable menopausal status. The patient can be categorized as normally menstruating, premenopausal, perimenopausal, possibly postmenopausal (give LNMP, LMP), or postmenopausal (give LNMP, LMP).

Psychological Response to Menopause

Determine the woman's perceptions of impending or actual menopause in relation to physical events, feelings, and relationships. Responses can range from denial of any effect, through active coping, to severe depression.

Patient's Knowledge About Menopause

Data from several studies indicate that many women do not know what to expect regarding menopause.[10,11] Complete and accurate information regarding menopause is essential to healthy and optimal functioning in the postmenopausal period.

Symptoms and Signs Related to Estrogen Deficiency

Vasomotor instability is expected in women aged 45 to 55. Other symptoms and signs are more apparent after age 60.

Risk for the Development of Osteoporosis

Only women at risk for osteoporosis and its associated complications should be considered for long-term estrogen therapy. (These risk factors are discussed in the next section.)

Safety of Short-term or Long-term Replacement Therapy

If estrogen replacement therapy (ERT) is being considered for the woman, an assessment of the indications and contraindications, risks, and benefits of ERT for the patient is needed.

Diagnostic Statements The following are examples of diagnostic statements:

Example 1: Normally menstruating 45-year-old woman (LMP 3/9/84, LNMP 3/9/84), knowledgeable about menopause, fears disruption of daily activities, no signs or symptoms of estrogen deficiency, low risk for osteoporosis, ERT not contraindicated nor indicated at present

Example 2: Premenopausal (LMP 4/6/84, LNMP 12/13/83), but probably close to menopause since menses are very irregular and accompanied by flooding, very fearful of menopause, has many misconceptions and dreads aging, has had several hot flashes beginning last week, possible contraindication to estrogen because of hypertension

Example 3: Ten years postmenopausal (LNMP 9/27/74), is noticing an acceleration of the changes accompanying aging, dislikes changes but is improving diet and rest habits to minimize them;

was on short-term estrogen therapy for 2 years when age 51 and 53 for hot flashes; no untoward effects then and no contraindications to estrogen therapy

DIFFERENTIAL DIAGNOSES

If the patient has night sweats consider possibilities of tuberculosis or hypothyroidism. Signs and symptoms in the case of tuberculosis include cough, fever, and hemoptysis. Patients with hypothyroidism also have fatigue, cold intolerance, constipation, dry hair, dry rough skin, hoarseness and periorbital edema. A tuberculin skin test (PPD) and chest x-ray assist in ruling out tuberculosis. Appropriate thyroid levels rule out hypothyroidism.

In patients experiencing severe vasomotor symptoms, consider the possibility of pheochromocytoma. The vasomotor symptoms related to pheochromocytoma also come in waves or attacks, but usually are accompanied by pounding headaches, skin pallor (rather than flushes) and marked elevation of blood pressure. Urine or blood tests for catecholamines establish the differential diagnosis.

Patients experiencing palpitation may need to be evaluated for cardiovascular problems. In this case, an ECG may be a useful diagnostic tool.

Evaluate patients with dyspareunia for the presence of vaginal infection by the appropriate wet mount or culture tests.

MANAGEMENT

ESTROGEN REPLACEMENT THERAPY

In the mid-1900s exogenous estrogen was widely used to treat the signs and symptoms of menopause. Many believed that exogenous estrogen would be the proverbial "fountain of youth" for all women. However, clinical and epidemiologic studies in the 1960s and 1970s indicated that exogenous estrogen was neither an innocuous nor always beneficial substance.

This section contains current guidelines for the use of estrogen with perimenopausal and postmenopausal women, the rationale for these guidelines, and discussions of the risks and benefits, and indications and contraindications of ERT. The phrase "estrogen replacement therapy" is used because of its common appearance in the literature. However, the notion of replacement implies abnormal deficit and thus is biased toward the belief that menopause is a hormone deficiency disease rather than a normal physiologic process.

Benefits

When exogenous estrogen first was marketed as a pharmacologic agent, it was used almost as a prophylactic agent against aging. As such, estrogen was an irregularly and slightly effective cosmetic agent; however, because exogenous estrogen is a potent pharmacologic agent, it must be used cautiously and only when specifically indicated. Estrogen is indicated in the following perimenopausal and postmenopausal problems:

Vasomotor instability is an estrogen deficiency problem for which estrogen therapy is of proven benefit. Specific indications for therapy and management are discussed later in this chapter.

Genital atrophy responds to ERT. Two specific symptoms respond well to estrogen: 1) the thinning of the epithelium of the vaginal wall, and 2) the changing pH of the vagina.

Osteoporosis is a serious disease of older women because of the sequelae of fractures and resultant immobility. It is characterized by a reduction of the quantity of bone without changes in its chemical composition. The process of osteoporosis is accelerated by the loss of ovarian function and is more prevalent in older women than older men. Studies indicate that ERT can arrest or retard bone loss if begun shortly (i.e., within 3 years) after menopause. It has not yet been definitely proven that early retardation of bone loss and long-term ERT will prevent the development of osteoporosis and its complications.

Risks

The primary risk of ERT is endometrial cancer. The association between administration of exogenous estrogen to middle-aged women and endometrial cancer was established through epidemiologic studies in the early 1970s.[5,22] Both studies showed a dramatic increase in endometrial cancer and parallelled a similar increase in estrogen sales. Since the research linking endometrial cancer and exogenous estrogens was reported, the sale of exogenous estrogen and the incidence of endometrial cancer have dropped concurrently.[8]

The risk of endometrial cancer due to exogenous estrogen can be reduced by using the lowest effective dose of estrogen, giving cyclic therapy, adding progestin to the regimen, and limiting the duration of therapy.[19]

Because breast cancer has been associated with exogenous estrogen administration in animals, its possible association with postmenopausal estrogen therapy has been studied. However, no increased incidence of breast cancer has been noted with increased estrogen usage. Women who are nulliparous, have a family history of breast cancer, or a past history of benign breast disease do have increased risk of breast cancer with the use of exogenous estrogen.[1,16]

Women receiving ERT have an increased incidence of symptomatic cholesterol chole-

lithiasis.[6] Exogenous estrogen reduces bile acid secretion, which results in increased bile cholesterol saturation and cholelithiasis.

Use of ERT may enhance the risk of heart disease.[8] Because of the increased incidence of heart disease after the menopause, and the unclear relationship between natural and exogenous estrogen and heart disease, the practitioner must be alert to new findings in this area.

Hypertension may be produced or exacerbated by ERT.[8] This problem is reversible after medication is discontinued.

Preliminary evidence suggests that the risk of thromboembolism doubles for postmenopausal women receiving ERT, as compared with nonusers.[20] The risk is higher with unconjugated steroids than with conjugated estrogens; however, this risk is not well documented. Until additional evidence is in, the practitioner should avoid prescribing ERT for women at risk for thromboembolic problems.

Estrogens can stimulate the growth of any estrogen-dependent tumor. Therefore, exogenous estrogens should be avoided or used cautiously in the presence of any estrogen-dependent tumor or lesion (e.g., uterine fibroids or endometriosis).

Indications

Short-term ERT is indicated in the following cases:

In the management of vasomotor instability symptoms that are moderate to severe or that disrupt the patient's daily functioning

In the management of atrophic vaginitis that has not responded to local therapy

Long-term ERT is indicated only in the prevention of osteoporosis and its sequelae. Because of the risks associated with long-duration exogenous estrogen administration,

ERT should only be given to women at risk for development of osteoporosis. Research has not yet provided data to clearly differentiate women at high risk versus low risk for osteoporosis. In general, frail white women seem to be at highest risk for osteoporosis. Other risk factors include immobilization, decreased activity, history of excessive alcohol consumption, malnutrition, early menopause, and use of corticosteroids. Osteoporosis can be noted on x-ray film. Although x-rays are not commonly used to screen candidates being considered for ERT, this technique (or one similar) may be more commonly used as a screening tool in the future.

Contraindications

Contraindications to the use of exogenous estrogen in postmenopause are because of estrogen's potential for stimulating existing malignant tumor growth, endometrial hyperplasia, and clot formation. Because estrogen is metabolized in the liver, any liver pathology would variably affect estrogen's utilization and clearance.

The following are consistently noted, absolute contraindications to the use of exogenous estrogen in the perimenopausal and later postmenopausal periods:

Breast disease
Previous breast cancer
Endometrial cancer
Undiagnosed vaginal bleeding
Significant endometrial hyperplasia
Acute liver disease
Chronic impaired liver function
Acute vascular thrombosis
Neuro-opthalmologic vascular disease

In addition, exogenous estrogens should be used with extreme caution and careful monitoring in patients with the following conditions:

Hypertension
Uterine fibroids
Familial hyperlipidemias
Migraine headaches
Chronic thrombophlebitis
Endometriosis
Gallbladder disease

Guidelines

The following guidelines are proposed for the practitioner in prescribing ERT:

Long-term therapy is not recommended for all women after menopause, with the exception of young women undergoing premature menopause.[20] The risks of ERT are too serious, the costs of ERT too high, and the group benefits too undocumented to consider standard use of ERT for all women. Costs include purchase of medication and payment for monitoring every 6 months. Additionally, all patients with unusual bleeding must be evaluated by endometrial biopsy, an expensive procedure. Additional costs to be considered are those of the complications and their treatment. The only documented potential therapeutic benefit for ERT is the prevention of osteoporosis. After an exhaustive analysis of the costs, risks, and benefits of ERT, Weinstein concluded that prophylactic use for the prevention of osteoporosis in women with intact uteri is not cost-effective, but that ERT was cost-effective in women with existing osteoporosis or previous hysterectomy.[21]

Women at risk for osteoporosis or with signs of osteoporosis are appropriate candidates for ERT. Other therapies can be considered for the prevention and control of osteoporosis in low-risk women. (See Management discussion in this chapter.)

The effectiveness of prophylactic use of ERT to prevent or retard the effects of normal aging on skin or other organs has not been demonstrated definitely. Its use as a placebo designed to heighten feelings of well-being and youth cannot be justified under any circumstances.

Short-term estrogen therapy for specific menopausal symptoms is acceptable.[20] Estrogens are effective in the treatment of vasomotor instability and atrophic vaginitis. All menopausal women do not experience these symptoms, and when they occur the symptoms are of limited duration. Treatment therefore should be directed toward the symptoms, not toward the control of menopause through lifelong estrogen replacement.

Although ERT is the only effective treatment of vasomotor instability, other therapies are available for the control of atrophic vaginitis.

Estrogen therapy should be given cyclically, using the lowest dosage compatible with effective treatment of symptoms.[8,15] The most serious complication of ERT is endometrial cancer. Estrogen can cause endometrial hyperplasia, which is a precursor of endometrial cancer. There is substantial evidence that cyclic administration of estrogen results in less endometrial hyperplasia than continuous administration and that lower doses result in less hyperplasia than higher doses.

In women with uteri, sequential addition of progestin during the last 5 to 10 days of estrogen ingestion is recommended.[3,8] The addition of progesterone at the end of cyclic estrogen administration replicates the physiology of the normal menstrual cycle and is less apt to induce endometrial hyperplasia than is cyclic administration of estrogens only.[23] Because effects of long-term progestin administration are unknown, the lowest, clinically effective dosages of progestin should be used. In addition, because the specific, protective effects of progestin are directed to the uterus, women without uteri do not need progestin.

Women receiving ERT should be assessed every 6 to 12 months to evaluate the effectiveness of therapy and to determine the presence of untoward effects. As was already elaborated, ERT can cause complications; the effects of therapy must be monitored regularly. This monitoring controls for the risks of therapy but substantially increases the cost of that therapy.

Women should be fully informed of the risks and benefits of ERT. An informed woman requesting long-term ERT should be considered for it provided that no contraindications are present and the patient agrees to regular examinations.

Because evidence regarding the long-term benefits of ERT is incomplete, a practitioner should consider objectively the request for ERT from a well-informed woman with no contraindications. The role of the practitioner is to inform, to assist in the consideration of appropriate alternatives, and to support the woman's choice of any appropriate alternative. Some practitioners require the woman to sign a consent form for the use of estrogen for prophylactic purposes.

Monitoring

The monitoring schedule shown opposite is recommended for women receiving both short- and long-term ERT.

Precautions

There is much individual variability in response to exogenous estrogen. Various women need more or less estrogen than others to effect the desired response. The practitioner should always attempt to determine and to use the lowest effective dosage to control symptoms. Prophylactic therapy should use the lowest recommended dosage. Symptoms of estrogen overdosage include breast swelling, abdominal bloating, increased leukorrhea, and edema.

Exogenous estrogen is associated with

Monitoring Schedule for Women on ERT

EVERY SIX MONTHS

History
    Follow-up of patient's symptoms and re-
        sponse to therapy
    Presence of bleeding
    Review of cardiovascular, gastrointestinal,
        respiratory, breast and lymphatic, and gen-
        itourinary symptoms
Physical
    Blood pressure
    Breast and lymphatic examination

Respiratory examination
Cardiovascular examination
Abdominal examination
Pelvic examination

EVERY YEAR

Pap smear
Cornification index, or another technique to
    assess estrogenic activity in the vagina
Endometrial biopsy

---

disturbed tryptophan metabolism resulting in increased xanthurenic acid secretion and pyridoxine (vitamin B_6) deficiency. Thus a vitamin preparation containing vitamin B_6 may be initiated for women receiving ERT. Symptoms of vitamin B_6 deficiency include: depression, emotional instability, irritability, fatigue, disturbances in concentration, insomnia, and decreased libido.

Women receiving cyclic estrogen and progestin therapy may have withdrawal bleeding, an important inconvenience of ERT. The dosages of estrogen and progestin can be reduced to avoid bleeding in some patients; however, it is unclear whether protection from hyperplasia occurs if periodic endometrial shedding does not occur.

Any unusual bleeding must be investigated immediately by endometrial biopsy. "Unusual bleeding" would be excessive or extended flow or bleeding during hormone ingestion rather than during withdrawal periods.

Estrogen Preparations

Three types of estrogen are commonly used in ERT. They are:

Conjugated Estrogens   Conjugated estrogens is a mixture containing the sodium of the water soluble esters of estrogen sub-

stances, similar to those excreted by pregnant mares. They may be derived naturally or synthetically. Estrone and estrified estrogens are the major components of conjugated estrogens.

Steroidal Estradiol Estrogens   Examples of steroidal estrogens are estradiol, ethinyl estradiol, and estradiol valerate. They can be derived naturally or synthetically.

Nonsteroidal Synthetic Estrogen   Examples of nonsteroidal synthetic estrogen are diethylstilbestrol (DES) and chlorotrianisene, and dienestrol.

Conjugated estrogen is the most commonly used postmenopausal estrogen in the United States. It is preferred over the other types because it is low in estrogenic activity and is thus least likely to cause endometrial cancer.

Steroidal estrogens have higher estrogenic activity than conjugated estrogens and thus are not indicated for long-term therapy. They are sometimes used for contraception in perimenopausal women for whom oral contraceptives are not contraindicated.

DES is not readily available because of past adverse publicity linking it to vaginal cancer. It is not indicated in perimenopause when some risk of pregnancy exists. DES may be the estrogen of choice in a young woman who has had a bilateral oophorectomy/hysterectomy, because of its high estrogenic activity.

Side-effects

Various side-effects result from estrogen therapy. The most common are breast discomfort, a feeling of tension in the legs, edema, uterine bleeding, weight gain, and nausea and other gastrointestinal complaints. The breast, leg, and uterine complaints may indicate overdosage. The gastrointestinal complaints may indicate an intolerance to a particular form of estrogen.

HOT FLASHES AND FLUSHES

If hot flashes are mild and do not disrupt a woman's daily activities, education regarding their etiology and limited duration provides reassurance that the symptoms are not indicative of pathology and will eventually clear. Methods of coping with the symptoms include wearing loose, absorbent, layered clothing and avoiding situations that may provoke embarrassing episodes of flashes.

Some evidence exists that adequate dietary intake of vitamins B and E can alleviate hot flashes.[4] In any case, a balanced diet can increase feelings of well-being.

The practitioner should attempt to initiate nonpharmacologic management of patients with moderate-to-severe vasomotor symptoms, and the practitioner should consider pharmacologic management if health education and guidance with coping are unsuccessful. Recommended regimens are 0.625 mg to 1.25 mg conjugated equine estrogen, 1 mg to 2 mg estradiol, or 0.01 mg to 0.02 mg ethinyl estradiol daily for 21 to 25 days per month, with progestin added for the last 7 to 10 days.

If estrogen therapy is contraindicated, medroxy-progesterone acetate or clonidine are sometimes considered.

Women on short-term as well as long-term ERT should be evaluated every 6 to 12 months. Any unusual bleeding should be immediately evaluated by endometrial biopsy. Treatment for vasomotor instability should be discontinued and reevaluated after 12 to 18 months, reevaluation consisting of withdrawal of the medication to determine if the condition still exists.

ATROPHIC VAGINITIS

At one time, it was believed that intravaginally applied estrogens had only local effects. Subsequent data, however, have demonstrated that topical intravaginal estrogen enters the bloodstream and reaches blood levels much higher than would be common with oral preparations. Intravaginal estrogen therefore is absolutely contraindicated in women with any contraindications to estrogen use. Atrophic vaginitis can be treated by the judicious use of vaginal creams containing estrogen or by oral administration of estrogen, using the same schedule recommended for the prevention or treatment of osteoporosis.

For those women in whom estrogen is contraindicated, maintenance of adequate hydration and use of lubricants during intercourse can prevent discomfort and trauma. The maintenance of regular, frequent sexual activity also can prevent extensive genital atrophy.

URINARY TRACT DISORDERS

Often, the postmenopausal woman who complains of burning on urination, but who has a normal urinalysis, is suffering from atrophic changes to the mucosa of the urethra and periurethral tissues. Short-term or intermittent cycles ERT can be considered for these women after a thorough evaluation for other pathology.

OSTEOPOROSIS

The relationships between normal post-menopausal bone loss and osteoporosis and between postmenopausal bone loss and fractures are still unclear. There are no definitive studies indicating that long-term ERT will significantly reduce the incidence of osteoporosis and its complications.[20]

The long-term ERT for the prevention of osteoporosis and resultant fractures is conjugated equine estrogen 0.625 mg daily or 0.02 mg to 0.05 mg of ethinyl estradiol daily on a schedule of 3 weeks on medication and 1 week off medication. If the woman has an intact uterus, the addition of a progestin during the last 10 days of estrogen administration is recommended. Commonly used progestins are: medroxyprogesterone acetate 5 mg to 10 mg, or norethindrone or norethindrone acetate 2.5 mg to 5 mg daily. Recent research indicates that estrogen doses are related to bone resorption. In a recent study investigators determined that there was a net loss of bone at dosages of ethanol estradiol below 0.015 mg and a net gain at doses above 0.025 mg. At doses between 0.015 mg and 0.025 mg, bone was neither gained nor lost.[7a]

An exercise program appropriate to age and ability, is recommended for all postmenopausal women for the prevention or control of osteoporosis. The amount of calcium deposited in the bone is determined by the activity it must support, therefore the more the bone is used, the denser it will become. Exercise also strengthens ligaments and increases the ability of musculoskeletal structures to withstand trauma. Exercise therapy should be adapted to the woman's capabilities and experience with exercise. Exercises appropriate for postmenopausal women are brisk walking, swimming, and bicycling.

Diets containing sufficient amounts of calcium and vitamin D can prevent excessive bone loss and possibly osteoporosis. If the woman is unwilling or unable to ingest foods containing minimum recommended amounts of calcium and vitamin D, supplementation is recommended. The recommended daily amounts for postmenopausal women are 1.5 gm of calcium and 400 units of vitamin D.

BIRTH CONTROL

The sexually active woman should use contraception for one year after the last menstrual period. Oral contraceptives are associated with increased risk of several problems after age 40; therefore, if possible, alternative acceptable methods of birth control should be considered for perimenopausal women.

HEALTH PROMOTION OF POSTMENOPAUSAL WOMEN

The interventions designed to promote and maintain perimenopausal and postmenopausal health of women should be emphasized. Because there is such a long period of postmenopause, enhancement of the quality of life during that time is important to the patient, and to society in general. Women generally lack sufficient information regarding menopause to provide adequate self-care. In addition, the number of myths and old wives' tales about menopause confuse and discourage premenopausal women. General health education and health education directed to the individual patient and groups of women are commonly used health interventions. Individually based instruction is directed to the woman's specific needs, problems, and risk factors. Written information distribution, group information sessions, or group peer-support sessions are good group education strategies. Clinical practices with access to audiovisual technology can use in-home or in-clinic transmission of information.

In addition to factual information regarding the processes and sequelae of menopause, the patient also needs information regarding possible interventions. Consumers need to be brought into the debate regarding long-term ERT. Because the risks and benefits of preventive ERT are not fully known, patients should be participants in decisions about the use of ERT.

Smoking, inappropriate diet, and inadequate exercise, all of which are major risk factors that increase in importance in the older age patient, should be a part of health education. Smoking is an unhealthy habit and is associated with osteoporosis as well as multiple other health problems affecting older women, including cancer and heart disease. The importance of diet and exercise have already been discussed.

The mental health needs in pre- and postmenopause are important. The perimenopausal years are the midlife crisis years. It is not unusual for both partners in a marriage to be simultaneously involved with significant adjustment. Responses to and methods of coping with changes in midlife are individual, and stereotyping problems or responses is not helpful. All women think about getting older and feel some loss, and these feelings and losses need to be dealt with by the health care practitioner in a preventive or therapeutic way. If they have caused the woman to become dysfunctional, a referral to a mental health care provider is indicated. In general, the woman who is active in satisfying personal, family, and work involvements will be able to make a healthy transition into later years. Women who have been sexually active before menopause are encouraged to continue sexual activity so long as it is satisfying to themselves and their partners. Such activity serves to maintain healthy relationships and may prevent or alleviate atrophic vaginal problems.

CONCLUSION

As more is learned about aging, the knowledge and practice underlying general and postmenopausal health care management of the older woman may change. The health care provider must be continuously alert for new findings in the field and incorporate these findings into clinical practice. Research, currently in progress, holds promise of resolving many of the controversies surrounding management of the postmenopausal woman. The risks and benefits of ERT will thus become clearer.

The psychosocial impact of menopause, however, will continue to be unique for every woman making the transition into postmenopause. Many women will continue to need guidance for the attainment of optimal health during this transition.

REFERENCES

1. Brinton LA, Hoover RN, Szklo M, et al: Menopausal estrogen use and risk of breast cancer. Cancer 47:2517–2522, 1980
2. Bungay GT, Vessey MP, McPherson CK: Study of symptoms in middle life with special reference to the menopause. Br Med J 281, No. 6234:181–183, 1980
3. Estrogen use and post menopausal women: A National Institutes of Health Consensus Development Conference. Ann Intern Med 91:921–922, 1979
4. Gelein JL, Heiple P: Aging. In Fogel CI, Woods NF: Health Care of Women: A Nursing Perspective. St. Louis, CV Mosby, 1981
5. Greenwald P, Caputo TA, Wolfgang PE: Endometrial cancer after menopause use of estrogens. Obstet Gynecol 50:239–243, 1977
6. Honore LH: Increased incidence of symptomatic cholesterol cholelithiasis in perimenopausal wom-

en receiving estrogen replacement therapy. J Reprod Med, 25, No. 4:187–189, 1980

7. Jaszmann LJB: Epidemiology of the climacteric syndrome. In Campbell S (ed): The Management of the Menopause and Postmenopausal Years. Baltimore, University Park Press, 1976

7a. Horsman A, Jones M, Francis R et al: The effect of estrogen dose on postmenopausal bone loss. N Engl J Med 309:1405–1407, 1983

8. Judd HL, Cleary RE, Creasman WT et al: Estrogen replacement therapy. Obstet Gynecol 58:267–275, 1981

9. Kaufman DW, Slone D, Rosenberg L et al: Cigarette smoking at natural menopause. American Journal of Public Health 70:420–422, 1980

10. Kresovich EAA: A comparison of attitudes toward menopause held by women during the three phases of the climacterium. Issues in Mental Health Nursing, 2, No. 3:59–69, 1980

11. LaRocco SA, Polit DF: Women's knowledge about the menopause. Nurs Res 29, No. 1:10–13, 1980

12. McArthur JW: The contemporary menopause. Primary Care 8, No. 1:141–164, 1981

13. Neugarten BL, Kraines RJ: "Menopausal symptoms" in women of various ages. Psychosom Med 271, No. 3:266–273, 1965

14. Notman M: Midlife concerns of women: implications of the menopause. Am J Psychiatry 136:1270–1273, 1979

15. Quigley MM: Postmenopausal oestrogen replacement therapy: An appraisal of risks and benefits. Drugs 22:153–159, 1981

16. Ross RK, Paganini–Hill A, Gerkins VR et al: A case-control study of menopausal estrogen therapy and breast cancer. JAMA 243:1635–1639, 1980

17. Schwarz BE: Does estrogen cause adenocarcinoma of the endometrium? In Pitkin KM, Scott JR (eds): Clinical Obstetrics and Gynecology. Hagerstown, Harper & Row, 1981

18. Severne L: Psycho-social aspects of the menopause. In Haspels AA, Musaph H: Psychosomatics in the Perimenopause. Baltimore, University Park Press, 1979

19. Silverberg SG, Majors FJ (eds): Estrogen and Cancer. New York, John Wiley & Sons, 1978

20. Utian WH: Estrogen replacement in the menopause. Obstet Gynecol Annu 8:369–391, 1979

21. Weinstein MC: Estrogen use in postmenopausal women—costs, risks, and benefits. New Engl J Med 303:308–316, 1980

22. Weiss NS, Szekeley DR, Austin DF: Increasing incidence of endometrial cancer in the United States. N Engl J Med 294:1259–1262, 1976

23. Whitehead MI, Townsend PT, Pryse–Davies J et al: Effects of estrogens and progestins on the biochemistry and morphology of the postmenopausal endometrium. N Engl J Med 307:1599–1605, 1981

BIBLIOGRAPHY

Beard RJ: The Menopause. Baltimore, University Park Press, 1976

Campbell S: Management of the Menopause and Postmenopausal Years. Baltimore, University Park Press, 1976

Christiansen C, Christensen MS, McNair P, et al: Prevention of early postmenopausal bone loss: Controlled 2-year study in 315 normal females. Eur J Clin Invest 10:273–279, 1980

Christiansen C, Christensen MS, Transbol I: Bone mass in postmenopausal women after withdrawal of oestrogen/gestagen replacement therapy. Lancet 1, No. 8210:459–461, 1981

Fogel CI, Woods NF: Health Care of Women: A Nursing Perspective. St. Louis, CV Mosby, 1981

Gambrell RD, Greenblatt RB: Hormone therapy for the menopause. Geriatrics 36, No. 7:53–61, 1981

Hailes, HD, Nelson, JB, Schneider, M, Rennie, GC, & Burger, HG: Conjugated equine oestrogen versus placebo. Med J Aus 2, No. 7:340–342, 1981

Haspels AA: Oestrogen therapy in the peri-menopause: a practical approach. Acta Endocrinol (Copenh) 233 (Suppl):57–61, 1980

Haspels AA, Musaph H: Psychosomatics in Peri-Menopause. Baltimore, University Park Press, 1979

Hutchinson TA, Polansky SM, Feinstein A: Postmenopausal oestrogens protect against fractures of hip and distal radius. Lancet 2, No. 8145:705–709, 1979

Johnson RE, Specht EE: The risk of hip fracture in postmenopausal females with and without estrogen drug exposure. American Journal of Public Health, 71:138–144, 1981

Jones HW, Jones GS: Novak's Textbook of Gynecology, 10th ed. Baltimore, Williams & Wilkins, 1981

Kauppila A, Janne O, Kivinen S et al: Postmenopausal hormone replacement with estrogen periodically supplemented with anti-estrogen. Am J Obstet Gynecol 140:787–792, 1981

Kemmann E, Jones JR: The female climacteric. Am Fam Phys 20, No. 5:140–151, 1979

Kistner RW: Gynecology: Principles and Practices, 3rd ed. Chicago, Year Book Medical Publishers, 1979

Lauritzen C: Selected aspects of endocrinology an epidemiology of the climacteric. Acta Obstet Gynecol Scand 65 (Suppl):11–18, 1977

Lind T, Cameron EC, Hunter WM, et al: A prospective, controlled trial of six forms of hormone replacement therapy given to postmenopausal women. Br J Obstet Gynaecol 86(Suppl 3):1–29, 1979

Meldrum DR, Davidson BJ, Tataryn IV, et al: Changes in circulating steroids with aging in postmenopausal women. Obstet Gynecol 57, No. 5:624 628, 1981

Mosher, BA, Whelan EM: Postmenopausal estrogen therapy: A review. Obstet Gynecol Surv 36:467–475, 1981

Paganini–Hill A, Ross RA, Gerkins VR et al: Menopausal estrogen therapy and hip fractures. Ann Intern Med 95:28–31, 1981

Rakoff AE: The female climacteric and the pros and cons of estrogen therapy. In Gold JJ, Josimovich JB (eds): Gynecologic Endocrinology, 3rd ed. Hagerstown, Harper & Row, 1980

Uphold CR, Susman EJ: Self-reported climacteric symptoms as a function of the relationships between marital adjustment and childrearing state. Nurs Res 30, No. 2:84–88, 1981

Vaughn TC, Hammond CB: Estrogen replacement therapy. Clin Obstet Gynecol 24, No. 1:253–283, 1981

Van Keep PM, Sorr DM, Greenblatt RB (eds): Female and Male Climacteric: Current Opinion 1978. Baltimore, University Park Press, 1979

Weideger, P: Menstruation and Menopause: The Physiology and Psychology, the Myth and the Reality. New York, Alfred A. Knopf, 1976

21

Chemical Dependency

Karen Kellam Smith

Chemical dependency is one of the major health problems in the United States. It knows no boundaries, cutting across all cultures, genders, ages, races, economic groups, intellectual levels, and religious groups. The scope of the problem is reflected by an estimated annual cost to the nation of $50 billion in health and medical expenses, diminished job productivity, motor vehicle accidents, and violent crimes.[31] This dollar value does not begin to reflect the psychological toll that millions of people are suffering presently as a result of living or associating with afflicted persons or of having the problem personally. Additionally, many innocent victims are suffering the consequences resulting from the chemically dependent person's intoxicated behavior.

The purpose of this chapter is to provide basic information about chemical dependency that can facilitate its prevention, early identification, and intervention. Frequently, the drug-dependent person is identified in a more advanced stage of the disorder rather than in early or middle stages. By this stage, the dependent person, the family, and society may have experienced extensive suffering and irreparable damage.

The nurse is a key health care provider who is in a strategic position to identify a chemical use problem since he or she has the most patient contact for the most extended period of time. The nurse's facilitation of earlier diagnosis and intervention of this problem can prevent the development of late stage complications and major life losses, since this is a chronic, progressive, and often fatal problem.

General concepts of the construct of chemical dependency are discussed, specifically those dependencies of the mood-altering type that are most problematic to society. The problematic mood-altering chemicals referred to in this chapter include sedatives, hypnotics and minor tranquilizers, opiates, narcotic analgesics, alcohol, cannabis (marijuana and hashish), stimulants (e.g., amphetamines, methylphenidate), cocaine, and hallucinogens (e.g., LSD, PCP, mescaline). Although caffeine and nicotine dependencies are the most prevalent in our culture, they do not produce the psychosocial problems for the person and for society that the more centrally acting, mood-altering chemicals do.

The chemical alcohol will be used primary as an example. Alcoholism is the most studied problem within the area of chemical dependency. Alcohol has been the most widely used drug, has been in existence the longest, and is the most easily accessible in our culture. The treatment of alcoholism is a paradigm of treatment for other dependencies. The biopsychosocial model for treating other dependencies has been derived from the treatment outcome research with alcoholism. Other mood-altering chemicals will be introduced as they relate to concepts being discussed.

In the past, the term *addiction* was used to describe extensive drug use problems. For clarification, however, the World Health Organization suggested that the term *dependence* be substituted, prefaced by the specific drug type, for example, "alcohol dependence."

Chemical Dependency

Chemical dependence can be defined as the use of a substance that interferes recurrently with the person's total quality of life, yet which the person continues to use in spite of the consequences of its use. Broad variables included in total quality of life are mental and physical health, social relationships, educational performance, economic aspects, legal aspects, and spiritual aspects.

The more socially problematic mood-altering chemicals referred to in this chapter are primarily those with high potential for physical or psychological dependence. A chemical dependency can have both these aspects of dependency simultaneously; however, they can occur independently. Usually psychological dependence occurs first, followed by the development of the physical dependence. In the early stage of chemical dependency, frequently the physical dependence is not developed or is imperceptible.

Psychological Characteristics

Psychological characteristics of a chemical dependency include the following: preoccupation with the drug and the securing of its supply, inability to abstain from using it regardless of repeated negative consequences of use, and psychological dependence on the chemical to do something for the person that cannot be done in and of oneself. Another psychological consequence includes the development of an emotional growth lag. Whenever a person develops a chemical dependency, he will have greater difficulty in successfully completing the present and succeeding stages of emotional growth and development. Clinically, there appears to be a correlation between the severity of the emotional growth lag and the time of onset of the dependency in the person's life; the earlier the onset and the more rapid the progression of the dependency, the more profound is the developmental arrest and the greater the disruption in the person's life. Conversely, the later the onset and the slower the progression of the dependency, the lesser the developmental arrest and the lesser the disruption it seems to create in the individual's life.

Physiological Characteristics

Physiological characteristics of a chemical dependency include blackouts or memory lapses, the development of tolerance, drug craving or hunger, difficulty in limiting the quantity of the chemical once the chemical use is initiated, and the development of a withdrawal syndrome on discontinuing use, or on decreasing the amount of the chemical used below the developed tolerance. Blackouts or memory lapses can occur with alcohol and other depressant drugs such as sedatives, minor tranquilizers, and cannabis (marijuana and hashish). These can be partial or complete. An example of a partial blackout is a person who remembers that a specific friend telephoned, but cannot remember any of the conversation. In a complete blackout (using the same example) the person has no memory of receiving the telephone call.

Tolerance

Tolerance is the necessity to increase chemical dose to obtain the desired effect that one achieved formerly at lower doses. This can occur with all mood-altering drugs. Because the body strives for homeostasis, the nervous tissue will adjust to the presence of a drug by countering its effect, rendering the organism relatively insensitive to the effects of the drug. Tolerance reflects the organism's tendency to maintain the "balance of power" in the relationship of different parts of the nervous system to one another. It is the result of the self-correcting mechanisms designed to maintain the body's homeostasis. Therefore, to achieve the desired effect, the person needs to ingest greater amounts of the drug to overcome the compensatory mechanisms now in existence.

Tolerance refers mainly to two different physiological events. The first is the need to increase the amount of a drug to obtain the desired effects. The second is the desensitization of the physiological systems to the effects of a drug. Both forms of tolerance contribute to the need for progressively increasing drug dosages.

Once tolerance to the drug is established, physical dependence can result, and is marked by the presence of withdrawal symptoms when the dose of the drug is decreased or the drug ingestion is stopped.[21] Thus, as the person's blood level of the drug falls below his tolerance, withdrawal symptoms can occur. This discomfort may be a contributing factor in the motivation to repeat the drug use. Ever-increasing amounts of the drug will be necessary to maintain the "status quo" as tolerance continues to accommodate upwards. Physical dependence, however, does not occur necessarily in every instance in which tolerance develops.

Withdrawal

Symptoms of withdrawal are drug-specific and are related to the drug-induced changes in the function of the cells. Usually withdrawal symptoms are the opposite of those changes that the drug-induced in the system. For example, barbiturates and benzodiazepines raise the seizure threshold and their withdrawal may precipitate seizures. Amphetamines produce euphoria but their withdrawal produces depression. The rebound effects produced by some drugs are referred to as *rebound hyperexcitability*.[11] These withdrawal phenomena are generally due to the exaggerated function of the systems previously suppressed by the drug. There is no one theoretical model that explains the mechanisms involved in producing the specific withdrawal syndromes of particular drugs.

Withdrawal syndromes can range from imperceptible to severe. Whether a withdrawal syndrome can be observed depends on the criteria of withdrawal symptoms, the sensitivity of techniques used to detect the withdrawal phenomena, and the rate at which the drug is removed from its site of action.[11]

Cross Tolerance

The ability of one drug to suppress the manifestations of physical dependence produced by another drug and to continue to maintain the physical dependent state is termed *cross tolerance*.[11] Cross tolerance between drugs can be partial or complete. Health care workers in the field of chemical dependency report that 20% to 40% of the patients seeking treatment for drug problems other than alcohol are experiencing sequelae of alcohol abuse or alcohol dependence concurrently.[18] For example, people dependent on alcohol can use sedatives to alleviate withdrawal symptoms from the cross tolerance between alcohol and other central nervous system (CNS) depressants. Other depressants include minor tranquilizers and cannabis. Such cross tolerance is not as complete between these drugs and opiates; however, opiate-dependent people use depressant drugs to modify or lessen withdrawal symptoms when opiate supplies are decreased or not obtainable.

Recruitment

Recruitment of one's chemical dependency is the process of activation of the disorder. The various levels of recruitment are low, moderate, and full. In low recruitment, a person who has alcoholism may begin to renew old drug-linked acquaintances, experience alcohol-related dreams, or forget to take disulfiram (Antabuse). In moderate recruitment, the person may begin to think consciously about using or actually begin to use small doses of alcohol or substitute other mood-altering chemicals. Full recruitment would be full activation of the dependency to the same or greater extent as before treatment, either with the drug of choice or with the substitute drug.

Recruitment can be initiated physiologically or psychologically. Psychological recruitment can occur through encounters with drug-linked cues, such as drug-related dreams, drug-using friends, places of use, memories, paraphernalia, and strongly drug-linked feelings. Physiological recruitment occurs mainly in two ways. One is by the use of other drugs that have central mood-altering properties or are cross tolerant with the drug group in which the person has a dependency. Many drugs prescribed for various conditions have ingredients that may be cross tolerant with the person's drug of dependence; therefore, patients who have dependencies and health care professionals treating or caring for such persons need to screen all drug ingredients carefully before accessing or prescribing. Such inadvertent chemical use would undermine recovery. Use of other mood-altering substances that are not cross tolerant are highly reinforcing. Persons who have dependencies are at risk when they attempt to use such substances. Either they get into difficulties with the chemical being substituted or they decide to return to their drug of choice at some point in the chemical use.

A second way the recruitment process is physiologically activated is by the phenomenon of *periodic affective disturbance*, or flare-up. (Alcoholics Anonymous refers to this phenomenon as a "dry drunk.") Minimal research has been conducted on this subject, and it remains poorly understood. Flare-ups have been observed in those persons recovering from depressant drug dependencies such as alcohol, sedatives, cannabis, and minor tranquilizers. They occur in the recovery process after the person has become chemically free. This phenomenon is most common in the first year of recovery; however, it has been reported to occur up to 7 years after recovery. It usually occurs abruptly and lasts an average of 2 days to 2 weeks. During this phenomenon, the person frequently describes the subjective symptoms as similar to those of withdrawal. This is a very uncomfortable and vulnerable time, and relapses in drug use frequently occur.

OVERVIEW

Chemical dependency, a pioneering field of knowledge, is a very complex phenomenon. More research is needed to understand clearly the mechanisms of dependence, its pathophysiology, and all the mind–body interrelationships and ramifications. Empirically, chemical dependence is a chronic, relapsing, progressive, and often fatal illness. People literally give their lives to it. Although there is no cure at this time, the disorder can be arrested by diagnosis, intervention, and treatment. The prognosis is more favorable the earlier the diagnosis can be established and the recovery process initiated. Often impediments to the diagnosis and recovery process are due to the complexities of the problem that are not clearly understood. Other impediments are the attitudes and values of the health care professionals toward psychoactive chemical use, the disorder, and the persons who are chemically dependent.

An overview of the complexities will consist of a discussion of dose variability, multiple dependencies, and the multifaceted nature of the problem. Furthermore, it will be helpful to reflect on societal attitudes and values in health care professionals which may impede the assessment and treatment process.

Chemical dependency is not dose-dependent; there are low-, medium-, and high-dose dependencies with all of the psychoactive chemicals. Therefore, the quantity of the chemical is not as relevant in assessing for chemical dependency as is what happens when the person uses the chemical, tries to stop, or decreases its use. For example, many social drinkers may actually drink more alcohol than a person who has alcoholism; however, social drinkers' use of alcohol is not interfering with the total quality of life. Other individuals may be taking 10 mg diazepam (Valium) per day, a low dose by therapeutic standards, and yet experience a major withdrawal syndrome when they stop it, whereas others may take 30 mg Valium per day and experience no withdrawal symptoms upon abstaining or decreasing the dose.[27,29,40] Furthermore, they do not experience any other interferences in the quality of life.

Multiple drug dependencies are common in persons who have chemical dependency; therefore, it is helpful for the nurse to understand chemical dependency as a substance use disorder rather than a single drug problem when making an assessment or caring for a recovering person. Frequently, a person with a drug use problem has experienced other dependencies in the past. Other dependencies can exist concurrently or can develop in the future.

Dependencies can be acquired innocently through prescribed drugs for existing conditions or through drug behaviors that contribute to further drug use problems. Two commonly observed drug behaviors are substituting either similarly acting chemicals for one's drug of choice or using chemicals that have opposing effects to counteract the effects of a drug previously consumed. Some people use other similar mood-altering substances to supplement the daily physical tolerance level. For example, a person who has alcoholism may use minor tranquilizers or marijuana throughout the day to meet sedative tolerance and to avoid detection from the smell of alcohol until after working hours when drinking can be resumed again safely. Another common drug behavior is the use of chemicals that have the opposite neurologic effects to help moderate the effects of the drug of choice. For example, a person who has a cocaine dependency may use a sedative like alcohol to modify the stimulation. The stimulant/sedative cycle becomes a vicious one. Usually the depressant causes the most problems, because these drugs remain in the body longer. The nurse may encounter people with both stimulant and sedative drug group dependencies simultaneously when they seek help for their drug problems. These people may not perceive a problem with the drug group they are using to moderate the effects of their drug of choice.

Chemical dependency is a multifaceted problem. Clinically, there appear to be many types of dependencies and many use patterns. Within the field of alcoholism, attempts have been made to describe the various types; however, clear criteria do not exist to distinguish between types. Alcoholism has two main subgroups. One group has an early onset and progresses rapidly to the more advanced stages. The other type begins later in life, usually in middle age, and progresses more slowly. These types are observed in persons with other drug dependencies. Frequently, such people have family histories that contain similar types of alcoholism. Even though people may have similar types of chemical dependency, each person brings to it the variables of age, sex, personality, physiological make-up, and experiences unique to one's sociocultural background, environment, education, and life experience.

Historical impediments to diagnosis and treatment are embedded in the culture. Many cultural attitudes, values, and rituals center on the social use of alcohol and other mood-altering chemicals that are considered "normal." In the United States, society values "normal" social use of mood-altering chemicals for convenience, relief, and pleasure; however, simultaneously, society abhors the destructive effects and negative conse-

quences of such chemicals and people who have problems with their use. This ambivalent societal attitude extends to professionals in hospitals, court rooms, and social agencies and is exemplified by the lack of response by professionals to identify alcoholism as a problem or to respond to its early detection. It has been estimated that 15% of the alcoholic population is receiving treatment for alcoholism; another 25% are somewhere being examined, probed, and treated for all types of emotional and physical conditions that are due to it; and the remaining 60% are not identified or treated in any way.[13]

Examining one's own drug use and one's own values in terms of the use of chemicals for other than medical purposes can be an uncomfortable process. It is helpful, however, for the nurse to explore her own feelings, values, and attitudes about chemical use and toward persons who have chemical use problems. This process of self-evaluation and clarification of values will help the nurse to become more effective with those persons with chemical use problems.

HISTORICAL PERSPECTIVES

Society has undergone widespread changes in attitudes, mores, and values related to drug-taking behavior. Some of these changes are a direct result of the advances in pharmacology. The advent of drugs for the treatment of mental illnesses has had far-reaching effects on the present-day psychoactive drug use in our culture. Barbiturates, bromides, narcotics, and anticholinergics were available in the 1940s for treatment of mental illness, but their actual restorative properties were minimal or nonexistent. The use of these drugs often was prohibitive because of severe side-effects, including the potential for addiction. The modern psychoactive drug era began in the 1950s with the development of major tranquilizers for the treatment of mental illness. In 1952, chlorpromazine and reserpine were introduced for the treatment of psychotic behavior. During this same decade, the introduction of meprobamate represented the advent of the drug "revolution" of minor tranquilizers to the general public. The benzodiazepines followed in the early 1960s and became the number one class of psychoactive drugs prescribed by American physicians. Since 1972, diazepam (Valium) was held to be "the most prescribed drug in America," and together with chlordiazepoxide hydrochloride (Librium), represented 68% of all psychoactive drug prescriptions in 1979.[8] With the widespread use of anti-anxiety drugs, the public's attitude toward drug-taking changed from taking a drug for restoration of mental health to one of taking a mood-altering drug into a healthy mind for instant "relief" or "pleasure." The use of drugs for pleasure evolved during the 1960s with the counterculture revolution. During the 1960s there was an increase in illegal drug use. Drug use involved educated persons whose primary reason was to alter mood and consciousness. Recreational drug use includes illegal drugs such as heroin, marijuana, cocaine, and illicit use of prescription drugs such as stimulants and depressants. Drug companies have capitalized on this societal attitude change and have provided a vast spectrum of mood-altering chemicals, available through legal prescriptions. Another expanding area for drug companies is the marketing of over-the-counter (OTC) drugs that have stimulating or sedating properties with FDA-approved ingredients and dosages. Additionally, this attitudinal change is reflected in the growth of clandestine laboratories that produce illegal look-alike drugs, which are then marketed on the street. One

inherent danger in the use of products from unregulated laboratories is their unknown ingredients and dosages (e.g., look-alike Quaaludes that have been analyzed and found to contain dangerous levels of a type of diazepam).

The outgrowth of society's attitudinal change toward psychoactive drug use is reflected in the increase of psychoactive chemical dependencies. The problem has become so widespread that it evoked a position statement on substance abuse by the American Psychiatric Association (APA). Because alcohol and drug abuse problems account for approximately 30% of total mental health problems in the United States, the APA urged psychiatrists and other physicians to address these issues at all levels: prevention, early identification, and treatment.[7]

MECHANISMS OF CHEMICAL DEPENDENCY

CAUSES

Although the development of chemical dependency has been attributed to many variables, no one causal theory provides a complete explanation; multiple factors may contribute to its development. Research in the field of alcoholism will be reviewed because it has been studied the most.

A social causal theory is the tension-reduction hypothesis, which posits that alcoholics drink to escape or to avoid anxiety generated by social stress. However, studies suggest that many alcoholics become more anxious and depressed during periods of prolonged drinking.[21] Overall, from the bulk of research literature, the tension-reduction model of alcohol consumption does not receive much support.[30]

The learning causal theory states that a person drinks in an alcoholic manner because of the highly reinforcing effects of the alcohol. The learning model operates on the premise that all behavior is learned; therefore, behavior can be extinguished or modified. Evidence reveals that the aversive stimulus produced by a severe disulfiram/alcohol reaction has not been sufficient to change the drinking behavior when the person is no longer ingesting disulfiram; however, used as an adjunct with supportive treatment and particularly in the first year of recovery, disulfiram has been shown to be highly correlated with favorable treatment outcomes.[15]

Another causal theory is the addictive personality theory. Although personality characteristics have been associated with alcoholism, their role in causation is unclear. Earlier studies were retrospective and suggested that alcoholics are oral-dependent, sociopathic, latently homosexual, premorbidly passive, and fearful of intimacy.[33] Prospective studies in which subjects have been studied before and after the development of alcoholism show that the retrospective studies' conclusions may be erroneous.[32] The prospective studies show that subjects had normal Minnesota Multiphasic Personality Inventories (MMPIs) and normal childhoods before the development of the disease.[33]

There is increasing evidence that genetic factors are associated with alcoholism.[16] A review of identical twin studies indicates growing evidence for the presence of a genetic factor contributing to drinking behavior; evidence for such a determinant of alcoholism remains inconclusive.[10]

Biologic studies continue to strive for the discovery of antecedents to the development and consequences of alcoholism. The interplay between genetic and biologic factors may influence alcohol metabolism and enzymatic mechanisms, which may have their expression in the development of tolerance and physical dependence on alcohol.[15]

ANATOMY AND PHYSIOLOGY

Because psychoactive chemicals have their primary effects on the nervous system, this section will be confined to an overview of that. Current information on brain function postulates that organized behavior is correlated with impulse transmission through intricate networks of neurons.[5] The nervous system is not interconnected structurally. It is interconnected functionally, primarily through chemical bridges called *synapses*.

The *neuron*, the basic functional unit, is a specialized cell designed to transmit information. The components of the neuron are the *dendrites*, which receive information; the *axon*, which carries the information; and the *nerve terminals*, which receive the information from the axons (Fig. 21-1). Information is transmitted by means of an electrical pulse; however, at the synapse the information is transmitted by chemicals called *neurotransmitters*.[21] Four important neurotransmitters in understanding drug use are norepinephrine, acetylcholine, dopamine, and serotonin.[21] It is believed that most mood-altering chemicals exert their action through effects on these neurotransmitters.

The area on the dendrite where a neurotransmitter is thought to have its effect is called a *receptor site*. The dynamics of receptor sites are one of the most active and controversial areas of neurobiology and the understanding of them is incomplete at this time. Receptor protein molecules are constituents of the cell membrane, and their structures are highly specific for a particular transmitter. They bind the neurotransmitter in a "lock-and-key" arrangement.[5] The association of transmitter to receptor is an equilibration process in which the transmitter

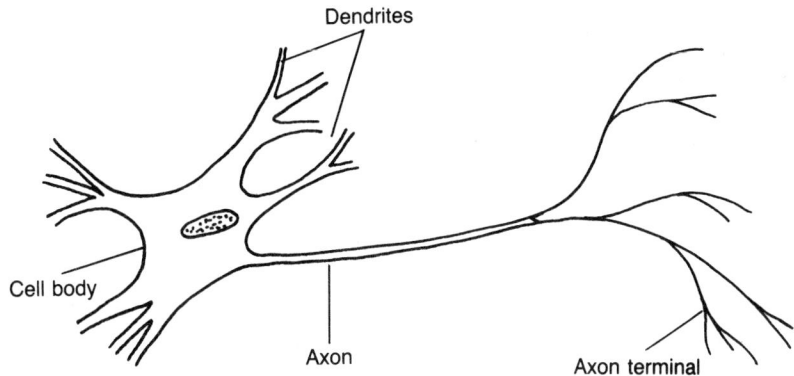

FIG. 21-1 The nerve cell.

molecules are constantly dissociating from the receptor, freeing it to be restimulated. In the cholinergic system, neurotransmitter action is terminated at the postsynaptic membrane by acetylcholinesterase. For catecholamines and indoleamines, termination of the transmitter action depends upon washout of the synaptic cleft by microcirculatory profusion, postsynaptic degradation, or re-uptake of the transmitter into a presynaptic neuron, the last being the most important.[5]

At the basic level in the nervous system there are functionally two types of synapses; *excitatory* synapses, in which the neurotransmitter acting at the receptor site makes it easier to elicit an electrical impulse in the axon; and *inhibitory* synapses, in which the neurochemical acting at the receptor site makes it less likely for an electrical impulse to be initiated in the axon. The effect that a drug has on this neuronal system is determined by a combination of the drug's action in the synaptic processes, its location, and its duration.[21]

The function of the cell body is to maintain neuronal integrity. The cell body synthesizes enzymes needed for the synthesis or degradation of specific transmitters. Each cell body also contains mechanisms in its membranes specifically to take up the appropriate neurotransmitter precursor from the surrounding environment. Together the precursor and enzymes are then transported down the axon to the nerve terminal. All uptake, synthetic, degradative, and release processes occur at the nerve terminal.[5] The terminal contains vesicles, which are specialized for the uptake, storage, and release of neurotransmitters. A normal, functioning nervous system depends on the regular manufacturing of these neurotransmitters in the neurons, their release as a result of the electrical impulse, and their breakdown or deactivation after they have had their effect on the dendrite. By changing one of these processes, information transmission is then modified or blocked.[21]

It is believed that psychoactive drugs affect the production, storage, deactivation, or action of neurotransmitters; for example, benzodiazepines exert their influence by binding to receptors. It is hypothesized that drugs that either mimic or block neurotransmission act at the receptor site. Some drugs have characteristics similar to the neurotransmitter; therefore, they can occupy the receptor and activate it. Other drugs prevent the transmitters from having an effect, since they occupy but do not activate the receptor site.

The neurotransmitters dopamine and norepinephrine are two catecholamines. Their distribution is specific to certain areas of the body. Norepinephrine is primarily in sympathetic nerves of both the peripheral nervous system and the CNS and acts locally on effector cells of vascular smooth muscle, adipose tissue, liver, heart, and brain as a neurotransmitter. Dopamine functions as a neurotransmitter in areas of the brain involved in coordinating motor activity, and it serves as a precursor of norepinephrine.[3] It also modulates sensory experience, may have mood-elevating effects, and inhibits prolactin release. The catecholamines in the brain are synthesized within CNS neurons, and circulating catecholamines do not cross the blood–brain barrier.[3] Norepinephrine and dopamine are either excitatory or inhibitory neurotransmitters, depending on the place of action.[20]

Serotonin, acetylcholine, and gamma-aminobutyric acid (GABA) are thought to act as neuroregulators that might be involved in the action of psychoactive drugs. Acetylcholine acts as an excitatory and inhibitory neurotransmitter; serotonin is probably an inhibitory transmitter.[21] Acetylcholine is a neurotransmitter in a number of systems, including neuromuscular junctions, postganglionic, parasympathetic, and preganglionic fibers of both the sympathetic and parasympathetic system. Less is known about its function as a neurotransmitter in the CNS. It is thought to be associated with arousal mechanisms, temperature regulation, and memory. It is highly likely to be identified as having a role in many illnesses. GABA is a relatively recently discovered transmitter, and much research is currently focused on its role.

Parts of the brain, such as the reticular activating system (RAS), the hypothalamus, the medial forebrain bundle, the periven-tricular system, the basal ganglia, and the cerebral cortex are of particular importance for the study of drug action and for understanding the effects of drugs on behavior. The RAS, located where the spinal cord connects with the brain, modulates incoming sensory information and outgoing motor impulses and regulates the degree of arousal and alertness that the person shows. The RAS receives electrical impulses from the sensory systems by way of branches of the sensory neurons. The RAS seems to be predominantly adrenergic, since high blood levels of adrenaline or noradrenaline result in its activation and thus the activation of the cerebral cortex. Sympathomimetic drugs activate the RAS; drugs that interrupt adrenergic synapses decrease the responsiveness of the RAS to sensory input. The hypothalamus primarily controls the autonomic nervous system and functions to integrate information from the body that is important to the maintenance of the organism. It also interfaces between the nervous system and the endocrine system. It acts to adjust the release of hormones for the purposes of homeostasis. Because of the rich blood supply to the hypothalamus, many drugs first enter the brain in high concentrations at this structure. Frequently the initial effects of such drugs cause changes in level of consciousness and mood. The medial forebrain bundle is a band of neurons on both sides of the hypothalamus and is a focus of pleasure in humans. The cerebral cortex is a part of the brain that is responsible for the analysis of incoming information and for the initiation of voluntary motor behavior. Speech, sensation, and movement centers are localized here. The cerebral cortex is the largest part of the brain and has receiving, output, and association areas, all of which are affected by psychoactive agents.

The nervous system is the primary site of

action of psychoactive drugs, most of which influence the functioning of the nervous system by modifying the production, release, action, or breakdown of the particular neurotransmitters with which they interact. The total effect of the nervous system/drug interaction becomes more complex when other variables are added. Some scientists believe that all experience, thoughts, and feelings are nothing more than electrical activity in some part of the brain, and therefore a person's experiences, thoughts, and feelings can be influenced and altered by modifying the electrical activity of neurons in the CNS.[21] However, to completely understand drug effects, individual behaviors must also be studied because these depend on unique factors in the person's personal history. Thus, the exact effect of the drugs becomes less predictable.

NURSING ASSESSMENT

People who have problems resulting from a chemical dependency rarely identify their chemical use as a problem. The development of a dependency is insidious. Generally, chemically dependent persons try many ways to understand and explain what is happening when the painful consequences from the drug use occur. During this process many reasons other than the chemical itself are given as the problem. Usually the person views the chemical as a positive influence that helps with coping with whatever has been identified as the problem. As one's self-esteem begins to erode, defense mechanisms are used to protect one's ego and one's use of the chemical. Mechanisms such as rationalization, justification, denial, projection, and minimization all serve this protective function. When questioned about the chemical use, the person employs these defenses along with avoidance or anger. As the nurse proceeds with the assessment, therefore, it is important to understand the purposes of these defenses for the chemically dependent person. In this way, the nurse can continue with the assessment and not be dissuaded by their presence. Whenever possible, interview a spouse or a significant other for additional documentation, since this gives a more accurate assessment picture of the person, the chemical use, and the effect of that use on the family and social system.[36]

The management plan needs to be structured to meet the highly individualized needs of each patient. Careful, detailed data collection is important to accurate diagnosis and treatment. The assessment information will be used throughout the person's course of treatment; therefore, it is important for the nurse to determine the following: how the patient understands his chemical use; the pattern of chemical use; how the patient perceives the chemical use to be interacting with his total quality of life; and what is personally meaningful. Understanding the patient's history and his perception of his drug use helps the nurse to develop an approach to assist the patient and family in reframing their perceptions of the chemical use problem.

SUBJECTIVE DATA

Demographic Variables

Identify age, sex, marital status, number and ages of children, present living situation, race, employment status, educational status, legal status, and religious preference.

Description of Chemical Use

When an individual has a dependency on one chemical, often others have existed or exist at present. The nurse must listen carefully for the possibility of multiple dependencies. Obtain a detailed history of chemical use and emotional problems including hospitalizations and treatment involved. Educational, job, and economic problems should be determined. What relationships or social problems arose from the chemical use? Whenever possible, a spouse or other family member should be interviewed in this regard (see chart pertaining to history).

Family History

Identify physical or mental diseases that run in the family, causes of death, and age at time of death of family members. A family tree diagram may be helpful to identify quickly these factors as well as any chemical use problems that individual family members may have had.

Describe the nature of family rela-

Information for History of Chemical Use

DETAILED HISTORY OF CHEMICAL USE

Ask if the following chemicals have been used:

Opiates/Analgesics Stimulants (Cocaine, amphetamines)
Minor Tranquilizers Hallucinogens
Alcohol   Marijuana/hashish

Identify the drug of choice in each of the drug groups.
Identify the overall drug of choice.
Identify specific names of drugs used in each of the groups.

Collect the following data for *each* chemical the patient has used in the past or is currently using.

The name of the chemical (use pharmaceutical names rather than street names to begin to reframe the chemical use in a health care context).
Age at first use
Age at which the chemical use was identified as a problem by the patient
The effect experienced with each chemical
Any adverse effects experienced
Routes of entry
Quantity over time (from onset of use to present)
Evidence of tolerance and persistence of tolerance
Blackouts
Use until unconscious
Evidence of loss of control:
    Using more of the chemical than planned

Inability to abstain from use in spite of recurring negative consequences
Overdose
Identification of withdrawal symptoms upon abstaining from the chemical or decreasing the amount of the chemical

HISTORY OF PREVIOUS CHEMICAL DEPENDENCY TREATMENT

Includes dates, treating personnel, and facilities

HOSPITALIZATIONS

Medical problems in which chemical use was a factor in the admission

HISTORY OF TREATMENT OF EMOTIONAL PROBLEMS

Instances in which chemical use was a contributing factor

LEGAL HISTORY

Collect information regarding legal problems as a result of chemical use.

Arrest for driving under the influence of liquor or other chemicals
Speeding tickets incurred while under the influence of chemicals
Felonies or misdemeanors
Divorce suit
Custody suit
Arrest (or being taken into custody) for disorderly behavior

Information for History of Chemical Use (continued)

Probation history
Jail or prison record
Abuse or neglect of child/spouse/significant other
Charges in relation to auto or other types of accidents or assaults
Bankruptcy
Involvement of protective services
Loss of children

EVIDENCE OF EDUCATIONAL PROBLEMS (as a result of chemical use)

Frequent tardiness or absence
Inability to complete assignments either on time or at all
Incomplete courses
History of withdrawal from courses or school
Inability to take as many class hours as in the past
Loss of interest or motivation to compete
Delinquent or disruptive behavior
Inability to concentrate, remember, or learn new material
Decline in grades and quality of work both objectively and subjectively
Failure to attain a grade-point average needed to pass a class, to advance to another grade level, or to stay in school

EVIDENCE OF JOB PROBLEMS (as a result of chemical use)

Frequently late or absent
Conflicts, verbal or physical, with other employees or administrators
A history of probationary periods at work
Decrease in the quality of performance
Decreased work output
Loss of jobs or promotions due to chemical use
Feelings of decreased competency or self-confidence
Decreased enthusiasm or interest in work
History of taking sick days before or after scheduled days off or vacation days

IDENTIFICATION OF ECONOMIC PROBLEMS (due to chemical use)

Unemployed
Receiving assistance through welfare, social services, or food stamps
Spouse, significant other, or children working to support patient
Moving back into parents' or relatives' home
Attempting to obtain or presently on Social Security disability
Extensive legal fees
Working extra jobs to support chemical use
Stealing or prostitution for money to support chemical use

RELATIONSHIPS/SOCIAL PROBLEMS

Whenever possible interview another family member

Decrease in the amount of time spent at home or with family
Marital discord or separation
Frequent family arguments/conflicts as disorder progresses
History of divorce and broken relationships
Progressive avoidance of social activities that do not center on chemical use
Inability to fulfill promises, obligations, or responsibilities
Verbal/emotional abuse of family members
Outbursts of violence or physical abuse
Signs of physical abuse or neglect in spouse or children (*e.g.,* bruises, vague or unexplained injuries, malnourished or unkempt appearance)
Evidence or signs of emotional problems in children: daydreaming, night terrors, bed wetting, stuttering, withdrawal, depression, school delinquency problems or drug problems
Estrangement from close friends, parents, or family members
Sexual abuse of family members
Decrease in sexual desire, frequency of sexual relations, or inability to perform sexually as in the past

tionships: family of origin and the nuclear family. Identify any history of abuse or neglect by the patient and which member of the family incurred this. This can be in the form of physical, verbal, emotional or sexual abuse.

Pertinent Medical History

Collect a complete list of all diseases, conditions, and surgeries with dates, physicians names, and hospitals where treatment was administered.

Present health status is important for the patient to describe, particularly of middle and late stage patients. It is common to have numerous physical and psychological complaints. Personal health is neglected frequently. Furthermore, many systems may be disrupted or affected by the chemical use.

Long-term chronic use of centrally depressant drugs produces sleep disturbances. Sleep laboratory research on most hypnotics has found them to lose their sleep-producing effect within 3 to 14 days of continuous use.[9] Carefully elicit information in this area for a clear understanding of the nature of the sleep. Helpful questions may be: How long does it take to fall asleep? What are the average hours of sleep per night? Does the individual dream? What is the general nature of the dreams? How does the person feel upon awakening? What has helped the person to induce sleep? Disturbed sleep as a result of chronic depressant use is characterized by difficulty in getting to sleep and staying asleep. Frequently there is an absence of dreaming, and when the person is in withdrawal from the chemical, the dreams have the quality of "night terrors" or are disjointed in nature. As the dependency progresses, sleep is often drug-induced and the person is literally "unconscious" as a result of the drug level in the blood. As the drug level is reduced throughout the night,

the person awakens abruptly and experiences difficulty falling asleep again. It is at this point that the person repeats the chemical use until sleep is induced. Because sleep is drug-induced, the person frequently complains of "stuporousness" or "sluggishness" upon awakening and experiences headache and difficulty in thinking clearly.

Psychiatric Problems

Collect a complete list of any emotional problems or psychiatric illnesses for which the person has received treatment. Include dates, types of treatment, treating professionals, and agencies in which treatment occurred.

Medications

Prescription Drugs, Past and Current Use Whenever possible, have the patient or family member bring in prescription bottles and record dates, drug names, dosages, refills, prescribing physician, and instructions. Ask the conditions for which these medications were prescribed, how long they were used, any untoward effects, and how frequently and how much was taken over time. With this line of questioning, the nurse is looking for ways to identify an increase in tolerance, escalation of dose, and the psychological dependence or valuing of the drug to produce an effect that the person feels cannot be achieved in and by oneself. Ascertain if there have been any previous dependencies and what drugs these include. Some less emotionally charged questions that elicit this type of information are suggested here:

Have you ever wanted to stop taking a drug and could not?
Do you think you ever took too many drugs?
Do you think you were ever habituated to any drug?
Which drug or drugs were these?

The identification of any additional centrally acting drugs or drugs with any mood-altering properties is strategic in treatment, management, and recovery from chemical dependency. This information is crucial in detoxification and the prevention of any medical, surgical, or psychiatric emergencies. Furthermore, this information is important in educating the patient about obstacles in recovery.

Regularly Used Over-The-Counter (OTC) Drugs OTC drugs are frequently overlooked but are important to determine in the overall clinical picture. Many of these chemicals contain depressants and stimulants, and therefore they may present a dependency problem for the person or may be an obstacle in the patient's detoxification and recovery. Many liquids contain high concentrations of alcohol. Decongestants have sedating or stimulating properties. Diet medications frequently contain stimulant or stimulantlike ingredients.

Because many people suffer from caffeinism, it is important to identify daily consumption of caffeine in all forms: soft drinks, coffee, Excedrin, No-Doz, tea, Midol, and so forth. Determine daily consumption of tobacco and history of use.

OBJECTIVE DATA

The presence of chemical dependency may be detected through physical signs found on physical examination. When conducting the examination, the nurse observes patients at various points in drug use, ranging from acute intoxication to fulminant withdrawal. In terms of recovery, attendance to the total person is an important factor in a patient's recovery process. Patients who use hospital medical outpatient departments show improvement in drinking reduction, which is thought to correlate with attention to phys-

ical health.[15] Furthermore, the patient's feeling of being physically sound appears to reinforce other treatment outcome predictors of family and job.[14]

A thorough physical and psychiatric examination is necessary to determine the person's baseline physical and mental health status. This is used as a guide throughout recovery. It is helpful for the chemically dependent person to become motivated and involved in the process toward achieving a goal of a better quality of life.

Physical Examination

Pertinent aspects of the physical examination include a general assessment of the total person and a careful assessment of the integumentary, gastrointestinal, cardiovascular, respiratory, and neurologic system (see Table 21-1 for a list of common medical problems associated with chemical dependency).

In the general assessment, characteristics that alert the nurse to the existence of a chemical dependency include the following:

Poor body hygiene
Unkempt appearance
Odors of chemicals (e.g., alcohol or marijuana)
Tremulousness
Impaired gait and coordination
Malnutrition or obesity
Discrepancy in apparent age as related to chronological age
Irritability or lethargy
Slurred speech or speech that is inappropriate in tone or pace
Any variations in vital signs

Obesity and malnutrition are common conditions in chemically dependent persons. With alcoholism, the ingestion of large amounts of various forms of alcohol directly accounts for a large calorie increase, which

TABLE 21-1
MEDICAL PROBLEMS ASSOCIATED WITH CHEMICAL DEPENDENCY

NEUROLOGIC	URINARY	GYNECOLOGIC/SEXUAL DYSFUNCTION	RESPIRATORY	GASTROINTESTINAL AND ACCESSORY ORGANS	DERMATOLOGIC	CARDIOVASCULAR
Concussion, subdural hematomas	Nephropathy	Amenorrhea	Sinus problems	Hepatitis	Abscesses, ulcerations	Hypertension
Headache	Trauma (hematuria)	Impotence	Impaired lung function	Cirrhosis	Hematomas	Palpitation
Blackout	Toxic cystitis	Decreased sexual desire	Aspiration pneumonia	Pancreatitis/ dysfunction	Puncture wounds	Arrhythmias
Delirium		Difficulty achieving orgasm or sustaining erection	Chronic obstructive pulmonary disease	Esophagitis/ esophageal varices	Lacerations	Heart enlargement
Peripheral neuropathy		Testicular atrophy	Lung cancer and tuberculosis	Gastritis	Psoriasis	Circulatory problems
Wernicke–Korsakoff syndrome		Gynecomastia in males		Hemorrhage/melena	Pruritis	Heart disease
Convulsion				Ulcers	Acne rosacea	
Sleep disturbance				Liver enlargement	Rhinophyma	
Organic brain syndrome, acute and chronic				Hiatal hernia	Spider angiomas	
				Hemorrhoids		

leads to excessive weight gain. Drugs that cause sedation and lead to decreased activity can account for weight gain. Observe patients for muscular wasting in the presence of both obesity and malnutrition. Severity and duration of neglect will be the most important variables causing evidence of malnutrition; however, this may not be clinically evident in those persons with chemical dependencies of lesser degree or duration, or for those who have been better at consistently attending to their general health. Vitamin deficiencies also may occur and produce characteristic abnormalities. Deficiencies of the B-complex vitamins are most common; deficiencies of vitamins A and C, serum protein, magnesium, and iron are also frequent.

Observe for the following variations in vital signs:

Increased pulse can be present in direct response to stimulants and hallucinogens or as a result of withdrawal from depressant drugs.

Hypertension, blood pressure over 140/90, or fluctuating blood pressure can reflect withdrawal from depressant drugs or the effect of stimulant drugs. There is evidence that three or more drinks per day increase the risk of hypertension.[22]

Elevated temperature in the absence of infection can result from toxic drug effects, such as from stimulants and hallucinogens, or as a result of withdrawal from depressant drugs.

Decreased respirations can represent the effect of depressant drugs and overdose of depressant drugs.

Decreased blood pressure, hypotension, slow pulse, bradycardia, and hypothermia can represent an overdose. Such symptoms can be due to a depressant effect on the medulla or to a direct effect on the myocardium, sympathetic ganglia, and vascular smooth muscle.[2,37]

Pay special attention to the outward appearance of the body because many signs of chemical dependency are directly observable. Skin inspection may reveal many external signs of chemical dependency. Proceed carefully with appraisal of skin texture, color, hydration, turgor, and any unusual markings or hair loss. Chronic chemical use can lead to infections. Contaminated injection technique and contents, poor personal hygiene, poor nutrition, and poor living conditions can lead to skin infections in the form of lesions, abscesses, inflammations, ulcerations and infestations. The skin also can reveal poor healing, the presence of injection marks, bruises in various stages from trauma, or scars or tattoos incurred during intoxication. Localized, reddened streaks, tender or hardened areas over veins can indicate phlebitis. There may be depressions over bony structures or evidence of old fractures that have been sustained from accidents, falls, or fights while intoxicated. Liver cell damage can be evident through jaundiced skin color, palmar erythema, and spider angiomas. Pallor, coolness, blanched areas, or cyanosis in extremities are indicative of poor circulation, which may be the result of sclerosed veins or cardiac changes because of alcoholism. Moist skin may reflect withdrawal from depressant drugs such as alcohol, opiates, and sedatives, or it may be the result of overdoses of other drug groups. Flushing of the face due to vasodilation is seen following the ingestion of alcohol. Reddened sclera can be observed following smoking marijuana or the ingestion of alcohol.

Consumption of large quantities of alcohol or other irritants contained in other mood-altering substances can produce a variety of gastrointestinal and accessory organ irritations or structural alterations. Head and neck cancers are more frequent in persons who smoke or drink heavily. Carefully inspect the oral cavity for the presence of lesions, inflammations, ulcerations, or masses. Palpate the neck area for any masses or nodules. Inspect closely for tenderness throughout the abdomen, enlargement of the liver, and the presence of hemorrhoids.

Problematic conditions in the cardiovascular system occur as the chemical dependency, particularly alcoholism, progresses to later stages. Abnormal signs and symptoms occur as the heart muscle becomes weakened and enlarged by fatty infiltration. Arrhythmias can occur as the result of chemically induced changes in the heart's electrical system; however, if detected early, these conditions can be reversible.

Respiratory changes can result from use of chemicals that are inhaled into nasal passages or the lungs. Sinus problems can result from chronic, nasally inhaled drugs such as cocaine. Cannabis produces similar pulmonary and cardiovascular conditions that tobacco use produces.

A comprehensive neurologic examination is necessary, focusing on the areas positive in the history. In particular, identify hyper-reflexia or hypo-reflexia, nystagmus, impaired coordination, ataxia, tremors, cogwheel rigidity, and clonus. In active states of the CNS, people may describe seeing things in the visual field such as lines or dots of light. All of the above signs and symptoms may be exhibited by people under the influence of various substances or in stages of withdrawal.

Paraclinical Data

Note that laboratory data may be negative in patients with severe problems of chemical use. Positive biologic data may be present only in later state dependencies. Due to the reparative capabilities of the liver, liver function changes often revert to normal within a day or two after stopping chemical use. Therefore, it is advisable to acquire blood specimens soon after admission (see Tables 21-2 to 21-7 for a consolidation of blood and urine profiles associated with chemical dependency.)

Mental Status Examination

Persons under the influence of drugs or in withdrawal will exhibit changes in the quality and quantity of affect. This is reflected in inappropriate, blunted, or limited range of affect. Mental confusion may be exemplified by disorientation to time, place, and person. Impaired concentration and cognition are observed in the patient's inability to focus on the content of the interview, or inaccuracy in adding, subtracting, or repeating a series of numbers forward and backward. The ability to abstract frequently is impaired, as re-

---

TABLE 21-2
BLOOD PROFILE ASSOCIATED WITH CHEMICAL DEPENDENCY

BLOOD TEST	RESULTS	DISCUSSION
Hemoglobin	Low	Anemias can result from nutritional deficiency or as a direct result of toxic effects from excessive drug use. Such effects can be in the form of malabsorption from the small bowel, damage to the liver, suppression of bone marrow, and chronic or acute blood loss. Various types of anemia can occur: hypochromic, normocytic, and macrocytic. Hemolytic anemia also can occur.
Platelets	Low	
RBC	Low	
WBC (without presence of infection)	Low	

TABLE 21-3
BLOOD PROFILE ASSOCIATED WITH CHEMICAL DEPENDENCY

BLOOD TEST	RESULTS	DISCUSSION
Vitamin B_1 (thiamine)	Low	Nutritional deficiency can be the result of diet or
Vitamin B_6 (folic acid)	Low	malabsorption from the small bowel as a result of direct
Vitamin B_{12}	Low	effect of drug use, particularly alcohol.
Ascorbic Acid	Low	Illnesses: Wernicke's encephalopathy, Korsakoff's
Amino Acids	Low	psychosis, anemias, dementia due to nutritional
Iron	Low	deficiencies and their effect on the brain

flected in more literal or concrete meaning given to parables. Irritability can be observed during the interview in which the patient expresses impatience, annoyance, or abruptness. Signs of stimulation are hyperalertness, hyperactivity, and distorted affect. A quality of mistrust and the degree of suspiciousness toward the nurse or interview may reflect the presence of paranoia. Memory impairment may be exhibited through contradictions in data or inability to retain information given in the interview.

The following are common emotional and psychiatric problems associated with chemical dependency:

Relationship problems
Anxiety, phobias, panic attacks
Delayed grief reactions
Insomnia
School or work problems
Sexual dysfunction
Sexual abuse
Suicidal thinking or attempts

TABLE 21-4
BLOOD PROFILE ASSOCIATED WITH CHEMICAL DEPENDENCY

BLOOD TEST	RESULTS	DISCUSSION
Blood glucose	Low/elevated	Blood metabolites and electrolytes may be abnormal,
Protein bound iodine	Low	primarily from inadequate nutrition or secondarily
Potassium	Low	from disturbed metabolism associated with
Chloride	Low	excessive chemical use. *Note:* If dehydration is
Magnesium	Low	present, blood specimens will reflect
Lactic acid	Elevated	hemoconcentration and values of the following
Uric acid	Elevated	will be increased: Na, K, Cl, Ca, phosphorus,
Calcium	Elevated	glucose, BUN, uric acid, cholesterol, total protein,
Phosphorus	Elevated	globulin, LDH, SGOT, creatine. If there is
Creatine		hemodilution, as in the case of patients who have
phosphokinase	Elevated	drunk large amounts of alcohol in the form of
Alkaline phosphatase	Elevated	hypotonic liquid (*e.g.,* beer), the following values
Triglycerides	Elevated	may be decreased: Na, K, Cl, Ca, phosphorus,
		BUN, uric acid, albumin, total proteins and
		cholesterol.[36]

TABLE 21-5
BLOOD PROFILE ASSOCIATED WITH CHEMICAL DEPENDENCY

BLOOD TEST	*RESULTS*	*DISCUSSION*
SGOT	Elevated	Hepatic abnormalities are related to excessive alcohol
LDH	Elevated	use, the presence of Laennec's cirrhosis, or serum
BSP	Elevated	hepatitis resulting from contaminated injections or
Bilirubin	Elevated	contents
Serum albumin to globulin ratio	Reversal	Myopathies of skeletal muscle will also be reflected by an increase in SGOT, LDH, and creatine phosphokinase

Depression
Paranoid states
Hallucinosis
Violence or crime
Adult or child abuse or neglect
Organic brain syndrome (acute or chronic)

The chemically dependent person may have abnormal electrocardiogram (ECG), electroencephalogram (EEG), and electro-myography (EMG) results. These abnormal results may be the result of a combination of nutritional deficiencies or direct effect of the excessive chemical use.[37] In earlier stages of the disease, these are usually reversible following detoxification and abstinence from the chemical use.

Because many signs and symptoms of chemical effects and withdrawal syndromes are similar, it is crucial to identify the chemicals involved. Identification of the chemicals is important to institute appropriate treatment and plan for the anticipation of emergencies precipitated by withdrawal, surgery, or implementation of other treatment regimens. Most hospital laboratories are equipped to run qualitative analyses on blood and urine specimens; some have more sophisticated quantitative analysis capabilities. Specimens need to be obtained at the time of admission or as soon as chemical effects are suspected. Urine specimens must be kept refrigerated to prevent drug deterioration. Blood analyses generally are more accurate, especially because there is less opportunity for deception by the patient. Many clinics, practitioners, emergency rooms, and hospitals have screening devices called breath analyzers to measure the amount of alcohol on the breath. A reading of 0.10% blood alcohol level represents legal intoxication. This reading in the absence of objec-

TABLE 21-6
URINE PROFILE ASSOCIATED WITH CHEMICAL DEPENDENCY

URINE TEST	*RESULTS*	*DISCUSSION*
Appearance		
Deviations:		
Green to yellow in color, brown approaching black	Bile	Liver disease
Red in color	Blood	Nephropathy
Brown to black	Blood (will turn black on standing)	Trauma (hematuria)

TABLE 21-7
URINE PROFILE ASSOCIATED WITH CHEMICAL DEPENDENCY

URINE TEST	RESULTS	DISCUSSION
Urobilinogen, bilirubin, and urobilin	Bile	Liver disease
Glucose	Present to various degrees	Alcoholics are prone to transient glycosuria.
Ketones	Present to various degrees	Ketones may be present in severe malnutrition.
Specific gravity	Low	Nephropathy can be associated with chemical dependency. This can be
Protein/albumin	Present to various degrees	the result of contaminated parenteral
Sediments:		injection or injectants or from
RBC	Present to various degrees	chronic ingestion of certain
WBC	Present to various degrees	analgesics, inhalation of
Casts	Present to various degrees	hydrocarbons, oral or parenteral amphetamine use, and heroin injection.
pH	Acid	As the use of the amphetamine increases and food intake decreases, urine becomes more acid.

tive signs of intoxication indicates a high tolerance to alcohol.

Administration of a Michigan Alcohol Screening Test (MAST; see test form) is currently the most widely used screening technique for the diagnosis of alcoholism.[6,23,24] This test consists of a series of 24 yes/no questions devised to provide a consistent, quantifiable, structured interview instrument for the detection of alcoholism. It has substantial reliability.[25] Each of the items is assigned a score between 0 and 5. Following administration, the weighted responses are totaled.

In validation studies a score of 0 to 3 is regarded as normal drinking; 4 is borderline or suggestive of alcoholism, and a score of 5 or more is indicative of established alcoholism.[25] Other studies indicate that false-positive scores may be obtained from young adults, college age, using a score of 5 or more as the critical level.[6] This population may engage in brief periods of excessive episodic drinking that may not be true alcoholism. As a result of such false positives, the use of the original criterion of 10 or above reduces the probability of diagnosing inappropriately.[6]

This instrument was designed to be a screening test and must be followed by a more thorough investigation for diagnosis of alcoholism to be made conclusively. However, research studies reveal that the MAST is highly reliable and valid in objectifying and quantifying patient data in a consistent manner to determine the presence of alcoholism. Other studies indicate that a score of 5 on the MAST represents an 81% chance that the individual has alcoholism and a score of 10 or more indicates alcoholism exists.[39]

NURSING DIAGNOSIS

The assessment section is comprehensive for the nurse to identify the problem and arrive at a diagnosis. Most nurses are in strategic positions to identify a chemical dependency problem in its earlier stages and facilitate referral of chemically dependent people to treatment sooner. The nurse's contribution is in early identification of the problem and referral of patients and family members to treatment agencies, self-help groups, and intervention specialists.

Michigan Alcoholism Screening Test (MAST)

POINTS		YES	NO
	0. Do you enjoy a drink now and then?		
(2)	*1. Do you feel you are a normal drinker? (By normal we mean you drink less than or as much as most other people.)		
(2)	2. Have you ever awakened the morning after some drinking the night before and found that you could not remember a part of the evening?		
(1)	3. Does your wife, husband, a parent, or other near relative ever worry or complain about your drinking?		
(2)	*4. Can you stop drinking without a struggle after one or two drinks?		
(1)	5. Do you ever feel guilty about your drinking?		
(2)	*6. Do friends or relatives think you are a normal drinker?		
(2)	*7. Are you able to stop drinking when you want to?		
(5)	8. Have you ever attended a meeting of Alcoholics Anonymous (AA)?		
(1)	9. Have you gotten into physical fights when drinking?		
(2)	10. Has your drinking ever created problems between you and your wife, husband, a parent, or other relative?		
(2)	11. Has your wife, husband (or other family members) ever gone to anyone for help about your drinking?		
(2)	12. Have you lost friends because of your drinking?		
(2)	13. Have you ever gotten into trouble at work or school because of drinking?		
(2)	14. Have you ever lost a job because of drinking?		
(2)	15. Have you ever neglected your obligations, your family, or your work for two or more days in a row because you were drinking?		
(1)	16. Do you drink before noon fairly often?		
(2)	17. Have you ever been told you have liver trouble? Cirrhosis?		
(2)	†18. After heavy drinking have you ever had delirium tremens (DTs) or severe shaking, or heard voices or seen things that really weren't there?		

DETERMINE THE PRESENCE OF A CHEMICAL DEPENDENCY

The following collection of subjective and objective data from the patient and closest significant other determines if a chemical dependency exists:

Has the chemical use had any effect on any aspect of the patient's life?

Has the patient continued using the chemical in spite of recurring negative consequences to himself or others?

Is there evidence of tolerance? Persistence of tolerance?

Is the MAST score 5 or above?

Are there physical withdrawal symptoms on abstaining from using or significantly

Michigan Alcoholism Screening Test (MAST) (continued)

POINTS		YES	NO
(5)	19. Have you ever gone to anyone for help about your drinking?	_____	_____
(5)	20. Have you ever been in a hospital because of drinking?	_____	_____
(2)	21. Have you ever been a patient in a psychiatric hospital or on a psychiatric ward of a general hospital where drinking was part of the problem that resulted in hospitalization?	_____	_____
(2)	22. Have you ever been seen at a psychiatric or mental health clinic or gone to any doctor, social worker, or clergyman for help with any emotional problem, where drinking was part of the problem?	_____	_____
(2)	‡23. Have you ever been arrested for drunk driving, driving while intoxicated, or driving under the influence of alcoholic beverages? (If yes, how many times? _____)	_____	_____
(2)	‡24. Have you ever been arrested, or taken into custody, even for a few hours, because of drunk behavior? (If yes, how many times? _____)	_____	_____

*Alcoholic response is negative.
†5 points for Delirium tremens
‡2 points for *each* arrest
Courtesy of Selzer ML

SCORING SYSTEM

In general, 5 points or more would place the subject in an "alcoholic" category. Four points would be suggestive of alcoholism, three points or less would indicate the subject was not alcoholic.

Programs using the above scoring system find it very sensitive at the five point level and it tends to find more people alcoholic than anticipated. However, it is a screening test and should be sensitive at its lower levels.

REFERENCES

Selzer ML: The Michigan Alcoholism Screening Test (MAST): The quest for a new diagnostic instrument. *Am J Psychiatr* 127:89–94, June 1971

Selzer ML, Vinokur A, van Rooijen L: A self-administered short version of the Michigan Alcoholism Screening Test (SMAST). *J Studies Alcohol* 36:117–26, 1975

Revised Aug 25, 1980

decreasing the amount of chemical in the absence of other chemical use?

If the answers to these questions are positive, the data supports a diagnosis of chemical dependency.[1,28,39]

FACTORS THAT INDICATE LIKELIHOOD OF SUCCESSFUL RECOVERY

Predictive variables for prognosis are employment, marital status, quality of marital interaction, state of maturity at admission, quality of socialization, and degree of social deviance.[20,26,39] Identify power sources that can be leverages to motivating the patient for treatment if a formal intervention is necessary. This information is helpful in planning for the multivariant treatment indicated to meet individual needs.

Obstacles to recovery include both psychological and physiological variables that can initiate the recruitment process. Psychological obstacles include experience with drug-linked cues such as: drug-using friends, drug-using places, drug paraphernalia, drug-related dreams, the anniversary of stopping drug use, memories of using drugs, and strong drug-linked feelings. Sensory experiences with one's drug of choice is highly reinforcing and can elicit the recruitment process. For example, if one has alcoholism, it can be highly recruiting to hear alcohol being poured or smell its aroma, see one's favorite beverage, or taste small amounts in foods or through sipping a small amount directly in a beverage.

Physiological variables include the actual use of one's drug of choice, the use of cross tolerant chemicals, the use of a mood-altering chemical that reminds one of the mood alteration resulting from one's drug of choice, experiencing a flare-up or periodic affective disturbance, and having the flu or other illness that may simulate the withdrawal process and remind one of withdrawing from one's drug of choice.

IS THE PATIENT A CANDIDATE FOR INPATIENT OR OUTPATIENT CHEMICAL DEPENDENCY TREATMENT?

Candidates for inpatient chemical dependency treatment centers can be determined by the presence of the following variables:[38]

Impending danger to self and others
Inability to abstain from use in spite of adequate outpatient treatment
Nonexistent or inadequate social support systems
A severe alcohol/Antabuse reaction
The presence of medical or psychiatric illness that is probably the result of the chemical use
Moderate-to-severe impairment in functioning
The need for an externally controlled environment to prevent drug use, coupled with an intensive focus on the chemical dependency for the purpose of breaking down denial and promoting internalization of the presence of dependency
A history of severe withdrawal syndrome (i.e., delirium tremens or convulsions)
Request by a patient for hospitalization

Inpatient programs vary from 2 weeks to 6 weeks, with the average program being 21 days.

Outpatient treatment is appropriate for most persons who have chemical dependency as long as the previously cited criteria for inpatient screening have been considered. Studies of outpatient treatment for alcoholism indicate that results are no better with inpatient than outpatient treatment.[19]

Outpatient treatment avoids the effects of institutionalization by keeping the person in a familiar environment with those who make up the support network. By recovering in a realistic environment, the patient learns to negotiate daily sobriety when confrontation occurs with the unique vulnerabilities and obstacles specific to his or her recovery. Furthermore, important positive internal and external controls can be identified more quickly, which facilitates sobriety and adds meaning to life. Outpatient treatment is more economical for the patient and employer by allowing employment to continue, and is more economical for the health care facility to provide. Criteria for success in outpatient treatment depend on the program's intensiveness, its thoroughness, and provision of regular and consistent monitoring of the patient's progress.[38]

For some patients whose dependencies are severe and later stage, the inpatient approach, combined with follow-up outpatient treatment programs, may not provide adequate intensity and length of controlled environment for a successful recovery; therefore, some patients may need a residential treatment program in which the person actually lives at the facility for several months in a recovery milieu.

DETERMINE IF FORMAL INTERVENTION IS NECESSARY

Following the discussion of the patient's diagnosis with the treatment team (nursing and medical staff, social worker, psychologist, and a consultant from a chemical dependency program), a plan of approach must be designed for discussing the diagnosis with the patient and family in preparation for treatment. If the patient rejects the diagnosis and is unwilling to participate in planning for treatment, it may be necessary for the treatment team to plan a formal intervention. The concept that "the patient must verbalize

a desire for treatment," indicating motivation as a predictor for successful long-term treatment outcome, has been misleading and does not correlate with successful treatment or long-term outcome.[17] Alcohol studies that have examined legal or economic coercion by legal forces, employers, spouse, children, relatives, and friends that have been employed to force people into treatment, have shown that such persons do as well or better than those who seek treatment voluntarily.[17] It is useful to determine coercive forces that have an impact on the person. These forces can be used at this time to motivate the person for treatment, as well as to enhance treatment throughout recovery. The above data lend support to the crisis production theory used by the intervention model. In this model, the treatment team and others actually can plan and produce a crisis that can force the person into treatment early in the course of the disease, rather than waiting for him to "hit bottom" and incur significant biopsychosocial losses. If the treatment team does not choose to do this, a referral can be made to a chemical dependency treatment facility that offers personnel who are skilled in this technique.

DETERMINE THE GOAL OF MANAGEMENT

The overall treatment goal for persons with chemical dependency is the improvement of the quality of life for both the patient and family through eventual abstinence from any drug with central depressant or mood-altering properties.[7] This requires a permanent change in the person's behavior, cognition, values, feelings, and attitudes regarding the chemical use. The latter three will take the longest to change.

In contracting for and setting goals for the treatment, the patient can have some latitude in the selection of the therapeutic modality: self-help group, frequency of attendance per week, or a formal treatment modality such as individual, group, marital, or family therapy (see examples listed). Such input depends on the particular program in which the patient is enrolled. However, the patient may not choose outpatient treatment if professional evaluation criteria warrant inpatient treatment. This must be the decision of the health care professional.

MANAGEMENT

At the present time there is no cure for chemical dependency. People will always have the problem once it has been activated; however, management is approached from the standpoint that the condition is highly treatable. It consists of abstaining from any mood-altering chemical use to keep the disorder inactive. The earlier it is diagnosed and treated, the more successful the treatment outcome, since in the earlier stage of the illness the person's denial system often is less developed and the support system still intact.[38] In addition, the symptom of "loss of control" is not as advanced. Relapses of chemical use

may be shorter and less intense, allowing the person to gain control easier and resume recovery.

Most nurses are not directly involved in the actual treatment programs for chemical dependency; however, most nurses are involved in primary and secondary prevention of chemical dependency and should be knowledgeable regarding the content of treatment programs. Primary prevention involves health teaching about drug groups and the risks involved in their use. Secondary prevention pertains to the identification and referral of chemically dependent persons. Nurses in all settings may be involved in the tertiary care of chemically dependent patients: assisting those who are in recovery to maintain that recovery process.

The nurse should identify cross-tolerant medications that may be prescribed inadvertently or purchased over the counter which would have a recruiting effect on the chemically dependent person. Patients who do require these medications for surgery, pain, or procedures need the health team's assistance in managing detoxification, carefully administering the medications, and switching to non-narcotic analgesics as soon as possible. Any indications of recruitment must be ad-

---

Examples of Specifically Designed Treatment Programs for Chemical Dependency

Inpatient treatment facilities
Outpatient treatment facilities
Residential treatment facilities

Treatment modalities available in most of these treatment facilities include

Individual
Group
Family
Marital

Self-help groups include the following:

Alcoholics Anonymous (AA)
Examples of specific-identity AA groups:
Physician   Women   Gay (male)
Nurse   Professor   Teen
Lawyer   Lesbian (female) Clergy/priest
Al-Anon (Self-help group for families of alcoholics)
Ala-Teen (Self-help group for children of alcoholics)
Narcotics Anonymous (NA)
Women for Sobriety

dressed while the patient is still hospitalized and appropriate referrals should be made at that time.

DETOXIFICATION

Once the diagnosis has been made and the appropriate treatment has been determined, the next step is to prepare the person for detoxification. The goal of detoxification is to help the person to stop using the chemical and withdraw safely. Most persons who have alcoholism can detoxify safely in their own environment; however, approximately 5% will require hospitalization for close supervision and medical management of the detoxification phase.[38] If the patient is ambulatory and presents an uncomplicated clinical picture, nondrug detoxification is less hazardous and just as effective as administering sedatives or tranquilizers.[38] Detoxification from other drug groups such as sedatives, opiates, and tranquilizers, requires a medical withdrawal regimen to prevent any untoward or severe withdrawal symptoms. This regimen consists of a carefully planned dose reduction. The goal is a safe withdrawal in which the patient is comfortable enough to comply with the withdrawal scheme, particularly on an outpatient basis.

Drug screening before the actual initiation of detoxification is necessary to identify any other drugs present that may interfere or impinge upon the detoxification phase, causing unexpected sequelae. Periodic screening may be necessary through the recovery period, especially if other drug use is suspected and the patient is unable to acknowledge it.

Opiate withdrawal is viewed by the public as the most life-threatening and frightening of the three major depressant drug groups: alcohol, opiates, and sedative hypnotics (this latter including the minor tranquilizers). Actually, opiate withdrawal is the least serious and most easily managed syndrome.[5] The opiate withdrawal syndrome, particularly for heroin and morphine, has been studied and described in detail. Abrupt withdrawal is rarely fatal in opiate-addicted persons who are in otherwise good health; however, the nature and severity of the withdrawal symptoms that appear when the opiate is discontinued will depend upon many variables such as the particular drug, the total daily dose used, the interval between doses, the duration of use, and the health and personality of the user.[11] Opiate withdrawal can be managed easily on a gradual dose-reduction schedule.

Sedatives, which include the minor tranquilizer group, should never be stopped abruptly.[29] Abrupt withdrawal from general depressants can be fatal; therefore, a gradual dose reduction is needed.[11] In addition, research has shown that severe health consequences, including severe withdrawal sequelae, have resulted in persons on therapeutic doses of benzodiazepines (i.e., diazepam, chlordiazepoxide, lorazepam) when the drug was stopped abruptly.

Withdrawal symptoms from sedative depressants is the opposite of the drug action; therefore, there will be a stimulation of the CNS in the withdrawal period. Nursing care includes regular measurement of vital signs such as blood pressure, pulse, respiration, and temperature, and measurement of neurologic reflexes. As withdrawal begins, the blood pressure rises, peaks about the middle of withdrawal, and then declines and stabilizes as the body reaches homeostasis. These time periods will vary with each drug. The neurologic reflexes show a similar rise in activity as the withdrawal peaks and then gradually decrease in activity as withdrawal finishes. Avoidance of stimulants like caffeine is helpful because these only add to the stimulation of the CNS and aggravate sleep disturbance. Many of these persons prefer not to eat due to a lack of appetite, nausea, and gastrointestinal discomfort. However, eating several small, well-balanced meals spread over the day keeps the person more comfortable. Hypoglycemia adds to the person's discomfort, irritability, and tremulousness.

During this phase the patient has difficulty with concentration and memory. Purposeful activities that require minimal concentration and exercise help to keep the person distracted from the discomfort of withdrawal without adding to the stimulation. Frequent verbal reassurance helps to decrease the patient's anxiety about what is happening. Periodic monitoring of the patient's vital signs is important to the patient's peace of mind. Although withdrawal seizures are not common in carefully regulated withdrawals, they do occur. The nurse must be alert for this condition without alarming the patient.

The use of disulfiram (Antabuse) for persons with alcoholism may be determined at this time. Disulfiram is not a cure for alcoholism, but can be used as an adjunct to supportive treatment.[12] When taken regularly disulfiram is stored in the tissues and serves as a protective barrier. This barrier allows the patient to make only one decision a day to "not drink" rather than many. If on impulse the person decides to drink, or forgets to take the daily dose, the protective barrier remains present for several days, allowing time for a change in decision.[12]

The adverse alcohol/Antabuse reaction includes the following symptoms: flushing, sweating, palpitations, dyspnea, hyperventilation, tachycardia, hypotension, nausea, and vomiting. Disulfiram blocks the metabolism of alcohol by inhibiting the breakdown of acetaldehyde by the enzyme aldehyde dehydrogenase; therefore, as one ingests alcohol in the presence of disulfiram, the level of acetaldehyde rises and a toxic reaction occurs. Emergency measures for a severe reaction include supportive measures to restore blood pressure and to treat shock, including administration of oxygen, and intravenous antihistamine or ephedrine sulfate.[4]

PATIENT EDUCATION

Education continues more fully once the person is through withdrawal. Memory and concentration are improved and the patient is able to think more clearly. Education includes nutritional concepts, learning about chemical dependency and obstacles to recovery, social interaction skills, and stress management concepts, such as condition relaxation. Educational groups help to provide the means for social interaction and peer support. Ongoing groups or individual therapy sessions help to continue the support and begin behavior modification and attitude changes necessary to achieve the goal of living chemically free. Many find this period a time for renewal of spiritual growth, which can lend further support to the internal commitment of a "new way of life." Church attendance and attendance at self-help groups such as AA can work together to provide a new social network to support sobriety. Within these groups one can find new activities and relationships that do not center on the use of psychoactive chemicals.

Early in the treatment program, when the person has first given up the psychoactive chemical, authorities advocate a combined confrontive, supportive, and directive approach to begin the process of acceptance of the disorder.[38,39] There are many ways the nurse can increase support for the client during the recovery process. The most strategic intervention in the area of support is the nurse's work with the family members and the significant others to increase their support of the patient. This support variable, particularly the support that comes from the quality of the marital relationship, is significant to the likelihood of success in recovery.

On an individual basis, through regular contacts with the patient, the nurse can provide support through the use of empathetic listening and genuine caring. In early recovery the patient is engaged in an intense struggle with the all-encompassing power of the chemical dependency itself. Acknowledgment of this struggle and positive reinforcement for the patient's efforts to remain chemically free is extremely valuable. Another critical area of support can be obtained through the regular attendance at group meetings with other recovering persons.

It is helpful that all three support areas be an integral part of the nursing contract with the patient. In early recovery, the nurse needs to intensify all support areas by increasing the patient's individual sessions, family contacts, and the required number of group meetings per week, until recovery is more stable.

Confrontive efforts are directed at helping the patient and family reframe the drug use. Breaking down the denial regarding the negative effects of the chemical use on one's total quality of life, one's loved ones, the employer, and society, and helping the patient to accept responsibility for the drug use, are vital in intervening in the power of the dependency. A primary goal in treatment, therefore, is to increase the conflict over using the drug. As long as one can continue to delude oneself that the substance use has had no effect on one's life or others, and to blame others or circumstances for the problem drug use, the person can continue to use it without feeling conflict. The relief from this conflict as it begins to develop comes from remaining chemically free. This relief

can become a powerful internal motivation for successful recovery. Furthermore, as one experiences an improved quality of life through remaining chemically free, one develops a greater understanding of what is sacrificed if one returns to drug use. Therefore, the accumulation of time living drug-free lends strength to the recovery. Success is promoted further through the increase of one's internal controls, which develop through the increasing conflict over using a chemical and the increasing ability to resist the decision to use it. Confrontive nursing intervention centers on assisting the patient to identify negative life-effects from the problem drug use, the meaning of relapse on the quality of life, the positive outcomes from remaining drug-free, and monitoring for activation of the recruitment process. This last is evidenced by behaviors or thoughts that the person is having in preparation for drug use or the reflection of positive feelings, attitudes, and values toward using it again.

Directive nursing interventions are centered on assisting the patient to plan strategies to remain drug-free. These are then entered in a nursing contract with the patient. The nurse must hold firm to the nursing contract, setting appropriate limitations and being consistent in following through on the agreed plan. For example, a patient with alcoholism, who is being treated in an outpatient setting, agrees to take Antabuse daily and to enter an inpatient alcohol treatment program if he stops the Antabuse and resumes drinking. The nurse must abide by the contract, remaining nonjudgmental but firm in its enforcement, and proceed to assist the patient in acquiring inpatient treatment if such a relapse in drinking occurs.

The psychoanalytic approach should be avoided since it has been shown repeatedly that treating patients who have chemical dependency on the premise that the abnormal drinking behavior is secondary to or symptomatic of an underlying psychopathology is not usually successful; it is often counterproductive.[33,38] Once stable sobriety has been achieved, the patient will have the same needs and capacity to benefit from psychotherapy as any other member of the population; however, early recovery is not the appropriate time for this.[33]

PATIENT REFERRAL

If the decision is made to refer the patient elsewhere for chemical dependency treatment, it is important to find a facility in which the staff are expert in alcohol and drug treatment. Any agency listed in the telephone book under drug or alcohol treatment must be licensed by the State Office of Substance Abuse and meet certain standards set by that agency. The National Council of Alcoholism, or a local council on alcoholism, is also listed in the Yellow Pages and provides information on local treatment facilities for the treatment of alcoholism. Important criteria for any agency or therapist include the following: a chemical-free philosophy, avoidance of prescribing psychoactive drugs during the long-term treatment, careful screening of any medication before prescribing for other conditions, the offer of disulfiram to most persons with alcoholism, planning for regular involvement of the family or significant others in the treatment, extensive use of self-help groups, regular follow-up outpatient treatment, and avoidance of insight-oriented psychotherapy until recovery is stable.

Many chemical dependency treatment facilities provide a program designed specifically for the treatment of families in addition to individual treatment for the member who has the chemical dependency. Such programs may designate a certain number of treatment hours to which one or several family members must commit themselves as their involvement in the treatment. This commitment may be a criterion for admission to the program.

The family treatment model is based on the following premise: "Chemical dependency is a family disease and a primary disease within each family member."[34] One study on alcoholism documented the following:

> Pathological drinking becomes integrated into the family system and leads to predictable, compulsive behavior, both in individual family members and in the interaction among them.[35]

As the disease insidiously develops, the family organization undergoes pathological changes that are directly related and parallel to the development of the disease. The growing dysfunction of the chemically dependent person affects each member of the family. Subsequently, each family member adapts to the pain of interacting with the dysfunctional member by developing behavior that causes the least amount of personal stress. These adaptations are dynamic and serve to keep the family in balance. These adaptations frequently are reflected in characteristic roles such as "the family hero, the chief enabler, the scapegoat, the mascot, and the lost child."[34] Although these roles and behaviors serve to keep the family in balance, they also allow the chemically dependent person to continue using the mood-altering drug.

This model of treatment serves a preventive function by treating the children of the chemically dependent family, who are more likely to develop the disease themselves. It has been reported in one study of persons with alcoholism that 52% of the sample were children of alcoholics.[35] Furthermore, it has been estimated that 15 million to 17 million children in this country have an alcoholic parent.[34] These figures do not reflect the number of children who have parents with other dependencies. By including such children in treatment, they become psychologically healthier by interrupting and changing the pathologic adaptations that may carry over into their adult lives with their families. The education they receive in treatment can increase their knowledge and awareness of the disease, which can serve to protect them from its development.

CONCLUSION

Chemical dependency is a complex, multifaceted problem that is chronic, relapsing, progressive, and fatal if allowed to follow its natural course. Although there is no cure, it is highly treatable. Its prognosis can be promising and is more favorable the earlier it is detected and treated. The nurse is in a strategic position for early detection of this problem. Research studies continue to seek possible cause-and-effect relationships with regard to the mechanisms of dependency. Neurobiology and physiology, genetics, pharmacology, and sociocultural aspects are critical areas under investigation that may hold the key to a more comprehensive understanding of chemical dependency.

REFERENCES

1. American Psychiatric Association: Diagnostic and Statistical Manual of Mental Disorders, 3rd ed. pp 163–179, Washington DC, American Psychiatric Association, 1980
2. Appleton WS, Davis JM: Practical Psychopharmacology. New York, Medcom, 1973
3. Axelrod J, Weinshilbaum R: Catecholamines. New Engl J Med 387:237–242, 1972
4. Ayerst Laboratories: Guidelines for Antabuse (Disulfiram) Users. New York, Ayerst Laboratories 1981
5. Barchas JD, Berger PA, Ciranello RD et al: Psychopharmacology, pp 3–64. New York, Oxford University Press, 1977
6. Brady JP, Foulks ET, Childres AR et al: The Michigan Alcoholism Screening Test as a Survey Instrument. J Operational Psychiatr 13, No. 1:27–31, 1982
7. Connelly JC et al: Position statement on substance abuse. Am J Psychiatr 138:874–875, June 1981
8. Department of Health, Education, and Welfare, Public Health Service, Food and Drug Administration: Prescribing of minor tranquilizers. FDA Drug Bull 10, No. 1:2–3, Feb 1980
9. Department of Health, Education, and Welfare, Public Health Service, Food and Drug Administration: Update on sedative hypnotics. FDA Drug Bull 10, No. 1: Feb 1980
10. Goodwin DW: Alcoholism and heredity. Arch Gen Psychiatr 36:57–61, Jan 1979
11. Jaffee JH, Gilman A (eds): The Pharmacological Basis of Therapeutics, 6th ed, pp 539–543. New York, MacMillan Publishing, 1980
12. Kwentus J, Major LF: Disulfiram in the treatment of alcoholism. J Studies on Alcohol 40, No. 5:428–444, 1979
13. Madden JS, Walker R, Kenzen WH (eds): Alcoholism and Drug Dependence: A Multidisciplinary Approach. New York, Plenum Press, 1977
14. Mayer J, Myerson DJ: Characteristics of outpatient alcoholics in relation to change in drinking, work and marital status during treatment. Quarterly J of Studies on Alcohol 31:889–897, 1970
15. Mayer J, Myerson DJ: Outpatient treatment of alcoholics: Effects on status, stability and nature of treatment. Quarterly J of Studies on Alcohol 32:620–627, 1971
16. Mendelson JH, Mello NK: Biologic concomitants of alcoholism. N Eng J Med 301:912–921, 1979
17. Mendelson JH, Mello NK (eds): The Diagnosis and Treatment of Alcoholism, p 155. New York, McGraw–Hill, 1979
18. Mirin SM, Weiss RD, Michael J: Alcohol abuse in patients dependent on other drugs. Psychiatr Annu 12, No. 4:430–433, Apr 1982
19. Polich JM, Armor DJ, Braiker HB: The course of alcoholism: Four years after treatment, R-2433, NIAAA. Santa Monica, Rand Corporation, 1980
20. Rae JB: The influence of the wives on the treatment of alcoholics: Follow-up study at two years. Br J Psychiatr 120:601–613, 1972
21. Ray O: Drugs, Society and Human Behavior, 2nd ed.

pp 2–12; 76–89; 108–110. St. Louis, CV Mosby, 1978

22. Scheig R: Alcohol use and the risk of medical illness. Research Monograph No. 5: Evaluation of the alcohol: Implications for research, theory and treatment, pp 251–257. US Dept of Health and Human Services, National Institute on Alcohol Abuse and Alcoholism. Washington, DC, U S Gov't Printing Office, 1981

23. Selzer ML: The Michigan alcohol screening test: The quest for a new diagnostic instrument. Am J Psychiatr 127, No. 12:89–94, June 1971

24. Selzer ML, Ehrlich NJ: A Screening Program to Detect Alcoholism in Traffic Offenders in the Prevention of Highway Injury, pp 45–50. In Selzer JL, Gikas WP, Huelke DF (eds): Ann Arbor, University of Michigan Highway Safety Research Institute, 1967

25. Selzer ML, Vinokur A, van Rooijen L: A self-administered short Michigan alcoholism screening test (SMAST). J Studies Alcohol 36, No. 1:117–126, 1975

26. Simpson DD, Savage JL, Lloyd MR: Evaluation of treatment of drug abuse during 1969 to 1972. Arch Gen Psychiatr 36:772–780, July 1979

27. Smith DE: Prescription Drugs and the Alcoholic: The Benzodiazepines: Therapeutic and Dependence Considerations, pp 42–48. Proceedings of the Eisenhower Medical Center and the California Society for the Treatment of Alcohol and Other Drug Dependencies Conference. Rancho Mirage, California, Winter 1981

28. Smith DE: Contemporary drug abuse patterns. Speech at the Health and Addiction Seminar. Park City, Utah, March 1982

29. Smith DE: Prescription drug abuse. Speech at the Health and Addiction Seminar. Park City, Utah, March 1982

30. Tarter RE, Suzerman AA (eds): Alcoholism: Interdisciplinary approaches to an enduring problem. Ready, MA, Addison–Wesley, 1976

31. US Department of Health, Education, and Welfare: The Alcohol Drug Abuse and Mental Health National Data Book, pp 80–938. Washington, DC, DHEW Publication, 1980

32. Vaillant GE: Natural history of male psychological health: VIII. Antecedents of alcoholism and "orality." Am J Psychiatr 137, No. 2:181–186, Feb 1980

33. Vaillant GE: Dangers of psychotherapy in the treatment of alcoholism. In Bean MH, Zenberg NE (eds): Dynamic Approaches to the Understanding and Treatment of Alcoholism, pp 36–49. New York, MacMillan, 1981

34. Wegscheider S: No One Escapes From a Chemically Dependent Family. Minneapolis, Johnson Institute, 1976

35. Wegscheider S: Another Chance, Hope and Health for the Alcoholic Family, pp 27–31. Palo Alto, CA, Science and Behavior Books, 1981

36. Weinberg JR: Assessing drinking problems by history. Postgrad Med 59, No. 4:87–90, April 1976

37. Westermeyer J: Primer on Chemical Dependency. Baltimore, Williams & Wilkins, 1976

38. Whitfield CL: Outpatient management of the alcoholic patient. Psychiatr Annu 12, No. 4:447–458, Apr 1982

39. Whitfield CL, Williams KH: Treatment of alcoholics. In Whitfield CL (ed): The Patient With Alcoholism and Other Drug Problems. Chicago, Year Book Medical Publishers (in press)

40. Winokur A et al: Withdrawal reaction for long-term low-dosage administration of diazepam. Arch Gen Psychiatr 37:101–105, Jan 1980

BIBLIOGRAPHY

Barchas JD, Berger PA, Ciranello RD et al: Psychopharmacology, pp 355–382. New York, Oxford University Press, 1977

Goldstein A: High on Research. Hollywood, Florida, The US Journal of Drug and Alcohol Dependence, Jan 1980

Goodwin DW, Schulsinger F, Knop J, et al: Alcoholism and depression in adopted-out daughters of alcoholics. Arch Gen Psychiatr 34:751–755, July 1977

Lieber CS: The metabolism of alcohol. Sci Am 234, No. 3:25–33, Mar 1976

Malasanos L, Barkauskas V, Moss M et al: Health Assessment. St. Louis, Missouri, CV Mosby, 1977

Oxford J et al: The cohesiveness of alcoholism-complicated marriages and its influence on treatment outcome. Br J Psychiatr 128:318–339, 1976

Schuckit MA, Goodwin DA, Winokur GA: A study of alcoholism in half-siblings. Am J Psychiatr 128:1132–1136, 1972

Vander AJ, Sherman JH, Luciano DS: Human Physiology: The Mechanisms of Body Function, 3rd ed, pp 144–190. New York, McGraw–Hill, 1980

Wegscheider S: Another Chance: Hope and Health for the Alcoholic Family, pp 17–31. Palo Alto, CA, Science and Behavior Books, 1981

Westermeyer J, Walker D: Approaches to treatment of alcoholism across cultural boundaries. Psychiatr Annu 12, No. 4:434–439, April 1982

Williams A: The student and the alcoholic patient. Nurs Outlook 27:470–472, 1979

Index

An *f* following a page number represents a figure; a *t* indicates tabular material.

diaphragmatic breathing, in dyspnea management, 432, 434
diaphragmatic disorders, and coughing, 436
diarrhea. *See* irritable bowel syndrome
diarrhea, 344–361
  in allergy to food, 454, 459
  in anxiety, 59
  assessment, 347–353
    history, 347–351, 350t
    laboratory studies, 351, 352–353t
    physical examination, 351
  body boundary and, 74
  bowel function, factors affecting, 339–344
  categories of, 351
  defined, 345
  dehydration with. *See also* dehydration
    and mental impairment, 5
    risks of, 353–354
  diagnosis, 351–355
  in fatigue, 110
  in headache, vascular, 187t
  management of, 355–360
  mechanisms of, 345–347, 347t
  with nausea and vomiting, diseases seen in, 391t
  nutritional alteration diagnosis, 397
diary
  diet
    in constipation management, 368
    in obesity, 482, 483
    in weight-reduction program, 489
  headache, 201, 202f
  symptom, in constipation management, 370
diazepam (Valium)
  and confusion, in elderly, 7t, 24
  dependency syndromes, 517
  history of, 517
  in low back pain management, acute conditions, 170
  mental status effects of, 7t
dienestrol, 507
diet. *See also* food allergies
  in Alzheimer's disease, 11
  in anxiety, physiological responses and, 59
  calcium deficiency, and confusion, 4
  and constipation, 360
    diagnostic consideration, 367
    management strategies, 369, 369t
  in depression
    assessment data, 45
    management considerations, 51
  in diarrhea
    assessment data, 353, 354
    as cause of, 348
    food allergies, 459
    management, 355–357, 358, 359
  in drug detoxification program, 540
  estrogens from, 496
  in fatigue, 110, 117

and headache
  prevention strategies, 201–203, 203t
  vascular, 187
and Hemoccult testing, 365
in low back pain management, 170
in menopause management, 508, 509
in nausea and vomiting
  as aggravating factor, 391t
  management considerations, 400
in osteoporosis management, 509
and pain, 126
and postmenopausal health, 510
potassium-containing food, 356
weight reduction program, 486–488
diet diary
  in obesity, 482, 483
  in weight-reduction program, 489
diethylstilbestrol, 507–508
digital examination, in diarrhea, 351
digitalis preparations
  mental status effects of, 6–7
  and skin rashes, 312
  and vertigo and dizziness, 234
  and vomiting, 379
dihydroergotamine mesylate (Hydergine), in confusion, 31–32
dimenhydrinate (Dramamine; Eldodram; Trav-arex)
  in motion sickness, 236–237
  in nausea and vomiting, 399
  in vertigo and dizziness, 231, 233
diphenhydramine hydrochloride (Benadryl)
  in allergic reactions, 468, 470–471
  in nausea and vomiting, 399
  in vertigo and dizziness, 231
diphenidol (Vontrol), in vertigo and dizziness, 231
diphenoxylate (Lomotil), in diarrhea, 357, 358
disability, and fatigue, 104f, 105
disbelief phase, in body image alterations, 85
discography, in low back pain, assessment data, 168
discomfort
  and constipation, diagnostic consideration, 367
  in fatigue, 104t, 105
disequilibrium, defined, 209
disk herniation, 159, 160. *See also* pain, low back
  assessment data, 166
  defined, 153
  management considerations, 172, 173
dismemberment, and body image, 80
disorganization, in fatigue, 104–105, 104t
disorientation, 29–30. *See also* confusion
displacement, in body image alterations, 83
distention. *See also* bloating; intestinal gas
  in anxiety
    assessment data, 63
    physiological responses and, 59
  in constipation, 363, 367
  with nausea and vomiting, diseases seen in, 395t
disulfiram (Antabuse), 516, 540

propoxyphene (Darvon), mental status effects of, 7t
propranolol (Inderal), in headache, 204
proprioception
  and balance, 209–210
  multiple sensory deficits, 219
prostaglandins
  and fever, 297
  in headache, migraine, 186
prostatectomy, 418
prostate disorders
  and incontinence, 408
    assessment of, 411–412
    surgical management in, 418
  low back pain with, 161
prostheses, in body image alterations, 82
protein levels, and decubitus ulcer formation, 315
proteins, digestion and absorption of, 339, 340
proteinuria, in dehydration, 394t
proteolytic enzymes, in wound management, 335
protrusion, spinal ligament, 160
pruritus
  in allergy, 459
  chemical mediators and, 450, 450t
  and decubitus ulcer formation, 316
  in drug dependency, 528t
  with rashes, 312, 313, 326–328
pseudodementia
  and confusion
    assessment data, 21
    management of, 23–24
  defined, 8
  treatment of, 9
pseudomembranous colitis, and diarrhea, 358
pseudomonal infections, 427
pseudoself, in depression, 40, 41
psoriasis, in drug dependency, 528t
psychiatric disorders
  with drug dependency, 526, 531–532
  impaired mobility with, 273t
  and self-induced infection, 302
psychoactive agents
  and confusion, 6, 7t
  and constipation, 364t
  in dementia, 24
  history of, 518–519
  in nausea and vomiting, 399
psychoanalytic approach, in drug dependency management, 541–542
psychoanalytic theory, of depression, 36–38
psychogenic cough, 436
psychogenic dyspnea, 423t, 425–426
psychogenic hyperventilation, 423t, 425
psychological characteristics, in chemical dependency, 514
psychological factors. See psychosocial factors
psychological support, in nausea and vomiting, 400
psychological testing
  in anxiety, 63–64

  in confusion, 16t, 21
  in confusion and dementia, 16t
  in drug dependency, 520
  in low back pain, 168
psychosocial factors
  in allergy, 454–456
  in anxiety
    management considerations, 67–68
    threat, 56–57
    unmet needs, 57–58, 58f
  in aphasia
    diagnostic considerations, 266
    impact of disorder, 261–262
    management considerations, 268–269
  in body image development, 77–79
  in bowel function
    culture, 341–342
    secondary gain, 344
    self-concept, 324
    stress, 343
    symptom meaning, 343–344
    toileting, 342
  chronic pain patient, 119
  communication deficits and. See aphasia; hearing impairment
  in confusion, 3f
    assessment data, 14t
    iatrogenic causes of, 8
    management considerations, 23–24
    psychological causes of, 8–9
  in constipation, 362, 362t
    assessment of, 366
    diagnostic consideration, 366–367
    history taking, 363–365
  in diarrhea, 349
    causes of, 348
    management strategies, 358, 359
  in drug dependency, 518
    history-taking, 524–525
    predictive variables for prognosis, 536
  in dyspnea, 423t, 425–426
  in fatigue
    assessment data, 108
    diagnosis, 111
    management considerations, 111–117
    mechanisms of, 105, 106, 107
  in headache, 189, 192
    assessment data, 193
    counseling, 203–204
    effects of disorder on health, 192–193
    migraine, 235
    muscle contraction, 183
    prevention strategies, 203
    triggers of, 187
  in hearing loss, 250, 256–257
  in hyperventilation syndrome, 219, 236
  in incontinence, urinary, 409
    diagnostic considerations, 413

receptive aphasia, 259
receptors
  macula, 210–211
  neurotransmitter, 520, 521
  pain mechanisms, 122
record-keeping
  in constipation management, 368, 370
  in dyspnea and cough management, 440
  in headache, 201, 202f
  in incontinence, in bladder retraining, 414–415, 415f
  pain patient, daily comfort log, 136, 137f
  in weight loss, 482, 483, 489
recreation, for mobility-impaired patient, 286–287
recruitment, in chemical dependency, 516
rectal examination
  in constipation, 365
  in diarrhea, 351
  in incontinence, 411
  in low back pain, 167
rectal fissure, and constipation, 362t, 363, 365
rectal prolapse, with constipation, 363
rectal temperature, in fever, 303
rectal tube, in constipation management, 370
rectocele, and incontinence, urinary, 408–409, 411
recurrence, defined, 537
redness, and decubitus ulcer formation, 324
referral
  in depression, 52
  for drug dependency treatment, 542–543
  in dyspnea, acute, 434
  in fatigue, 117
  in headache, 196
  pain patient, 133, 144–145
reflexes
  acoustic neurinoma and, 218
  bladder emptying, 406, 416
  in confusion, 20–21
  in constipation, 365
  defecation, 340
  in drug dependency, 530
  gastrocolic, 340, 444
  in headache, secondary, 190t
  immobilization and, 281
  in low back pain
    assessment data, 166
    nerve root disorders and, 158, 163, 163t
  in nausea and vomiting, 396t
  in vertigo and dizziness, 224, 225
  vomiting, 376–379, 377–378f
reflex neurogenic bladder, 408f
reflux esophagitis, 382, 390t
regression, and incontinence, urinary, 409
regurgitation
  defined, 373
  with gastritis and cancer, 384
  in gastrointestinal disorders, 382, 383, 384, 390t
rehabilitation

in aphasia
  residual dysfunctions, 261
  support during, 269
in body image alterations, 81, 82, 93, 100–101
in hearing loss, 245–246, 250, 256
reinforcement, in behavior modification, 30–31
relapsing fever, defined, 300
relationships, See also psychosocial factors
  and fatigue, mechanisms in, 106, 107
  in low back pain, assessment data, 165
relaxation techniques
  in anxiety management, 69
  in diarrhea management, 360
  in headache management, 198, 199
  in low back pain management, 176
  in pain management. See also holistic techniques
    chronic disorders, 139
    low back, 176
religion, in anxiety management, 67–68
remittent fever, defined, 300
renal disease. See kidney disorders
renal failure
  in dehydration, 394t
  and fatigue, 106
renal function. See also kidneys
  and confusion, 14t, 18
  in dehydration, acid–base disorders, 381–382, 381f
  in fluid loss, 382
  hypothermia and, 4
  in normal fluid balance, 379
renal stones, immobilization and, 275
repetitiveness, in dementia, 29
repression, in body image alterations, 83
reserpine, 519
reserve fibers, 341
respiration(s). See also dyspnea
  in anxiety
    assessment data, 63
    differential diagnosis, 64
    levels affecting, 60, 61t
  drugs effects on
    assessment of, 528t, 529
    confusion, 6–8, 7t
  in fatigue, 105, 110
    assessment data, 109
    associated signs and symptoms, 111, 112t
  in fever, 300
  in nausea and vomiting
    abnormal findings, diseases seen in, 395t
    for control of, 376, 402
  sighing, 426
respiratory alkalosis, hyperventilation and, 219, 425
respiratory disorders. See also chronic obstructive pulmonary disease; coughing; dyspnea; respiratory infections
  and confusion
    as cause of, 5
    assessment data, 18

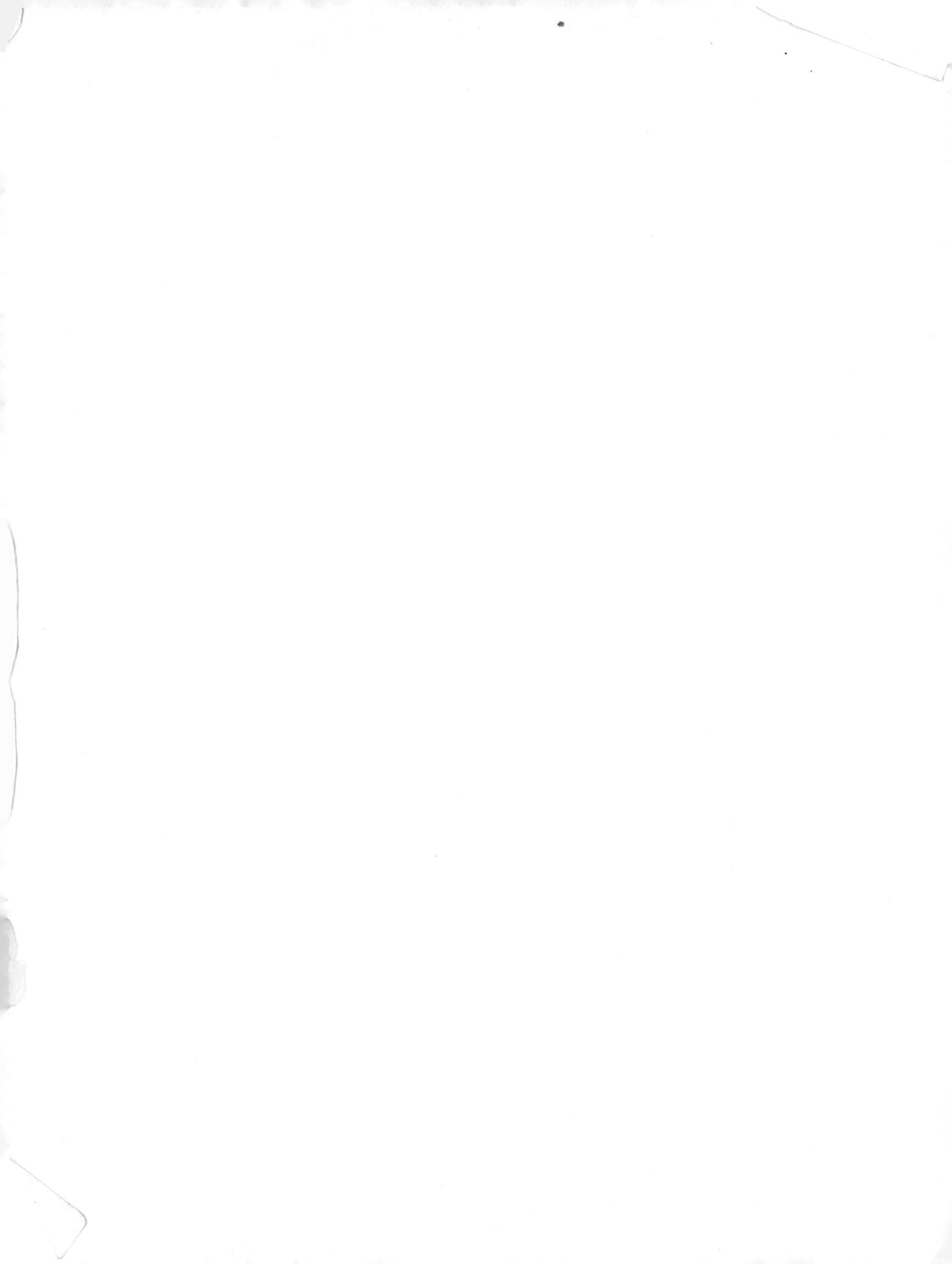